Topics in Bone Biology

Felix Bronner • Mary C. Farach-Carson
Helmtrud I. Roach[†]
Editor

Felix Bronner • Mary C. Farach-Carson
Series Editors

Bone-Metabolic Functions and Modulators

[†]Deceased

Springer

Editors
Felix Bronner, Ph.D.
Department of Reconstructive Sciences
Department of BioStructure
and Function
Department of Pharmacology
University of Connecticut Health Center
Farmington, CT, USA

Helmtrud I. Roach
University of Southampton
General Hospital
Southampton
United Kingdom

Mary C. Farach-Carson, Ph.D.
Department of Biochemistry
and Cell Biology
Rice University
Houston, Texas, USA

ISBN 978-1-4471-2744-4 ISBN 978-1-4471-2745-1 (eBook)
DOI 10.1007/978-1-4471-2745-1
Springer Dordrecht Heidelberg New York London

Library of Congress Control Number: 2012939625

Printed on acid-free paper

Springer is part of Springer Science+Business Media (www.springer.com)

Contents

Contributors

Manasi Agrawal, M.B.B.S. Internal Medicine, Maimonides Medical Center, Brooklyn, NY, USA

Shitij Arora, M.D. Internal Medicine, Wyckoff Heights Medical Center, Brooklyn, NY, USA

Mary F. Barbe, Ph.D. Department of Anatomy and Cell Biology, Temple School of Medicine, Philadelphia, PA, USA

Felix Bronner, Ph.D., Dr (H.C.) Reconstructive Sciences, The University of Connecticut Health Center, Farmington, CT, USA

David A. Bushinsky, M.D. Department of Medicine, University of Rochester School of Medicine, Rochester, NY, USA

Graziana Colaianni, Ph.D. The Mount Sinai Bone Program, Mount Sinai School of Medicine, New York, NY, USA

Jillian Cornish, Ph.D. Department of Medicine, University of Auckland, Auckland, New Zealand

Marie B. Demay, M.D. Endocrine Unit, Department of Medicine, Massachusetts General Hospital, Harvard Medical School, Boston, MA, USA

Linda A. DiMeglio, M.D., M.P.H. Department of Pediatrics, Indiana University School of Medicine, Indianapolis, IN, USA

Paul M. Epstein, Ph.D. Department of Cell Biology, University of Connecticut Health Center, Farmington, CT, USA

Mary C. Farach-Carson, Ph.D. Department of Biochemistry and Cell Biology, Rice University, Houston, TX, USA

Kathleen C. Horner, Ph.D. Faculté des Sciences et Techniques, INSERM, CRN2M, Université Paul Cézanne, Marseille, Cedex, France

Jameel Z. Iqbal, M.D., Ph.D. Department of Pathology and Lab Medicine, University of Pennsylvania, Philadelphia, PA, USA

Nancy S. Krieger, Ph.D. Department of Medicine, University of Rochester School of Medicine, Rochester, NY, USA

Adrian D. LeBlanc, Ph.D. Division of Space Life Sciences, Universities space Research Association, Houston, TX, USA

T. John Martin, M.D., D.Sc. Bone Cell Biology and Disease, St. Vincent's Institute of Medical Research, Fitzroy, VIC, Australia

Paul D. Miller, M.D., FACP Department of Medicine, Colorado Center for Bone Research, Lakewood, CO, USA

Faryal S. Mirza, M.D. Division of Endocrinology and Metabolism, Department of Medicine, University of Connecticut Health Center, Farmington, CT, USA

Dorit Naot, Ph.D. Department of Medicine, University of Auckland, Auckland, New Zealand

Kong Wah Ng, M.D. Department of Endocrinology and Diabetes, St. Vincent's Institute Hospital, Fitzroy, VIC, Australia

Roberto Pacifici, M.D. Division of Endocrinology, Metabolism and Lipids, Department of Medicine, Emory University, Atlanta, GA, USA

Nicola C. Partridge, Ph.D. Department of Basic Science and Craniofacial Biology, New York University College of Dentistry, New York, NY, USA

Steven N. Popoff, Ph.D. Department of Anatomy and Cell Biology, Temple School of Medicine, Philadelphia, PA, USA

Ling Qin, Ph.D. Department of Orthopaedic Surgery, Perelman School of Medicine, University of Pennsylvania, Philadelphia, PA, USA

G. David Roodman, M.D., Ph.D. Department of Medicine, Director of Hematology/Oncology, Indiana University, Indianapolis, Indiana, USA

VA Pittsburgh Health Care System, Research and Development, Pittsburgh, PA, USA

Clifford J. Rosen, M.D. Clinical and Translational Research, Maine Medical Center Research Institute, Scarborough, ME, USA

Victor S. Schneider, M.D. Office of the Chief Health and Medical Officer, NASA, Washington, DC, USA

Frederick R. Singer, M.D. Endocrine/Bone Disease Program, John Wayne Cancer Institute, St. John's Health Center, Santa Monica, CA, USA

Elisabeth R. Spector, B.S. Bone and Mineral Lab, Wyle Laboratories, Houston, TX, USA

Paula H. Stern, Ph.D. Department of Molecular Pharmacology and Biological Chemistry, Northwestern University Feinberg School of Medicine, Chicago, IL, USA

René St-Arnaud, Ph.D. Departments of Medicine, Surgery, and Human Genetics, McGill University, Montreal, QC, Canada

Genetics Unit, Shriners Hospital for Children, Montreal, QC, Canada

Li Sun, M.D., Ph.D. The Mount Sinai Bone Program, Mount Sinai School of Medicine, New York, NY, USA

Pamela Taxel, M.D. Department of Endocrinology and Metabolism, University of Connecticut Health Center, Farmington, CT, USA

Sumithra K. Urs, Ph.D. Center for Molecular Medicine, Maine Medical Center Research Institute, Scarborough, ME, USA

M. Neale Weitzmann, Ph.D. Division of Endocrinology, Metabolism and Lipids, Department of Medicine, Emory University, Atlanta, GA, USA

Mone Zaidi, M.D., Ph.D., F.R.C.P. The Mount Sinai Bone Program, Department of Medicine, Mount Sinai School of Medicine, New York, NY, USA

Liam Zakko, M.D. Yale Department of Medicine, Yale New Haven Hospital, New Haven, CT, USA

Acronym/Abbreviation

AAA-ATP	Adenosine triphosphatases associated with diverse cellular activities
AC	Adenylyl cyclase
(ACD)-BMCs	Adherent cell depleted bone marrow cells
ACTH	Adrenocorticotropic hormone, adrenocorticotropin
adrb2	Beta 2 adrenergic receptors
AF1,2	Activation function 1,2
Ags	Antigens
AG	Artificial gravity
2-AG	2-arachidonylglycerol
AGE	Advanced glycation end product
AIDS	Acquired immunodeficiency syndrome
ALP	Alkaline phosphatase
ALS	Acid labile subunit
AMPA	Alpha amino-3-hydroxy-5-methyl-4-isoxazolepropionic acid receptor
AMPK	Adenosine monophosphate protein kinase
AP	Activator protein
AR	Androgen receptor
ARED	Advanced resistive exercise device
AS-MVNP	Antisense-measles virus nucleocapsid protein
ATF-1	cAMP-dependent activating transcription factor 1
ATF4	Activating transcription factor 4
ATP	Adenosine-5'-triphosphate
AUF1	AU-rich element RNA binding protein 1
AVP	Arginine vasopressin
Bcl-2	B-cell lymphoma-2
BM	Bone marrow
BMAD	Bone mineral apparent density
BMC	Bone mineral content
BMCs	Bone marrow cells
BMD	Bone mineral density
BMI	Body mass index
BMP	Bone morphogenetic protein
Botox-A	OnabotulinumtoxinA
BPN	Bisphosphonates

BPPV	Benign paroxysmal positional vertigo
Brg1	Brahma-related gene 1
Brm	Brahma (ATP-dependent helicase)
BSAP	Bone specific alkaline phosphatase
BSP	Bone sialoprotein
BTM	Bone turnover markers
BW	Body weight
cAMP	Cyclic 3′, 5′-adenosine monophosphate
CaR	Calcium sensing receptor
CART	Cocaine and amphetamine regulated transcript
CB1,2	Cannabinoid receptor type 1,2
CBP	cAMP response element binding protein (CREB) binding protein
CD	Cluster of differentiation
CD44	Hyaluronic acid receptor
CDV	Canine distemper virus
C/EBP	CCAAT enhancer-binding protein site
CF	Cystic fibrosis
CFTR	CF transmembrane conductance regulator
CFU-GM	Colony forming unit-granulocyte macrophage
CGH	Comparative genomic hybridization
cGMP	Cyclic GMP
CGRP α, β	Calcitonin gene-related peptide α, β
CKD	Chronic kidney disease
CKD-MBD	Chronic kidney disease-metabolic bone disease
CLR	Calcitonin receptor-like receptor
CNS	Central nervous system
Col1	Collagen type 1
COX(−2)	Cyclooxygenase(−2)
CNGC	Cyclic nucleotide gated channels
CP	Cerebral palsy
cPTH	Continuous infusion of PTH
Cre	Bacteriophage P1 Cre recombinase
CRE	cAMP response element
CREB	cAMP-response element-binding protein
CREM	cAMP-response element modulator
CRH	Corticotrophin-releasing hormone
CRPS	Complex regional pain syndrome
CSF	Colony stimulating factor; cerebral spinal fluid
CTR	Calcitonin receptor
CTS	Carpal tunnel syndrome
CTX	Carboxy-terminal collagen crosslinks
CYP2R1	Cytochrome P450 2R1, vitamin D 25-hydroxylase
CYP27B1	Cytochrome P450 27B1, 25-hydroxyvitamin D-1α-hydroxylase
CYP27A1	Cytochrome P450 27A1
CYP2C11	Cytochrome P450 2C11
CYP2D5	Cytochrome P450 2D5

CYP2J2	Cytochrome P450 2J2
CYP24A1	Cytochrome P450 24A1, 25-hydroxyvitamin D-24-hydroxylase
CYP3A4	Cytochrome P450 3A4
3-D	Three-dimensional
DAG	Diacylglycerol
db/db	Leptin receptor-deficient
DBP	Vitamin D binding protein
DβH	Dopamine-beta-hydroxylase
DECIDE	Determining efficacy: comparison of initiating denosumab vs. AlEndronate phase III clinical trial
DEFEND	DEnosumab FortifiEs boNe density phase III clinical trial
DEXA (DXA)	Dual energy X-ray absorptiometry
DHEA	Dihydroepiandrostenedione
Dkk (1)	Dickkopf (1)
DMD	Duchenne muscular dystrophy
Dmp-1	Dentin matrix acidic phosphoprotein 1
DNMT1,3B	DNA methyltransferase 1,3B
DRIP	D receptor interacting proteins
DRIP/TRAP	Vitamin D receptor interacting protein/TR –associated protein
dsRNA	Double stranded RNA
Dvl	Dishevelled
ECD	Extracellular domain
E15.5	Embryonic day (15.5)
EPAC	Exchange protein activated by cAMP
Erk	Extracellular signal related kinase
EST	Expressed sequence tags
FDA	Food and Drug Administration
FEV	Forced expiratory volume
FGF(23)	Fibroblast growth factor (23)
FE	Finite element
Fos	FBJ murine osteosarcoma viral oncogene homolog
FREEDOM	Fracture Reduction Evaluation of Denosumab in Osteoporosis
FSH	Follicle stimulating hormone
FSHR	FSH receptor
G	Gravitational constant
GAP	GTPase activating protein
GC-B	Guanylyl cyclase B
GDI	Guanine nucleotide dissociation inhibitor
GEF	Guanine nucleotide exchange factor
GH	Growth hormone
GIO	Glucocorticoid-induced osteoporosis
GLAST	GLutamate ASpartate Transporter
GLT-1	Glutamate transporter

Glu	Glutaminergic or glutamate
GluR	Glutamate receptor
GM-CSF	Granulocyte-macrophage colony stimulating factor
GMFCS	Gross Motor Function Classification System
GnRH	Gonadotropin releasing hormone
GPCR	G protein-coupled receptor
GR α, β	Glucocorticoid receptor α, β
GRK2	G protein-coupled receptor kinase 2
GSK3β	Glycogen synthase kinase 3 beta
GTP	Guanosine triphosphate
HA	Hypothalamic amenorrhea
HAART	Highly-active anti-retroviral therapy
HAT	Histone acetyltransferase
HDAC(4)	Histone deacetylases(4)
HDT	Head down tilt
HH	Hypogonadotrophic hypogonadism
HO	Heterotopic ossification
HIV	Human immunodeficiency virus
HRT	Hormone replacement therapy
HHM	Humoral hypercalcemia of malignancy
HSC	Hematopoietic stem cell
11βHSD	11 beta-hydroxysteroid dehydrogenase
$5\text{-HT}_{2B}R$	5-hydroxytryptamine (serotonin) receptor
HVDRR	Hereditary vitamin D resistant rickets
Hz	Hertz
IBMPFD	Inclusion body myopathy, Paget's disease, frontotemporal dementia
IBMX	3-isobutyl-1-methylxanthine
ICAM-1	Intercellular adhesion molecule 1
ICER	Inducible cAMP early repressor
ICTP	Serum carboxy-terminal 1-telopeptide
IDDM	Insulin dependent diabetes mellitus
IFN β,γ	Interferon beta, gamma
IGD	Isolated GnRH deficiency
IGF –1	Insulin-like growth factor –1
IGFBP	Insulin-like growth factor binding protein
Ihh	Indian hedgehog
IHH	Idiopathic hypogonadotropic hypogonadism
IKK	Inhibitor kappa kinase
IκBα	Inhibitor kappa alpha
IκBβ	Inhibitor kappa beta
IκBε	Inhibitor kappa epsilon
IκBγ	Inhibitor kappa gamma
IL-1,2,4,6,10	Interleukin-1,2,4,6,10
IL-1R	Interleukin-1 receptor
INSL3	Insulin like factor 3
IP3	Inositol trisphosphate

iPTH	Intermittent infusion of PTH
IR	Immunoreactive
IRED	Interim resistive exercise device
ISS	International space station
IU	International units
I.V.	Intravenous
JAG1	Jagged1
JNK	c-jun–terminal kinase
Jun	Jun proto-oncogene
kD	KiloDalton
KDIGO	Kidney disease: improving global outcomes
KDOQI	Kidney diseases outcomes quality initiative
KO	Knockout
KS	Klinefelter syndrome
KSRP	KH-type splicing regulatory protein
LAT 1	L-type amino acid transporter 1
LBM	Lean body mass
LH	Luteinizing hormone
LID	Liver IGF-1 deficient
LPS	Lipopolysaccharide
LRP (Lrp) 5	LDL-receptor related protein 5
MAPK, MAP	Mitogen-activated protein kinase
MARRS	Membrane-associated rapid response steroid binding protein
MBD(4)	Methyl-CpG-binding domain protein(4)
MCP-1	Monocyte chemoattractant protein-1
MCSF	Macrophage colony stimulating factor
MCT8	Monocarboxylate transporter 8
Met	Metabolic acidosis
MGP	Matrix gla protein
MicroCT	Microcomputerized tomography
MIP-1a	Macrophage inflammatory protein-1
MK801	(5*S*,10*R*)-(+)-5-Methyl-10,11-dihydro -5*H*-dibenzo[*a*,*d*]cyclohepten-5,10-imine maleate, a NMDA receptor antagonist
MKP-1	Mitogen activated kinase phosphatase-1
MLC	Myosin light chain
MMP (13)	Matrix metalloproteinase (13)
MRI	Magnetic resonance imaging
MrOS	Osteoporotic fractures in men study
MV	Measles virus
NADPH	Nicotinamide adenine dinucleotide phosphate
NASA	National Aeronautics and Space Administration
NBQX	2,3-dioxo-6-nitro-1,2,3,4-tetrahydrobenzo[*f*] quinoxaline-7-sulfonamide, a AMPA/kainic acid receptor antagonist

NCoR	Nuclear receptor co-repressor
NEFA	Non-esterified fatty acid
NEMO	NFκB essential modulator
NFATc1	Nuclear factor of activated T cells-1
NFκB	Nuclear factor kappa B
NGF	Nerve growth factor
NHERF-1	Na^+/H^+ exchanger regulatory factor 1
NIDDM	Non-insulin dependent diabetes mellitus
NIH	National Institutes of Health
NK1 receptor	Neurokinin 1 receptor
NMDA	N-methyl-D-aspartic acid
NO	Nitric oxide
NPR2	Natriuretic peptide receptor 2
Npt2a	Sodium phosphate co-transporter gene 2a
NPY	Neuropeptide-y
NSAID	Nonsteroidal anti-inflammatory drug
NSF	National Science Foundation
NTX	N-terminal telopeptide of type I collagen
OCIL	Osteoclast inhibitory lectin
ob/ob	Obese leptin deficient mice
OBs	Osteoblasts
OCs	Osteoclasts
ODF	Osteoclast differentiation factor
OGR1	Ovarian G-protein coupled receptor 1
$1(\alpha),25(OH)_2D$	1α,25-dihydroxyvitamin D
25(OH)D	25-hydroxyvitamin D
$1,24,25(OH)_3D$	1,24,25-trihydroxyvitamin D
$24\text{-oxo-}1,23,25(OH)_3D$	24-oxo-1,23,25- trihydroxyvitamin D
$24,25(OH)_2D$	24,25- dihydroxyvitamin D
$23,25(OH)_2D$	23,25- dihydroxyvitamin D
$23,25,26(OH)_3D$	23,25,26- trihydroxyvitamin D
OMIM	Online Mendelian Inheritance in Man
ON	Osteonectin
ONJ	Osteonecrosis of the jaw
OP	Osteopontin
OPG	Osteoprotegerin
OPGL	Osteoprotegerin ligand
OT	Oxytocin
PAPP-A	Pregnancy associated plasma protein- A
PBEF	Pre-B-cell-enhancing factor
PBM	Peak bone mass
PCAF	p300/CBP-associated factor
PDB	Paget's disease of bone
PDDR	Pseudo vitamin D deficiency rickets
PDE	Cyclic nucleotide phosphodiesterase
PDZ domain	Post synaptic density protein (PSD95), Drosophila disc large tumor suppressor (DlgA), and zonula occludens-1 protein (zo-1) domain

PEA-3	Polyoma enhancer activator-3
PECAM-1	Platelet endothelial cell adhesion molecule-1
PGE_2	Prostaglandin E_2
Phex	Phosphate-regulating neutral endopeptidase
PICP	C-terminal propeptide of type I procollagen
PINP	N-terminal propeptide of type I procollagen
PKA	Protein kinase A
PKC	Protein kinase C
PKG	cGMP dependent protein kinase
PLA_2	Phospholipase A_2
PLC	Phospholipase C
PLD	Phospholipase D
PMO	Postmenopausal osteoporosis
PPARγ	Peroxisome proliferator-activated receptor gamma
PPR	PTH/PTHrP receptor
Prkg2	cGMP dependent protein kinase gene
PRL	Prolactin
PRLR	Prolactin receptor
PTH	Parathyroid hormone
PTH1R, PTHRc1	Parathyroid hormone 1 receptor
PTHrP	Parathyroid hormone-related protein
PVN	Parventricular nucleus
QCT	Quantitative computerized tomography
RA	Rheumatoid arthritis
RAMPs	Receptor activity modifying proteins
RANK	Receptor activator of NF-κB
RANKL	Receptor activator of NF-κB ligand
Ras	Protein superfamily of small GTPases
RD	Runt domain-binding sequence
RelA	V-rel reticuloendotheliosis viral oncogene homolog A
Rho	Rho family of GTPases, a subfamily of the Ras superfamily
RhoA	Member of the Rho family of GTPases
rhPTH	Recombinant human parathyroid hormone
ROCK	Rho-associated kinase
RSD	Reflex sympathetic dystrophy
RTA	Renal tubular acidosis
Runx2	Runt-related transcription factor 2
RXFP2	Relaxin family peptide 2
RXR	Retinoid X receptor
SBE	Smad binding element
SCI	Spinal cord injury

SCs	Stromal cells
Sfrp(4)	Secreted frizzled-related protein(4)
SHPT	Secondary hyperparathyroidism
siRNA	Silencing RNA
SMRT	Silencing mediator of retinoid and thyroid receptors
SNP	Single nucleotide polymorphism
SNS	Sympathetic nervous system
Sox9	SRY (sex determining region Y)-box 9
SPA	Single photon absorptiometry
SQ	Subcutaneous
SRC	Steroid receptor coactivator
STAND	Study of Transition from Alendronate to Denosumab phase III clinical trial
SULT2A	Sulfotransferase 2A
SyK	Spleen tyrosine kinase
T3	Triiodothyronin
T4	Thyroxin
TBI	Traumatic brain injury
TFIIB	Transcription factor IIB
Tg	Transgenic
TGFβ	Transforming growth factor beta
Th17	T helper 17 cells
TIP39	Tuberoinfundibular peptide of 39 residues
TLR	Toll like receptors
TNF(α)	Tumor necrosis factor(α)
TPH 1	Tryptophan synthase 1
TPTD	Teriparatide
TRα,β	Thyroid receptor alpha,beta
TRAF	TNF receptor-associated factor
TRANCE	TNF-related activation-induced cytokine
TRAP	Tartrate-resistant acid phosphatase
TRE	Thyroid response element
TRH	Thyrotropin-releasing hormone
TRPV5,6	Transient receptor potential vanilloid cation channel subfamily V member 5,6
TSH	Thyroid-stimulating hormone
TZD	Thiazolidinedione
UNR	Upstream of N-ras
USDA	United States Department of Agriculture
vBMD	Volumetric bone mineral density
VCAM-1	Vascular cell adhesion molecule 1
VCP	Valine-containing protein
VDIR	VDR interacting repressor
VDR	Vitamin D receptor
VDRE	Vitamin D response element

VEGF	Vascular endothelial growth factor
vTBMD	Volumetric tibial bone mineral density
WBV	Whole body vibration
Wnt	Wingless-type MMTV integration site family
WINAC	WSTF including nucleosome assembly complex
WSTF	Williams Syndrome transcription factor
XT-44	1-n-butyl-3-n-propylxanthine
XT-611	3,4-dipropyl-4,5,7,8-tetrahydro-3H-imidazo [1,2-i]-purin-5-one

Parathyroid Hormone and Parathyroid-Hormone-Related Protein: Normal Function, Diseases, and Emerging Therapeutics

1

Ling Qin and Nicola C. Partridge

Keywords
Parathyroid hormone • Parathyroid-hormone-related protein • Calcium homeostasis • Phosphate homeostasis • Hypercalcemia • Teriparatide

1.1 Introduction

Parathyroid hormone (PTH) and parathyroid-hormone-related protein (PTHrP) are two predominant members of the PTH family of peptides with major roles in calcium homeostasis and bone formation. PTH was discovered in the acid extracts of parathyroid glands which were capable of restoring the blood calcium level in the parathyroidectomized dog [24]. The existence of PTHrP and its close resemblance to PTH was first suggested by Fuller Albright in 1941 and later discovered and isolated from lung [88, 129] and renal carcinomas [128] in 1987. PTHrP is overexpressed in certain tumors and is the major pathogenic factor for humoral hypercalcemia of malignancy (HHM), a condition that is characterized by hypercalcemia caused by the secretion of the calcemic factor from tumors. The past two decades have witnessed an explosion in the knowledge of the biological function of these peptides at the molecular level and their use as therapeutics or as targets in certain diseases. This chapter will review their functions in bone.

1.2 PTH/PTHrP Polypeptide Family

In mammals, PTH is encoded by a single-copy gene that consists of three exons and two introns. PTH is synthesized as a prepropeptide with a 25-amino-acid presequence that facilitates passage through the membrane of the endoplasmic reticulum [48], a 6-amino-acid prosequence for delivery of the molecule to secretory vesicles [67], and an 84-amino-acid mature peptide. The PTH molecules from different mammalian species exhibit extensive sequence homology (Fig. 1.1). Chicken PTH, the only avian PTH isolated thus far, contains 88 amino acids derived from a 119-amino-acid prepropeptide [68]. Compared to its mammalian homologues, chicken PTH has two deletions in the

L. Qin, Ph.D.
Department of Orthopaedic Surgery, Perelman School of Medicine, University of Pennsylvania, 424D Stemmler Hall, 36th Street & Hamilton Walk, Philadelphia, PA 19104, USA

N.C. Partridge, Ph.D. (✉)
Department of Basic Science and Craniofacial Biology, New York University College of Dentistry, 345 E. 24th Street, Room 902A, New York, NY 10010, USA
e-mail: ncp234@nyu.edu

F. Bronner et al. (eds.), *Bone-Metabolic Functions and Modulators*, Topics in Bone Biology,
DOI 10.1007/978-1-4471-2745-1_1, © Springer-Verlag London 2012

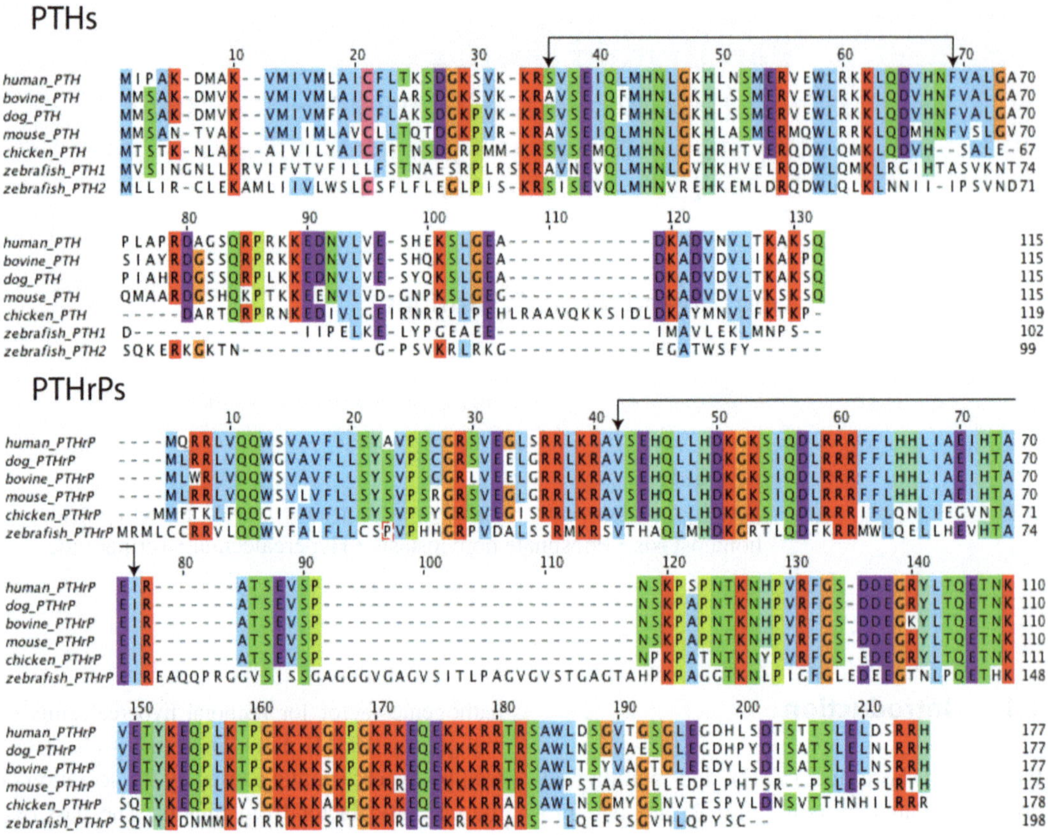

Fig. 1.1 Multiple sequence alignment of PTH and PTH prepropeptides showing the conservation among different species. Conserved residues are *shaded*. *Horizontal bars* above each sequence with two *arrows* indicate the beginning residue and the end residue of PTH (1–34) and PTHrP (1–36)

hydrophobic middle portion with an insertion of amino acids near the C-terminus. Fish lack a parathyroid gland, but two forms of PTH have been found in puffer fish [26], zebra fish [41], and elephant shark [81]. Interestingly, the N-terminal PTH (1–34), which is associated with most of the biological actions of the PTH molecule, shows high homology throughout all species.

The human PTHrP gene is much more complicated than human PTH. It consists of eight exons and at least three promoters and produces three forms of mRNA through alternative mRNA splicing that code for mature proteins of 139, 141, or 173 amino acids with identical sequences within the first 139 amino acids [97]. Similar to PTH, human PTHrP is synthesized as a prepropeptide with a 24-amino-acid presequence and a 12-amino-acid prosequence. The similarity between the gene structures of PTHrP and PTH and the location of the two genes on related chromosomes in the human (short arm of chromosome 11 for PTH and short arm of chromosome 12 for PTHrP) may be because these two genes have arisen from the same ancestral gene through gene duplication. There is high-sequence homology among all vertebrate PTHrPs (Fig. 1.1). Recently, two forms of PTHrP gene were discovered in puffer fish, with 63% sequence similarity [18]. PTHrP is indeed a polyhormone. Posttranslational processing of mammalian PTHrP yields at least three mature fragments with distinct biological functions [97]: N-terminal 1–36, structurally related to PTH and acting through PTH1R; a middle region 38–94, with a nuclear localization sequence [58] and with a possible role in regulating placental calcium transport [19, 71]; and C-terminal 107–139,

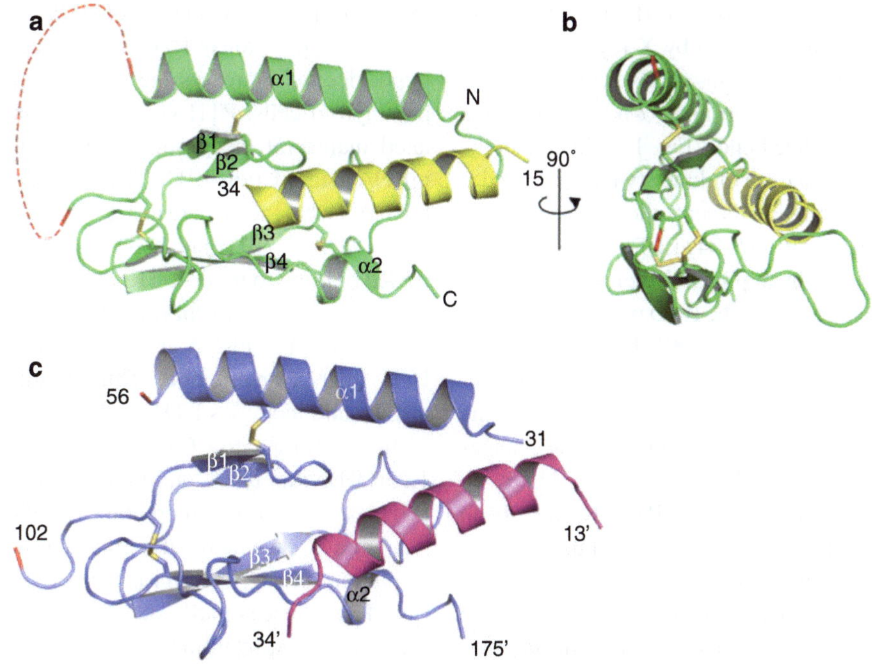

Fig. 1.2 The crystal structures of PTH (15–34)/PTH1R N-terminal extracellular domain (ECD, 29–187) complex (**a** and **b**) and PTHrP (12–34)/PTH1R ECD complex (**c**). In (**a, b**), ECD is shown in *green* and PTH in *yellow*. In (**c**), ECD is shown in *slate blue* and PTHrP in *magenta*. The disulfide bonds are depicted as *sticks*. Residues 57–101 of PTH1R are either designated as a *dashed red line* in (**a**) or missing in (**c**) due to their disordered structure (**a, b** – reproduced with permission from Pioszak and Xu [100]. Copyright (2008) National Academy of Sciences, U.S.A.; **c** – reproduced with permission from Pioszak et al. [99]. © 2009 The American Society for Biochemistry and Molecular Biology)

named osteostatin because of its inhibition of osteoclastic bone resorption [25, 32]. Our chapter will focus on PTHrP (1–36) because it is the most studied in bone metabolism. PTHrP's homology to PTH only lies in its N-terminal 13 amino acids of mature peptide, which are involved in activation of the receptor shared with PTH, that is, PTH1R. This sharing explains why PTHrP mimics PTH in inducing bone resorption, renal phosphate wasting, and hypercalcemia of malignancy. The receptor-binding domain of PTHrP (amino acids 18–34) has little similarity with the primary sequence of PTH, but the peptides share a common α-helical secondary structure (Fig. 1.2).

1.3 PTH and PTHrP Receptors

The N-terminal sequences of both PTH and PTHrP bind with equal affinity to PTH1R, a highly expressed receptor in bone and kidney, where it mediates the effects of PTH and PTHrP on calcium and phosphate metabolism. The receptor has low levels of expression in other tissues, such as skin, brain, muscle, heart, placenta, etc., where it mediates the autocrine and paracrine effects of PTHrP [22]. PTH1R is a member of class B of the large family of G-protein-coupled receptors (GPCRs) whose characteristic feature is the long extracellular N-terminal domain that consists of about 160 amino acids that function in ligand binding. The crystal structure of PTH1R has not yet been resolved, but its seven transmembrane domains are believed to be arranged in a circular or oval configuration, a common feature for those GPCRs whose structures have been resolved. These include rhodopsin, the adenosine A2A receptor, and β 1 and β 2 adrenoceptors [57]. The transmembrane domains of PTH1R are connected by three extracellular and three intracellular loops and the receptor has a C-terminal intracellular tail of about 130 amino acids. Recently, the structure of the extracellular domain (ECD) of human PTH1R has been analyzed by X-ray crystallography. The structure contains an N-terminal α-helix, four β-strands, a C-terminal α-helix, and three conserved disulfide bonds (Fig. 1.2). Interestingly, the ECD is in the form of dimers when no ligand is present. PTH binding disrupts the oligomerization [98]. In the PTH (15–34)/ECD complex, PTH docks as a straight amphipathic helix into a central hydrophobic groove in the ECD of PTH1R, resembling a hot dog in a bun [100] (Fig. 1.2a, b). The helix of PTHrP in the PTHrP (12–34)/ECD complex is gently curved and unwound at the C-terminus, with corresponding structural changes in the ECD [99] (Fig. 1.2c).

Another PTH receptor, PTH2R, has been identified in the brain, on the basis of its sequence homology to PTH1R (about 50% in human) [136]. Although PTH, but not PTHrP, activates PTH2R, strong pharmacological evidence suggests that tuberoinfundibular peptide of 39 residues (TIP39), a peptide sharing similarity to both PTH and PTHrP, is the endogenous ligand for PTH2R [137]. An additional receptor, PTH3R, has been identified in fish. This receptor has high affinity toward PTHrP [112, 113].

1.4 Normal Functions of PTH in Bone Metabolism

1.4.1 PTH Synthesis and Secretion from Parathyroid Gland

PTH is synthesized in the chief cells of the parathyroid gland. The calcium-sensing receptor (CaR), another GPCR member, is expressed on the plasma membrane of the gland cells and is the major regulator of PTH synthesis and secretion. The CaR senses extracellular Ca^{2+} levels by binding the ion in the extracellular Venus flytrap domain. When serum Ca^{2+} is low, PTH, stored in secretory vesicles, is exocytosed promptly (within seconds and minutes). Small changes in Ca^{2+} lead to large changes in PTH [30]. The amount of PTH secreted bears a steep inverse sigmoidal relationship with the ionized serum calcium concentration. To correct long-term hypocalcemia, the intracellular degradation of PTH is inhibited and gene expression of PTH is increased. Chronic hypocalcemia increases the size and number of parathyroid cells. PTH gene expression is regulated mainly at the posttranscriptional level by mRNA degradation [91]. The half-life of PTH mRNA is balanced between a stabilizing complex (AUF1/UNR) and a destabilizing protein KSRP binding to the 3′-UTR. A low calcium diet results in an increase in the interaction between AUF1 and PTH mRNA and a decrease in KSRP-PTH mRNA interaction. This stabilizes PTH mRNA and increases PTH production.

In addition to Ca^{2+}, serum phosphate, $1,25(OH)_2$vitamin D_3, and FGF23 also modulate PTH expression and secretion. The hyperphosphatemia of chronic renal failure is accompanied by parathyroid hyperplasia and hyperparathyroidism. This effect is partly due to phosphate binding to calcium, resulting in a decrease of serum calcium, which in turn stimulates PTH secretion, synthesis, and parathyroid cell proliferation. It is also partly due to the direct effect of phosphate stabilizing the PTH mRNA through a similar AUF1/KSRP mechanism [91]. The vitamin D_3 receptor, together with its ligand $1,25(OH)_2$vitamin D_3, binds to negative regulatory elements in the PTH gene promoter and blocks the transcription of PTH [69, 92]. Therefore, deficiency of vitamin D_3 or of $1,25(OH)_2$vitamin D_3 is associated with PTH overproduction. FGF23 acts directly on its receptor, FGFR1c, along with the coreceptor α-Klotho on the parathyroid. This inhibits PTH secretion and decreases PTH mRNA levels [8]. In addition, studies with α-Klotho null mice suggest that α-Klotho stimulates PTH secretion in a FGF-independent manner by binding with Na^+, K^+-ATPase [56].

1.4.2 PTH Regulation of Serum Calcium and Phosphate Homeostasis

Extracellular ionized calcium plays a key role in many biological processes, such as synaptic function, smooth muscle contractility, and cell signal transduction. It is normally strictly maintained at a concentration of 1.1–1.3 mM, with PTH as the principal regulator of calcium homeostasis. PTH is secreted from the chief cells of the parathyroid gland in response to a drop in serum calcium, and it acts directly on bone and kidney and indirectly on the small intestine via 1,25(OH)$_2$vitamin D$_3$. As a result, serum calcium levels are shortly restored to normal.

Via mechanisms as yet not fully understood, PTH stimulates calcium release from bone from a pool of calcium that turns over rapidly and then from a pool that turns over more slowly [130]. PTH1R is abundantly expressed in osteoblast lineage cells, but not in osteoclasts. Under physiological conditions, the major function of PTH is to stimulate osteoclast formation and activity, resulting in bone degradation and release of calcium into plasma. In the kidney, PTH stimulates calcium reabsorption at the distal tubule by regulating the level and activities of two calcium transporter proteins, TRPV5, a highly selective calcium channel that moves Ca^{2+} from the tubular lumen across the apical membrane into the tubular cells, and NCX1, a sodium/calcium exchanger that moves Ca^{2+} across the basolateral membrane into the blood stream [138]. In addition, PTH activates the mitochondrial 25-hydroxyvitamin D-1-α-hydroxylase in the proximal tubular cells [38], which converts 25-(OH)$_2$vitamin D$_3$ into 1,25(OH)$_2$vitamin D$_3$. This, in turn, increases intestinal calcium absorption and thus raises serum calcium levels.

Phosphate is required for many cellular functions, such as nucleic acid synthesis, membrane lipid synthesis, intracellular signaling, and energy metabolism. PTH also plays an important role in maintaining serum phosphorus concentrations by regulating phosphate reabsorption. As discussed above, hyperphosphatemia stimulates PTH secretion. PTH binding to its receptor PTH1R on the renal proximal tubules quickly removes two sodium-dependent phosphate cotransporters, NaPi-IIa and NaPi-IIc, from the apical and basolateral membranes by endocytosis [5, 118]. The extent of Pi reabsorption is determined largely by the abundance of these two cotransporters and thus PTH stimulates phosphate excretion.

1.4.3 Hyperparathyroidism

Overexpression of PTH leads to hyperparathyroidism. Primary hyperparathyroidism is a relatively common endocrine disease, with an incidence of 1 in 500–1,000, and is usually caused by a benign adenoma of the parathyroid and, less commonly, by hyperplasia or, rarely, by carcinoma of the parathyroid glands. The oversecretion of PTH in these diseases leads to hypercalcemia and affects the skeleton, kidney, and the gastrointestinal tract. Secondary hyperparathyroidism refers to excessive secretion of PTH by the parathyroid glands in response to hypocalcemia. In patients with chronic renal failure, secondary hyperparathyroidism is usually associated with defective phosphorus excretion and impaired 1,25(OH)$_2$vitamin D$_3$ synthesis. If left untreated, the patients will develop tertiary hyperparathyroidism with hypercalcemia due to parathyroid gland hyperplasia. Currently, type II calcimimetics, small molecules that interact with the CaR, are used to treat hyperparathyroidism. Calcimimetics increase receptor sensitivity toward extracellular calcium by shifting the PTH-Ca^{2+} dose–response curve to the left. This reduces serum PTH and calcium concentrations [49]. One agent, cinacalcet HCl, has received regulatory approval for treatment of hyperparathyroidism in chronic kidney disease and parathyroid carcinoma.

1.5 Functions of PTHrP in Normal Bone Metabolism and Bone Cancer

PTHrP is expressed in almost all tissues and plays paracrine and autocrine roles locally. It has a nuclear localization sequence (NLS) and is thought to have a nuclear intracrine role [35]. Because it does not circulate, PTHrP rarely acts as an endocrine factor. One exception is HHM, a condition where tumors act as secretory glands and PTHrP, released from the tumors, mimics PTH acting on bone and kidney to raise serum calcium levels. PTHrP regulates many physiological processes and therefore is essential for life. In addition to its skeletal actions (see below), normal physiological roles for PTHrP have been demonstrated, in embryonic and fetal development, in skin, mammary gland, smooth muscle and vascular system, pancreas, central nervous system, kidney, etc. PTHrP regulates cell proliferation, differentiation, survival, and calcium transport in a cell-type-specific manner [97].

1.5.1 Bone Development

Most of the mammalian skeleton, except for much of the craniofacial skeleton, forms through the process of endochondral ossification consisting of two steps: mesenchymal cell proliferation followed by chondrocyte differentiation to form a cartilage anlagen that then is replaced by bone. In long bones, this process involves two distinct sites, the primary and secondary ossification centers. These are separated by the growth plate, a polarized plate of chondrocytes. To achieve longitudinal growth, growth plate chondrocytes first proliferate rapidly, then expand their cell volume, finally differentiating into mineralized hypertrophic chondrocytes. The cartilage extracellular matrix at the chondro-osseous junction is then degraded and remodeled into bone tissue.

PTHrP is a most important regulator of growth plate development during endochondral ossification. It is expressed mainly in the perichondrial region, made up of immature and proliferating chondrocytes at the ends of long bones. PTHrP, through its receptor on chondrocytes, stimulates their proliferation, but blocks differentiation into hypertrophic chondrocytes. Phosphorylation of Sox9 [53] and downregulation of Runx2 [47] in chondrocytes may mediate action by PTHrP on chondrocyte differentiation inasmuch as these two transcription factors are essential for chondrocyte differentiation. Indian hedgehog (Ihh) is a major stimulator of PTHrP expression in the growth plate [140]. It is expressed and secreted by prehypertrophic and hypertrophic chondrocytes just after chondrocytes cease proliferation [11]. Therefore, PTHrP and Ihh constitute a negative feedback loop that determines the length of the proliferative chondrocyte zone and the uniformity of chondrocyte structure within the growth plate. In addition, PTHrP increases the expression of Bcl-2, an anti-apoptotic factor, in prehypertrophic chondrocytes and blocks chondrocyte apoptosis [2].

Animal models have confirmed the significant role played by PTHrP/PTH1R in growth plate development. Targeted disruption of the PTHrP gene in embryonic mice is lethal and causes widespread abnormalities in endochondral bone development that result from accelerated chondrocyte differentiation and premature hypertrophy in the cartilage [1, 64]. PTH1R null mice exhibit a similar bone phenotype with accelerated chondrocyte differentiation [76]. On the other hand, mice, overexpressing PTHrP [142] or in which PTH1R is constitutively active in proliferating chondrocytes [116], have shorter and thicker limbs. The changes in the limbs are the result of decelerated, not accelerated, terminal chondrocyte differentiation and of delayed mineralization. Similar human mutations have been linked to Jansen-type human metaphyseal chondrodysplasia, a disease characterized by delayed skeletal maturation [115].

1.5.2 Bone Remodeling

PTHrP has important anabolic functions in bone formation. PTHrP is expressed by early osteoblastic lineage cells, but its expression is diminished in the more differentiated bone lining osteoblasts and osteocytes [65, 82]. Adult PTH null mice exhibit increased trabecular bone volume with diminished bone turnover and increased skeletal PTHrP expression [86, 87]. Interestingly, this increase in bone mass is reversed by knocking out one allele of PTHrP in PTH null mice, suggesting that PTHrP is required to maintain bone mass [87]. Decreased bone volume and defective bone formation are observed in PTHrP heterozygous and osteoblast-specific PTHrP knockout mice [85].

1.5.3 The Role of PTHrP in Cancer Bone Metastasis

In addition to its role as an endocrine factor that is secreted from tumors and responsible for hypercalcemia in HHM, PTHrP is also a major mediator of osteolysis induced by tumors that have metastasized to bone. Solid cancers, such as breast, lung, and prostate cancers, frequently metastasize to bone. Osteolytic metastasis is much more common than osteoblastic metastasis and leads to the most severe complications, including bone pain, pathological fractures, hypercalcemia, and/or nerve compression. PTHrP secreted from tumors has a paracrine or autocrine effect in stimulating tumor growth, adhesion, and survival [27, 123, 124]. Breast tumors express more PTHrP at the bone metastasis site than at the primary or other metastasis sites [139]. Tumor-produced PTHrP acts on osteoblasts and increases their expression of receptor activator of NF-kB ligand (RANKL), a key mediator for activating the osteoclast receptor RANK on hematopoietic precursor cells. PTHrP also decreases expression of osteoprotegerin (OPG), a soluble decoy receptor for RANKL. It thus stimulates osteoclast formation. Increased bone resorption from bone matrix releases transforming growth factor beta (TGFβ), a potent stimulator for tumor PTHrP production, therefore constituting a "vicious cycle" that establishes tumor colonies in the bone environment [89]. In murine models, administration of neutralizing antibodies against PTHrP reduced bone destruction due to metastasis of the tumors [45] and lowered serum calcium in HHM [74]. Two small molecules that transcriptionally block PTHrP secretion from tumors have reduced osteolytic lesions in bone metastasis and alleviated hypercalcemia in HHM [40]. These results point to a promising treatment for PTHrP-related tumors.

1.6 Signaling Pathways Activated by PTH1R

1.6.1 Canonical G-Protein-Dependent Pathways

PTH1R belongs to the family of GPCRs, and activation of the receptor by PTH or PTHrP initiates a cascade of intracellular signaling pathways primarily through heterotrimeric G proteins (Gαβγ). The major Gα protein responsible for PTH1R signal transduction is the stimulatory $G\alpha_s$. Binding to PTH1R induces a conformational change in $G\alpha_s$ and leads to exchange of GDP for GTP with concomitant release of $G\alpha_s$ and Gβγ from the ligand-receptor complex. The activated GTP-bound $G\alpha_s$ then binds to and activates adenylate cyclase on the cell membrane and stimulates the formation of cyclic 3′, 5′-adenosine monophosphate (cAMP). In turn, cAMP binds the regulatory subunits of protein kinase A (PKA) to release the catalytic subunits of the enzyme. The catalytic subunits of PKA phosphorylate proteins on serine or threonine residues in the recognition sequence R-X-X-S and cause changes in structure and function of several proteins, particularly in transcription factors such as Runx2 [121] and cAMP-response element-binding protein (CREB) [96]. Alternatively, ligand binding with PTH1R also leads to activation of $G\alpha_q$. This stimulates the activity of phospholipase Cβ to break down phosphatidylinositolbisphosphate to diacylglycerol (DAG) and 1,4,5-inositol trisphosphate. As a result, cytosolic Ca^{2+} is increased and protein kinase C (PKC) is activated [21]. In addition, PTH1R activates $G_{12/13}$. This stimulates RhoA/Rho kinase and phospholipase D (PLD) activities in osteoblastic cells [126].

Currently, cAMP-PKA is the main route to transduce PTH/PTH1R signaling in osteoblasts because most PTH-regulated genes and the major physiological actions of PTH and PTHrP are mediated through this pathway. PTH (1–34) and PTH (1–31), a truncated PTH analog that activates cAMP/PKA but not the PKC pathway, differentially regulate some 1,000 genes in bone after PTH injection into rats. Only about 40 genes are regulated by PTH (3–34), which activates PLC/PKC and induces intracellular calcium signaling, but not the cAMP/PKA pathway [78]. In some cases, the PLC pathway seems to have effects that are the opposite of cAMP signaling. For example, while the effects of PTHrP on growth plate development are largely considered to be mediated by the PTH1R/cAMP pathway, mice with PTH1R mutant DSEL, which abrogates PLC but not cAMP signaling, display skeletal phenotypes, such as expansion of proliferating chondrocytes and a delay in chondrocyte maturation, effects that are similar to those in mice with elevated PTH1R activity in chondrocytes [46]. Interestingly, the Na^+/H^+ exchanger regulatory factor 1 (NHERF-1), a cytoplasmic scaffolding protein, binds to the C-terminal intracellular tail of PTH1R through its PDZ domain and shifts the PTH1R signaling from the PKA to the PKC pathway [84]. In kidney cells, the PTH-mediated inhibition of phosphate uptake utilizes both PKA and PKC pathways, with the latter largely NHERF-1 dependent [83].

As is true for most GPCRs, signaling through PTH1R is attenuated by rapid receptor desensitization. This involves phosphorylation by G-protein-coupled receptor kinase 2 (GRK2), arrestin recruitment, and subsequent endocytosis and receptor degradation. Surprisingly, PTH (1–34) bound PTH1R is still associated with Gαs and adenylyl cyclases and generates a sustained cAMP signal after it is internalized into endosomes. However, PTHrP (1–36) action is restricted to the cell surface, and its signaling is attenuated rapidly [33]. Moreover, even though the two ligands have similar affinity toward PTH1R, they have selectivity for a distinct conformation of PTH1R, with the response relatively greater with PTH (1–34) [28]. On the basis of these findings, the two ligands may exert distinctly different biological functions through the same receptor. Recently, a novel mechanism of PTH1R endocytosis was proposed that the TGF type II receptor is able to directly phosphorylate the cytoplasmic domain of PTH1R and facilitate the PTH-induced endocytosis of the PTH1R-TbRII complex [105].

1.6.2 Noncanonical G-Protein-Independent Pathways

Recent evidence suggests that PTH1R regulates Wnt signaling in a G-protein-independent manner. Wnt signaling is a central regulator of skeletal modeling and remodeling. In the canonical Wnt pathway, Wnt binds to its receptor frizzled and coreceptors (Lrp5/6) and recruits axin to the plasma membrane. This causes dissociation of a large cytoplasmic complex which, without Wnt, targets β-catenin for degradation. In the presence of Wnt, stabilized β-catenin accumulates in the nucleus and, together with TCF/LEF transcription factors, enhances gene expression [44]. PTH action on osteoblasts differentially regulates the expression, mostly through the cAMP/PKA pathway, of a number of key components of the Wnt pathway, such as β-catenin [75, 134], Dickkopf (Dkk)-1 [75], sclerostin [66], secreted frizzled-related protein 4 (sfrp4, [102]), and Wnt4 [9], among others. These effects stimulate Wnt signaling. PTH can also influence the Wnt pathway by forming a ternary PTH/PTH1R/Lrp6 complex followed by phosphorylation of Lrp6, and recruitment of axin to Lrp6 and stabilization of β-catenin [141]. Alternatively, PTH1R has a Dishevelled (Dvl)-interacting domain in its C-terminal intracellular tail and recruits Dvl from the cytoplasm in response to PTH activation [111]. Dvl is an adaptor protein that connects the Wnt receptor frizzled to axin. Therefore, PTH activates β-catenin directly in a frizzled- and Lrp-independent manner. In addition, PTH can stimulate Erk1/2 activation in a G-protein-independent pathway that recruits β-arrestins to the plasma membrane and forms scaffolding complexes in association with PTH1R [42]. The β-arrestin2-dependent PTH1R pathway contributes to increased bone mineral density in vivo [43].

1.6.3 PTH1R-Related Human Diseases

Defective PTH1R signaling causes two rare human diseases. Blomstrand chondrodysplasia is a perinatal lethal disease associated with mutations of the PTH1R so that it cannot bind to ligands and cannot activate downstream Gs pathways [62, 63]. The chondrodysplasia is characterized by highly advanced skeletal maturation with thickened cortical bone and marked reduction of resting and proliferating chondrocytes in the growth plate of long bones [13]. The second rare disease is Jansen's metaphyseal chondrodysplasia. It displays the opposite skeletal phenotype with abnormal growth plate elongation and a delay in chondrocyte maturation. Moreover, these patients have hypercalcemia and hypophosphatemia, conditions that mimic PTH actions.

Jansen's chondrodysplasia is an autosomal dominant disease that results from activating mutants of the PTH1R that lead to a ligand-independent accumulation of cAMP [115]. Another mutation in the PTH/PTHrP receptor gene, R150C, leads to a low degree of constitutive activity and appears to be responsible for some forms of enchondromatosis (Ollier's disease) [50].

1.7 Transcriptional Regulation by PTH1R

The involvement of transcriptional events in PTH action on osteoblastic cells was initially established by studying the UMR 106-01 rat osteosarcoma cell line. This cell line displays many osteoblastic markers including PTH1R, type I collagen synthesis, and high alkaline phosphatase. When treated with PTH, UMR cells typically decrease collagen synthesis and begin producing collagenase-3 (matrix metalloproteinase-13, MMP-13; [95, 106]). Northern blots and nuclear run-on assays with PTH-treated UMR cells have shown a hundredfold increase in the rate of synthesis of MMP-13 mRNA with the steady state levels of mRNA increased 180-fold at 4 h [117]. mRNA levels decline to approximately 30% of maximum by 8 h. The induction of MMP-13 transcription occurred only after a lag period of 1 h and was completely abolished by cycloheximide. This suggests that PTH effects on the MMP-13 gene in UMR cells are secondary responses that depend on expression of other genes.

A comprehensive analysis of changes in the profile of gene expression in UMR cells treated with 10^{-8} M rat PTH (1–34) was conducted in our laboratory with the aid of DNA microarray analysis [102]. One hundred twenty-five known genes and thirty unknown expressed sequence tags (ESTs) were found to have at least twofold expression changes after PTH treatment at 4, 12, and 24 h. The mechanisms by which PTH affected expression of a number of these genes and others identified from the in vivo microarrays (amphiregulin [104], IL-18 [107], Jagged1, syndecan-4, MKP-1 [101], Wnt-4 [9], MCP-1 [79]) were subsequently investigated in our laboratory; the bulk of them were by transcription, were primary events and were regulated by the PKA pathway implicating phosphorylation of CREB or similar proteins (e.g., ATF4) as their major mechanism of regulation. Yu et al. [146] have shown that PTH regulates ATF4, which then stimulates Osterix transcription.

Another gene regulated by PTH is that encoding bone sialoprotein (BSP), a major noncollagenous protein. In primary cultures of embryonic osteoblasts, this gene was shown to increase nearly fourfold after PTH treatment; cotransfection of a bsp promoter/reporter construct with a plasmid encoding the inhibitor of cAMP-dependent protein kinase abolished PTH-induced bsp transcription and also decreased basal transcription. PKC stimulates bsp expression independently of PTH because inhibitors of PKC have no effect on PTH induction of bsp expression [144]. Subsequently, two cAMP response elements (CREs) have been identified in the promoter of bsp. These are required for PTH stimulation of bsp transcription. The hormone increases the amount of phospho-CREB associated with these elements [3].

The discussion which follows will concentrate on PTH transcriptional activation of the MMP-13 gene, a complex secondary response gene. Activation involves changes in chromatin structure, two sets of transcription factors, Runx2 and Fos/Jun, and many steps of phosphorylation by PKA. In UMR cells, PTH induces MMP-13 transcription primarily through activation of cAMP and the PKA signaling pathway, rather than through PKC or calcium signaling, and this response requires expression of other genes. A series of deletion and point mutants of the MMP-13 promoter region have been generated to identify the PTH-responsive region and the primary response factors that convey the hormonal signal and bind to this region of the MMP-13 gene. The minimum PTH regulatory region is within 148 bp upstream of the transcriptional start site [119]. This region contains several consensus transcription factor recognition sequences, including SBE (Smad binding element), C/EBP (CCAAT enhancer-binding protein site), RD (runt domain-binding sequence), p53,

PEA-3 (polyoma enhancer activator-3), and AP (activator protein)-1 and AP-2. The AP-1 site is a major target for the Fos and Jun families of oncogenic transcription factors. The RD site is a target for runt homology domain-containing proteins, specifically Runx2. Mice containing a targeted disruption of the Runx2 gene die at birth and lack both skeletal ossification and mature osteoblasts [31, 70, 93]. These mutant mice also do not express MMP-13 during fetal development. MMP-13 is therefore one of the target genes regulated by Runx2 [61].

Additional experiments on the MMP-13 promoter have shown that both native AP-1 and RD sites and their corresponding binding proteins, AP-1 and Runx2-related proteins, are involved in PTH regulation of MMP-13 transcription. With the aid of gel-shift analysis, we have shown [119] that treatment with PTH enhanced binding of Fos and Jun proteins at the AP-1 site, even though the level of Runx2 binding to the RD site did not change. PTH induces PKA-mediated posttranslational phosphorylation of Runx2 and leads to enhanced MMP-13 promoter activity in UMR cells [120, 121].

PTH treatment transiently increases the mRNA expression of the AP-1 protein subunits c-fos and c-jun [23]. Both mRNA species are maximally induced within 30 min, well before the MMP-13 transcription rate reaches maximum at 2 h. PTH is responsible for PKA-dependent phosphorylation of CREB at serine 133 [135]. Once phosphorylated, CREB binds a CRE in the c-fos promoter and activates its transcription [96].

Runx2 binds to the RD sequence in promoter regions and regulates the expression of many bone-specific and bone-related genes, including osteocalcin [31], osteopontin [114], and MMP-13 [119]. Runx2 functions as a coactivator or corepressor of transcription, depending on which factors it binds with at promoter regions. At the MMP-13 promoter in osteoblastic cells, Runx2 binds histone deacetylase-4 (HDAC4), causing a repression of transcription under basal conditions [125]. After PTH treatment, through PKA-dependent pathways, HDAC4 dissociates from Runx2, which is then free to recruit the histone acetyltransferase (HAT), p300, to activate transcription [15]. PTH stimulates HDAC4 gene expression, an effect that feeds back to repress MMP-13 transcription. PCAF (another HAT) is a downstream transcriptional coactivator of PTH that is required for MMP-13 transcription to occur after PTH treatment of UMR 106-01 cells or of primary rat osteoblasts. The HAT activity of PCAF is stimulated by the acetylation of lysine residues in the C-terminus. This may involve autoacetylation or be brought about by p300, but not by CREB-binding protein (CBP). PTH increases the acetylation of PCAF, with the involvement of p300. In addition, PTH stimulation of MMP-13 promoter activity requires the HAT activities of both p300 and PCAF [77]. These findings suggest a model for PTH-regulation of genes that have a runt domain in their promoter region (Fig. 1.3).

1.8 PTH and PTHrP as Therapeutic Agents

1.8.1 PTH as an Anabolic Treatment for Osteoporosis

Even though PTH's physiological function is to regulate calcium and phosphate homeostasis and elevation of PTH in primary hyperparathyroidism leads to bone destruction, current interest in the study of PTH in the bone field focuses on its anabolic action through intermittent administration to increase bone mass, particularly in trabecular bone. This anabolic effect of PTH was first reported in the 1930s [7, 122], but was largely neglected due to the apparent contradiction between the physiological and pathological roles of PTH until the 1970s when clinical trials with PTH began in osteoporosis patients. In the 1980s, Tam et al. identified the differential effects of pulsatile and continuous administration of PTH on net bone apposition [131]. In 2002, the Food and Drug Administration (FDA) in the Unites States approved teriparatide, a recombinant human PTH (1–34), for the treatment of osteoporosis in postmenopausal women and men who are at high risk for fracture (20 μg daily injection for less than 2 years). Intact human PTH (1–84) is approved and available in Europe.

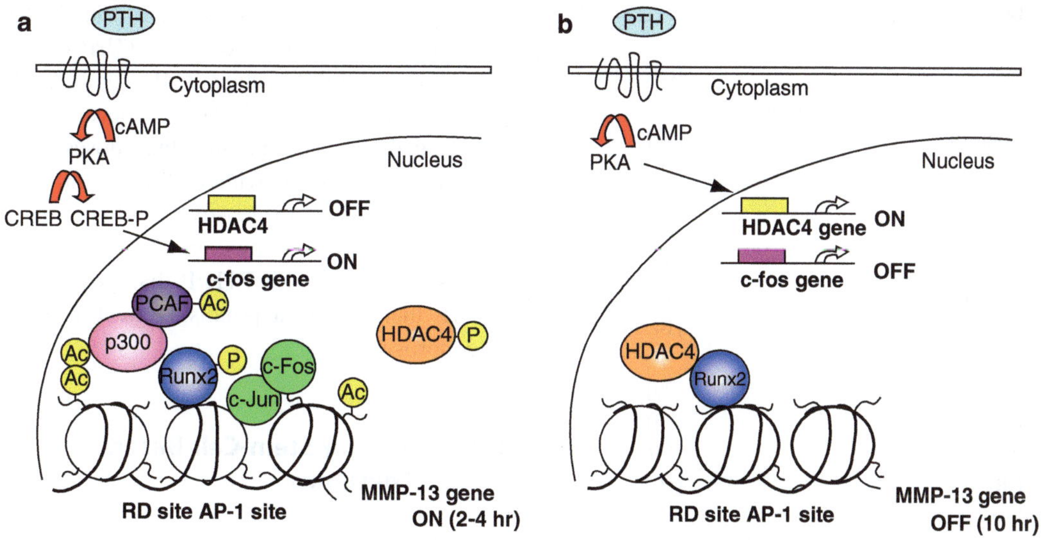

Fig. 1.3 Mechanisms of PTH regulation of transcription of the MMP-13 gene in osteoblastic cells. (**a**) PTH acting though PTH1R elicits activation of adenyl cyclase, production of cAMP, and activation of PKA. PKA initiates all the subsequent steps shown here. It phosphorylates CREB, which activates transcription of c-fos. It phosphorylates HDAC4 and Runx2, which are bound to the runt site of the MMP-13 promoter, causing their dissociation. With HDAC4 dissociated from Runx2 and trafficked to the cytoplasm, Runx2 is free to recruit the HATs, p300, and PCAF. This recruitment of p300 to Runx2 stimulates the acetylation of the corecruited PCAF. At about the same time (1 h after PTH stimulation), the Fos-Jun heterodimer binds to the AP-1 site of the MMP-13 promoter and interacts with Runx2 and p300/PCAF. This then leads to acetylation of the histones in this area of the promoter and induction of transcription of the MMP-13 gene. (**b**) PTH at later times, also acting through PKA, stimulates HDAC4 transcription. Newly synthesized HDAC4 reassociates with the MMP-13 promoter, deacetylating the histones and shutting off transcription of the gene encoding MMP-13

Compared to the more popular antiresorptive agents, such as estrogen, selective estrogen modulators, and bisphosphonates, intermittent injection of PTH as an anabolic agent stimulates both bone formation and resorption with the effect on formation greater than on resorption, leading to a net gain in bone mass [103]. PTH injection exerts most of its effects on trabecular bone, with significant increases in trabecular bone volume, connectivity, and improvement in the plate-like microarchitecture [59, 109]. At cortical sites, PTH typically does not increase bone density, but tends to increase porosity. PTH increases periosteal bone mass and enlarges the cross-sectional area. This strengthens cortical bone [16, 94]. Because PTH stimulates RANKL expression and inhibits OPG expression [39], injection with PTH markedly increases osteoclastogenesis and bone resorption. Clinical trials have shown that the anabolic effects of PTH are impaired by concurrent antiresorptive agent treatment [12, 36, 37]. In other words, bone resorption is necessary for PTH-induced bone formation. Possibly this involves a TGFβ1-mediated mechanism. TGFβ1 is a chemotactic factor for bone marrow mesenchymal stem cells [133], the progenitors for osteoblasts. Inhibition of TGFβ1 release from bone matrix by an antiresorptive agent impairs the PTH-stimulated recruitment of mesenchymal stem cells [143]. Monocyte chemoattractant protein-1 (MCP-1), a chemokine highly upregulated by PTH in vivo and involved in osteoclast migration and differentiation [79], is also required for mediating PTH's anabolic actions in a murine model [132].

Extensive investigations have been carried out to understand the cellular and molecular mechanisms by which intermittent injection of PTH increases osteoblast numbers. Multiple cellular mechanisms, including activation of bone lining cells, stimulation of osteoblast differentiation, and prevention of osteoblast apoptosis, contribute to the anabolic action of PTH [60, 103].

Table 1.1 A list of genes that mediate PTH's anabolic effects

Genes	References
Ligands, cytokines, growth factors	
Sclerostin	[72]
IGF-1	[10]
Interleukin 18	[107]
MCP-1	[132]
Fgf-2	[55]
TGF-β1	[143]
Sfrp1	[14, 145]
Transcription factors	
c-fos	[29]
Runx2	[73]
ATF4	[146]
CREM	[80]
Others	
Bcl-2	[90]
Connexin43	[20]
β-arrestin2	[34]

At the molecular level, the activation by PTH of distinct pathways indicates that Gas/cAMP/PKA is the major route for its anabolic action [4, 110]. PTH has profound effects on gene expression with hundreds of genes either upregulated or downregulated in osteoblastic cultures [102] or in osteoblast-rich rat trabecular bone [78]. The PTH-regulated genes have broad functions, stimulating growth factors and cytokines, signal transducers, structural molecules, transcription factors, transporters, and enzymes. This indicates that PTH influences many processes in osteoblasts. Identification of genes that respond to PTH and study of knockout mouse models of some of these genes together confirm that the anabolic action of PTH requires the expression of many genes (Table 1.1).

1.8.2 PTHrP as an Anabolic Treatment for Osteoporosis

Because PTHrP shares the same receptor with PTH, PTHrP (1–36) has been investigated as a potential anabolic agent to treat osteoporosis. PTHrP is effective in increasing bone mass and bone strength in ovariectomized rats [127]. Subsequent clinical studies have found that 3 months of daily injections of PTHrP (1–36) increased the lumbar spine BMD significantly [52]. In contrast to PTH, PTHrP appears to be a pure anabolic agent because high doses stimulate bone formation without effects on bone resorption markers [51]. Adverse effects, such as nausea, muscle cramps, and hypercalcemia, are less common with PTHrP than with PTH. PTHrP therefore is a promising treatment for osteoporosis.

1.8.3 PTH for Stem-Cell-Based Therapies

In adult bone marrow, hematopoietic stem cells (HSCs) are found in the endosteal niche, located at the surface of bone where quiescent HSCs come in contact with osteoblasts [17, 148]. Since intermittent injection of PTH greatly increases osteoblast number, it is not surprising that PTH has a strong effect on the HSC pool. This effect has been investigated intensively to manipulate this pool for therapeutic usage. It has been demonstrated that PTH signaling expands the HSC pool by increasing expression of Jagged1 in osteoblasts and activating the Notch pathway in HSC [17]. In addition, animal models have shown that PTH treatment contributes to (1) mobilize HSCs into the peripheral circulation, (2) protect and expand the HSC pool in bone marrow during chemotherapy cycles, and (3) expand exogenous stem cells delivered to the niche by a bone marrow transplantation protocol [108]. A phase I study showed that PTH enhances HSC mobilization in patients undergoing autologous stem cell transplantation who failed prior stem cell mobilization when on a standard protocol [6]. Moreover, PTH treatment of myocardial infarction in a murine model has demonstrated significantly improved survival and myocardial function because HSC progenitor cells were mobilized to the ischemic heart and enhanced neovascularization [54, 147]. Together with the well-known hypotensive and vasodilatory effect of PTH/PTHrP [97], PTH is a promising treatment for cardiovascular diseases.

Conclusion

PTH and PTHrP have classical roles on calcium and phosphate metabolism. PTHrP has this role in the fetus and in diseases such as HHM. PTHrP plays an important paracrine and autocrine role as a local factor, particularly in the regulation of growth plate formation and endochondral ossification. It does this by stimulating proliferation of chondrocytes and blocking their differentiation to hypertrophic chondrocytes. In tumor metastasis to bone, PTHrP can be produced by the tumor and perpetuate the "vicious cycle" of osteolysis and tumor growth. Apart from its classical effect to stimulate bone breakdown, PTH has the paradoxical effect of stimulating bone formation, its anabolic effect. Because of this, it is now used as teriparatide to treat osteoporosis. The mechanism is still unknown, but many genes seem to be involved in this action. PTHrP may be an excellent alternative to PTH treatment of osteoporosis. PTH may also be a treatment option to mobilize stem cells. Overall, exciting possibilities exist for research and therapy for both PTH and PTHrP.

References

1. Amizuka N, Warshawsky H, Henderson JE, Goltzman D, Karaplis AC. Parathyroid hormone-related peptide-depleted mice show abnormal epiphyseal cartilage development and altered endochondral bone formation. J Cell Biol. 1994;126:1611–23.
2. Amling M, Neff L, Tanaka S, Inoue D, Kuida K, Weir E, Philbrick WM, Broadus AE, Baron R. Bcl-2 lies downstream of parathyroid hormone-related peptide in a signaling pathway that regulates chondrocyte maturation during skeletal development. J Cell Biol. 1997;136:205–13.
3. Araki S, Mezawa M, Sasaki Y, Yang L, Li Z, Takai H, Nakayama Y, Ogata Y. Parathyroid hormone regulation of the human bone sialoprotein gene transcription is mediated through two cAMP response elements. J Cell Biochem. 2009;106:618–25.
4. Armamento-Villareal R, Ziambaras K, Abbasi-Jarhomi SH, Dimarogonas A, Halstead L, Fausto A, Avioli LV, Civitelli R. An intact N terminus is required for the anabolic action of parathyroid hormone on adult female rats. J Bone Miner Res. 1997;12:384–92.
5. Bacic D, Lehir M, Biber J, Kaissling B, Murer H, Wagner CA. The renal Na+/phosphate cotransporter NaPi-IIa is internalized via the receptor-mediated endocytic route in response to parathyroid hormone. Kidney Int. 2006;69:495–503.
6. Ballen KK, Shpall EJ, Avigan D, Yeap BY, Fisher DC, McDermott K, Dey BR, Attar E, McAfee S, Konopleva M, Antin JH, Spitzer TR. Phase I trial of parathyroid hormone to facilitate stem cell mobilization. Biol Blood Marrow Transplant. 2007;13:838–43.
7. Bauer W, Aub JC, Albright F. Studies of calcium and phosphorus metabolism: V. A study of the bone trabeculae as a readily available reserve supply of calcium. J Exp Med. 1929;49:145–62.
8. Ben-Dov IZ, Galitzer H, Lavi-Moshayoff V, Goetz R, Kuro-o M, Mohammadi M, Sirkis R, Naveh-Many T, Silver J. The parathyroid is a target organ for FGF23 in rats. J Clin Invest. 2007;117:4003–8.
9. Bergenstock MK, Partridge NC. Parathyroid hormone stimulation of noncanonical Wnt signaling in bone. Ann N Y Acad Sci. 2007;1116:354–9.
10. Bikle DD, Sakata T, Leary C, Elalieh H, Ginzinger D, Rosen CJ, Beamer W, Majumdar S, Halloran BP. Insulin-like growth factor I is required for the anabolic actions of parathyroid hormone on mouse bone. J Bone Miner Res. 2002;17:1570–8.
11. Bitgood MJ, McMahon AP. Hedgehog and Bmp genes are coexpressed at many diverse sites of cell-cell interaction in the mouse embryo. Dev Biol. 1995;172:126–38.
12. Black DM, Greenspan SL, Ensrud KE, Palermo L, McGowan JA, Lang TF, Garnero P, Bouxsein ML, Bilezikian JP, Rosen CJ. The effects of parathyroid hormone and alendronate alone or in combination in postmenopausal osteoporosis. N Engl J Med. 2003; 349:1207–15.
13. Blomstrand S, Claesson I, Save-Soderbergh J. A case of lethal congenital dwarfism with accelerated skeletal maturation. Pediatr Radiol. 1985;15:141–3.
14. Bodine PV, Seestaller-Wehr L, Kharode YP, Bex FJ, Komm BS. Bone anabolic effects of parathyroid hormone are blunted by deletion of the Wnt antagonist secreted frizzled-related protein-1. J Cell Physiol. 2007;210:352–7.
15. Boumah CE, Lee M, Selvamurugan N, Shimizu E, Partridge NC. Runx2 recruits p300 to mediate parathyroid hormone's effects on histone acetylation and transcriptional activation of the matrix metalloproteinase-13 gene. Mol Endocrinol. 2009;23: 1255–63.
16. Burr DB, Hirano T, Turner CH, Hotchkiss C, Brommage R, Hock JM. Intermittently administered human parathyroid hormone(1–34) treatment increases intracortical bone turnover and porosity without reducing bone strength in the humerus of ovariectomized cynomolgus monkeys. J Bone Miner Res. 2001;16:157–65.
17. Calvi LM, Adams GB, Weibrecht KW, Weber JM, Olson DP, Knight MC, Martin RP, Schipani E, Divieti P, Bringhurst FR, Milner LA, Kronenberg HM, Scadden DT. Osteoblastic cells regulate the haematopoietic stem cell niche. Nature. 2003;425:841–6.

18. Canario AV, Rotllant J, Fuentes J, Guerreiro PM, Rita Teodosio H, Power DM, Clark MS. Novel bioactive parathyroid hormone and related peptides in teleost fish. FEBS Lett. 2006;580:291–9.
19. Care AD, Abbas SK, Pickard DW, Barri M, Drinkhill M, Findlay JB, White IR, Caple IW. Stimulation of ovine placental transport of calcium and magnesium by mid-molecule fragments of human parathyroid hormone-related protein. Exp Physiol. 1990;75:605–8.
20. Chung DJ, Castro CH, Watkins M, Stains JP, Chung MY, Szejnfeld VL, Willecke K, Theis M, Civitelli R. Low peak bone mass and attenuated anabolic response to parathyroid hormone in mice with an osteoblast-specific deletion of connexin43. J Cell Sci. 2006;119: 4187–98.
21. Civitelli R, Reid IR, Westbrook S, Avioli LV, Hruska KA. PTH elevates inositol polyphosphates and diacylglycerol in a rat osteoblast-like cell line. Am J Physiol. 1988;255:E660–7.
22. Clemens TL, Cormier S, Eichinger A, Endlich K, Fiaschi-Taesch N, Fischer E, Friedman PA, Karaplis AC, Massfelder T, Rossert J, Schluter KD, Silve C, Stewart AF, Takane K, Helwig JJ. Parathyroid hormone-related protein and its receptors: nuclear functions and roles in the renal and cardiovascular systems, the placental trophoblasts and the pancreatic islets. Br J Pharmacol. 2001;134:1113–36.
23. Clohisy JC, Scott DK, Brakenhoff KD, Quinn CO, Partridge NC. Parathyroid hormone induces c-fos and c-jun messenger RNA in rat osteoblastic cells. Mol Endocrinol. 1992;6:1834–42.
24. Collip JB. Extraction of a parathyroid hormone which will prevent or control parathyroid tetany and which regulates the level of blood calcium. J Biol Chem. 1925;63:395–438.
25. Cornish J, Callon KE, Nicholson GC, Reid IR. Parathyroid hormone-related protein-(107–139) inhibits bone resorption in vivo. Endocrinology. 1997; 138:1299–304.
26. Danks JA, Ho PM, Notini AJ, Katsis F, Hoffmann P, Kemp BE, Martin TJ, Zajac JD. Identification of a parathyroid hormone in the fish Fugu rubripes. J Bone Miner Res. 2003;18:1326–31.
27. DaSilva J, Gioeli D, Weber MJ, Parsons SJ. The neuroendocrine-derived peptide parathyroid hormone-related protein promotes prostate cancer cell growth by stabilizing the androgen receptor. Cancer Res. 2009;69:7402–11.
28. Dean T, Vilardaga JP, Potts Jr JT, Gardella TJ. Altered selectivity of parathyroid hormone (PTH) and PTH-related protein (PTHrP) for distinct conformations of the PTH/PTHrP receptor. Mol Endocrinol. 2008;22:156–66.
29. Demiralp B, Chen HL, Koh AJ, Keller ET, McCauley LK. Anabolic actions of parathyroid hormone during bone growth are dependent on c-fos. Endocrinology. 2002;143:4038–47.
30. Diaz R, El-Hajj GF, Brown E. Regulation of parathyroid function. In: Fray JGS, editor. Handbook of physiology. New York: Oxford University Press; 1998. p. 607–62.
31. Ducy P, Zhang R, Geoffroy V, Ridall AL, Karsenty G. Osf2/Cbfa1: a transcriptional activator of osteoblast differentiation. Cell. 1997;89:747–54.
32. Fenton AJ, Kemp BE, Kent GN, Moseley JM, Zheng MH, Rowe DJ, Britto JM, Martin TJ, Nicholson GC. A carboxyl-terminal peptide from the parathyroid hormone-related protein inhibits bone resorption by osteoclasts. Endocrinology. 1991;129:1762–8.
33. Ferrandon S, Feinstein TN, Castro M, Wang B, Bouley R, Potts JT, Gardella TJ, Vilardaga JP. Sustained cyclic AMP production by parathyroid hormone receptor endocytosis. Nat Chem Biol. 2009;5: 734–42.
34. Ferrari SL, Pierroz DD, Glatt V, Goddard DS, Bianchi EN, Lin FT, Manen D, Bouxsein ML. Bone response to intermittent parathyroid hormone is altered in mice null for {beta}-Arrestin2. Endocrinology. 2005;146: 1854–62.
35. Fiaschi-Taesch NM, Stewart AF. Minireview: parathyroid hormone-related protein as an intracrine factor – trafficking mechanisms and functional consequences. Endocrinology. 2003;144:407–11.
36. Finkelstein JS, Hayes A, Hunzelman JL, Wyland JJ, Lee H, Neer RM. The effects of parathyroid hormone, alendronate, or both in men with osteoporosis. N Engl J Med. 2003;349:1216–26.
37. Finkelstein JS, Wyland JJ, Lee H, Neer RM. Effects of teriparatide, alendronate, or both in women with postmenopausal osteoporosis. J Clin Endocrinol Metab. 2010;95:1838–45.
38. Fraser DR, Kodicek E. Regulation of 25-hydroxycholecalciferol-1-hydroxylase activity in kidney by parathyroid hormone. Nat New Biol. 1973;241: 163–6.
39. Fu Q, Jilka RL, Manolagas SC, O'Brien CA. Parathyroid hormone stimulates receptor activator of NFkappa B ligand and inhibits osteoprotegerin expression via protein kinase A activation of cAMP-response element-binding protein. J Biol Chem. 2002;277: 48868–75.
40. Gallwitz WE, Guise TA, Mundy GR. Guanosine nucleotides inhibit different syndromes of PTHrP excess caused by human cancers in vivo. J Clin Invest. 2002;110:1559–72.
41. Gensure RC, Ponugoti B, Gunes Y, Papasani MR, Lanske B, Bastepe M, Rubin DA, Juppner H. Identification and characterization of two parathyroid hormone-like molecules in zebrafish. Endocrinology. 2004;145:1634–9.
42. Gesty-Palmer D, Chen M, Reiter E, Ahn S, Nelson CD, Wang S, Eckhardt AE, Cowan CL, Spurney RF, Luttrell LM, Lefkowitz RJ. Distinct beta-arrestin- and G protein-dependent pathways for parathyroid hormone receptor-stimulated ERK1/2 activation. J Biol Chem. 2006;281:10856–64.
43. Gesty-Palmer D, Flannery P, Yuan L, Corsino L, Spurney R, Lefkowitz RJ, Luttrell LM. A beta-arrestin-biased agonist of the parathyroid hormone receptor (PTH1R) promotes bone formation independent of G protein activation. Sci Transl Med. 2009;1:1ra1.

44. Gordon MD, Nusse R. Wnt signaling: multiple pathways, multiple receptors, and multiple transcription factors. J Biol Chem. 2006;281:22429–33.
45. Guise TA, Yin JJ, Taylor SD, Kumagai Y, Dallas M, Boyce BF, Yoneda T, Mundy GR. Evidence for a causal role of parathyroid hormone-related protein in the pathogenesis of human breast cancer-mediated osteolysis. J Clin Invest. 1996;98:1544–9.
46. Guo J, Chung UI, Kondo H, Bringhurst FR, Kronenberg HM. The PTH/PTHrP receptor can delay chondrocyte hypertrophy in vivo without activating phospholipase C. Dev Cell. 2002;3:183–94.
47. Guo J, Chung UI, Yang D, Karsenty G, Bringhurst FR, Kronenberg HM. PTH/PTHrP receptor delays chondrocyte hypertrophy via both Runx2-dependent and -independent pathways. Dev Biol. 2006;292:116–28.
48. Habener JF, Potts Jr JT, Rich A. Pre-proparathyroid hormone. Evidence for an early biosynthetic precursor of proparathyroid hormone. J Biol Chem. 1976;251:3893–9.
49. Hebert SC. Therapeutic use of calcimimetics. Annu Rev Med. 2006;57:349–64.
50. Hopyan S, Gokgoz N, Poon R, Gensure RC, Yu C, Cole WG, Bell RS, Juppner H, Andrulis IL, Wunder JS, Alman BA. A mutant PTH/PTHrP type I receptor in enchondromatosis. Nat Genet. 2002;30:306–10.
51. Horwitz MJ, Tedesco MB, Garcia-Ocana A, Sereika SM, Prebehala L, Bisello A, Hollis BW, Gundberg CM, Stewart AF. Parathyroid hormone-related protein for the treatment of postmenopausal osteoporosis: defining the maximal tolerable dose. J Clin Endocrinol Metab. 2010;95:1279–87.
52. Horwitz MJ, Tedesco MB, Gundberg C, Garcia-Ocana A, Stewart AF. Short-term, high-dose parathyroid hormone-related protein as a skeletal anabolic agent for the treatment of postmenopausal osteoporosis. J Clin Endocrinol Metab. 2003;88:569–75.
53. Huang W, Chung UI, Kronenberg HM, de Crombrugghe B. The chondrogenic transcription factor Sox9 is a target of signaling by the parathyroid hormone-related peptide in the growth plate of endochondral bones. Proc Natl Acad Sci USA. 2001;98:160–5.
54. Huber BC, Fischer R, Brunner S, Groebner M, Rischpler C, Segeth A, Zaruba MM, Wollenweber T, Hacker M, Franz WM. Comparison of parathyroid hormone and G-CSF treatment after myocardial infarction on perfusion and stem cell homing. Am J Physiol Heart Circ Physiol. 2010;298:H1466–71.
55. Hurley MM, Okada Y, Xiao L, Tanaka Y, Ito M, Okimoto N, Nakamura T, Rosen CJ, Doetschman T, Coffin JD. Impaired bone anabolic response to parathyroid hormone in Fgf2–/– and Fgf2+/– mice. Biochem Biophys Res Commun. 2006;341:989–94.
56. Imura A, Tsuji Y, Murata M, Maeda R, Kubota K, Iwano A, Obuse C, Togashi K, Tominaga M, Kita N, Tomiyama K, Iijima J, Nabeshima Y, Fujioka M, Asato R, Tanaka S, Kojima K, Ito J, Nozaki K, Hashimoto N, Ito T, Nishio T, Uchiyama T, Fujimori T. Alpha-Klotho as a regulator of calcium homeostasis. Science. 2007;316:1615–8.
57. Jaakola VP, Ijzerman AP. The crystallographic structure of the human adenosine A2A receptor in a high-affinity antagonist-bound state: implications for GPCR drug screening and design. Curr Opin Struct Biol. 2010;20:401–14.
58. Jans DA, Thomas RJ, Gillespie MT. Parathyroid hormone-related protein (PTHrP): a nucleocytoplasmic shuttling protein with distinct paracrine and intracrine roles. Vitam Horm. 2003;66:345–84.
59. Jiang Y, Zhao JJ, Mitlak BH, Wang O, Genant HK, Eriksen EF. Recombinant human parathyroid hormone (1–34) [teriparatide] improves both cortical and cancellous bone structure. J Bone Miner Res. 2003;18:1932–41.
60. Jilka RL. Molecular and cellular mechanisms of the anabolic effect of intermittent PTH. Bone. 2007;40:1434–46.
61. Jimenez MJ, Balbin M, Lopez JM, Alvarez J, Komori T, Lopez-Otin C. Collagenase 3 is a target of Cbfa1, a transcription factor of the runt gene family involved in bone formation. Mol Cell Biol. 1999;19:4431–42.
62. Jobert AS, Zhang P, Couvineau A, Bonaventure J, Roume J, Le Merrer M, Silve C. Absence of functional receptors for parathyroid hormone and parathyroid hormone-related peptide in Blomstrand chondrodysplasia. J Clin Invest. 1998;102:34–40.
63. Karaplis AC, He B, Nguyen MT, Young ID, Semeraro D, Ozawa H, Amizuka N. Inactivating mutation in the human parathyroid hormone receptor type 1 gene in Blomstrand chondrodysplasia. Endocrinology. 1998;139:5255–8.
64. Karaplis AC, Luz A, Glowacki J, Bronson RT, Tybulewicz VL, Kronenberg HM, Mulligan RC. Lethal skeletal dysplasia from targeted disruption of the parathyroid hormone-related peptide gene. Genes Dev. 1994;8:277–89.
65. Kartsogiannis V, Moseley J, McKelvie B, Chou ST, Hards DK, Ng KW, Martin TJ, Zhou H. Temporal expression of PTHrP during endochondral bone formation in mouse and intramembranous bone formation in an in vivo rabbit model. Bone. 1997;21:385–92.
66. Keller H, Kneissel M. SOST is a target gene for PTH in bone. Bone. 2005;37:148–58.
67. Kemper B, Habener JF, Rich A, Potts Jr JT. Microtubules and the intracellular conversion of proparathyroid hormone to parathyroid hormone. Endocrinology. 1975;96:903–12.
68. Khosla S, Demay M, Pines M, Hurwitz S, Potts Jr JT, Kronenberg HM. Nucleotide sequence of cloned cDNAs encoding chicken preproparathyroid hormone. J Bone Miner Res. 1988;3:689–98.
69. Kim MS, Fujiki R, Murayama A, Kitagawa H, Yamaoka K, Yamamoto Y, Mihara M, Takeyama K, Kato S. 1Alpha,25(OH)2D3-induced transrepression by vitamin D receptor through E-box-type elements in the human parathyroid hormone gene promoter. Mol Endocrinol. 2007;21:334–42.
70. Komori T, Yagi H, Nomura S, Yamaguchi A, Sasaki K, Deguchi K, Shimizu Y, Bronson RT, Gao YH, Inada M, Sato M, Okamoto R, Kitamura Y, Yoshiki S, Kishimoto T.

Targeted disruption of Cbfa1 results in a complete lack of bone formation owing to maturational arrest of osteoblasts. Cell. 1997;89:755–64.
71. Kovacs CS, Lanske B, Hunzelman JL, Guo J, Karaplis AC, Kronenberg HM. Parathyroid hormone-related peptide (PTHrP) regulates fetal-placental calcium transport through a receptor distinct from the PTH/PTHrP receptor. Proc Natl Acad Sci USA. 1996;93:15233–8.
72. Kramer I, Loots GG, Studer A, Keller H, Kneissel M. Parathyroid hormone (PTH)-induced bone gain is blunted in SOST overexpressing and deficient mice. J Bone Miner Res. 2010;25:178–89.
73. Krishnan V, Moore TL, Ma YL, Helvering LM, Frolik CA, Valasek KM, Ducy P, Geiser AG. Parathyroid hormone bone anabolic action requires Cbfa1/Runx2-dependent signaling. Mol Endocrinol. 2003;17:423–35.
74. Kukreja SC, Shevrin DH, Wimbiscus SA, Ebeling PR, Danks JA, Rodda CP, Wood WI, Martin TJ. Antibodies to parathyroid hormone-related protein lower serum calcium in athymic mouse models of malignancy-associated hypercalcemia due to human tumors. J Clin Invest. 1988;82:1798–802.
75. Kulkarni NH, Halladay DL, Miles RR, Gilbert LM, Frolik CA, Galvin RJ, Martin TJ, Gillespie MT, Onyia JE. Effects of parathyroid hormone on Wnt signaling pathway in bone. J Cell Biochem. 2005;95: 1178–90.
76. Lanske B, Karaplis AC, Lee K, Luz A, Vortkamp A, Pirro A, Karperien M, Defize LH, Ho C, Mulligan RC, Abou-Samra AB, Juppner H, Segre GV, Kronenberg HM. PTH/PTHrP receptor in early development and Indian hedgehog-regulated bone growth. Science. 1996;273:663–6.
77. Lee M, Partridge NC. Parathyroid hormone activation of matrix metalloproteinase-13 transcription requires the histone acetyltransferase activity of p300 and PCAF and p300-dependent acetylation of PCAF. J Biol Chem. 2010;285:38014–22.
78. Li X, Liu H, Qin L, Tamasi J, Bergenstock M, Shapses S, Feyen JH, Notterman DA, Partridge NC. Determination of dual effects of parathyroid hormone on skeletal gene expression in vivo by microarray and network analysis. J Biol Chem. 2007;282:33086–97.
79. Li X, Qin L, Bergenstock M, Bevelock LM, Novack DV, Partridge NC. Parathyroid hormone stimulates osteoblastic expression of MCP-1 to recruit and increase the fusion of pre/osteoclasts. J Biol Chem. 2007; 282:33098–106.
80. Liu F, Lee SK, Adams DJ, Gronowicz GA, Kream BE. CREM deficiency in mice alters the response of bone to intermittent parathyroid hormone treatment. Bone. 2007;40:1135–43.
81. Liu Y, Ibrahim AS, Tay BH, Richardson SJ, Bell J, Walker TI, Brenner S, Venkatesh B, Danks JA. Parathyroid hormone gene family in a cartilaginous fish, the elephant shark (*Callorhinchus milii*). J Bone Miner Res. 2010;25:2337–47.
82. Lomri A, de Pollak C, Sebag M, Goltzman D, Kremer R, Marie PJ. Expression of parathyroid hormone-related peptide (PTHrP) and PTH/PTHrP receptor in newborn human calvaria osteoblastic cells. Eur J Endocrinol. 1997;136:640–8.
83. Mahon MJ, Cole JA, Lederer ED, Segre GV. Na+/H+ exchanger-regulatory factor 1 mediates inhibition of phosphate transport by parathyroid hormone and second messengers by acting at multiple sites in opossum kidney cells. Mol Endocrinol. 2003;17:2355–64.
84. Mahon MJ, Donowitz M, Yun CC, Segre GV. Na(+)/H(+) exchanger regulatory factor 2 directs parathyroid hormone 1 receptor signalling. Nature. 2002;417:858–61.
85. Miao D, He B, Jiang Y, Kobayashi T, Soroceanu MA, Zhao J, Su H, Tong X, Amizuka N, Gupta A, Genant HK, Kronenberg HM, Goltzman D, Karaplis AC. Osteoblast-derived PTHrP is a potent endogenous bone anabolic agent that modifies the therapeutic efficacy of administered PTH 1–34. J Clin Invest. 2005; 115:2402–11.
86. Miao D, He B, Lanske B, Bai XY, Tong XK, Hendy GN, Goltzman D, Karaplis AC. Skeletal abnormalities in Pth-null mice are influenced by dietary calcium. Endocrinology. 2004;145:2046–53.
87. Miao D, Li J, Xue Y, Su H, Karaplis AC, Goltzman D. Parathyroid hormone-related peptide is required for increased trabecular bone volume in parathyroid hormone-null mice. Endocrinology. 2004;145:3554–62.
88. Moseley JM, Kubota M, Diefenbach-Jagger H, Wettenhall RE, Kemp BE, Suva LJ, Rodda CP, Ebeling PR, Hudson PJ, Zajac JD, et al. Parathyroid hormone-related protein purified from a human lung cancer cell line. Proc Natl Acad Sci USA. 1987;84: 5048–52.
89. Mundy GR. Mechanisms of bone metastasis. Cancer. 1997;80:1546–56.
90. Nagase Y, Iwasawa M, Akiyama T, Ogata N, Kadono Y, Nakamura M, Oshima Y, Yasui T, Matsumoto T, Masuda H, Bouillet P, Nakamura K, Tanaka S. Antiapoptotic molecule Bcl-2 is essential for the anabolic activity of parathyroid hormone in bone. Ann N Y Acad Sci. 2010;1192:330–7.
91. Naveh-Many T. Minireview: the play of proteins on the parathyroid hormone messenger ribonucleic acid regulates its expression. Endocrinology. 2010;151: 1398–402.
92. Okazaki T, Igarashi T, Kronenberg HM. 5′-flanking region of the parathyroid hormone gene mediates negative regulation by 1,25-(OH)2 vitamin D3. J Biol Chem. 1988;263:2203–8.
93. Otto F, Thornell AP, Crompton T, Denzel A, Gilmour KC, Rosewell IR, Stamp GW, Beddington RS, Mundlos S, Olsen BR, Selby PB, Owen MJ. Cbfa1, a candidate gene for cleidocranial dysplasia syndrome, is essential for osteoblast differentiation and bone development. Cell. 1997;89:765–71.
94. Parfitt AM. Parathyroid hormone and periosteal bone expansion. J Bone Miner Res. 2002;17:1741–3.

95. Partridge NC, Jeffrey JJ, Ehlich LS, Teitelbaum SL, Fliszar C, Welgus HG, Kahn AJ. Hormonal regulation of the production of collagenase and a collagenase inhibitor activity by rat osteogenic sarcoma cells. Endocrinology. 1987;120:1956–62.
96. Pearman AT, Chou WY, Bergman KD, Pulumati MR, Partridge NC. Parathyroid hormone induces c-fos promoter activity in osteoblastic cells through phosphorylated cAMP response element (CRE)-binding protein binding to the major CRE. J Biol Chem. 1996;271:25715–21.
97. Philbrick WM, Wysolmerski JJ, Galbraith S, Holt E, Orloff JJ, Yang KH, Vasavada RC, Weir EC, Broadus AE, Stewart AF. Defining the roles of parathyroid hormone-related protein in normal physiology. Physiol Rev. 1996;76:127–73.
98. Pioszak AA, Harikumar KG, Parker NR, Miller LJ, Xu HE. Dimeric arrangement of the parathyroid hormone receptor and a structural mechanism for ligand-induced dissociation. J Biol Chem. 2010;285: 12435–44.
99. Pioszak AA, Parker NR, Gardella TJ, Xu HE. Structural basis for parathyroid hormone-related protein binding to the parathyroid hormone receptor and design of conformation-selective peptides. J Biol Chem. 2009;284:28382–91.
100. Pioszak AA, Xu HE. Molecular recognition of parathyroid hormone by its G protein-coupled receptor. Proc Natl Acad Sci USA. 2008;105:5034–9.
101. Qin L, Li X, Ko JK, Partridge NC. Parathyroid hormone uses multiple mechanisms to arrest the cell cycle progression of osteoblastic cells from G1 to S phase. J Biol Chem. 2005;280:3104–11.
102. Qin L, Qiu P, Wang L, Li X, Swarthout JT, Soteropoulos P, Tolias P, Partridge NC. Gene expression profiles and transcription factors involved in parathyroid hormone signaling in osteoblasts revealed by microarray and bioinformatics. J Biol Chem. 2003;278:19723–31.
103. Qin L, Raggatt LJ, Partridge NC. Parathyroid hormone: a double-edged sword for bone metabolism. Trends Endocrinol Metab. 2004;15:60–5.
104. Qin L, Tamasi J, Raggatt L, Li X, Feyen JH, Lee DC, Dicicco-Bloom E, Partridge NC. Amphiregulin is a novel growth factor involved in normal bone development and in the cellular response to parathyroid hormone stimulation. J Biol Chem. 2005;280: 3974–81.
105. Qiu T, Wu X, Zhang F, Clemens TL, Wan M, Cao X. TGF-beta type II receptor phosphorylates PTH receptor to integrate bone remodelling signalling. Nat Cell Biol. 2010;12:224–34.
106. Quinn CO, Scott DK, Brinckerhoff CE, Matrisian LM, Jeffrey JJ, Partridge NC. Rat collagenase. Cloning, amino acid sequence comparison, and parathyroid hormone regulation in osteoblastic cells. J Biol Chem. 1990;265:22342–7.
107. Raggatt LJ, Qin L, Tamasi J, Jefcoat Jr SC, Shimizu E, Selvamurugan N, Liew FY, Bevelock L, Feyen JH, Partridge NC. Interleukin-18 is regulated by parathyroid hormone and is required for its bone anabolic actions. J Biol Chem. 2008;283:6790–8.
108. Rashidi N, Adams GB. The influence of parathyroid hormone on the adult hematopoietic stem cell niche. Curr Osteoporos Rep. 2009;7:53–7.
109. Recker RR, Bare SP, Smith SY, Varela A, Miller MA, Morris SA, Fox J. Cancellous and cortical bone architecture and turnover at the iliac crest of postmenopausal osteoporotic women treated with parathyroid hormone 1–84. Bone. 2009;44:113–9.
110. Rixon RH, Whitfield JF, Gagnon L, Isaacs RJ, Maclean S, Chakravarthy B, Durkin JP, Neugebauer W, Ross V, Sung W, Willick GE. Parathyroid hormone fragments may stimulate bone growth in ovariectomized rats by activating adenylyl cyclase. J Bone Miner Res. 1994;9:1179–89.
111. Romero G, Sneddon WB, Yang Y, Wheeler D, Blair HC, Friedman PA. Parathyroid hormone receptor directly interacts with dishevelled to regulate beta-Catenin signaling and osteoclastogenesis. J Biol Chem. 2010;285:14756–63.
112. Rotllant J, Guerreiro PM, Redruello B, Fernandes H, Apolonia L, Anjos L, Canario AV, Power DM. Ligand binding and signalling pathways of PTH receptors in sea bream (*Sparus auratus*) enterocytes. Cell Tissue Res. 2006;323:333–41.
113. Rubin DA, Juppner H. Zebrafish express the common parathyroid hormone/parathyroid hormone-related peptide receptor (PTH1R) and a novel receptor (PTH3R) that is preferentially activated by mammalian and fugufish parathyroid hormone-related peptide. J Biol Chem. 1999;274:28185–90.
114. Sato M, Morii E, Komori T, Kawahata H, Sugimoto M, Terai K, Shimizu H, Yasui T, Ogihara H, Yasui N, Ochi T, Kitamura Y, Ito Y, Nomura S. Transcriptional regulation of osteopontin gene in vivo by PEBP2alphaA/CBFA1 and ETS1 in the skeletal tissues. Oncogene. 1998;17:1517–25.
115. Schipani E, Langman CB, Parfitt AM, Jensen GS, Kikuchi S, Kooh SW, Cole WG, Juppner H. Constitutively activated receptors for parathyroid hormone and parathyroid hormone-related peptide in Jansen's metaphyseal chondrodysplasia. N Engl J Med. 1996;335:708–14.
116. Schipani E, Lanske B, Hunzelman J, Luz A, Kovacs CS, Lee K, Pirro A, Kronenberg HM, Juppner H. Targeted expression of constitutively active receptors for parathyroid hormone and parathyroid hormone-related peptide delays endochondral bone formation and rescues mice that lack parathyroid hormone-related peptide. Proc Natl Acad Sci USA. 1997;94:13689–94.
117. Scott DK, Brakenhoff KD, Clohisy JC, Quinn CO, Partridge NC. Parathyroid hormone induces transcription of collagenase in rat osteoblastic cells by a mechanism using cyclic adenosine 3′,5′-monophosphate and requiring protein synthesis. Mol Endocrinol. 1992;6:2153–9.

118. Segawa H, Yamanaka S, Onitsuka A, Tomoe Y, Kuwahata M, Ito M, Taketani Y, Miyamoto K. Parathyroid hormone-dependent endocytosis of renal type IIc Na-Pi cotransporter. Am J Physiol Renal Physiol. 2007;292:F395–403.
119. Selvamurugan N, Chou WY, Pearman AT, Pulumati MR, Partridge NC. Parathyroid hormone regulates the rat collagenase-3 promoter in osteoblastic cells through the cooperative interaction of the activator protein-1 site and the runt domain binding sequence. J Biol Chem. 1998;273:10647–57.
120. Selvamurugan N, Pulumati MR, Tyson DR, Partridge NC. Parathyroid hormone regulation of the rat collagenase-3 promoter by protein kinase A-dependent transactivation of core binding factor alpha1. J Biol Chem. 2000;275:5037–42.
121. Selvamurugan N, Shimizu E, Lee M, Liu T, Li H, Partridge NC. Identification and characterization of Runx2 phosphorylation sites involved in matrix metalloproteinase-13 promoter activation. FEBS Lett. 2009;583:1141–6.
122. Selye H. On the stimulation of new bone-formation with parathyroid extract and irradiated ergosterol. Endocrinology. 1932;16:547–58.
123. Shen X, Falzon M. PTH-related protein upregulates integrin alpha6beta4 expression and activates Akt in breast cancer cells. Exp Cell Res. 2006;312:3822–34.
124. Shen X, Mula RV, Li J, Weigel NL, Falzon M. PTHrP contributes to the anti-proliferative and integrin alpha6beta4-regulating effects of 1,25-dihydroxyvitamin D(3). Steroids. 2007;72:930–8.
125. Shimizu E, Selvamurugan N, Westendorf JJ, Olson EN, Partridge NC. HDAC4 represses matrix metalloproteinase-13 transcription in osteoblastic cells, and parathyroid hormone controls this repression. J Biol Chem. 2010;285:9616–26.
126. Singh AT, Gilchrist A, Voyno-Yasenetskaya T, Radeff-Huang JM, Stern PH. G alpha12/G alpha13 subunits of heterotrimeric G proteins mediate parathyroid hormone activation of phospholipase D in UMR-106 osteoblastic cells. Endocrinology. 2005;146:2171–5.
127. Stewart AF, Cain RL, Burr DB, Jacob D, Turner CH, Hock JM. Six-month daily administration of parathyroid hormone and parathyroid hormone-related protein peptides to adult ovariectomized rats markedly enhances bone mass and biomechanical properties: a comparison of human parathyroid hormone 1–34, parathyroid hormone-related protein 1–36, and SDZ-parathyroid hormone 893. J Bone Miner Res. 2000;15:1517–25.
128. Strewler GJ, Stern PH, Jacobs JW, Eveloff J, Klein RF, Leung SC, Rosenblatt M, Nissenson RA. Parathyroid hormonelike protein from human renal carcinoma cells. Structural and functional homology with parathyroid hormone. J Clin Invest. 1987;80:1803–7.
129. Suva LJ, Winslow GA, Wettenhall RE, Hammonds RG, Moseley JM, Diefenbach-Jagger H, Rodda CP, Kemp BE, Rodriguez H, Chen EY, Hudson PJ, Martin TJ, Wood WI. A parathyroid hormone-related protein implicated in malignant hypercalcemia: cloning and expression. Science. 1987;237:893–6.
130. Talmage RV, Elliott JR. Removal of calcium from bone as influenced by the parathyroids. Endocrinology. 1958;62:717–22.
131. Tam CS, Heersche JN, Murray TM, Parsons JA. Parathyroid hormone stimulates the bone apposition rate independently of its resorptive action: differential effects of intermittent and continuous administration. Endocrinology. 1982;110:506–12.
132. Tamasi J, Shimizu E, Benton N, Johnson J, Morrison NA, Partridge NC. The anabolic action of parathyroid hormone on bone is mediated by monocyte chemoattractant protein-1. J Bone Miner Res. 2010;25:S94.
133. Tang Y, Wu X, Lei W, Pang L, Wan C, Shi Z, Zhao L, Nagy TR, Peng X, Hu J, Feng X, Van Hul W, Wan M, Cao X. TGF-beta1-induced migration of bone mesenchymal stem cells couples bone resorption with formation. Nat Med. 2009;15:757–65.
134. Tobimatsu T, Kaji H, Sowa H, Naito J, Canaff L, Hendy GN, Sugimoto T, Chihara K. Parathyroid hormone increases beta-catenin levels through Smad3 in mouse osteoblastic cells. Endocrinology. 2006; 147:2583–90.
135. Tyson DR, Swarthout JT, Partridge NC. Increased osteoblastic c-fos expression by parathyroid hormone requires protein kinase A phosphorylation of the cyclic adenosine 3′,5′-monophosphate response element-binding protein at serine 133. Endocrinology. 1999;140:1255–61.
136. Usdin TB, Gruber C, Bonner TI. Identification and functional expression of a receptor selectively recognizing parathyroid hormone, the PTH2 receptor. J Biol Chem. 1995;270:15455–8.
137. Usdin TB, Wang T, Hoare SR, Mezey E, Palkovits M. New members of the parathyroid hormone/parathyroid hormone receptor family: the parathyroid hormone 2 receptor and tuberoinfundibular peptide of 39 residues. Front Neuroendocrinol. 2000;21: 349–83.
138. van Abel M, Hoenderop JG, van der Kemp AW, Friedlaender MM, van Leeuwen JP, Bindels RJ. Coordinated control of renal Ca(2+) transport proteins by parathyroid hormone. Kidney Int. 2005;68:1708–21.
139. Vargas SJ, Gillespie MT, Powell GJ, Southby J, Danks JA, Moseley JM, Martin TJ. Localization of parathyroid hormone-related protein mRNA expression in breast cancer and metastatic lesions by in situ hybridization. J Bone Miner Res. 1992;7:971–9.
140. Vortkamp A, Lee K, Lanske B, Segre GV, Kronenberg HM, Tabin CJ. Regulation of rate of cartilage differentiation by Indian hedgehog and PTH-related protein. Science. 1996;273:613–22.
141. Wan M, Yang C, Li J, Wu X, Yuan H, Ma H, He X, Nie S, Chang C, Cao X. Parathyroid hormone signaling through low-density lipoprotein-related protein 6. Genes Dev. 2008;22:2968–79.

142. Weir EC, Philbrick WM, Amling M, Neff LA, Baron R, Broadus AE. Targeted overexpression of parathyroid hormone-related peptide in chondrocytes causes chondrodysplasia and delayed endochondral bone formation. Proc Natl Acad Sci USA. 1996;93: 10240–5.
143. Wu X, Pang L, Lei W, Lu W, Li J, Li Z, Frassica FJ, Chen X, Wan M, Cao X. Inhibition of sca-1-positive skeletal stem cell recruitment by alendronate blunts the anabolic effects of parathyroid hormone on bone remodeling. Cell Stem Cell. 2010;7:571–80.
144. Yang R, Gerstenfeld LC. Signal transduction pathways mediating parathyroid hormone stimulation of bone sialoprotein gene expression in osteoblasts. J Biol Chem. 1996;271:29839–46.
145. Yao W, Cheng Z, Shahnazari M, Dai W, Johnson ML, Lane NE. Overexpression of secreted frizzled-related protein 1 inhibits bone formation and attenuates parathyroid hormone bone anabolic effects. J Bone Miner Res. 2010;25:190–9.
146. Yu S, Franceschi RT, Luo M, Fan J, Jiang D, Cao H, Kwon TG, Lai Y, Zhang J, Patrene K, Hankenson K, Roodman GD, Xiao G. Critical role of activating transcription factor 4 in the anabolic actions of parathyroid hormone in bone. PLoS One. 2009;4:e7583.
147. Zaruba MM, Huber BC, Brunner S, Deindl E, David R, Fischer R, Assmann G, Herbach N, Grundmann S, Wanke R, Mueller-Hoecker J, Franz WM. Parathyroid hormone treatment after myocardial infarction promotes cardiac repair by enhanced neovascularization and cell survival. Cardiovasc Res. 2008;77:722–31.
148. Zhang J, Niu C, Ye L, Huang H, He X, Tong WG, Ross J, Haug J, Johnson T, Feng JQ, Harris S, Wiedemann LM, Mishina Y, Li L. Identification of the haematopoietic stem cell niche and control of the niche size. Nature. 2003;425:836–41.

Vitamin D: Normal Function, Metabolism, Diseases, and Emerging Therapeutics

2

René St-Arnaud and Marie B. Demay

Keywords
Vitamin D • Vitamin D hydroxylases • Vitamin D receptor • Rickets
Cytochrome p450 enzymes

2.1 Overview of Vitamin D Metabolism

Vitamin D is produced in the skin upon exposure to ultraviolet light (sunlight). It is activated in two steps to function as a key regulator of mineral ion homeostasis. Vitamin D becomes bound to the vitamin D binding protein, DBP, in the circulation and is transported to the liver where the enzyme vitamin D 25-hydroxylase (CYP2R1) adds a hydroxyl group on carbon 25 to produce 25-hydroxyvitamin D [25(OH)D].

R. St-Arnaud, Ph.D.
Departments of Medicine,
Surgery, and Human Genetics, McGill University,
Montreal, QC, Canada

Genetics Unit, Shriners Hospital for Children,
1529 Cedar Avenue, Montreal, QC,
H3G 1A6, Canada
e-mail: rst-arnaud@shriners.mcgill.ca

M.B. Demay, M.D. (✉)
Endocrine Unit, Department of Medicine,
Massachusetts General Hospital,
Harvard Medical School,
Their 11, 50 Blossom St, Boston, MA 02114, USA

When the 25(OH)D metabolite enters the bloodstream, it also becomes bound to DBP. In the kidney, it is further hydroxylated, gaining hormonal bioactivity. Hydroxylation at position 1α by the enzyme 25-hydroxyvitamin D-1α-hydroxylase (CYP27B1) converts 25(OH)D to 1α,25-dihydroxyvitamin D [$1,25(OH)_2D$; calcitriol], the active, hormonal form of vitamin D. Upon reaching target tissues, $1,25(OH)_2D$ binds to its specific receptor, the vitamin D receptor (VDR). This step enhances or inhibits the transcription of vitamin D target genes that carry out the physiological actions of $1,25(OH)_2D$: mineral homeostasis, skeletal homeostasis, and cellular differentiation.

When exposed to sunlight, both plants and animals synthesize vitamin D. Vitamin D_2 (ergocalciferol) is generated in yeast; vitamin D_3 (cholecalciferol) is produced in fish and mammals. There are only small structural differences in the chemical structure of the two compounds: a double bond between carbons C22 and C23 and a methyl group at position C24 (Fig. 2.1a). These differences do not greatly affect function or metabolism in mammals. Vitamin D is the generic term which will be used without subscript hereafter in the text.

F. Bronner et al. (eds.), *Bone-Metabolic Functions and Modulators*, Topics in Bone Biology,
DOI 10.1007/978-1-4471-2745-1_2,

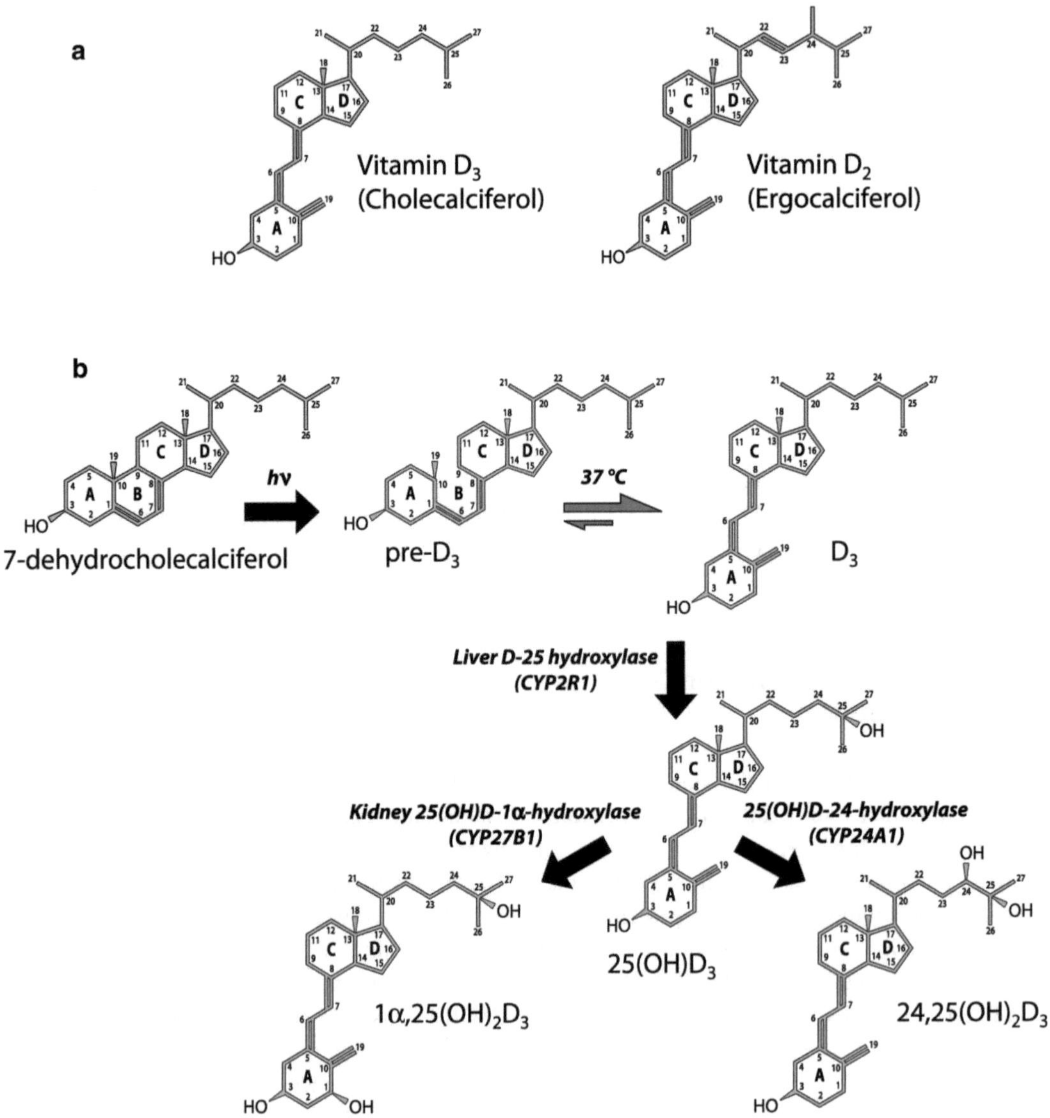

Fig. 2.1 Structure and metabolism of vitamin D. (**a**) Structure of vitamin D_3 (cholecalciferol) and vitamin D_2 (ergocalciferol). Plants and yeast synthesize vitamin D_2; fish and mammals synthesize vitamin D_3. The small differences in the chemical structure of the two compounds do not significantly affect function or metabolism. The open cyclopentanoperhydrophenanthrene core identifies vitamin D metabolites as secosteroids and not steroids. (**b**) Metabolism: Vitamin D is produced endogenously in the skin upon exposure to ultraviolet light (*hν*). It is transported to the liver where the enzyme vitamin D 25-hydroxylase (CYP2R1) adds an hydroxyl group to carbon 25 to produce 25-hydroxyvitamin D [25(OH) D]. The 25(OH)D metabolite is further hydroxylated at position 1α by the enzyme 25-hydroxyvitamin D-1α-hydroxylase (CYP27B1) to yield 1α,25-dihydroxyvitamin D [1,25$(OH)_2$D; calcitriol], the active, hormonal form of vitamin D

2.2 Vitamin D Status

In humans, 80% of the vitamin D requirement can be produced in the skin upon exposure to sunlight. The rest must be acquired through dietary sources such as fish, plants, and grains.

Ultraviolet B photons penetrate the epidermis and photolyze 7-dehydrocholesterol into previtamin D through cleavage of the B ring of the steroid nucleus. This step yields the characteristic secosteroid structure. Previtamin D is an unstable compound that is rapidly converted to a more thermodynamically stable molecule, vitamin D [86]. Vitamin D then exits the keratinocyte cells and enters the dermal capillary bed, where it is bound to the gamma globulin, vitamin D binding protein (DBP). In the circulation, vitamin D is transported to the liver where the cytochrome P450 enzyme vitamin D 25-hydroxylase (CYP2R1) adds a hydroxyl group on carbon 25 to produce 25-hydroxyvitamin D [25(OH)D] (Fig. 2.1b).

25(OH)D levels are used clinically to indicate individual vitamin D status [94]. The reliability of the assays used to measure 25(OH)D levels has greatly improved, in part because of the availability of standard reference compounds from the US National Institute of Standards and Technology [89, 225]. Individuals vary considerably with regard to their endogenous production of vitamin D, the amount converted to 25(OH)D, and the degree of vitamin D catabolism. The levels of 25(OH)D measured in a population level vary widely. It is not surprising, therefore, that a specific 25(OH) D level to define optimal vitamin D status has not yet been agreed upon. Nevertheless, by using the 25(OH)D to PTH "inflection point" [43, 87] or other criteria such as liver 25-hydroxylase enzyme kinetics and saturation [75], it is now agreed that values below 30–32 ng/ml (75 nmol/l) of 25(OH) D are low [17]. Vitamin D deficiency, associated with 25(OH)D concentrations of 10 ng/ml or under, leads to calcium malabsorption, bone hypomineralization (rickets/osteomalacia), and myopathy. Various terms have been used to describe the clinical situation when 25(OH)D levels are between 10 and 30 ng/ml, for example, vitamin D insufficiency, "inadequacy," or simply "low vitamin D status." It appears that low vitamin D status as defined by levels of 25(OH)D between 30 and 32 ng/ml is extremely common worldwide [67, 87, 119, 163].

If 25(OH)D plasma concentrations above 30 ng/ml are considered optimal, at what concentration does vitamin D toxicity occur? Conditions that characterize vitamin D toxicity are hypercalcemia, hypercalciuria, and soft tissue mineralization, but there is as yet no clear-cut definition of the toxic level. A valid suggestion is to use as the reference value for high 25(OH)D levels the concentrations measured in highly sun-exposed individuals without supplementation (thus representing maximal cutaneous production). Using this criterion, high 25(OH)D values are in the 70–80 ng/ml range (175–200 nmol/l) [13, 88].

Optimal vitamin D status is important for overall health [17], inasmuch as the hormone modulates mineral homeostasis and bone biology, muscle function, contributes to preventing falls, and plays a role in immune function. Epidemiological studies have linked poor vitamin D status with the risk of cancer and cardiovascular disease.

2.3 Hepatic 25-Hydroxylation

All vitamin D hydroxylases characterized to date belong to the superfamily of cytochrome P450 enzymes. They are heme-containing, mixed function oxidases that use molecular oxygen as a terminal electron acceptor. They require the accessory electron transfer proteins, adrenodoxin and adrenodoxin reductase, to accept reducing equivalents from nicotinamide adenine dinucleotide phosphate (NADPH) and stereospecifically hydroxylate vitamin D metabolites.

Kinetic studies using the perfused rat have revealed two 25-hydroxylase activities: a microsomal (endoplasmic reticulum) high-affinity, low-capacity enzyme and a mitochondrial low-affinity, high-capacity form [65]. With the aid of an elegant expression-based screening strategy, the microsomal, high-affinity vitamin D 25-hydroxylase was recently identified as CYP2R1 [34]. CYP2R1 exhibits several characteristics that strongly support its role as the physiologically relevant 25-hydroxylase enzyme: it is a microsomal cytochrome P450, expressed primarily in liver and testis [34]. It can hydroxylate vitamin D_2 and vitamin D_3 at physiologically relevant substrate concentrations [34], exhibits specificity toward vitamin D as a substrate, and does not metabolize cholesterol or 7-dehydrocholesterol [212]. Finally, a mutation in CYP2R1 has been identified in a patient with vitamin D-dependent rickets, type IA [30, 33, 58].

Another cytochrome P450 that hydroxylates vitamin D at position 25 is the bifunctional CYP27A1. This enzyme derives its name because it 27-hydroxylates the side-chains of cholesterol-derived intermediates that are involved in bile acid biosynthesis [157]. The physiological relevance of CYP27A1 as a vitamin D 25-hydroxylase has been considered controversial. Indeed, in mice with a disrupted *Cyp27a1* gene, bile acid synthesis is reduced, but their vitamin D metabolite levels are normal [187]. Patients with the inherited disease cerebrotendinous xanthomatosis, caused by mutations in *CYP27A1* [25, 194], have a normal vitamin D metabolism and no obvious deficiency of 25(OH)D or $1,25(OH)_2D$ [114]. CYP27A1 is a mitochondrial enzyme [5, 26]. It is likely that CYP2R1 is the physiologically relevant enzyme at normal, nanomolar vitamin D concentrations, but that is backed up by CYP27A when substrate concentrations rise to high nanomolar or low micromolar. Other P450 enzymes (CYP2C11, CYP2D5, CYP2J2, CYP3A4) have vitamin D 25-hydroxylase activity in vitro [2, 71, 90, 180], but whether they are involved in vitamin D metabolism remains to be determined.

2.4 Renal 1α-Hydroxylation

25(OH)D must be further hydroxylated to attain hormonal bioactivity (Fig. 2.1b). Hydroxylation takes place in the convoluted and straight portions of the proximal kidney tubule. Hydroxylation at position 1α by the mitochondrial cytochrome P450 enzyme, 25-hydroxyvitamin D-1α-hydroxylase (CYP27B1) converts 25(OH)D to 1α,25-dihydroxyvitamin D [$1,25(OH)_2D$], the active, hormonal form of vitamin D.

CYP27B1 also belongs to the class of the mixed-function oxidases. The *CYP27B1* cDNA was cloned from rat and mouse kidney, as well as from human keratinocytes and kidney [61, 204, 210, 217]. The cDNAs from all species examined to date show high sequence similarity. The human *CYP27B1* cDNA is 2,469 bp in length and codes for a deduced protein of 508 amino acids that contains an adrenodoxin-binding domain and a heme-binding domain.

The cloning of *CYP27B1* cDNAs rapidly led to the cloning of the *CYP27B1* gene in various species. The gene exists as a single copy in the human genome and contains nine exons spanning 5 kb of sequence. The adrenodoxin-binding domain is encoded by sequences contained in exons 6 and 7, while the heme-binding domain is contained in exon 8 [62, 166]. The human gene has been localized to chromosome 12 [62], then mapped to 12q13.1–13.3 by fluorescence in situ hybridization (FISH) [109, 210, 239]. The chromosomal location provided further circumstantial evidence that mutations in the gene were responsible for the hereditary disease, pseudovitamin D deficiency rickets (PDDR), also termed vitamin D dependency rickets type I, since the disease had been previously mapped to this locus by linkage analysis [115, 116]. Incontrovertible proof that mutations in *CYP27B1* caused PDDR was provided by the characterization of *CYP27B1* mutations in patients with the disease (reviewed in [130, 171]). Animal models of the disease have been engineered by gene-targeting technology [41, 167].

The main tissue site of *CYP27B1* expression is the proximal tubule of the renal cortex [237]. Expression of the enzyme has also been reported: osteoblasts [175], keratinocytes [61], and cells of the lymphohematopoietic system [183]. The identification of these extrarenal sites of expression of *CYP27B1* has led investigators to hypothesize that local production of $1,25(OH)_2D$ could play an autocrine or paracrine role in the differentiation or function of these cells. In the kidney, the expression of the *CYP27B1* gene is subject to complex regulation by parathyroid hormone, calcitonin, calcium, phosphorus, and $1,25(OH)_2D$ itself [159, 160].

2.5 24-Hydroxylation

In target cells, $1,25\text{-}(OH)_2D$ induces the expression of the gene encoding the key effector of its catabolic breakdown: 25-hydroxyvitamin D-24-hydroxylase (CYP24A1) [126, 158]. This ensures attenuation of the $1,25\text{-}(OH)_2D$ biological signal inside target cells and helps regulate vitamin D homeostasis. Catabolism of 1,25$(OH)_2$D occurs through CYP24A1-mediated modification of the secosteroid's aliphatic side chain (Fig. 2.2). The main substrates for the hydroxylation reactions catalyzed by CYP24A1 are 25(OH)D and 1,25$(OH)_2$D. In the first case, the reaction leads to the formation of 24,25$(OH)_2$D, a metabolite that circulates in the bloodstream. In the second instance, the initial, short-lived enzymatic product is 1,24,25$(OH)_3$D. The specificity of the catalytic reaction is determined by substrate orientation within the active site of the enzyme, where the target carbon atom must be in close proximity to the heme-oxyferryl center. Interestingly, the CYP24A1 enzyme hydroxylates both the C23 and the C24 side-chain carbons of 25(OH)D or of 1,25$(OH)_2$D [192]. The relative level of C23- and C24-hydroxylase activity appears to be species specific. The structural basis of this altered specificity has been examined with the aid of sequence alignment and site-directed mutagenesis [174]. C24 hydroxylation leads to side-chain cleavage and oxidation to a carboxylic acid (C24 oxidation pathway), while hydroxylation at carbon 23 results in side-chain lactone formation (C23 hydroxylation pathway).

The C24 oxidation catabolic pathway can be induced in a number of vitamin D target cells [137, 185, 220] and comprises five enzymatic steps (Fig. 2.2): it begins with 24-hydroxylation of 1,25$(OH)_2$D to yield 1,24,25$(OH)_3$D which is then ketonized to 24-oxo-1,25$(OH)_2$D. Carbon 23 is hydroxylated to generate 24-oxo-1,23,25$(OH)_3$D, which is metabolized by oxidative cleavage of the carbon–carbon bond between C23 and C24 to produce 24,25,26,27-tetranor-1,23$(OH)_2$D. This C23 alcohol converts to calcitroic acid, the excretory product of 1,25$(OH)_2$D in bile.

When the initial substrate is 25(OH)D, the metabolic intermediates are 24,25$(OH)_2$D, 24-oxo-25(OH)D, 24-oxo-23,25$(OH)_2$D, 24,25,26,27-tetranor-23(OH)D, and finally calcitroic acid.

All steps of the C23-hydroxylation pathway are catalyzed by the recombinant human CYP24A1 enzyme: from 25(OH)D to 23,25$(OH)_2$D, then 23,25,26$(OH)_3$D, followed by conversion to 25(OH)D-26,23-lactol, and finally 25(OH) D-26,23-lactone [192].

When the initial substrate is 1,25$(OH)_2$D, the metabolic intermediates are 1,23,25$(OH)_3$D, 1,23,25,26$(OH)_4$D, 1,25$(OH)_2$D-26,23-lactol, and finally 1,25$(OH)_2$D-26,23-lactone (Fig. 2.2).

The biological activity of the C23-hydroxylation metabolites is unclear, but the terminal 1,25$(OH)_2$-D-derived product, 1,25$(OH)_2$D-26,23-lactone, could act as a VDR antagonist [95, 219].

2.6 Vitamin D Receptor (VDR)

The biological effects of 1,25$(OH)_2$D are mediated by a nuclear receptor, the VDR (reviewed in [74]). The VDR belongs to the subfamily of nuclear hormone receptors, which also includes the receptors for retinoic acid, retinoid X, and thyroid hormone. The members of the subfamily are characterized by three isoforms (α, β, and γ), but only one nuclear VDR has been isolated. As in other members of the nuclear receptor superfamily, the principal domains of the VDR are involved in DNA binding, ligand binding, dimerization, and transcriptional activation (Fig. 2.3). These domains are highly conserved in vertebrates [8, 118]. The DNA-binding domain is the most highly conserved, with more than 90% of the amino acid sequence conserved across vertebrate species [118]. Unlike most nuclear hormone receptors that contain a substantial amino terminal transactivation domain (activation function 1 or AF1), the human VDR has a very short N-terminal region with two zinc fingers creating the DNA-binding domain. Sequences of amino acid residues 24–90 within the DNA-binding domain are responsible for DNA binding and for nuclear localization and contribute to heterodimerization. The region of the VDR carboxy terminal and the DNA-binding domain contain residues that are involved in hormone binding, heterodimerization, transactivation, and interactions with nuclear receptor coactivators (Fig. 2.3) (for review, see [74]).

The 1,25$(OH)_2$D hormone has the highest binding affinity for the VDR, whereas the affinity

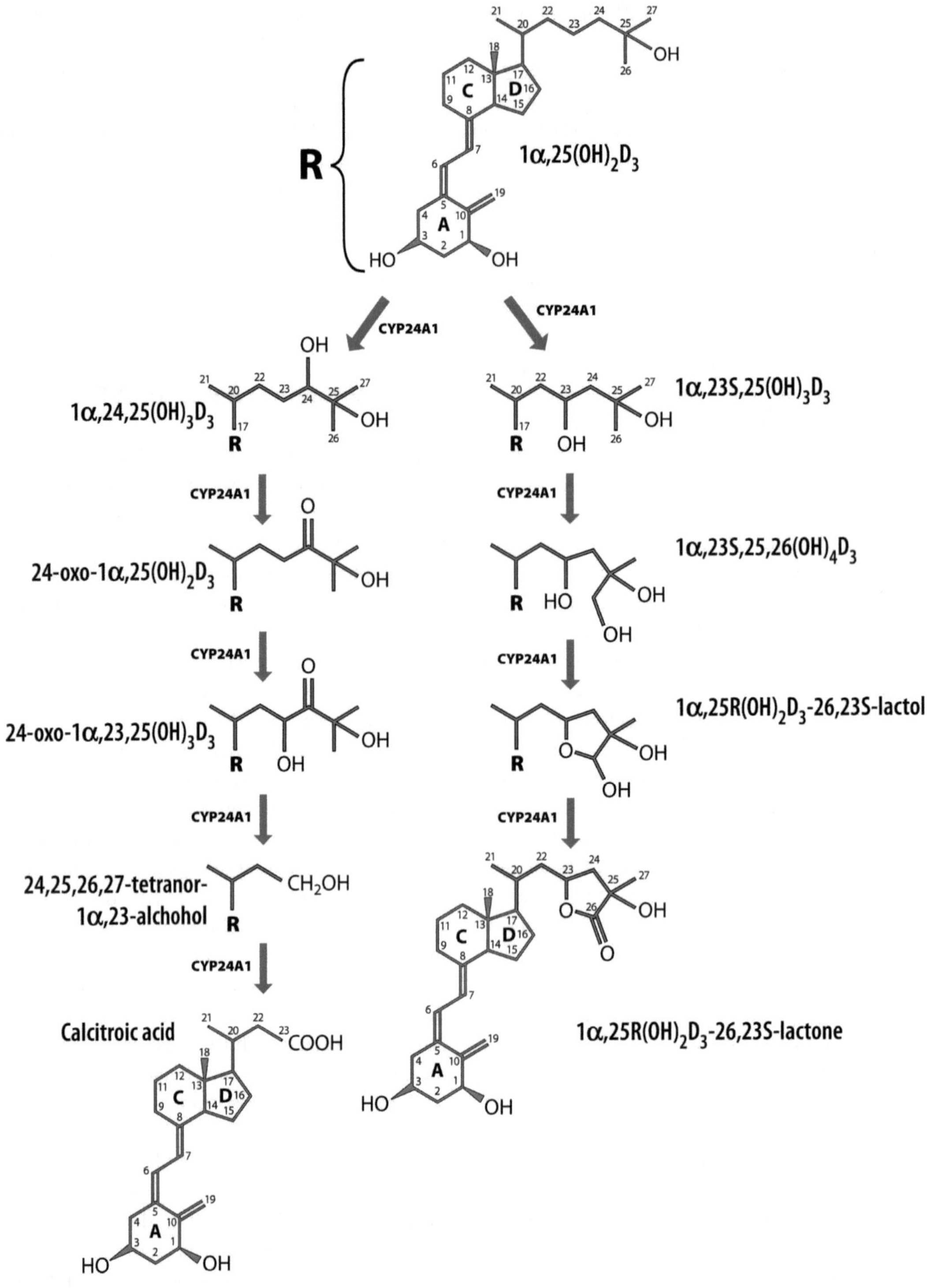

Fig. 2.2 Enzymatic pathways catalyzed by CYP24A1. The C24-oxidation pathway products are shown on the left; the C23-hydroxylation products are depicted at the right. Only the products of $1,25(OH)_2D$ are represented; refer to the text for 25(OH)D products

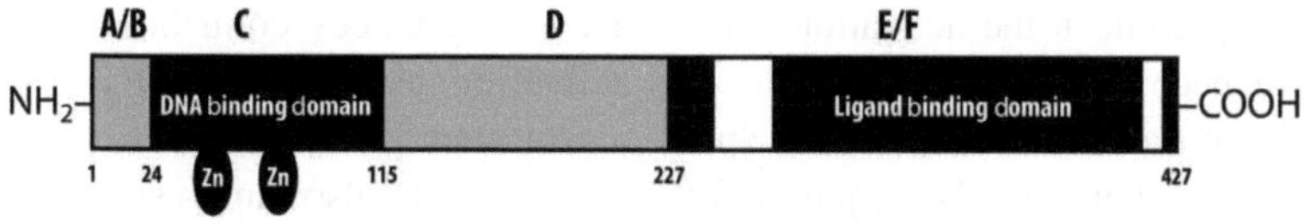

Fig. 2.3 Functional domains in the vitamin D receptor. Schematic view of the vitamin D receptor. The 427-amino-acid protein can be separated into domains: *A*/*B*, *C*, *D*, and *E*/*F*. The DNA-binding zinc finger motifs are depicted below the DNA-binding domain *C*. The *white* regions represent helices within the *E*/*F* domain that are important for transcriptional activation

of 25(OH)D for the receptor is some 1,000-fold less. Additional ligands for the VDR are curcumin or some polyunsaturated fatty acids [73]. The functional significance of these lower-affinity ligands remains to be determined. One VDR ligand of physiological relevance is the bile acid, lithocholic acid [127], formed by dehydroxylation of chenodeoxycholic acid by the action of gut bacteria [84]. Lithocholic acid is hepatotoxic and carcinogenic in several species [84]. In humans, however, it is detoxified by sulfation and conjugation with taurine or glycine [84]. The proposed mechanism involves activation of the VDR through lithocholic acid binding, which leads to expression of the sulfotransferase gene *SULF2A* that encodes the enzyme responsible for the detoxification of lithocholic acid [223]. Lithocholic acid induces its own sulfation in both the colonic enterocyte and the hepatocyte. Detoxification of lithocholic acid may involve other nuclear receptors like CAR, the constitutive androstane receptor [106, 188].

1,25(OH)$_2$D binding by the VDR leads to receptor phosphorylation and promotes heterodimerization, high-affinity binding to DNA response elements, and recruitment of nuclear receptor coactivators [73]. An amphipathic alpha-helical region at the C terminus (residues 416–422), referred to as the activating function 2 or AF2 region, is critical for transactivation and recruitment of nuclear receptor coactivators.

Nuclear receptor coactivators provide a critical link between ligand-activated nuclear receptors and basal transcription. The best characterized nuclear receptor coactivators belong to the SRC/p160 (steroid receptor coactivator) family [141, 161]. The members of this family interact with nuclear receptors *via* an alpha-helical LXXLL motif that binds to an alpha helical region in the distal carboxy terminal region (416–422) of the VDR. It is postulated that ligand binding by the VDR results in a conformational change, exposing residues to the carboxy terminal of the DNA-binding domain residues (224–246, 255–278, and 416–422). The residues in turn bind SRC-1. Mutagenesis of the sequences impairs transactivation in the setting of normal hormone binding and heterodimerization with RXR [112]. SRC-1 knockout mice exhibit abnormal responses to some nuclear receptors, but action of 1,25-dihydroxyvitamin D action in vivo is not impaired.

In addition to interacting with general transcription factors, including TFIIB and TATA-binding protein [216], SRC-1 family members have histone acetyl transferase activity [208]. The activity of this enzyme increases access to the general transcriptional apparatus by remodeling chromatin, thereby modifying the repressive effects of nucleosomes on gene expression. SRC/p160 family members form complexes with CBP/p300, which also provides histone acetyl transferase activity [12]. Although CBP/p300 binds to nuclear receptors with low affinity, its interactions with SRC-1 family members link CBP/p300 to nuclear receptors and other proteins that mediate gene regulation by nuclear receptors.

A multimeric complex, whose isolation is due to interaction with the hormone-binding domain of the VDR and of the D receptor interacting proteins, plays a crucial role in direct recruitment of the transcriptional machinery. The complex enhances VDR-mediated transactivation in a cell-free system [177] and is essential for ligand-dependent transactivation [176]. Binding of liganded VDR to the DRIP complex enhances binding to RNA polymerase II; this suggests that binding is critical to mediate transcriptional activation [35]. Several components of the DRIP complex are also present in the activation complexes that have been purified with the aid of nonnuclear receptor transactivators, such as Sp1. Transactivation may, therefore, be required for transcriptional activation.

Corepressors such as NCoR and SMRT also interact with nuclear hormone receptors, and their actions are thought to be responsible for the transcription-repressing activities of unliganded receptors for triiodothyronine and retinoic acid. The corepressors stabilize chromatin by deacetylation of histones. In contrast, $1,25(OH)_2D$ recruits SMRT and NCoR to the promoters of target genes. The ligand-bound VDR promotes binding of the corepressors to RXR, whereas the RXR ligand induces corepressor release from the heterodimer [196].

Hairless, a protein that was first characterized as a thyroid hormone receptor corepressor, binds the VDR and represses VDR-mediated transcription whether or not the ligand is present [91]. What this interaction brings about has not been established. Absence of functional VDR or of the Hairless protein is associated with alopecia in humans and mice [1, 135]. Follicle homeostasis therefore seems to require the combined action of the Hairless protein with the VDR.

The DNA sequence for VDR binding consists of direct repeat hexameric response elements that are separated by three bases on target genes that have been upregulated by $1,25(OH)_2D$ [49, 222]. These response elements have been identified in genes for osteocalcin [48, 164], osteopontin [155], $\alpha_V\beta_3$ integrin [29, 142], and *CYP24A1* [101, 156].

With the advent of chromatin immunoprecipitation and analyses of DNA sequences that bind the VDR in the context of intact chromatin, a complicated regulatory network has been unveiled. Studies of the *CYP24A1* gene, which is induced by $1,25(OH)_2D$, have demonstrated that, in addition to the two vitamin D response elements (VDREs) located near the proximal promoter, the VDR/RXR heterodimer also binds a cluster of potential enhancers in the intergenic region, 50–69 kilobase pairs downstream from the human gene and 35–45 kilobase pairs downstream from the mouse gene. These sequences contribute to transcriptional activation by $1,25(OH)_2D$ and to coregulator recruitment [144].

The VDR also suppresses the expression of several genes. The study of these transcriptional repression events has unveiled novel mechanisms of VDR action. The sequences that are responsible for $1,25(OH)_2D$-mediated transcriptional repression of the *CYP27B1* gene bind a basic helix-loop transcription factor known as the VDR-interacting repressor (VDIR) [148]. When the VDIR binds this response element, transactivation is initiated. The liganded VDR-RXR heterodimer interacts with VDIR to dissociate the histone acetyl transferase p300/CBP and to recruit the histone deacetylase nuclear receptor corepressor HDAC, with the *CYP27B1* gene repressed as a result. Similar interactions of the VDIR with sequences in the PTH and PTHrP promoters have been implicated in transcriptional gene repression by the liganded VDR [104]. Recently, an epigenetic modification has been identified as contributing to the PTH control of *CYP27B1* expression. It seems that PTH treatment induces active demethylation of CpG sites within the *CYP27B1* promoter [105]. This activates the DNA glycosylase, MBD4 [77], which, due to PTH action, is phosphorylated through protein kinase C. The glycosylase lyses the methylated DNA and via a base-excision repair process leads to DNA demethylation and transcriptional derepression [105]. On the other hand, treatment with $1,25(OH)_2D$ induces methylation by activating the DNA methyltransferases, DNMT1 and DNMT3B [105]. The identification of this methylation switching at the DNA level is a novel concept in the hormonal control of gene transcription.

In addition to binding histone acetyl transferases and deacetylases, VDR interacts with chromatin-remodeling complexes that rearrange nucleosomes in an energy-dependent fashion and thereby render chromosomal DNA accessible to transcription factors. The VDR binds a multimeric complex with ATP-dependent chromatin remodeling activity known as WINAC (WSTF Including Nucleosome Assembly Complex). The complex derives its name in part from the

Williams syndrome transcription factor (WSTF), a protein that is mutated in a congenital disorder characterized by abnormal vitamin D metabolism, vascular lesions, developmental delay, and atypical facies. The VDR binds directly to WSTF which, in turn, binds to the ATP-dependent chromatin-remodeling enzymes Brg1 and Brm [107]. In addition to promoting ligand-dependent transactivation by the VDR, the WINAC complex is also required for transrepression of the CYP27B1 gene by the liganded VDR. Transrepression requires the bromodomain of WSTF that interacts with acetylated histones.

2.7 Endocrine Role of 1α, 25-Dihydroxyvitamin D in Calcium Homeostasis

$1,25(OH)_2D$ promotes intestinal calcium absorption. Several proteins present in the brush border of the intestinal cell membrane, including the Ca/Mg ATPase, brush border alkaline phosphatase, and intestinal calcium-binding protein, are induced by $1,25(OH)_2D$. In addition, two calcium channels, expressed in the intestine, TRPV5 and TRPV6 [82, 170] promote entry of calcium into the enterocyte. The interactions of these with parathyroid hormone are discussed in Chap. 1 of this volume. Both TRPV5 and TRPV6 are induced by $1,25(OH)_2D$. However, TRPV5 is expressed primarily in the kidney, and mice lacking TRPV5 exhibit renal calcium wasting with enhanced intestinal calcium absorption, due to a compensatory increase in $1,25(OH)_2D$ [83]. $1,25(OH)_2D$ is also a potent inducer of the gene encoding calbindin D_{9K}, a protein that binds calcium ions and is thought to play a role in transcellular calcium transport. Studies in vitamin-D-deficient animals have demonstrated that calbindin D_{9K} levels are increased early and dramatically after injection of vitamin D metabolites and correlate with an increase in active transport of calcium across the intestine [229]. However, mice lacking both TRPV6, the predominant intestinal calcium channel, and calbindin D_{9K} still exhibit increases in calcium transport in response to $1,25(OH)_2D$ [16]. These results suggest that additional proteins or pathways are involved in $1,25(OH)_2D$-regulated intestinal calcium absorption. Two proteins thought to form paracellular calcium channels, claudin 2 and claudin 12, are also induced by $1,25(OH)_2D$ [63], and thus paracellular as well as transcellular calcium transport may be modulated by $1,25(OH)_2D$.

2.8 Paracrine/Autocrine Role of 1α, 25-Dihydroxyvitamin D

$1,25(OH)_2D$ may have effects unrelated to mineral ion homeostasis. Consistent with these observations, the VDR is expressed in several tissues including skin, breast, prostate, pancreas, colon, muscle, and immune cells. Studies of the immunomodulatory effects of vitamin D metabolites have demonstrated that activation of Toll-like receptors (TLRs) induces *CYP27B1* in cells of the macrophage lineage. Coupled with the increase in VDR expression that is also observed, this leads to a dramatic enhancement in local autocrine signaling by $1,25(OH)_2D$, which in turn induces the synthesis of antimicrobial peptides such as cathelicidin [240] that play a role in host defense to microbes, including mycobacteria [120]. Interestingly, the promoter of the human antimicrobial peptide cathelicidin contains functional vitamin D response elements [69, 227, 230]. Treatment with $1,25(OH)_2D$ induces transcription of cathelicidin in human keratinocytes, monocytes, neutrophils, and human cell lines [227, 230]. The TLR-mediated upregulation of the expression of the VDR and *CYP27B1* provokes the intracrine $1,25(OH)_2D$-dependent induction of cathelicidin and increased microbicidal activity of the macrophages [120]. In addition to demonstrating the importance of the VDR in immune function, this model system makes clear that conversion of vitamin D to $1,25(OH)_2D$ is critical in target tissues.

VDR-mediated signaling also regulates chondrocyte differentiation or function in the context of normal vitamin D endocrine actions. Masuyama et al. [138] targeted the VDR gene with loxP sites and crossed mice with the floxed allele producing transgenic mice that express the Cre recombinase under the control of the type II collagen promoter and enhancer. This led to inactivation of the VDR gene in proliferating chondrocytes. Growth plate structure was not affected in 15-day-old mutant mice (chondrocyte-specific VDR-KO). A surprising finding is the increase in bone volume in mutant newborn and 15-day-old mice. This phenotype is transient, inasmuch as adult chondrocyte-specific VDR-KO mice did not manifest it [138]. After ruling out that the augmented bone volume was caused by increases in osteoblast-mediated bone formation, the authors examined the interesting possibility that defects in vascular invasion and/or osteoclastogenesis could be responsible for the observed phenotype. Immunodetection of endothelial cells in developing tibiae of chondrocyte-specific VDR-KO mutant mice revealed the number of invading blood vessels in the growth plate had decreased, and vascular endothelial growth factor (VEGF) mRNA levels were significantly reduced in the growth plates of mutant newborn [138]. The number of osteoclasts and RANKL expression also decreased. Elegant cell culture studies have shown that 1,25(OH)$_2$D induced RANKL expression in chondrocytes in a VDR-dependent manner, thus confirming earlier findings [214].

To complete the phenotypic assessment of the mice with chondrocyte-specific inactivation of the VDR, the authors analyzed the blood of the mutant mice before weaning and detected an increase in circulating phosphate and 1,25(OH)$_2$D levels. These changes plateaued when the mice got older. These changes were surprising considering that the mutation targeted the VDR gene in chondrocytes and should not have affected the function of vitamin D. Investigation has revealed that in chondrocyte-specific VDR-KO mice, the renal expression of the appropriate phosphate cotransporter *Npt2a* has increased, as have the *Cyp27b1* mRNA levels [138]. The impact of a localized mutation on the regulation of gene expression in a distant tissue as the kidney suggests that an endocrine regulator is involved. FGF23 is an obvious candidate, because this phosphaturic factor inhibits renal expression of *Npt2a* and *Cyp27b1* [121, 189]. The expression of FGF23 is reduced in the metaphysis of chondrocyte-specific VDR mutant mice. Chondrocytes do not express FGF23 [138]. Rather, expression of FGF23 in osteoblasts is regulated by a chondrocyte-derived secreted factor whose expression requires VDR activity [138]. These findings have established that the genomic action of 1,25(OH)$_2$D on bone is direct. In other words, VDR signaling in chondrocytes is necessary for vascular invasion to occur in time and osteoclastogenesis to take place during development.

However, the source of the 1,25(OH)$_2$D ligand activating VDR-mediated signaling in chondrocytes remained undetermined. Because the CYP27B1 enzyme that synthesizes 1,25(OH)$_2$D is expressed in chondrocytes, local production of 1,25(OH)$_2$D could play an autocrine or paracrine role in the differentiation of these cells and explain the partial rescue of the phenotype when mineral homeostasis is corrected [42]. To test this hypothesis, mutant mice that do not express the *Cyp27b1* gene in chondrocytes were generated. In these mice, the hypertrophic zone of the growth plate was increased at the embryonic age of 15.5 days. At the same time, bone mass was increased in the long bones, as was the chondrocytic expression of the differentiation markers Indian Hedgehog and PTH/PTHrP receptor. VEGF mRNA levels were decreased, as was PECAM-1 immunostaining. This suggests vascularization was delayed [150]. These findings agree with the phenotype of chondrocyte-specific VDR-ablated mice [138] and give support to an autocrine/paracrine role of 1,25(OH)$_2$D in endochondral ossification and chondrocyte development.

2.9 Nonclassical Effects

Some actions of 1,25(OH)$_2$D are too rapid to be mediated by transcriptional mechanisms. These include activation of second messengers [14, 38], voltage-dependent calcium channels [14, 38, 44, 54], and the induction of vitamin D metabolites that bind the nuclear VDR with very low affinity, and have specific biological effects. These comprise the effect of 24,25(OH)$_2$D on growth plate chondrocyte maturation [197, 200].

Studies in mice lacking the VDR DNA binding and AF1 domains have shown that intracellular calcium does not increase rapidly in response to $1,25(OH)_2D$, a response that seems to require an intact nuclear VDR [53]. ERp60/ERp57/GRp58 is also known as the membrane-associated rapid response steroid binding (MARRS) protein that binds vitamin D metabolites. Detailed mechanistic studies have identified pathways that act downstream of the $1,25(OH)_2D$/Erp60 interaction in growth zone chondrocytes. $1,25(OH)_2D$ binding to ERp60 [153] induces protein kinase Cα signaling that is mediated by phospholipase A_2 (PLA_2) activation and the PLA_2-activating protein [198, 199]. Many of the signaling molecules involved are found in specialized regions of the plasma membrane called lipid rafts or caveolae. A major scaffolding component of these structures is caveolin-1 [203, 224]. Interestingly, caveolin-1-deficient growth zone chondrocytes do not respond to $1,25(OH)_2D$. Therefore, the membrane-mediated effects of $1,25(OH)_2D$ seem to require caveolae and caveolin-1 [22]. Even though most of these studies were conducted in vitro (or ex vivo), the physiological relevance of these findings is emerging, inasmuch as caveolin-1 deficiency results in altered growth plate structure [22]. The functional relevance of ERp60-mediated signaling derives support from the finding that VDR-deficient growth zone chondrocytes respond to $1,25-(OH)_2D$, but that their response is blocked by antibodies against ERp60 [21]. Further demonstration of the physiological role of ERp60 in mediating effects of $1,25(OH)_2D$ and other vitamin D metabolites will require studies with mice that lack this protein [102].

2.10 Vitamin D Deficiency Rickets

Vitamin D metabolism is affected by inadequate exposure to sunlight, inadequate dietary intake of the vitamin, malabsorption of dietary vitamin D, impaired hepatic 25-hydroxylation, and defects in renal 1α-hydroxylation and in receptor function. Three types of hereditary disorders are associated with vitamin D endocrine system.

The prime metabolic consequence of vitamin D deficiency is reduced net intestinal absorption of calcium [28, 46]. Calcium malabsorption leads to a fall in plasma calcium, which may result in secondary hyperparathyroidism, a condition that in turn is characterized by a reduction in renal tubular reabsorption of phosphate, hypophosphatemia, and a lowering of the calcium X phosphate product. Ultimately because the supply of the relevant ions is reduced, deposition of mineral in osteoid is impaired, which triggers the development of the rachitic and/or osteomalacic phenotype.

2.10.1 Vitamin D Deficiency Rickets Type IA

Chang et al. [33] have reported a single case of mutations in both alleles of CYP2R1, the microsomal hepatic 25-hydroxylase [34]. The patient had low serum calcium, low levels of 25(OH)D, and rickets [30]. This rare disorder, termed vitamin D deficiency rickets type IA, demonstrates that 25-hydroxylase deficiency causes a hereditary defect in vitamin D metabolism.

2.10.2 Pseudovitamin D Deficiency Rickets (PDDR)

PDDR (also referred to as vitamin-D-dependent rickets type I) is characterized by failure to thrive, hypotonia, and growth retardation. Affected babies lie supine because of severe muscle weakness and bone pain. At this age, gross skeletal deformities are rare; however, if diagnosis and treatment are delayed, the spine and long bones develop severe deformities together with generalized muscle weakness simulating myopathy. Motor problems translate into regression in head control and ability to stand. In some patients, the initial event is generalized convulsions, tremulations, and Bravais-Jacksonian fits or tetany. Pathological fractures may happen. The onset in most cases occurs early during the third trimester of life; the patients look healthy at birth.

Physical examination reveals a small, hypotonic child with wide anterior fontanel, frontal bossing and frequent craniotabes, and softenings near sutures. Tooth eruption is delayed; erupted teeth show evidence of enamel hypoplasia. A rachitic rosary is either visible or palpable. In limbs, widening of the metaphyseal areas is evidenced by enlargement of wrists and ankles; there is a variable degree of bowing of long bone diaphyses. Deformities of the thorax may interfere with ventilation and predispose to pulmonary infection; infant death by pulmonary infection is not infrequent when the diagnosis is either missed or confused with a neurological or respiratory condition or made too late. A positive Chvostek sign reflects nerve irritability, a consequence of a fall in serum calcium.

The x-ray features include diffuse osteopenia (mild to severe hypomineralization of the skeleton) and classic rachitic metaphyseal changes: fraying, cupping, widening, and fuzziness of the zone of provisional calcification. These changes are best detected in the most active growth plates, namely, the distal ulna, the femur, and the proximal and distal tibia. Changes in the diaphyses may not be evident when metaphyseal changes are first detected, but will appear a few weeks later as rarefaction, coarse trabeculation, cortical thinning, and subperiosteal erosion.

Hypocalcemia is the main biochemical feature in PDDR. A rapid decrease in serum calcium may give rise to tetany and convulsions, which may occur prior to any radiological evidence of rickets. Prolonged hypocalcemia triggers secondary hyperparathyroidism and hyperaminoaciduria [7]. Urinary calcium excretion is very low, whereas fecal calcium is high because of impaired intestinal calcium absorption.

Serum phosphate concentrations may be normal or low. When present, hypophosphatemia results from the combination of impaired intestinal absorption and increased urinary loss induced by secondary hyperparathyroidism. Serum alkaline phosphatase activity is consistently elevated, and its increase precedes the appearance of clinical symptoms.

Patients with PDDR have normal serum levels of 25(OH)D after exposure to sunlight or on intake of small doses of vitamin D. With higher intake, 25(OH)D will go up [47]. Serum levels of $1,25(OH)_2D$ are low to undetectable in untreated patients [47, 202]. This is evident immediately after birth, months before any clinical evidence of rickets appears. Even when patients are treated with high doses of vitamin D, the circulating levels of 25(OH)D increase significantly, but concentrations of $1,25(OH)_2D$ may not reach the normal range. These features of vitamin D metabolites have helped understand that the defective activity of the CYP 27B1 enzyme constitutes the metabolic abnormality in PDDR.

PDDR is inherited as a simple autosomal trait [201]. Heterozygotes have no phenotypic abnormalities [7]. Because PDDR has a relatively high incidence in the French-Canadian population, it has been possible to obtain a fair amount from kindred and to map the locus of PDDR to the region of band 14 on the long arm of chromosome 12 (12q 13–14) [115, 116]. The ultimate proof that mutations in the *CYP27B1* gene were responsible for the PDDR phenotype required identification of the mutations in PDDR patients and carriers of the disease. The first identification of the mutation was reported by Fu et al. in 1997 [61]; several additional mutations in various ethnic groups have since been published [103, 108, 109, 206, 226, 228, 239]. These findings have unequivocally established the genetic basis of PDDR as the presence of inactivating mutation(s) in the *CYP27B1* gene.

2.10.3 Treatment of PDDR

High doses of vitamin D_2 have been used to treat PDDR initially, causing the levels of 25(OH)D to increase sharply. High concentrations of 25(OH)D bind to the VDR and induce normalization of calcium homeostasis. However, the risk of overdose under these conditions is high because vitamin D accumulates in fat and muscle, and the therapeutic doses approach toxic doses, ultimately placing the patient at risk for nephrocalcinosis and impaired renal function. The use of $25(OH)D_3$ as a therapeutic agent in PDDR has been reported [11]. The mechanism of action is likely to be similar to the one just described for vitamin D_2. The low availability and high cost of the metabolite have not encouraged its wide use as long-term therapy for PDDR.

The treatment of choice is lifelong replacement therapy with $1,25(OH)_2D_3$ [47, 68] which results in rapid and complete correction of the abnormal phenotype, eliminating hypocalcemia, secondary hyperparathyroidism, and radiographic evidence of rickets. Strikingly, the myopathy disappears within days after initiation of therapy. The restoration of bone mineral content is equally rapid and with the bone structure healing [47]. Correction of tooth enamel hypoplasia is only partial. An important aspect of treatment is to ensure adequate calcium intake during the bone healing phase is assured by frequent monitoring of urinary calcium excretion. It should be noted that hypercalciuria is common as a result of treatment with $1,25(OH)_2D_3$, particularly during the first year of administration. A typical initial dose is 1–2 μg/day, with maintenance dose varying between 0.5 and 1 μg/day. High levels of calcium excretion may amplify the pattern of calcium deposition in the kidney; therefore, frequent renal imaging and assessment of renal function are essential.

Before $1,25(OH)_2D_3$ became available from commercial sources, investigators used the monohydroxylated analog $1\alpha(OH)D_3$ [182], which only requires liver hydroxylation at position 25 to become the hormonally active metabolite. It should be remembered that the 25-hydroxylation step is not affected by the PDDR mutation. Response to treatment with $1\alpha(OH)D_3$ is rapid, with healing of rickets in 7–9 weeks. On a weight basis, $1\alpha(OH)D_3$ is about half as potent as $1,25(OH)_2D_3$; this nullifies any possible economic advantage in favor of the monohydroxylated compound.

2.10.4 Hereditary Vitamin-D-Resistant Rickets (HVDRR)

Many of the clinical findings in patients with HVDRR (also termed vitamin-D-dependent rickets type II) are identical to those described for PDDR, including bone pain, muscle weakness, hypotonia, and occasional convulsions [132]. Children are often growth retarded and often have hypoplasia of the teeth. The radiological features of rickets are present. Many children with HVDRR have sparse body hair, and some have total scalp and body alopecia, sometimes even including eyebrows and eyelashes. Hair loss may already be evident at birth or occur during the first months of life. Patients with alopecia generally have resistance to vitamin D. In families that have a history of the disease, the absence of scalp hair in newborns can be the first diagnostic sign for HVDRR. Alopecia in an animal model of HVDRR has been shown due to a defect in epithelial-mesenchymal communication, required for normal hair cycling [37, 117, 190, 191].

Serum parameters include low concentrations of calcium and phosphate, while alkaline phosphatase activity is high in HVDRR. With secondary hyperparathyroidism, the difference concerns circulating levels of vitamin D metabolites. The serum levels of 25(OH)D are normal, but those of $1,25(OH)_2D$ are elevated. This distinguishes HVDRR from PDDR, where $1,25(OH)_2D$ concentrations are depressed. Patients with HVDRR are resistant to supraphysiologic doses of all compounds used in vitamin D therapy. This is the result of mutations in the VDR that render the receptor less functional than the wild type. It has been possible to engineer animal models of HVDRR by inactivating the VDR gene through gene targeting (reviewed in [20]).

HVDRR follows an autosomal recessive pattern of inheritance. Parents of patients who are heterozygous for the mutation show no symptoms and have normal bone development. In many cases, parental consanguinity is associated with the disease. Families often have several affected children, with boys and girls affected equally. Close to 30 mutations including missense, nonsense, and frameshift mutations have been described in HVDRR patients [130, 131].

2.10.5 Treatment of HVDRR

Large doses of vitamin D and vitamin D metabolites have been used to overcome the target organ resistance to vitamin D. Patients with HVDRR without alopecia are generally more responsive to treatment with high doses of vitamin D preparations than patients with alopecia [135]. Doses have ranged from 5,000 to 40,000 IU/day for vitamin D, 20–200 μg/day for 25(OH)D, and 17–20 μg/day for $1,25(OH)_2D$ [23, 136, 242]. The reason high doses of vitamin D metabolites are effective is the molecular basis of HVDRR. When the resistance to vitamin D is caused by VDR mutations that moderately decrease the affinity of the receptor for its ligand, such as the H305Q or I314S mutations [129, 234], high doses of the hormone can apparently overcome the low-affinity binding defect and achieve adequate VDR occupancy to mediate normal $1,25(OH)_2D$ responses. A few HVDRR patients with alopecia have been treated successfully with vitamin D metabolites [10, 31, 78, 92, 113, 215, 221].

When vitamin D therapy has proven ineffective, intensive calcium therapy is the alternate treatment of choice. Some success has been achieved with high doses of oral calcium [193]. To bypass the defect in calcium absorption, long-term high-dose calcium infusions are indicated. These are usually given at night over a period of several months. Rapid disappearance of bone pains has been documented, along with gradual decrease in calcemia and parathyroid function, followed by improvement of rickets, and gains in body weight and height [9, 18, 80, 231]. The syndrome may recur when the i.v. infusions are discontinued [9]. After the serum calcium normalizes and radiological control of the rickets has been achieved with i.v. calcium infusions, high-dose oral calcium therapy is effective in maintaining normocalcemia [80]. This two-step calcium protocol (i.v. infusions followed by high oral doses) appears to be the preferred therapeutic approach.

Spontaneous improvement in the disease of HVDRR patients has been reported [32, 78, 79]. When rickets heal spontaneously, this typically occurs at 7–15 years of age, but is not associated with the onset of puberty. Spontaneous recovery does not appear to be related to treatment, as therapy is often ineffective and improvement may occur after treatment is discontinued. The patients appear to remain normocalcemic without therapy and show no evidence of rickets or osteomalacia. Spontaneous improvement has been reported for both ligand-binding-positive and ligand-binding-negative HVDRR patients [32, 78, 79]. Alopecia may persist even if the rickets has healed [32, 78, 79]. It is not uncommon for children to "outgrow" genetic diseases, as the organism seems to be able to compensate for the loss of VDR function after skeletal growth has been completed. Compensation is not true in the case of the hair follicle [117].

2.11 Current and Emerging Therapeutics

2.11.1 Vitamin D Analog

In addition to its role in mineral homeostasis, $1,25(OH)_2D$ regulates growth, differentiation, and apoptosis of many cell types. The broad functions of the vitamin D hormone and its possible role in cancer [66] have raised interest whether $1,25(OH)_2D$ or suitable analogs can serve as anti-proliferative agents in psoriasis or cancer [45]. $1,25(OH)_2D$ targets many proliferation-related pathways, including inhibition of cell-cycle progression, induction of apoptosis, as well as reduction of angiogenesis [45]. Because the anti-proliferative effects of $1,25(OH)_2D$ are markedly reduced in tumors that have been derived from VDR-deficient mice [243], it is apparent VDR mediates these effects.

An in-depth discussion of the chemical structures, biochemical properties, and metabolism of vitamin D analogs is beyond the scope of this chapter. For more information on analogs, the reader is referred to two recent reviews [24, 97]. One class of clinically relevant vitamin D analogs are 1α-hydroxy-D2 [165] and 1α-hydroxy-D3 [15]. Both compounds are activated following hepatic 25-hydroxylation. 1α(OH)D3 is used to treat osteoporosis and occasionally pseudovitamin D deficiency rickets [162, 182]. Doxercalciferol

[1α(OH)D2] is approved for treating secondary hyperparathyroidism [24, 60].

The pharmaceutical industry has spent much effort in an effort to develop vitamin D analogs with reduced calcemic properties. Many of these are based on the structure of 1,25$(OH)_2$D and involve modifications of the side chain of the nucleus. Paricalcitol (19-Nor-1α,25$(OH)_2D_2$), an analog that lacks the 19-methylene group, is used to manage secondary hyperparathyroidism [24, 133]. Other analogs intended for the treatment of hyperproliferative diseases like psoriasis include 22-oxacalcitriol (OCT; maxacalcitol) where oxygen atom carbon replaces carbon 22 [149, 154], and calcipotriol, a compound with a double bond in C22–C23, and a 24-hydroxyl group, and a cyclopropane ring in the side chain of 1,25$(OH)_2$D [27, 111].

Analogs that lack the conventional secosteroid vitamin D structure are the substituted biphenyls with a spatial separation of the A-ring and side-chain hydroxyl groups needed for positioning within the ligand-binding pocket of the VDR [19, 125]. These and other analogs are still in development [97].

2.11.2 CYP24A1 as a Candidate Oncogene

The bioactivity of 1,25$(OH)_2$D and analogs is regulated by catabolic pathways in the target tissues. The effects of the vitamin D compounds may therefore be restricted by the activity of CYP24A1. This is relevant for the intended clinical use of vitamin D compounds, as in cancer treatment. Indeed, *CYP24A1* has increased expression in human tumors. The assessment of the expression or possible amplification of *CYP24A1* may therefore have clinical relevance for oncotherapy with vitamin D analogs.

The human *CYP24A1* gene maps to the 20q13.2–20q13.3 chromosomal region [72]. The 20q region is of particular significance in cancer research, as it shows gains or amplifications in a number of adenocarcinoma types [3, 64, 110, 143, 207, 218, 232, 233]. With the aid of comparative genomic hybridization (CGH), three studies have examined aberrations of chromosome 20 in breast cancer, prostate cancer, and gastric adenocarcinomas [3, 232, 236]. The chromosome region where *CYP24A1* is located was found amplified in each type of cancer. *CYP24A1* could therefore very well be an oncogene [3].

Terming CYP24A1 an oncogene may be going too far. Yct CYP24A1 is overexpressed in breast tumors [3], esophageal cancers [146], cutaneous squamous carcinomas [147, 184], ovarian cancers [4], colon adenocarcinomas [4, 39], and primary lung tumors [4]. The expression of the CYP24A1 gene is also elevated in a variety of human cancer cell lines such as esophagus [146], colon [39], lung [98, 168], and prostate [124, 145]. In several of these model systems, the growth inhibition induced by 1,25$(OH)_2$D is inversely proportional to the level of *CYP24A1* expression or to CYP24A1 activity [4, 145, 146, 168, 238]. These findings help explain the poor prognosis of *CYP24A1*-overexpressing cancers [146].

Preclinical model systems may also provide clues to the underlying mechanisms. While there is no evidence that mice deficient in *Cyp24al* develop spontaneous cancers [209], the distal mouse chromosome 2, which is one of the largest regions of conserved synteny between mouse and human autosomes, corresponds to the human chromosome 20q [128], which is amplified in mouse islet carcinomas [81]. More interestingly, DNA-methylation-based epigenetic changes at the *Cyp24al* gene promoter are responsible for the differential response to 1,25$(OH)_2$D by tumor-derived endothelial cells, compared with hormone endothelial cells [36]. The finding that aberrant DNA hypermethylation targets the *Cyp24al* locus to effect endothelial cell responses suggests that endothelial cells may be a target of vitamin D in the tumor microenvironment. This in turn may lead to novel therapeutic interventions.

There has also been recent interest in the putative association between gene pathway polymorphisms and cancer risk [140]. Human *CYP24A1* gene contains 12 exons and several single nucleotide polymorphisms (SNPs) [50, 85, 186]. Because SNPs are within noncoding regions, they may not exert a functional effect. However, SNP characterized in the *CYP24A1* promoter may modulate expression of the CYP24A1 protein [186]. Studies are needed to establish the risk associations and to determine the functional significance of the sequence variations.

2.11.3 CYP24A1 in Chronic Kidney Disease

Chronic kidney disease (CKD) is increasing worldwide, because of aging of the population and the increase in the incidence of obesity with complications of hypertension and adult-onset diabetes [169]. Stages 3 and 4 of CKD are characterized by progressively decreasing kidney function. Patients with severe CKD (stage 5) require regular dialysis or kidney transplant for survival [151]. With declining renal function, kidney failure patients experience declining 1,25(OH)$_2$D levels. This in turn causes hypocalcemia and leads to the development of secondary hyperparathyroidism (SHPT) [52, 134, 195]. Patients with SHPT due to renal failure also develop bone disorders, characterized by disorganized bone remodeling and by loss of bone strength and integrity, with associated morbidity [122, 205, 211]. Untreated, SHPT of renal failure is associated with increased mortality due to cardiovascular calcification and associated ischemic events [70, 178, 179].

Treatment with vitamin D analogs has been advocated [51, 152] so as to normalize PTH levels and blood calcium and to maintain bone health and cardiovascular integrity [59, 60, 133, 139].

Recent results suggest that in CKD, *CYP24A1* expression may be elevated [76, 241] as a result of kidney damage and replacement with vitamin D analogs because CYP24A1 inactivates vitamin D and analogs. Elevation in *CYP24A1* expression may contribute to vitamin D insufficiency and exacerbate SHPT in CKD patients. On the basis of these findings, treatment of CKD patients may benefit from the availability of specific inhibitors of CYP24A1 [172].

2.11.4 CYP24A1 Inhibitors

It has long been surmised that inhibition of CYP24A1 activity would enhance the effect of 1,25(OH)$_2$D. It now appears that CYP24A1 inhibitors may help in the clinical management of chronic kidney disease. The first inhibitors were antifungal imidazole derivatives, such as ketoconazole and liarozole. They lack specificity and inhibit steroidogenesis by interfering with the cytochrome P450 enzyme systems [123]. This feature could prove beneficial in the treatment of prostate cancer [124].

The prominent phytoestrogen in soy, genistein, inhibits CYP24A1 in cultured cells [55–57, 181, 235] and in the mouse [100]. It appears to inhibit *CYP24A1* expression (at the transcriptional level) [55] and the activity of the CYP24A1 protein [56]. Phytoestrogens have a beneficial effect on cancers [93, 96]. Their effect on vitamin D metabolic pathways suggests that part of their antitumorigenic effects may be mediated by vitamin D [100]. This also raises the possibility that inhibition of CYP24A1 can be effected in part by nutritional means [40, 213].

In the effort to synthesize vitamin D analogs with low calcemic activity, potent inhibitors of CYP24A1 have been identified [172]. These include sulfone [173] and sulfoximine [99] derivatives of 1,25(OH)$_2$D. The 16,23-diene-25sulfone analog (compound CTA018/MT2832) [172] is particularly interesting from a therapeutic standpoint as it exhibits a dual mechanism of action, acting as a potent and low-calcemic inhibitor of CYP24A1, and is a potent activator of VDR-mediated transcription [172]. The compound exhibits an adequate pharmacokinetic and pharmacodynamic profile; it suppresses elevated PTH without affecting calcemia or phosphatemia in a preclinical rodent model of CKD [172]. This new class of analogs with a dual mechanism of action may prevent secondary hyperparathyroidism in late-stage chronic kidney disease without leading to acquired resistance to vitamin D analog therapy caused by induction of CYP24A1. It is possible that further refinement modifying the crystal structure of the enzyme could lead to additional properties of CYP24A1 [6].

Conclusion

Notwithstanding decades of studies of the metabolism and mechanism of its action, vitamin D continues to be a focus of research. The studies linking low vitamin D status with a multitude of conditions suggest that optimization of vitamin D levels is a global health issue, and that it is of interest to develop more specific and efficient vitamin D analogs, as well as inhibitors of CYP24A1. There is need to develop an animal model to assess the potential role of CYP2R1 as a vitamin D-25-hydroxylase in vivo. Understanding of the autocrine/paracrine role of $1,25(OH)_2D$ in macrophages and chondrocytes has grown, but the contribution of nonendocrine pathways in osteoblasts or keratinocytes remains to be determined. At the molecular level, the study of VDR-dependent gene regulation has highlighted previously unrecognized mechanisms of transcriptional control. The activation of the VDR by unconventional ligands needs study, as does the putative biological role of the membrane molecules that may mediate the activity of vitamin D and metabolites in given tissues.

References

1. Ahmad W, Faiyaz ul Haque M, Brancolini V, Tsou HC, ul Haque S, Lam H, Aita VM, Owen J, de Blaquiere M, Frank J, Cserhalmi-Friedman PB, Leask A, McGrath JA, Peacocke M, Ahmad M, Ott J, Christiano AM. Alopecia universalis associated with a mutation in the human hairless gene. Science. 1998;279:720–4.
2. Aiba I, Yamasaki T, Shinki T, Izumi S, Yamamoto K, Yamada S, Terato H, Ide H, Ohyama Y. Characterization of rat and human CYP2J enzymes as vitamin D 25-hydroxylases. Steroids. 2006;71:849–56.
3. Albertson DG, Ylstra B, Segraves R, Collins C, Dairkee SH, Kowbel D, Kuo WL, Gray JW, Pinkel D. Quantitative mapping of amplicon structure by array CGH identifies CYP24 as a candidate oncogene. Nat Genet. 2000;25:144–6.
4. Anderson MG, Nakane M, Ruan X, Kroeger PE, Wu-Wong JR. Expression of VDR and CYP24A1 mRNA in human tumors. Cancer Chemother Pharmacol. 2006;57:234–40.
5. Andersson D, Davis DL, Dahlback H, Jornvall H. Cloning, structure and expression of the mitochondrial cytochrome P-450 sterol 26-hydroxylase, a bile acid biosynthetic enzyme. J Biol Chem. 1989;264:8222–9.
6. Annalora AJ, Goodin DB, Hong WX, Zhang Q, Johnson EF, Stout CD. Crystal structure of CYP24A1, a mitochondrial cytochrome P450 involved in vitamin D metabolism. J Mol Biol. 2010;396:441–51.
7. Arnaud C, Maijer R, Reade T, Scriver CR, Whelan DT. Vitamin D dependency: an inherited postnatal syndrome with secondary hyperparathyroidism. Pediatrics. 1970;46:871–80.
8. Baker AR, McDonnell DP, Hughes M, Crisp TM, Mangelsdorf DJ, Haussler MR, Pike JW, Shine J, O'Malley BW. Cloning and expression of full-length cDNA encoding human vitamin D receptor. Proc Natl Acad Sci USA. 1988;85:3294–8.
9. Balsan S, Garabedian M, Larchet M, Gorski AM, Cournot G, Tau C, Bourdeau A, Silve C, Ricour C. Long-term nocturnal calcium infusions can cure rickets and promote normal mineralization in hereditary resistance to 1,25-dihydroxyvitamin D. J Clin Invest. 1986;77:1661–7.
10. Balsan S, Garabedian M, Liberman UA, Eil C, Bourdeau A, Guillozo H, Grimberg R, Le Deunff MJ, Lieberherr M, Guimbaud P, Broyer M, Marx SJ. Rickets and alopecia with resistance to 1,25-dihydroxyvitamin D: two different clinical courses with two different cellular defects. J Clin Endocrinol Metab. 1983;57:803–11.
11. Balsan S, Garabedian M, Lieberherr M, Gueris J, Ulmann A, et al. Serum 1,25-dihydroxyvitamin D concentrations in two different types of pseudo-deficiency rickets. In: Norman AW, Schaefer K, Herrath DV, editors. Vitamin D: basic research and its clinical application. Berlin: Walter de Gruyter; 1979. p. 1143–9.
12. Bannister A, Kouzarides T. The CBP coactivator is a histone acetyl transferease. Nature. 1996;384:641–3.
13. Barger-Lux MJ, Heaney RP. Effects of above average summer sun exposure on serum 25-hydroxyvitamin D and calcium absorption. J Clin Endocrinol Metab. 2002;87:4952–6.
14. Barsony J, Marx S. Rapid accumulation of cyclic GMP near activated vitamin D receptors. Proc Natl Acad Sci USA. 1991;88:1436–40.
15. Barton DH, Hesse RH, Pechet MM, Rizzardo E. A convenient synthesis of 1-hydroxy-vitamin D 3. J Am Chem Soc. 1973;95:2748–9.
16. Benn BS, Ajibade D, Porta A, Dhawan P, Hediger M, Peng JB, Jiang Y, Oh GT, Jeung EB, Lieben L, Bouillon R, Carmeliet G, Christakos S. Active intestinal calcium transport in the absence of transient receptor potential vanilloid type 6 and calbindin-D9k. Endocrinology. 2008;149:3196–205.
17. Binkley N, Ramamurthy R, Krueger D. Low vitamin D status: definition, prevalence, consequences, and correction. Endocrinol Metab Clin North Am. 2010;39:287–301. Table of contents.
18. Bliziotes M, Yergey AL, Nanes MS, Muenzer J, Begley MG, Vieira NE, Kher KK, Brandi ML, Marx SJ. Absent intestinal response to calciferols in hereditary resistance to 1,25-dihydroxyvitamin D: documentation and effective therapy with high dose

intravenous calcium infusions. J Clin Endocrinol Metab. 1988;66:294–300.
19. Boehm MF, Fitzgerald P, Zou A, Elgort MG, Bischoff ED, Mere L, Mais DE, Bissonnette RP, Heyman RA, Nadzan AM, Reichman M, Allegretto EA. Novel nonsecosteroidal vitamin D mimics exert VDR-modulating activities with less calcium mobilization than 1,25-dihydroxyvitamin D3. Chem Biol. 1999;6: 265–75.
20. Bouillon R, Van Cromphaut S, Carmeliet G. Intestinal calcium absorption: molecular vitamin D mediated mechanisms. J Cell Biochem. 2003;88:332–9.
21. Boyan BD, Sylvia VL, McKinney N, Schwartz Z. Membrane actions of vitamin D metabolites 1alpha,25(OH)2D3 and 24R,25(OH)2D3 are retained in growth plate cartilage cells from vitamin D receptor knockout mice. J Cell Biochem. 2003;90:1207–23.
22. Boyan BD, Wong KL, Wang L, Yao H, Guldberg RE, Drab M, Jo H, Schwartz Z. Regulation of growth plate chondrocytes by 1,25-dihydroxyvitamin D3 requires caveolae and caveolin-1. J Bone Miner Res. 2006;21:1637–47.
23. Brooks MH, Bell NH, Love L, Stern PH, Orfei E, Queener SF, Hamstra AJ, DeLuca HF. Vitamin-D-dependent rickets type II. Resistance of target organs to 1,25-dihydroxyvitamin D. N Engl J Med. 1978;298: 996–9.
24. Brown AJ, Slatopolsky E. Drug insight: vitamin D analogs in the treatment of secondary hyperparathyroidism in patients with chronic kidney disease. Nat Clin Pract Endocrinol Metab. 2007;3:134–44.
25. Cali JJ, Hsieh CL, Francke U, Russell DW. Mutations in the bile acid biosynthetic enzyme sterol 27-hydroxylase underlie cerebrotendinous xanthomatosis. J Biol Chem. 1991;266:7779–83.
26. Cali JJ, Russell DW. Characterization of human sterol 27-hydroxylase. A mitochondrial cytochrome P-450 that catalyzes multiple oxidation reactions in bile acid biosynthesis. J Biol Chem. 1991;266:7774–8.
27. Calverley MJ. Synthesis of MC930, a biologically active vitamin D metabolite analogue. Tetrahedron. 1987;43:4609–19.
28. Canadillas S, Rodriguez-Benot A, Rodriguez M. More on the bone-kidney axis – lessons from hypophosphataemia. Nephrol Dial Transplant. 2007;22: 1521–3.
29. Cao X, Ross FP, Zhang L, MacDonald PN, Chappel J, Teitelbaum SL. Cloning of the promoter for the avian integrin β_3 subunit gene and its regulation by 1,25-dihydroxyvitamin D_3. J Biol Chem. 1993;268:27371–80.
30. Casella SJ, Reiner BJ, Chen TC, Holick MF, Harrison HE. A possible genetic defect in 25-hydroxylation as a cause of rickets. J Pediatr. 1994;124:929–32.
31. Castells S, Greig F, Fusi MA, Finberg L, Yasumura S, Liberman UA, Eil C, Marx SJ. Severely deficient binding of 1,25-dihydroxyvitamin D to its receptors in a patient responsive to high doses of this hormone. J Clin Endocrinol Metab. 1986;63:252–6.
32. Chen TL, Hirst MA, Cone CM, Hochberg Z, Tietze HU, Feldman D. 1,25-dihydroxyvitamin D resistance, rickets, and alopecia: analysis of receptors and bioresponse in cultured fibroblasts from patients and parents. J Clin Endocrinol Metab. 1984;59: 383–8.
33. Cheng JB, Levine MA, Bell NH, Mangelsdorf DJ, Russell DW. Genetic evidence that the human CYP2R1 enzyme is a key vitamin D 25-hydroxylase. Proc Natl Acad Sci USA. 2004;101:7711–5.
34. Cheng JB, Motola DL, Mangelsdorf DJ, Russell DW. De-orphanization of Cytochrome P450 2R1: a microsomal vitamin D 25-hydroxylase. J Biol Chem. 2003;278:38084–93.
35. Chiba N, Suldan Z, Freedman LP, Parvin J. Binding of liganded vitamin D receptor to the vitamin D receptor interacting protein coactivator complex induces interaction with RNA polymerase II holoenzyme. J Biol Chem. 2000;275:10719–22.
36. Chung I, Karpf AR, Muindi JR, Conroy JM, Nowak NJ, Johnson CS, Trump DL. Epigenetic silencing of CYP24 in tumor-derived endothelial cells contributes to selective growth inhibition by calcitriol. J Biol Chem. 2007;282:8704–14.
37. Cianferotti L, Cox M, Skorija K, Demay MB. Vitamin D receptor is essential for normal keratinocyte stem cell function. Proc Natl Acad Sci USA. 2007;104:9428–33.
38. Civitelli R, Kim YS, Gunsten SL, Fujimori A, Huskey M, Avioli LV, Hruska KA. Nongenomic activation of the calcium message system by vitamin D metabolites in osteoblast-like cells. Endocrinology. 1990;127: 2253–62.
39. Cross HS, Bises G, Lechner D, Manhardt T, Kallay E. The vitamin D endocrine system of the gut – its possible role in colorectal cancer prevention. J Steroid Biochem Mol Biol. 2005;97:121–8.
40. Cross HS, Kallay E, Lechner D, Gerdenitsch W, Adlercreutz H, Armbrecht HJ. Phytoestrogens and vitamin D metabolism: a new concept for the prevention and therapy of colorectal, prostate, and mammary carcinomas. J Nutr. 2004;134:1207S–12.
41. Dardenne O, Prud'homme J, Arabian A, Glorieux FH, St-Arnaud R. Targeted inactivation of the 25-hydroxyvitamin D(3)-1(alpha)- hydroxylase gene (CYP27B1) creates an animal model of pseudovitamin D- deficiency rickets. Endocrinology. 2001;142:3135–41.
42. Dardenne O, Prud'homme J, Hacking SA, Glorieux FH, St-Arnaud R. Correction of the abnormal mineral ion homeostasis with a high-calcium, high-phosphorus, high-lactose diet rescues the PDDR phenotype of mice deficient for the 25-hydroxyvitamin D-1alpha-hydroxylase (CYP27B1). Bone. 2003;32: 332–40.
43. Dawson-Hughes B, Heaney RP, Holick MF, Lips P, Meunier PJ, Vieth R. Estimates of optimal vitamin D status. Osteoporos Int. 2005;16:713–6.
44. de Boland AR, Nemere I, Norman AW. Ca^{2+}-Channel agonist bay K8644 mimics $1,25(OH)_2$-vitamin D_3 rapid enhancement of Ca^{2+} transport in chick perfused duodenum. Biochem Biophys Res Commun. 1990;166:217–22.

45. Deeb KK, Trump DL, Johnson CS. Vitamin D signalling pathways in cancer: potential for anticancer therapeutics. Nat Rev Cancer. 2007;7:684–700.
46. DeLuca HF. Overview of general physiologic features and functions of vitamin D. Am J Clin Nutr. 2004;80: 1689S–96.
47. Delvin EE, Glorieux FH, Marie PJ, Pettifor JM. Vitamin D dependency: replacement therapy with calcitriol. J Pediatr. 1981;99:26–34.
48. Demay MB, Gerardi JM, DeLuca HF, Kronenberg HM. DNA sequences in the rat osteocalcin gene that bind the 1,25-dihydroxyvitamin D_3 receptor and confer responsiveness to 1,25-dihydroxyvitamin D_3. Proc Natl Acad Sci USA. 1990;87:369–73.
49. Demay MB, Kiernan MS, DeLuca HF, Kronenberg HM. Characterization of 1,25-dihydroxyvitamin D3 receptor interactions with target sequences in the rat osteocalcin gene. Mol Endocrinol. 1992;6:557–62.
50. Dong LM, Ulrich CM, Hsu L, Duggan DJ, Benitez DS, White E, Slattery ML, Farin FM, Makar KW, Carlson CS, Caan BJ, Potter JD, Peters U. Vitamin D related genes, CYP24A1 and CYP27B1, and colon cancer risk. Cancer Epidemiol Biomarkers Prev. 2009;18:2540–8.
51. Drueke TB. Which vitamin D derivative to prescribe for renal patients. Curr Opin Nephrol Hypertens. 2005;14:343–9.
52. Elder G. Pathophysiology and recent advances in the management of renal osteodystrophy. J Bone Miner Res. 2002;17:2094–105.
53. Erben RG, Soegiarto DW, Weber K, Zeitz U, Lieberherr M, Gniadecki R, Moller G, Adamski J, Balling R. Deletion of deoxyribonucleic acid binding domain of the vitamin D receptor abrogates genomic and nongenomic functions of vitamin D. Mol Endocrinol. 2002;16:1524–37.
54. Farach-Carson MC, Sergeev I, Norman AW. Nongenomic actions of 1,25-dihydroxyvitamin D_3 in rat osteosarcoma cells: structure-function studies using ligand analogs. Endocrinology. 1991;129: 1876–84.
55. Farhan H, Cross HS. Transcriptional inhibition of CYP24 by genistein. Ann N Y Acad Sci. 2002;973: 459–62.
56. Farhan H, Wahala K, Adlercreutz H, Cross HS. Isoflavonoids inhibit catabolism of vitamin D in prostate cancer cells. J Chromatogr B Analyt Technol Biomed Life Sci. 2002;777:261–8.
57. Farhan H, Wahala K, Cross HS. Genistein inhibits vitamin D hydroxylases CYP24 and CYP27B1 expression in prostate cells. J Steroid Biochem Mol Biol. 2003;84:423–9.
58. Fraser D, Kooh SW, Kind HP, Holick MF, Tanaka Y, DeLuca HF. Pathogenesis of hereditary vitamin-D-dependent rickets. An inborn error of vitamin D metabolism involving defective conversion of 25-hydroxyvitamin D to 1 alpha,25-dihydroxyvitamin D. N Engl J Med. 1973;289:817–22.
59. Frazao JM, Chesney RW, Coburn JW. Intermittent oral 1alpha-hydroxyvitamin D2 is effective and safe for the suppression of secondary hyperparathyroidism in haemodialysis patients. 1alphaD2 Study Group. Nephrol Dial Transplant. 1998;13 Suppl 3:68–72.
60. Frazao JM, Elangovan L, Maung HM, Chesney RW, Acchiardo SR, Bower JD, Kelley BJ, Rodriguez HJ, Norris KC, Robertson JA, Levine BS, Goodman WG, Gentile D, Mazess RB, Kyllo DM, Douglass LL, Bishop CW, Coburn JW. Intermittent doxercalciferol (1alpha-hydroxyvitamin D(2)) therapy for secondary hyperparathyroidism. Am J Kidney Dis. 2000;36: 550–61.
61. Fu GK, Lin D, Zhang MY, Bikle DD, Shackleton CH, Miller WL, Portale AA. Cloning of human 25-hydroxyvitamin D-1 alpha-hydroxylase and mutations causing vitamin D-dependent rickets type 1. Mol Endocrinol. 1997;11:1961–70.
62. Fu GK, Portale AA, Miller WL. Complete structure of the human gene for the vitamin D 1alpha- hydroxylase, P450c1alpha. DNA Cell Biol. 1997;16: 1499–507.
63. Fujita H, Sugimoto K, Inatomi S, Maeda T, Osanai M, Uchiyama Y, Yamamoto Y, Wada T, Kojima T, Yokozaki H, Yamashita T, Kato S, Sawada N, Chiba H. Tight junction proteins claudin-2 and -12 are critical for vitamin D-dependent Ca^{2+} absorption between enterocytes. Mol Biol Cell. 2008;19:1912–21.
64. Fukushige S, Waldman FM, Kimura M, Abe T, Furukawa T, Sunamura M, Kobari M, Horii A. Frequent gain of copy number on the long arm of chromosome 20 in human pancreatic adenocarcinoma. Genes Chromosomes Cancer. 1997;19:161–9.
65. Fukushima M, Suzuki Y, Tohira Y, Nishii Y, Suzuki M. 25-Hydroxylation of 1alpha-hydroxyvitamin D3 in vivo and in perfused rat liver. FEBS Lett. 1976;65: 211–4.
66. Garland CF, Garland FC. Do sunlight and vitamin D reduce the likelihood of colon cancer? Int J Epidemiol. 1980;9:227–31.
67. Ginde AA, Liu MC, Camargo Jr CA. Demographic differences and trends of vitamin D insufficiency in the US population, 1988–2004. Arch Intern Med. 2009;169:626–32.
68. Glorieux FH. Calcitriol treatment in vitamin D-dependent and vitamin D-resistant rickets. Metabolism. 1990;39(suppl):10–2.
69. Gombart AF, Borregaard N, Koeffler HP. Human cathelicidin antimicrobial peptide (CAMP) gene is a direct target of the vitamin D receptor and is strongly up-regulated in myeloid cells by 1,25-dihydroxyvitamin D3. FASEB J. 2005;19:1067–77.
70. Goodman WG, Goldin J, Kuizon BD, Yoon C, Gales B, Sider D, Wang Y, Chung J, Emerick A, Greaser L, Elashoff RM, Salusky IB. Coronary-artery calcification in young adults with end-stage renal disease who are undergoing dialysis. N Engl J Med. 2000;342: 1478–83.
71. Gupta RP, Hollis BW, Patel SB, Bell NH. CYP3A4 is a human microsomal vitamin D-25-hydroxylase. J Bone Miner Res. 2004;19(4):680–8. Epub 2003.

72. Hahn CN, Baker E, Laslo P, May BK, Omdahl JL, Sutherland GR. Localization of the human vitamin D 24-hydroxylase gene (CYP24) to chromosome 20q13.2->q13.3. Cytogenet Cell Genet. 1993;62: 192–3.
73. Haussler MR, Haussler CA, Bartik L, Whitfield GK, Hsieh JC, Slater S, Jurutka PW. Vitamin D receptor: molecular signaling and actions of nutritional ligands in disease prevention. Nutr Rev. 2008;66: S98–112.
74. Haussler MR, Whitfield GK, Haussler CA, Hsieh JC, Thompson PD, Selznick SH, Dominguez CE, Jurutka PW. The nuclear vitamin D receptor: biological and molecular regulatory properties revealed. J Bone Miner Res. 1998;13:325–49.
75. Heaney RP, Armas LA, Shary JR, Bell NH, Binkley N, Hollis BW. 25-Hydroxylation of vitamin D3: relation to circulating vitamin D3 under various input conditions. Am J Clin Nutr. 2008;87:1738–42.
76. Helvig C, Kharebov A, Petkovich M, Ryder K, Ireland B, Cuerrier D. The role of CYP24-mediated catabolism on vitamin D status and responsiveness in a rodent model of CKD. J Bone Miner Res. 2009. Vol 24 (Suppl. 1): Available at URL: http://www.asbmr.org/Meetings/AnnualMeeting/AbstractDetail.aspx?aid=df1f0fcc-a9c8-4c14-9ab6-587adcf72123.
77. Hendrich B, Hardeland U, Ng HH, Jiricny J, Bird A. The thymine glycosylase MBD4 can bind to the product of deamination at methylated CpG sites. Nature. 1999;401:301–4.
78. Hirst MA, Hochman HI, Feldman D. Vitamin D resistance and alopecia: a kindred with normal 1,25-dihydroxyvitamin D binding, but decreased receptor affinity for deoxyribonucleic acid. J Clin Endocrinol Metab. 1985;60:490–5.
79. Hochberg Z, Benderli A, Levy J, Vardi P, Weisman Y, Chen T, Feldman D. 1,25-Dihydroxyvitamin D resistance, rickets, and alopecia. Am J Med. 1984;77: 805–11.
80. Hochberg Z, Tiosano D, Even L. Calcium therapy for calcitriol-resistant rickets. J Pediatr. 1992;121:803–8.
81. Hodgson G, Hager JH, Volik S, Hariono S, Wernick M, Moore D, Nowak N, Albertson DG, Pinkel D, Collins C, Hanahan D, Gray JW. Genome scanning with array CGH delineates regional alterations in mouse islet carcinomas. Nat Genet. 2001;29:459–64.
82. Hoenderop J, VanDerKemp A, Hartog A, VandeGraaf S, Van Os C, Willems P, Bindels R. Molecular identification of the apical Ca^{2+} channel in 1,25-dihydroxyvitamin D-responsive epithelia. J Biol Chem. 1999;274:8375–8.
83. Hoenderop JG, van Leeuwen JP, van der Eerden BC, Kersten FF, van der Kemp AW, Merillat AM, Waarsing JH, Rossier BC, Vallon V, Hummler E, Bindels RJ. Renal Ca^{2+} wasting, hyperabsorption, and reduced bone thickness in mice lacking TRPV5. J Clin Invest. 2003;112:1906–14.
84. Hofmann AF. Detoxification of lithocholic acid, a toxic bile acid: relevance to drug hepatotoxicity. Drug Metab Rev. 2004;36:703–22.
85. Holick CN, Stanford JL, Kwon EM, Ostrander EA, Nejentsev S, Peters U. Comprehensive association analysis of the vitamin D pathway genes, VDR, CYP27B1, and CYP24A1, in prostate cancer. Cancer Epidemiol Biomarkers Prev. 2007;16: 1990–9.
86. Holick MF. Photobiology of vitamin D. In: Feldman D, Glorieux FH, Pike JW, editors. Vitamin D. San Diego: Academic Press; 1997. p. 33–9.
87. Holick MF, Siris ES, Binkley N, Beard MK, Khan A, Katzer JT, Petruschke RA, Chen E, de Papp AE. Prevalence of vitamin D inadequacy among postmenopausal North American women receiving osteoporosis therapy. J Clin Endocrinol Metab. 2005;90:3215–24.
88. Hollis BW. Circulating 25-hydroxyvitamin D levels indicative of vitamin D sufficiency: implications for establishing a new effective dietary intake recommendation for vitamin D. J Nutr. 2005;135:317–22.
89. Hollis BW. Assessment and interpretation of circulating 25-hydroxyvitamin D and 1,25-dihydroxyvitamin D in the clinical environment. Endocrinol Metab Clin North Am. 2010;39:271–86. Table of contents.
90. Hosseinpour F, Ibranovic I, Tang W, Wikvall K. 25-Hydroxylation of vitamin D3 in primary cultures of pig hepatocytes: evidence for a role of both CYP2D25 and CYP27A1. Biochem Biophys Res Commun. 2003;303:877–83.
91. Hsieh JC, Sisk JM, Jurutka PW, Haussler CA, Slater SA, Haussler MR, Thompson CC. Physical and functional interaction between the vitamin D receptor and hairless corepressor, two proteins required for hair cycling. J Biol Chem. 2003;278:38665–74.
92. Hughes MR, Malloy PJ, Kieback DG, Kesterson RA, Pike JW, Feldman D, O'Malley BW. Point mutations in the human vitamin D receptor gene associated with hypocalcemic rickets. Science. 1988;242: 1702–5.
93. Ingram D, Sanders K, Kolybaba M, Lopez D. Case-control study of phyto-oestrogens and breast cancer. Lancet. 1997;350:990–4.
94. Standing Committee on the Scientific Evaluation of Dietary Reference Intakes, Food and Nutrition Board and Institute of Medicine Staff. Dietary reference intakes for calcium, phosphorus, magnesium, vitamin D, and fluoride. Washington, D.C.: National Academy Press; 1997.
95. Ishizuka S, Kurihara N, Reddy SV, Cornish J, Cundy T, Roodman GD. (23S)-25-Dehydro-1{alpha}-hydroxyvitamin D3–26,23-lactone, a vitamin D receptor antagonist that inhibits osteoclast formation and bone resorption in bone marrow cultures from patients with Paget's disease. Endocrinology. 2005; 146:2023–30.
96. Jacobsen BK, Knutsen SF, Fraser GE. Does high soy milk intake reduce prostate cancer incidence? The Adventist Health Study (United States). Cancer Causes Control. 1998;9:553–7.
97. Jones G. Vitamin D analogs. Endocrinol Metab Clin North Am. 2010;39:447–72. Table of contents.

98. Jones G, Ramshaw H, Zhang A, Cook R, Byford V, White J, Petkovich M. Expression and activity of vitamin D-metabolizing cytochrome P450s (CYP1alpha and CYP24) in human nonsmall cell lung carcinomas. Endocrinology. 1999;140:3303–10.
99. Kahraman M, Sinishtaj S, Dolan PM, Kensler TW, Peleg S, Saha U, Chuang SS, Bernstein G, Korczak B, Posner GH. Potent, selective and low-calcemic inhibitors of CYP24 hydroxylase: 24-sulfoximine analogues of the hormone 1alpha,25-dihydroxyvitamin D(3). J Med Chem. 2004;47:6854–63.
100. Kallay E, Adlercreutz H, Farhan H, Lechner D, Bajna E, Gerdenitsch W, Campbell M, Cross HS. Phytoestrogens regulate vitamin D metabolism in the mouse colon: relevance for colon tumor prevention and therapy. J Nutr. 2002;132:3490S–3.
101. Kerry DM, Dwivedi PP, Hahn CN, Morris HA, Omdahl JL, May BK. Transcriptional synergism between vitamin D-responsive elements in the rat 25-hydroxyvitamin D3 24-hydroxylase (CYP24) promoter. J Biol Chem. 1996;271:29715–21.
102. Khanal RC, Nemere I. The ERp57/GRp58/1,25D3-MARRS receptor: multiple functional roles in diverse cell systems. Curr Med Chem. 2007;14: 1087–93.
103. Kim CJ, Kaplan LE, Perwad F, Huang N, Sharma A, Choi Y, Miller WL, Portale AA. Vitamin D 1alpha-hydroxylase gene mutations in patients with 1alpha-hydroxylase deficiency. J Clin Endocrinol Metab. 2007;92:3177–82.
104. Kim MS, Fujiki R, Murayama A, Kitagawa H, Yamaoka K, Yamamoto Y, Mihara M, Takeyama K, Kato S. 1Alpha,25(OH)2D3-induced transrepression by vitamin D receptor through E-box-type elements in the human parathyroid hormone gene promoter. Mol Endocrinol. 2007;21:334–42.
105. Kim MS, Kondo T, Takada I, Youn MY, Yamamoto Y, Takahashi S, Matsumoto T, Fujiyama S, Shirode Y, Yamaoka I, Kitagawa H, Takeyama K, Shibuya H, Ohtake F, Kato S. DNA demethylation in hormone-induced transcriptional derepression. Nature. 2009;461:1007–12.
106. Kitada H, Miyata M, Nakamura T, Tozawa A, Honma W, Shimada M, Nagata K, Sinal CJ, Guo GL, Gonzalez FJ, Yamazoe Y. Protective role of hydroxysteroid sulfotransferase in lithocholic acid-induced liver toxicity. J Biol Chem. 2003;278: 17838–44.
107. Kitagawa H, Fujiki R, Yoshimura K, Mezaki Y, Uematsu Y, Matsui D, Ogawa S, Unno K, Okubo M, Tokita A, Nakagawa T, Ito T, Ishimi Y, Nagasawa H, Matsumoto T, Yanagisawa J, Kato S. The chromatin-remodeling complex WINAC targets a nuclear receptor to promoters and is impaired in Williams syndrome. Cell. 2003;113:905–17.
108. Kitanaka S, Murayama A, Sakaki T, Inouye K, Seino Y, Fukumoto S, Shima M, Yukizane S, Takayanagi M, Niimi H, Takeyama K, Kato S. No enzyme activity of 25-hydroxyvitamin D3 1alpha-hydroxylase gene product in pseudovitamin D deficiency rickets, including that with mild clinical manifestation. J Clin Endocrinol Metab. 1999;84:4111–7.
109. Kitanaka S, Takeyama K, Murayama A, Sato T, Okumura K, Nogami M, Hasegawa Y, Niimi H, Yanagisawa J, Tanaka T, Kato S. Inactivating mutations in the 25-hydroxyvitamin D3 1alpha-hydroxylase gene in patients with pseudovitamin D-deficiency rickets. N Engl J Med. 1998;338:653–61.
110. Korn WM, Yasutake T, Kuo WL, Warren RS, Collins C, Tomita M, Gray J, Waldman FM. Chromosome arm 20q gains and other genomic alterations in colorectal cancer metastatic to liver, as analyzed by comparative genomic hybridization and fluorescence in situ hybridization. Genes Chromosomes Cancer. 1999;25:82–90.
111. Kragballe K, Gjertsen BT, De Hoop D, Karlsmark T, van de Kerkhof PC, Larko O, Nieboer C, Roed-Petersen J, Strand A, Tikjob G. Double-blind, right/left comparison of calcipotriol and betamethasone valerate in treatment of psoriasis vulgaris. Lancet. 1991;337:193–6.
112. Kraichely D, Collins J, DeLisle R, MacDonald PN. The autonomous transactivation domain in helix H3 of the vitamin D receptor is required for transactivation and coactivator interaction. J Biol Chem. 1999;274:14352–8.
113. Kudoh T, Kumagai T, Uetsuji N, Tsugawa S, Oyanagi K, Chiba Y, Minami R, Nakao T. Vitamin D dependent rickets: decreased sensitivity to 1,25-dihydroxyvitamin D. Eur J Pediatr. 1981;137:307–11.
114. Kuriyama M, Fujiyama J, Kubota R, Nakagawa M, Osame M. Osteoporosis and increased bone fractures in cerebrotendinous xanthomatosis. Metabolism. 1993;42:1497–8.
115. Labuda M, Labuda D, Korab-Laskowska M, Cole DE, Zietkiewicz E, Weissenbach J, Popowska E, Pronicka E, Root AW, Glorieux FH. Linkage disequilibrium analysis in young populations: pseudo-vitamin D-deficiency rickets and the founder effect in French Canadians. Am J Hum Genet. 1996;59:633–43.
116. Labuda M, Morgan K, Glorieux FH. Mapping autosomal recessive vitamin D dependency type I to chromosome 12q14 by linkage analysis. Am J Hum Genet. 1990;47:28–36.
117. Li YC, Amling M, Pirro AE, Priemel M, Meuse J, Baron R, Delling G, Demay MB. Normalization of mineral ion homeostasis by dietary means prevents hyperparathyroidism, rickets, and osteomalacia, but not alopecia in vitamin D receptor-ablated mice. Endocrinology. 1998;139:4391–6.
118. Li YC, Bergwitz C, Juppner H, Demay M. Cloning and characterization of the vitamin D receptor from *Xenopus laevis*. Endocrinology. 1997;138:2347–53.
119. Lips P, Hosking D, Lippuner K, Norquist JM, Wehren L, Maalouf G, Ragi-Eis S, Chandler J. The prevalence of vitamin D inadequacy amongst women with osteoporosis: an international epidemiological investigation. J Intern Med. 2006;260:245–54.
120. Liu PT, Stenger S, Li H, Wenzel L, Tan BH, Krutzik SR, Ochoa MT, Schauber J, Wu K, Meinken C,

Kamen DL, Wagner M, Bals R, Steinmeyer A, Zugel U, Gallo RL, Eisenberg D, Hewison M, Hollis BW, Adams JS, Bloom BR, Modlin RL. Toll-like receptor triggering of a vitamin D-mediated human antimicrobial response. Science. 2006;311:1770–3.
121. Liu S, Gupta A, Quarles LD. Emerging role of fibroblast growth factor 23 in a bone-kidney axis regulating systemic phosphate homeostasis and extracellular matrix mineralization. Curr Opin Nephrol Hypertens. 2007;16:329–35.
122. Llach F, Fernandez E. Overview of renal bone disease: causes of treatment failure, clinical observations, the changing pattern of bone lesions, and future therapeutic approach. Kidney Int. 2003; 64(Suppl):S113–9.
123. Loose DS, Kan PB, Hirst MA, Marcus RA, Feldman D. Ketoconazole blocks adrenal steroidogenesis by inhibiting cytochrome P450-dependent enzymes. J Clin Invest. 1983;71:1495–9.
124. Lou YR, Qiao S, Talonpoika R, Syvala H, Tuohimaa P. The role of vitamin D3 metabolism in prostate cancer. J Steroid Biochem Mol Biol. 2004;92:317–25.
125. Ma Y, Khalifa B, Yee YK, Lu J, Memezawa A, Savkur RS, Yamamoto Y, Chintalacharuvu SR, Yamaoka K, Stayrook KR, Bramlett KS, Zeng QQ, Chandrasekhar S, Yu XP, Linebarger JH, Iturria SJ, Burris TP, Kato S, Chin WW, Nagpal S. Identification and characterization of noncalcemic, tissue-selective, nonsecosteroidal vitamin D receptor modulators. J Clin Invest. 2006;116:892–904.
126. Makin G, Lohnes D, Byford V, Ray R, Jones G. Target cell metabolism of 1,25-dihydroxyvitamin D3 to calcitroic acid. Evidence for a pathway in kidney and bone involving 24-oxidation. Biochem J. 1989;262:173–80.
127. Makishima M, Lu TT, Xie W, Whitfield GK, Domoto H, Evans RM, Haussler MR, Mangelsdorf DJ. Vitamin D receptor as an intestinal bile acid sensor. Science. 2002;296:1313–6.
128. Malas S, Peters J, Abbott C. The genes for endothelin 3, vitamin D 24-hydroxylase, and melanocortin 3 receptor map to distal mouse chromosome 2, in the region of conserved synteny with human chromosome 20. Mamm Genome. 1994;5:577–9.
129. Malloy PJ, Eccleshall TR, Gross C, Van Maldergem L, Bouillon R, Feldman D. Hereditary vitamin D resistant rickets caused by a novel mutation in the vitamin D receptor that results in decreased affinity for hormone and cellular hyporesponsiveness. J Clin Invest. 1997;99:297–304.
130. Malloy PJ, Feldman D. Genetic disorders and defects in vitamin d action. Endocrinol Metab Clin North Am. 2010;39:333–46. Table of contents.
131. Malloy PJ, Hochberg Z, Tiosano D, Pike JW, Hughes MR, Feldman D. The molecular basis of hereditary 1,25-dihydroxyvitamin D3 resistant rickets in seven related families. J Clin Invest. 1990;86:2071–9.
132. Malloy PJ, Pike JW, Feldman D. The vitamin D receptor and the syndrome of hereditary 1,25- dihydroxyvitamin D-resistant rickets. Endocr Rev. 1999;20:156–88.
133. Martin KJ, Gonzalez EA, Gellens M, Hamm LL, Abboud H, Lindberg J. 19-Nor-1-alpha-25-dihydroxyvitamin D2 (Paricalcitol) safely and effectively reduces the levels of intact parathyroid hormone in patients on hemodialysis. J Am Soc Nephrol. 1998;9:1427–32.
134. Martinez I, Saracho R, Montenegro J, Llach F. The importance of dietary calcium and phosphorous in the secondary hyperparathyroidism of patients with early renal failure. Am J Kidney Dis. 1997;29: 496–502.
135. Marx SJ, Bliziotes MM, Nanes M. Analysis of the relation between alopecia and resistance to 1,25-dihydroxyvitamin D. Clin Endocrinol. 1986;25:373–81.
136. Marx SJ, Spiegel AM, Brown EM, Gardner DG, Downs Jr RW, Attie M, Hamstra AJ, DeLuca HF. A familial syndrome of decrease in sensitivity to 1,25-dihydroxyvitamin D. J Clin Endocrinol Metab. 1978;47:1303–10.
137. Masuda S, Strugnell S, Calverley MJ, Makin HL, Kremer R, Jones G. In vitro metabolism of the antipsoriatic vitamin D analog, calcipotriol, in two cultured human keratinocyte models. J Biol Chem. 1994;269:4794–803.
138. Masuyama R, Stockmans I, Torrekens S, Van Looveren R, Maes C, Carmeliet P, Bouillon R, Carmeliet G. Vitamin D receptor in chondrocytes promotes osteoclastogenesis and regulates FGF23 production in osteoblasts. J Clin Invest. 2006;116:3150–9.
139. Maung HM, Elangovan L, Frazao JM, Bower JD, Kelley BJ, Acchiardo SR, Rodriguez HJ, Norris KC, Sigala JF, Rutkowski M, Robertson JA, Goodman WG, Levine BS, Chesney RW, Mazess RB, Kyllo DM, Douglass LL, Bishop CW, Coburn JW. Efficacy and side effects of intermittent intravenous and oral doxercalciferol (1alpha-hydroxyvitamin D(2)) in dialysis patients with secondary hyperparathyroidism: a sequential comparison. Am J Kidney Dis. 2001;37:532–43.
140. McCullough ML, Bostick RM, Mayo TL. Vitamin D gene pathway polymorphisms and risk of colorectal, breast, and prostate cancer. Annu Rev Nutr. 2009; 29:111–32.
141. McKenna N, Xu J, Nawaz Z, Tsai S, Tsai M, O'Malley B. Nuclear receptor coactivators: multiple enzymes, multiple complexes, multiple functions. J Steroid Biochem Molec Biol. 1999;69:3–12.
142. Medhora MM, Teitelbaum S, Chappel J, Alvarez J, Mimura H, Ross FP, Hruska K. 1α,25-dihydroxyvitamin D_3 up-regulates expression of the osteoclast integrin $\alpha_v\beta_3$. J Biol Chem. 1993;268:1456–61.
143. Meijer GA, Hermsen MA, Baak JP, van Diest PJ, Meuwissen SG, Belien JA, Hoovers JM, Joenje H, Snijders PJ, Walboomers JM. Progression from colorectal adenoma to carcinoma is associated with non-random chromosomal gains as detected by comparative genomic hybridisation. J Clin Pathol. 1998;51:901–9.
144. Meyer MB, Goetsch PD, Pike JW. A downstream intergenic cluster of regulatory enhancers contributes

to the induction of CYP24A1 expression by 1alpha,25-dihydroxyvitamin D3. J Biol Chem. 2010; 285:15599–610.

145. Miller GJ, Stapleton GE, Hedlund TE, Moffat KA. Vitamin D receptor expression, 24-hydroxylase activity, and inhibition of growth by 1alpha,25-dihydroxyvitamin D3 in seven human prostatic carcinoma cell lines. Clin Cancer Res. 1995;1: 997–1003.
146. Mimori K, Tanaka Y, Yoshinaga K, Masuda T, Yamashita K, Okamoto M, Inoue H, Mori M. Clinical significance of the overexpression of the candidate oncogene CYP24 in esophageal cancer. Ann Oncol. 2004;15:236–41.
147. Mitschele T, Diesel B, Friedrich M, Meineke V, Maas RM, Gartner BC, Kamradt J, Meese E, Tilgen W, Reichrath J. Analysis of the vitamin D system in basal cell carcinomas (BCCs). Lab Invest. 2004;84: 693–702.
148. Murayama A, Kim MS, Yanagisawa J, Takeyama K, Kato S. Transrepression by a liganded nuclear receptor via a bHLH activator through co-regulator switching. EMBO J. 2004;23:1598–608.
149. Murayama E, Miyamoto K, Kubodera N, Mori T, Matsunaga I. Synthetic studies of vitamin D3 analogues. VIII. Synthesis of 22-oxavitamin D3 analogues. Chem Pharm Bull(Tokyo). 1986; 34:4410–3.
150. Naja RP, Dardenne O, Arabian A, St Arnaud R. Chondrocyte-specific modulation of Cyp27b1 expression supports a role for local synthesis of 1,25-dihydroxyvitamin D3 in growth plate development. Endocrinology. 2009;150:4024–32.
151. National Kidney Foundation. K/DOQI clinical practice guidelines for chronic kidney disease: evaluation, classification, and stratification. Am J Kidney Dis. 2002;39:S1-266.
152. National Kidney Foundation. K/DOQI clinical practice guidelines for bone metabolism and disease in chronic kidney disease. Am J Kidney Dis. 2003;42: S1-201.
153. Nemere I, Farach-Carson MC, Rohe B, Sterling TM, Norman AW, Boyan BD, Safford SE. Ribozyme knockdown functionally links a 1,25(OH)2D3 membrane binding protein (1,25D3-MARRS) and phosphate uptake in intestinal cells. Proc Natl Acad Sci USA. 2004;101:7392–7.
154. Nishii Y, Sato K, Kobayashi T. The development of vitamin D3 analogues for the treatment of osteoporosis. Osteoporos Int. 1993;3 Suppl 1:190–3.
155. Noda M, Vogel RL, Craig AM, Prahl J, DeLuca HF, Denhardt DT. Identification of a DNA sequence responsible for binding of the 1,25-dihydroxyvitamin D_3 receptor and 1,25-dihydroxyvitamin D_3 enhancement of mouse secreted phosphoprotein 1 (Spp-1 or osteopontin) gene expression. Proc Natl Acad Sci USA. 1990;87:9995–9.
156. Ohyama Y, Ozono K, Uchida M, Shinki T, Kato S, Suda T, Yamamoto O, Noshiro M, Kato Y. Identification of a vitamin D-responsive element in the 5′-flanking region of the rat 25-hydroxyvitamin D3 24-hydroxylase gene. J Biol Chem. 1994;269: 10545–50.
157. Okuda KI, Usui E, Ohyama Y. Recent progress in enzymology and molecular biology of enzymes involved in vitamin D metabolism. J Lipid Res. 1995;36:1641–52.
158. Omdahl JL, Bobrovnikova EA, Choe S, Dwivedi PP, May BK. Overview of regulatory cytochrome P450 enzymes of the vitamin D pathway. Steroids. 2001; 66:381–9.
159. Omdahl JL, Bobrovnikova EV, Annalora A, Chen P, Serda R. Expression, structure-function, and molecular modeling of vitamin D P450s. J Cell Biochem. 2003;88:356–62.
160. Omdahl JL, Morris HA, May BK. Hydroxylase enzymes of the vitamin D pathway: expression, function, and regulation. Annu Rev Nutr. 2002;22: 139–66.
161. Onate S, Tsai S, Tsai M, O'Malley B. Sequence and characterization of a coactivator for the steroid hormone receptor superfamily. Science. 1995;270: 1354–7.
162. Orimo H, Shiraki M, Hayashi T, Nakamura T. Reduced occurrence of vertebral crush fractures in senile osteoporosis treated with 1 alpha (OH)-vitamin D3. Bone Miner. 1987;3:47–52.
163. Orwoll E, Nielson CM, Marshall LM, Lambert L, Holton KF, Hoffman AR, Barrett-Connor E, Shikany JM, Dam T, Cauley JA. Vitamin D deficiency in older men. J Clin Endocrinol Metab. 2009;94: 1214–22.
164. Ozono K, Liao J, Kerner SA, Scott RA, Pike JW. The vitamin D-responsive element in the human osteocalcin gene: association with a nuclear proto-oncogene enhancer. J Biol Chem. 1990;265:21881–8.
165. Paaren HE, Hamer DE, Schnoes HK, DeLuca HF. Direct C-1 hydroxylation of vitamin D compounds: convenient preparation of 1alpha-hydroxyvitamin D3, 1alpha, 25-dihydroxyvitamin D3, and 1alpha-hydroxyvitamin D2. Proc Natl Acad Sci USA. 1978;75:2080–1.
166. Panda DK, Al Kawas S, Seldin MF, Hendy GN, Goltzman D. 25-hydroxyvitamin D 1alpha-hydroxylase: structure of the mouse gene, chromosomal assignment, and developmental expression. J Bone Miner Res. 2001;16:46–56.
167. Panda DK, Miao D, Tremblay ML, Sirois J, Farookhi R, Hendy GN, Goltzman D. Targeted ablation of the 25-hydroxyvitamin D 1alpha -hydroxylase enzyme: evidence for skeletal, reproductive, and immune dysfunction. Proc Natl Acad Sci USA. 2001;98: 7498–503.
168. Parise RA, Egorin MJ, Kanterewicz B, Taimi M, Petkovich M, Lew AM, Chuang SS, Nichols M, El-Hefnawy T, Hershberger PA. CYP24, the enzyme that catabolizes the antiproliferative agent vitamin D, is increased in lung cancer. Int J Cancer. 2006; 119:1819–28.
169. Patel UD, Young EW, Ojo AO, Hayward RA. CKD progression and mortality among older patients with diabetes. Am J Kidney Dis. 2005;46:406–14.

170. Peng J, Chen X, Berger U, Vassilev P, Tsukaguchi H, Brown E, Hediger M. Molecular cloning and characterization of a channel-like transporter mediating intestinal calcium absorption. J Biol Chem. 1999;274:22739–46.
171. Portale AA, Miller WL. Human 25-hydroxyvitamin D-1alpha-hydroxylase: cloning, mutations, and gene expression. Pediatr Nephrol. 2000;14:620–5.
172. Posner GH, Helvig C, Cuerrier D, Collop D, Kharebov A, Ryder K, Epps T, Petkovich M. Vitamin D analogues targeting CYP24 in chronic kidney disease. J Steroid Biochem Mol Biol. 2010;121(1–2):13–9.
173. Posner GH, Wang Q, Han G, Lee JK, Crawford K, Zand S, Brem H, Peleg S, Dolan P, Kensler TW. Conceptually new sulfone analogues of the hormone 1alpha, 25-dihydroxyvitamin D(3): synthesis and preliminary biological evaluation. J Med Chem. 1999;42:3425–35.
174. Prosser DE, Kaufmann M, O'Leary B, Byford V, Jones G. Single A326G mutation converts human CYP24A1 from 25-OH-D3–24-hydroxylase into -23-hydroxylase, generating 1alpha,25-(OH)2D3–26,23-lactone. Proc Natl Acad Sci USA. 2007;104:12673–8.
175. Puzas JE, Turner RT, Howard GA, Brand JS, Baylink DJ. Synthesis of 1,25-dihydroxycholecalciferol and 24,25- dihydroxycholecalciferol by calvarial cells. Characterization of the enzyme systems. Biochem J. 1987;245:333–8.
176. Rachez C, Lemon B, Suldan Z, Bromleigh B, Gamble M, Naar N, Erdjument-Bromage H, Tempst P, Freedman LP. Ligand-dependent transcription activation by nuclear receptors requires the DRIP complex. Nature. 1999;398:824–8.
177. Rachez C, Suldan Z, Ward J, Chang CP, Burakov D, Erdjument-Bromage H, Tempst P, Freedman LP. A novel protein complex that interacts with the vitamin D3 receptor in a ligand-dependent manner and enhances VDR transactivation in a cell-free system. Genes Dev. 1998;12:1787–800.
178. Raggi P, Boulay A, Chasan-Taber S, Amin N, Dillon M, Burke SK, Chertow GM. Cardiac calcification in adult hemodialysis patients. A link between end-stage renal disease and cardiovascular disease? J Am Coll Cardiol. 2002;39:695–701.
179. Raggi P, Kleerekoper M. Contribution of bone and mineral abnormalities to cardiovascular disease in patients with chronic kidney disease. Clin J Am Soc Nephrol. 2008;3:836–43.
180. Rahmaniyan M, Patrick K, Bell NH. Characterization of recombinant CYP2C11: a vitamin D 25-hydroxylase and 24-hydroxylase. Am J Physiol Endocrinol Metab. 2005;288:E753–60.
181. Rao A, Woodruff RD, Wade WN, Kute TE, Cramer SD. Genistein and vitamin D synergistically inhibit human prostatic epithelial cell growth. J Nutr. 2002;132:3191–4.
182. Reade TM, Scriver CR, Glorieux FH, Nogrady B, Delvin E, Poirier R, Holick F, DeLuca HF. Response to crystalline 1alpha-hydroxyvitamin D3 in vitamin D dependency. Pediatr Res. 1975;9:593–9.
183. Reichel H, Bishop JE, Koeffler HP, Norman AW. Evidence for 1,25-dihydroxyvitamin D3 production by cultured porcine alveolar macrophages. Mol Cell Endocrinol. 1991;75:163–7.
184. Reichrath J, Rafi L, Rech M, Mitschele T, Meineke V, Gartner BC, Tilgen W, Holick MF. Analysis of the vitamin D system in cutaneous squamous cell carcinomas. J Cutan Pathol. 2004;31:224–31.
185. Reinhardt TA, Horst RL. Self-induction of 1,25-dihydroxyvitamin D3 metabolism limits receptor occupancy and target tissue responsiveness. J Biol Chem. 1989;264:15917–21.
186. Roff A, Wilson RT. A novel SNP in a vitamin D response element of the CYP24A1 promoter reduces protein binding, transactivation, and gene expression. J Steroid Biochem Mol Biol. 2008;112:47–54.
187. Rosen H, Reshef A, Maeda N, Lippoldt A, Shpizen S, Triger L, Eggertsen G, Bjorkhem I, Leitersdorf E. Markedly reduced bile acid synthesis but maintained levels of cholesterol and vitamin D metabolites in mice with disrupted sterol 27-hydroxylase gene. J Biol Chem. 1998;273:14805–12.
188. Saini SP, Sonoda J, Xu L, Toma D, Uppal H, Mu Y, Ren S, Moore DD, Evans RM, Xie W. A novel constitutive androstane receptor-mediated and CYP3A-independent pathway of bile acid detoxification. Mol Pharmacol. 2004;65:292–300.
189. Saito H, Kusano K, Kinosaki M, Ito H, Hirata M, Segawa H, Miyamoto K, Fukushima N. Human fibroblast growth factor-23 mutants suppress Na+-dependent phosphate co-transport activity and 1alpha,25-dihydroxyvitamin D3 production. J Biol Chem. 2003;278:2206–11.
190. Sakai Y, Demay MB. Evaluation of keratinocyte proliferation and differentiation in vitamin D receptor knockout mice. Endocrinology. 2000;141:2043–9.
191. Sakai Y, Kishimoto J, Demay MB. Metabolic and cellular analysis of alopecia in vitamin D receptor knockout mice. J Clin Invest. 2001;107:961–6.
192. Sakaki T, Sawada N, Komai K, Shiozawa S, Yamada S, Yamamoto K, Ohyama Y, Inouye K. Dual metabolic pathway of 25-hydroxyvitamin D3 catalyzed by human CYP24. Eur J Biochem FEBS. 2000;267:6158–65.
193. Sakati N, Woodhouse NJ, Niles N, Harfi H, de Grange DA, Marx S. Hereditary resistance to 1,25-dihydroxyvitamin D: clinical and radiological improvement during high-dose oral calcium therapy. Horm Res. 1986;24:280–7.
194. Salen G, Shefer S, Cheng FW, Dayal B, Batta AK, Tint GS. Cholic acid biosynthesis: the enzymatic defect in cerebrotendinous xanthomatosis. J Clin Invest. 1979;63:38–44.
195. Salusky IB. Are new vitamin D analogues in renal bone disease superior to calcitriol? Pediatr Nephrol. 2005;20:393–8.
196. Sanchez-Martinez R, Zambrano A, Castillo AI, Aranda A. Vitamin D-dependent recruitment of corepressors to vitamin D/retinoid X receptor heterodimers. Mol Cell Biol. 2008;28:3817–29.

197. Schwartz Z, Brooks B, Swain L, Del Toro F, Norman A, Boyan B. Production of 1,25-dihydroxyvitamin D3 and 24,25-dihydroxyvitamin D3 by growth zone and resting zone chondrocytes is dependent on cell maturation and is regulated by hormones and growth factors. Endocrinology. 1992;130:2495–504.
198. Schwartz Z, Graham EJ, Wang L, Lossdorfer S, Gay I, Johnson-Pais TL, Carnes DL, Sylvia VL, Boyan BD. Phospholipase A2 activating protein (PLAA) is required for 1alpha,25(OH)2D3 signaling in growth plate chondrocytes. J Cell Physiol. 2005;203:54–70.
199. Schwartz Z, Shaked D, Hardin RR, Gruwell S, Dean DD, Sylvia VL, Boyan BD. 1alpha,25(OH)2D3 causes a rapid increase in phosphatidylinositol-specific PLC-beta activity via phospholipase A2-dependent production of lysophospholipid. Steroids. 2003;68:423–37.
200. Schwartz Z, Sylvia VL, Luna MH, DeVeau P, Whetstone R, Dean DD, Boyan BD. The effect of 24R,25-(OH)(2)D(3) on protein kinase C activity in chondrocytes is mediated by phospholipase D whereas the effect of 1alpha,25-(OH)(2)D(3) is mediated by phospholipase C. Steroids. 2001;66: 683–94.
201. Scriver CR. Vitamin D dependency. Pediatrics. 1970;45:361–3.
202. Scriver CR, Reade TM, DeLuca HF, Hamstra AJ. Serum 1,25-dihydroxyvitamin D levels in normal subjects and in patients with hereditary rickets or bone disease. N Engl J Med. 1978;299:976–9.
203. Shaul PW, Anderson RG. Role of plasmalemmal caveolae in signal transduction. Am J Physiol. 1998;275:L843–51.
204. Shinki T, Shimada H, Wakino S, Anazawa H, Hayashi M, Saruta T, DeLuca HF, Suda T. Cloning and expression of rat 25-hydroxyvitamin D3–1alpha-hydroxylase cDNA. Proc Natl Acad Sci USA. 1997;94:12920–5.
205. Slatopolsky E, Gonzalez E, Martin K. Pathogenesis and treatment of renal osteodystrophy. Blood Purif. 2003;21:318–26.
206. Smith SJ, Rucka AK, Berry JL, Davies M, Mylchreest S, Paterson CR, Heath DA, Tassabehji M, Read AP, Mee AP, Mawer EB. Novel mutations in the 1alpha-hydroxylase (P450c1) gene in three families with pseudovitamin D-deficiency rickets resulting in loss of functional enzyme activity in blood-derived macrophages. J Bone Miner Res. 1999;14:730–9.
207. Sonoda G, Palazzo J, du Manoir S, Godwin AK, Feder M, Yakushiji M, Testa JR. Comparative genomic hybridization detects frequent overrepresentation of chromosomal material from 3q26, 8q24, and 20q13 in human ovarian carcinomas. Genes Chromosomes Cancer. 1997;20:320–8.
208. Spencer T, Jenster G, Burcin M, Allis C, Zhou J, Mizzen C, McKenna NJ, Onate S, Tsai S, Tsai M, O'Malley B. Steroid receptor coactivator-1 is a histone acetyltransferase. Nature. 1997;389:194–8.
209. St-Arnaud R, Arabian A, Travers R, Barletta F, Raval-Pandya M, Chapin K, Depovere J, Mathieu C, Christakos S, Demay MB, Glorieux FH. Deficient mineralization of intramembranous bone in vitamin D-24-hydroxylase-ablated mice is due to elevated 1,25-dihydroxyvitamin D and not to the absence of 24,25-dihydroxyvitamin D. Endocrinology. 2000; 141:2658–66.
210. St-Arnaud R, Messerlian S, Moir JM, Omdahl JL, Glorieux FH. The 25-hydroxyvitamin D 1-alpha-hydroxylase gene maps to the pseudovitamin D-deficiency rickets (PDDR) disease locus. J Bone Miner Res. 1997;12:1552–9.
211. Steddon SJ, Fan SL, Cunningham J. New prospects for the management of renal bone disease. Nephron Clin Pract. 2005;99:c1–7.
212. Strushkevich N, Usanov SA, Plotnikov AN, Jones G, Park HW. Structural analysis of CYP2R1 in complex with vitamin D3. J Mol Biol. 2008;380:95–106.
213. Swami S, Krishnan AV, Moreno J, Bhattacharyya RB, Peehl DM, Feldman D. Calcitriol and genistein actions to inhibit the prostaglandin pathway: potential combination therapy to treat prostate cancer. J Nutr. 2007;137:205S–10.
214. Takamoto M, Tsuji K, Yamashita T, Sasaki H, Yano T, Taketani Y, Komori T, Nifuji A, Noda M. Hedgehog signaling enhances core-binding factor a1 and receptor activator of nuclear factor-kappaB ligand (RANKL) gene expression in chondrocytes. J Endocrinol. 2003;177:413–21.
215. Takeda E, Kuroda Y, Saijo T, Naito E, Kobashi H, Yokota I, Miyao M. 1 alpha-hydroxyvitamin D3 treatment of three patients with 1,25-dihydroxyvitamin D-receptor-defect rickets and alopecia. Pediatrics. 1987;80:97–101.
216. Takeshita A, Yen P, Misiti S, Cardona G, Liu Y, Chin W. Molecular cloning and properties of a full-length putative thyroid hormone receptor coactivator. Endocrinology. 1996;137:3594–7.
217. Takeyama K, Kitanaka S, Sato T, Kobori M, Yanagisawa J, Kato S. 25-Hydroxyvitamin D3 1alpha-hydroxylase and vitamin D synthesis. Science. 1997;277:1827–30.
218. Tanner MM, Grenman S, Koul A, Johannsson O, Meltzer P, Pejovic T, Borg A, Isola JJ. Frequent amplification of chromosomal region 20q12-q13 in ovarian cancer. Clin Cancer Res. 2000;6: 1833–9.
219. Toell A, Gonzalez MM, Ruf D, Steinmeyer A, Ishizuka S, Carlberg C. Different molecular mechanisms of vitamin D(3) receptor antagonists. Mol Pharmacol. 2001;59:1478–85.
220. Tomon M, Tenenhouse HS, Jones G. Expression of 25-hydroxyvitamin D3–24-hydroxylase activity in Caco-2 cells. An in vitro model of intestinal vitamin D catabolism. Endocrinology. 1990;126:2868–75.
221. Tsuchiya Y, Matsuo N, Cho H, Kumagai M, Yasaka A, Suda T, Orimo H, Shiraki M. An unusual form of vitamin D-dependent rickets in a child: alopecia and marked end-organ hyposensitivity to biologically active vitamin D. J Clin Endocrinol Metab. 1980;51: 685–90.

222. Umesono K, Murakami KK, Thompson CC, Evans RM. Direct repeats as selective response elements for the thyroid hormone, retinoic acid and vitamin D_3 receptors. Cell. 1991;65:1255–66.
223. Uppal H, Saini SP, Moschetta A, Mu Y, Zhou J, Gong H, Zhai Y, Ren S, Michalopoulos GK, Mangelsdorf DJ, Xie W. Activation of LXRs prevents bile acid toxicity and cholestasis in female mice. Hepatology. 2007;45:422–32.
224. van Deurs B, Roepstorff K, Hommelgaard AM, Sandvig K. Caveolae: anchored, multifunctional platforms in the lipid ocean. Trends Cell Biol. 2003; 13:92–100.
225. Wagner D, Hanwell HE, Vieth R. An evaluation of automated methods for measurement of serum 25-hydroxyvitamin D. Clin Biochem. 2009;42: 1549–56.
226. Wang JT, Lin CJ, Burridge SM, Fu GK, Labuda M, Portale AA, Miller WL. Genetics of vitamin D 1alpha-hydroxylase deficiency in 17 families. Am J Hum Genet. 1998;63:1694–702.
227. Wang TT, Nestel FP, Bourdeau V, Nagai Y, Wang Q, Liao J, Tavera-Mendoza L, Lin R, Hanrahan JW, Mader S, White JH. Cutting edge: 1,25-dihydroxyvitamin D3 is a direct inducer of antimicrobial peptide gene expression. J Immunol. 2004;173:2909–12.
228. Wang X, Zhang MY, Miller WL, Portale AA. Novel gene mutations in patients with 1alpha-hydroxylase deficiency that confer partial enzyme activity in vitro. J Clin Endocrinol Metab. 2002;87:2424–30.
229. Wasserman RH, Fullmer CS. Calcium transport proteins, calcium absorption, and vitamin D. Ann Rev Physiol. 1983;45:375–90.
230. Weber G, Heilborn JD, Chamorro Jimenez CI, Hammarsjo A, Torma H, Stahle M. Vitamin D induces the antimicrobial protein hCAP18 in human skin. J Invest Dermatol. 2005;124:1080–2.
231. Weisman Y, Bab I, Gazit D, Spirer Z, Jaffe M, Hochberg Z. Long-term intracaval calcium infusion therapy in end-organ resistance to 1,25-dihydroxyvitamin D. Am J Med. 1987;83:984–90.
232. Weiss MM, Snijders AM, Kuipers EJ, Ylstra B, Pinkel D, Meuwissen SG, van Diest PJ, Albertson DG, Meijer GA. Determination of amplicon boundaries at 20q13.2 in tissue samples of human gastric adenocarcinomas by high-resolution microarray comparative genomic hybridization. J Pathol. 2003; 200:320–6.
233. Werner M, Mattis A, Aubele M, Cummings M, Zitzelsberger H, Hutzler P, Hofler H. 20q13.2 amplification in intraductal hyperplasia adjacent to in situ and invasive ductal carcinoma of the breast. Virchows Arch. 1999;435:469–72.
234. Whitfield GK, Selznick SH, Haussler CA, Hsieh JC, Galligan MA, Jurutka PW, Thompson PD, Lee SM, Zerwekh JE, Haussler MR. Vitamin D receptors from patients with resistance to 1,25-dihydroxyvitamin D3: point mutations confer reduced transactivation in response to ligand and impaired interaction with the retinoid X receptor heterodimeric partner. Mol Endocrinol. 1996;10:1617–31.
235. Wietzke JA, Welsh J. Phytoestrogen regulation of a Vitamin D3 receptor promoter and 1,25-dihydroxyvitamin D3 actions in human breast cancer cells. J Steroid Biochem Mol Biol. 2003;84: 149–57.
236. Wolter H, Gottfried HW, Mattfeldt T. Genetic changes in stage pT2N0 prostate cancer studied by comparative genomic hybridization. BJU Int. 2002;89:310–6.
237. Yamagata M, Kimoto A, Michigami T, Nakayama M, Ozono K. Hydroxylases involved in vitamin D metabolism are differentially expressed in murine embryonic kidney: application of whole mount in situ hybridization. Endocrinology. 2001;142: 3223–30.
238. Yee SW, Campbell MJ, Simons C. Inhibition of vitamin D3 metabolism enhances VDR signalling in androgen-independent prostate cancer cells. J Steroid Biochem Mol Biol. 2006;98:228–35.
239. Yoshida T, Monkawa T, Tenenhouse HS, Goodyer P, Shinki T, Suda T, Wakino S, Hayashi M, Saruta T. Two novel 1alpha-hydroxylase mutations in French-Canadians with vitamin D dependency rickets type I. Kidney Int. 1998;54:1437–43.
240. Zasloff M. Antimicrobial peptides of multicellular organisms. Nature. 2002;415:389–95.
241. Zehnder D, Quinkler M, Eardley KS, Bland R, Lepenies J, Hughes SV, Raymond NT, Howie AJ, Cockwell P, Stewart PM, Hewison M. Reduction of the vitamin D hormonal system in kidney disease is associated with increased renal inflammation. Kidney Int. 2008;74:1343–53.
242. Zerwekh JE, Glass K, Jowsey J, Pak CY. An unique form of osteomalacia associated with end organ refractoriness to 1,25-dihydroxyvitamin D and apparent defective synthesis of 25-hydroxyvitamin D. J Clin Endocrinol Metab. 1979;49:171–5.
243. Zinser GM, McEleney K, Welsh J. Characterization of mammary tumor cell lines from wild type and vitamin D3 receptor knockout mice. Mol Cell Endocrinol. 2003;200:67–80.

3 Gonadal Hormones, Diseases, and Emerging Therapeutics

Faryal S. Mirza, Liam Zakko, and Pamela Taxel

Key words
Gonadal hormones • Androgens • Hypogonadism • Testosterone • Estrogen
Klinefelter syndrome

3.1 Introduction

Gonadal steroids play a critical role in bone metabolism throughout life. Not only are they essential for normal bone mass accrual and development during adolescence, but they also are critical in the maintenance of bone health through adult and senior life. In this chapter, discussion of normal gonadal hormone synthesis will be reviewed, and commonly encountered disease states and therapies will be considered for both men and women. We will initiate the discussion with disorders that occur at the level of the target organs, the testes and ovaries, and then consider defects of the pituitary and hypothalamus. Discussion will focus on common disorders of primary and secondary hypogonadism in men and women, including their diagnosis and therapeutic strategies for treatment of these diseases.

3.2 Sex Steroid Biosynthesis and Normal Feedback Mechanism

3.2.1 Androgens

Testosterone is the principal androgen produced in men. It is a steroid hormone with a four ring structure, made mainly in the Leydig cells, which are located in the interstitium of the testis. The classical biological effects of androgens are primarily mediated by binding to the androgen receptor, which leads to gene expression by regulating the transcription of a number of androgen-responsive genes. Synthesis of testosterone by enzymatic steps begins with cholesterol predominantly formed by de novo synthesis from acetate, preformed cholesterol from intracellular cholesterol ester stores or extracellular supply from

F.S. Mirza, M.D.
Division of Endocrinology and Metabolism, Department of Medicine, University of Connecticut Health Center, 263 Farmington Avenue, Farmington, CT 06030, USA
e-mail: fmirza@uchc.edu

L. Zakko, M.D.
Yale Department of Medicine, Yale New Haven Hospital, 333 Cedar St, New Haven, CT 06520, USA

P. Taxel, M.D. (✉)
Division of Endocrinology and Metabolism, Department of Medicine, University of Connecticut Health Center, 263 Farmington Avenue, Farmington, CT 06030, USA
e-mail: taxel@nso.uchc.edu

F. Bronner et al. (eds.), *Bone-Metabolic Functions and Modulators*, Topics in Bone Biology,
DOI 10.1007/978-1-4471-2745-1_3, © Springer-Verlag London 2012

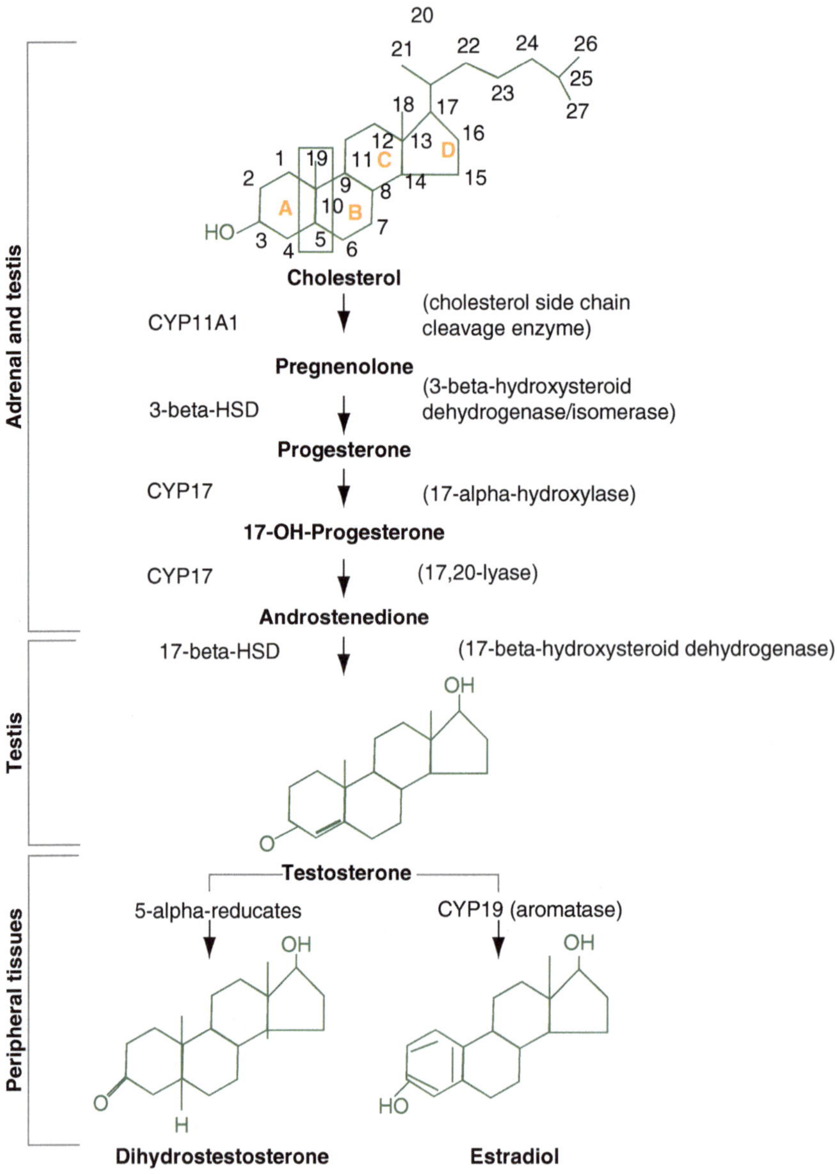

Fig. 3.1 Testosterone and estradiol formation and metabolism (Reproduced with permission from Griffin and Wilson [35]. Copyright © 2011 UpToDate, Inc. For more information, visit www.uptodate.com)

circulating low-density lipoproteins [38]. Two multifunctional cytochrome P-450 complexes are involved (Fig. 3.1). In addition, extragonadal biosynthesis of testosterone and dihydrotestosterone from the circulating weak adrenal androgen precursor dehydroepiandrostenedione (DHEA) within specific tissues has been described, although the net contribution of adrenal androgens to circulating testosterone levels is small. Secretion of testosterone is primarily governed by luteinizing hormone (LH) through its regulation of the cholesterol to pregnenolone conversion within Leydig cell mitochondria.

3.2.2 Estrogens

Estradiol and progesterone are the main sex steroids made by the ovaries in women. The levels of the sex steroids are extremely low in prepubertal females and increase after menarche, under the influence of pituitary gonadotropins, with the initiation of the menstrual cycle. The main source of estradiol is the ovary, with a small amount produced in the peripheral tissues from circulating androgens. The synthesis of estradiol involves the synthesis of androgens from cholesterol by the same mechanisms described above for androgen synthesis in males (Fig. 3.1). The main source of androgens in women is the adrenal gland (DHEA and androstenedione) and the ovaries (androstenedione and testosterone). During follicular growth, theca cells, which express the enzymes needed to convert cholesterol into androgens, synthesize testosterone and androstenedione that are converted to estradiol and estrone by the aromatase enzyme present in granulosa cells. In premenopausal women, more than 95% of the estradiol is synthesized this way, with a small amount made in the peripheral tissues from estrone.

3.3 GnRH, FSH, and LH Secretion and Normal Hypothalamic-Pituitary Feedback Mechanism

The hypothalamus normally signals the pituitary via a portal vascular system as well as via neural pathways. The preoptic area and the arcuate nucleus of the hypothalamus contain neurons that secrete gonadotropin-releasing hormone (GnRH) in a pulsatile fashion, termed the GnRH pulse generator. Regulation of GnRH release is complex and can be modulated by a variety of factors including several hormones, neurotransmitters, and cytokines. Kisspeptin, a neuropeptide, and its receptor, KISS 1R (also called GPR54), has been shown to be important for normal hypothalamic GnRH processing or secretion [35].

The initiation and maintenance of the reproductive axis in humans requires pulsatile secretion of GnRH from the hypothalamus, which leads to synthesis and secretion of luteinizing hormone (LH) and follicle-stimulating hormone (FSH) from the anterior pituitary. This, in turn, initiates intragonadal testosterone production and spermatogenesis as well as systemic testosterone secretion and ultimately virilization. The pulsatility of GnRH secretion is critical for the stimulation of LH and FSH release, while, incontrast, continuous administration of GnRH or GnRH agonists can be used therapeutically to inhibit LH and FSH release.

LH and FSH are each composed of two glycoprotein chains that contain alpha and beta subunits. While both hormones share the same alpha subunit, their unique beta subunits convey distinct immunologic and functional characteristics to these two hormones. The amount of LH and FSH released depends upon the frequency and magnitude of GnRH pulses as well as age of the individual. LH interacts with Leydig cell membrane receptors in the testes to stimulate adenyl cyclase and the formation and release of cyclic adenosine monophosphate (cAMP). cAMP then activates a protein kinase through a series of incompletely understood intermediate steps to initiate testosterone synthesis [25]. Similarly, FSH interacts with receptors on the Sertoli cell membrane [104] to stimulate cAMP and activate protein kinase. The development of normal spermatogenesis involves both FSH as well as testosterone, likely functioning in a synergistic manner [23].

In women, with the onset of puberty, hypothalamic secretion of GnRH in a pulsatile manner results in the secretion of FSH and LH in a cyclic fashion by the pituitary gland, which in turn regulates the synthesis and release of ovarian steroids. GnRH secretion also is regulated by dopamine, serotonin, -endorphin, and norepinephrine. The cyclic variation in the levels of the gonadotropins during the menstrual cycle induces maturation of one ovum each month. The menstrual cycle begins with the onset of vaginal bleeding each month and ends just before the onset of bleeding the next month. The median duration of the menstrual cycle is 28 days, although it varies considerably in individuals from 21 to 40 days. The normal menstrual cycle is divided into the earlier follicular or proliferative phase and the later luteal or secretory phase. The luteal phase is typically 14 days in length, while the follicular phase is relatively more variable in length.

FSH and LH made by the gonadotropes bind to a transmembrane G protein–coupled receptor in the ovary, activating the G-stimulatory (G_s) subunit, which then interacts with adenylate cyclase to increase levels of cyclic cAMP, ultimately leading to the activation of protein kinase A, thereby stimulating ovarian hormone production. cAMP also serves as a second messenger mediating the upregulation of steroidogenic acute regulatory protein and the cytochrome P450 enzyme system, increasing the ovarian production of estradiol and progesterone [1]. FSH regulates ovarian follicle development and stimulates ovarian estrogen production. LH is responsible for ovulation and corpus luteum formation and for progesterone and estrogen production by the corpus luteum during the early and mid-luteal phases of the menstrual cycle. Activation of the LH receptors in theca cells stimulates androstenedione production, providing the substrate for the enzymatic conversion to 17-estradiol that is mediated by the enzyme aromatase in granulosa cells [66].

3.4 Normal Hypothalamic-Pituitary Feedback Mechanism

Adequate concentrations of testosterone, estradiol, and progesterone are required to serve as negative feedback to decrease FSH and LH release at both the level of the hypothalamus and pituitary. Testosterone can be converted to estradiol through an aromatase step (via CYP19 in the brain, gonads, adipose, skin, blood vessels or bone), but the two hormones are thought to regulate gonadotropin secretion independently. Nonetheless, regulation of FSH secretion in men has been shown to be more dependent on estradiol than it is on testosterone [38], but dihydrotestosterone, a nonaromatizable androgen, also can inhibit LH, suggesting that aromatization of testosterone to estrogen is not absolutely critical for LH feedback and secretion [88]. Another important factor in the feedback loop of FSH and LH is inhibin, a glycoprotein consisting of two disulfide-linked subunits, alpha and beta. Inhibin is produced by germ cells, specifically by the Sertoli cells in males and the ovarian follicle in females, with production beginning at the time of puberty. The beta subunit exists in two forms; thus, inhibin A and inhibin B are recognized forms of this hormone. FSH and androgen are required for normal secretion of inhibin, which influences FSH synthesis and secretion more so than it does that of LH. In men, inhibin B is the most important form of the hormone, and an inverse relationship exists between inhibin B and FSH levels [35].

3.5 Peak Bone Mass

Peak bone mass (PBM) is the maximal amount of bone mineral acquired during skeletal growth and the consolidation after the attainment of final height. PBM is influenced by hormonal status, normal menarche, and presence of a regular menstrual cycle [24]. Adolescence and young adulthood are periods of rapid bone mass gain. Approximately 40% of PBM is achieved during the puberty period [96], and up to 90% of PBM is acquired by the age of 18 years in girls and by 20 years in boys [39]. The final formation of PBM occurs by approximately 25–30 years of age [90]. Overall, young men have approximately 30% higher PBM than do young women, although African American women tend to achieve higher PBM than do Caucasian women [96]. These differences in PBM may be seen as early as childhood and adolescence. Genetic factors contribute significantly to PBM with up to 60–80% effect as determined by intraclass correlations for monozygotic twins [46]. Hence, environmental factors that can be manipulated to produce higher PBM can contribute only 20–40%. Nutritional factors such as calcium intake and vitamin D deficiency may also contribute to the differences in PBM [82]. Calcium deficiencies in young people can account for a 5–10% reduction in PBM and can increase the risk for hip fracture later in life. Moderate physical activity contributes positively to PBM [30, 105], but excessive exercise in pubertal women can cause hypothalamic amenorrhea and hypoestrogenism and thus adversely affect PBM [46]. Several hormones including estrogen and androgen have significant effects on the attainment of PBM, although other hormones such as growth hormone (GH) and insulin-like growth factor 1 (IGF-1) also influence PBM formation [43].

3.6 Role of Testosterone in Bone Development

Skeletal growth is influenced by genetics, hormonal status, nutritional and mechanical factors. With regard to hormonal influences, testosterone was traditionally believed to play the major role in male skeletal development. Data from animal studies in the 1990s led to the concept that androgens in males stimulate periosteal bone formation. This notion also was confirmed by studies in rats and mice with mutations or manipulations of the androgen receptor [14]. Clinically, evidence of higher PBM acquisition seen in puberty in men compared with women seemed to confirm these data. Additionally, men gain more bone during growth than women and also have lesser decline in bone with aging. No sharp decline occurs in midlife, as there is no male equivalent of menopause. Observations of hypogonadal men and patients with androgen insensitivity also support androgen action as the major factor in the male bone phenotype. Thus, attainment of PBM at the end of puberty, the overall larger and stronger male skeleton, and the maintenance of male bone mass throughout life have been attributed to the actions of androgens.

Interestingly, recent evidence has confirmed that estrogen is essential for the accretion and consolidation of male bone health; thus, androgens and estrogens are no longer considered to be pure male and female hormones. Men convert androgens, C19 steroids secreted from the testes as well as the adrenals, into estrogen via an aromatization step. The adrenal glands also secrete androgens such as DHEA, and these also can be converted into estrone by aromatase. Estrogens so produced will activate the estrogen receptor alpha (ERα) or beta (ERβ). Several "experiments of nature" have demonstrated the importance of estrogen in the acquisition of PBM in men. Individuals with genetic defects in the estrogen receptor or in aromatase [15, 67, 94] demonstrated osteoporosis and increased bone turnover. In several observational studies, bone loss and fracture risk have been associated with estrogen exposure, particularly in older men [60]. Thus, the traditional models of male and female bone health are much more complex than they were when originally conceived, and a significant body of evidence from observational and clinical investigations has demonstrated the importance of estrogens in male bone health. A more detailed discussion of this topic can be found elsewhere [50].

3.7 Role of Estrogen in Female Bone Development

The predominant gonadal steroid influencing attainment of PBM and its preservation in women is estrogen, the synthesis of which increases with the onset of puberty. Estrogen has complex effects on the skeleton, which are beyond the scope of this chapter and have been discussed elsewhere [18]. The antiresorptive effects of estrogen predominate, although it also influences bone formation. Bone remodeling is a process that begins at conception and continues throughout life. Consisting of cycles of bone formation and bone resorption, remodeling involves the basic multicellular unit, which consists of the osteoclasts, osteoblasts, and bone-embedded osteocytes within the bone-remodeling cavity. Remodeling is crucial for the well-being of the skeletal system. Estrogens or androgens contribute to the sexual dimorphism seen in the male and female skeleton by their actions exerted during fetal development [20]. Short-term exposure to exogenous estrogen during fetal life affects bone growth and development in postnatal life, suggesting that an imprinting mechanism acts on bone cell programming early in skeletal development [63]. Skeletal development also is influenced by the effects of the sex steroids on the initiation of the pubertal growth spurt and the closure of the epiphyses at the end of puberty. Sex steroids also have direct effects on chondrocytes in growth plates and influence linear growth of long bones [12].

Estrogens and androgens also decrease the number of remodeling cycles by slowing the birth rate of osteoclasts and osteoblasts from their respective progenitors residing in bone marrow.

Osteoclasts are derived from hematopoietic progenitors of the myeloid lineage, stimulated by colony-forming unit-granulocyte/macrophage (CFU-GM) and CFU-M. Osteoblasts, as well as the hematopoiesis-supporting stromal cells and adipocytes of the bone marrow, are derived from mesenchymal stem cells. More important, the development of osteoclasts depends on a network of autocrine and paracrine factors produced by stromal and osteoblastic cells. Estrogen has been shown to suppress receptor activator nuclear factor kappa-B ligand (RANKL) production by osteoblastic, T-, and B-cells [26], which binds to its receptor, RANK on osteoclast lineage cells resulting in growth and proliferation of osteoclasts and an increase in their bone-resorbing capability. Estrogen also increases the secretion of osteoprotegrin (OPG) [40], a soluble, decoy receptor that neutralizes RANKL [40, 94]. These effects of estrogen reduce formation of osteoclasts from hematopoietic and mesenchymal lineage cells. Estrogen also reduces the production of additional bone-resorbing cytokines such as interleukin (IL)-1 [75], IL-6, tumor necrosis factor-α (TNF-α), macrophage-colony stimulating factor (M-CSF) [101], and prostaglandins from osteoblasts and bone marrow mononuclear cells, thereby modulating osteoclastic activity in a paracrine fashion [61]. Evidence is increasing to show that bone-resorbing cytokines are potential candidates for mediating the bone loss that occurs following estrogen deficiency such as occurs as a result of menopause. Both IL-1 and M-CSF production are increased in estrogen-deficient model systems [75, 101], which can be inhibited using specific antagonists [3, 51, 52]. Additionally, the bone-resorptive effects of TNF-α are well documented and can be reversed using a soluble type I TNF receptor [53]. Several studies have shown that IL-6 plays a key role in mediating bone loss following estrogen or androgen deficiency [31, 45].

Sex steroids also have direct effects on osteoclast lineage cells. Estrogen and androgens both induce apoptosis of these cells [42, 54], and both sex steroids suppress RANKL-induced osteoclast differentiation by blocking RANKL/M-CSF-induced activator protein-1-dependent transcription through a reduction of c-Jun activity. The latter is due both to reduced c-Jun expression and to decreased phosphorylation [41, 93, 98]. Moreover, estrogen and androgens inhibit the activity of mature osteoclasts through direct, receptor-mediated mechanisms [74, 77]. Estrogen also reduces the life span of osteoclasts by stimulating the production of TGF-β by nearby osteoblastic cells [73], which induces apoptosis of osteoclasts [42]. Imai et al. have shown that estrogens directly control the function and life span of mature osteoclasts by downregulation of bone resorption–related genes and induction of the proapoptotic Fas ligand, respectively [43].

At the cellular level, estrogen prolongs the life span of the osteoblast by inhibiting osteoblast apoptosis [54]. Sex steroid effects on osteoblast apoptosis appear to be mediated by activation of the Src/Shc/ERK signaling pathway [54] along with downregulation of JNK, leading to alterations in the activity of key transcription factors, including Elk-1, CCAAT-enhancer-binding protein-β (C/EBPβ), cyclic adenosine monophosphate response element binding protein (CREB), and c-Jun/cFos [55]. Provocative studies also indicate that 4-estren-3α,17β-diol, a synthetic ligand for the ER that does not affect classical transcription, may protect against bone loss following ovariectomy in mice solely by activating these nongenotropic pathways [54].

Recent evidence also suggests that osteocytes are a target for estrogen action. Estrogen withdrawal associated with GnRH therapy induces apoptosis of osteocytes in iliac bone [102]. Furthermore, estrogen treatment inhibits osteocyte apoptosis induced by pro-apoptotic stimuli [54]. Because osteocytes are involved in mechanosensing and transducing loading responses [78], these effects of estrogen deficiency could potentially impair the skeletal response to loading. Our group (unpublished data) and others [65] have shown that treatment of postmenopausal women with estrogen decreases serum sclerostin levels, the effects of which on bone density need to be explored further. Ongoing studies are examining the effect of antisclerostin antibodies on bone density. Estrogen also may regulate progenitor cell differentiation along the osteoblast rather than toward the adipocyte lineage. Using primary mouse bone marrow cells, Dang et al. [21] showed that estradiol stimulates the differentiation of these progenitor cells into osteoblasts and concurrently inhibited adipocyte formation. Estradiol also stimulates the mRNA expression of the osteoblast differentiation "master gene," Runx2 through ER alpha receptor and may play a key role in osteoblast differentiation [48].

To summarize, in either primary or secondary sex steroid deficiency, loss of transcriptional effects of estrogen may be responsible for the increased osteoclastogenesis and osteoblastogenesis and an increased rate of bone remodeling. Conversely, loss of nongenotropic antiapoptotic effects on mature osteoblasts and osteocytes and an opposite effect on the life span of mature osteoclasts may create an imbalance between bone formation and resorption and lead to a progressive loss of bone mass and strength.

Therefore, prolonged hypoestrogenism in young women, whether primary or secondary, is associated with an increased risk for osteopenia and osteoporosis [64]. We will discuss the effects of primary gonadal failure resulting in hypoestrogenemia and its effects on bone density here along with discussion of the two common causes of secondary gonadal failure, namely, hypothalamic amenorrhea (HA) and anorexia nervosa (AN). The risk for osteopenia and osteoporosis and fracture risk is approximately three times higher for individuals with anorexia nervosa or gonadal dysgenesis than it is in healthy young women [6]. Six months' amenorrhea caused by hypoestrogenism is regarded as an indication for bone densitometry examination [32]. The discussion of menopause-related hypogonadism is beyond the scope of this chapter and will not be discussed in detail here.

3.8 Defining Hypogonadism

Hypogonadism in males refers to the failure of the testes to produce adequate testosterone and/or normal spermatogenesis or in females, the failure of the ovaries to produce estrogen. This chapter will primarily focus on testosterone and estrogen deficiency and not on infertility. Hypogonadism is considered primary when there is failure of hormone production from the testes or ovaries in response to pituitary gonadotropins, LH and FSH. When hypogonadism is attributed to failure of stimulation from the hypothalamus (lack of or decreased GnRH) or the pituitary (FSH, LH), then it is deemed secondary. Many secondary disorders are common to both men and women and can include pituitary defects such as adenomas or craniopharyngiomas, autoimmune hypophysitis, hyperprolactinemia, infarction, trauma, and infiltrative diseases such as hemochromatosis or sarcoidosis. See Table 3.1 for major causes of primary and secondary causes of hypogonadism in men and women.

3.8.1 Primary Male Hypogonadism

In young men, genetic defects can cause primary hypogonadism including Klinefelter syndrome (KS) and cryptorchidism or undescended testes, a common congenital anomaly of the male genitourinary tract. A discussion of KS follows below. Other possible etiologies of primary testicular failure include acquired disorders such as orchitis, testicular torsion, orchidectomy from various diseases such a prostate or testicular cancers (if bilateral surgery) and testicular trauma due to surgery, radiation, or chemotherapy. History and physical examination are often the most accurate way to diagnose the etiology of acquired primary hypogonadism, especially when coupled with laboratory evaluation including serum testosterone, FSH, and LH levels for confirmation. Androgen replacement therapy in these disorders should follow guidelines described below.

3.8.2 Klinefelter Syndrome

KS is a chromosomal abnormality found in males, with a usual karyotype 47, XXY a result of meiotic nondisjunction of sex chromosomes during gametogenesis. Mosaic 46, XY/47, XXY forms account for 10% of the population of this disease and result from abnormal mitosis in the zygote. Other karyotypes with larger numbers of X

Table 3.1 Primary vs. secondary hypogonadism in men and women

Men	Women
Primary testicular failure (hypergonadotropic hypogonadism)	*Primary ovarian failure (hypergonadotropic hypogonadism)*
I. Genetic or congenital defects	I. Genetic or congenital defects
(a) Klinefelter syndrome or other seminiferous tubular dysgenesis variants	(a) Chromosomal (gonadal dysgenesis) Turner syndrome
(b) Biosynthetic defects (male pseudohermaphroditism, 17 α-hydroxylase deficiency)	(b) Single-gene disorders
(c) LH resistance	
(d) Cryptorchidism or anorchia	
(e) Testicular biosynthetic defects	
II. Acquired	II. Acquired
(a) Orchitis	(a) Infectious
(b) Testicular torsion or trauma	(b) Autoimmune
(c) Chemotherapeutic agents	(c) Premature menopause
(d) Radiation or surgery	(d) Iatrogenic
	(e) Environmental
Secondary testicular failure (Hypogonadotropic hypogonadism)	*Secondary ovarian failure (hypogonadotropic hypogonadism)*
I. Congenital	I. Congenital
(a) Kallmann syndrome	(a) Idiopathic hypogonadotropic hypogonadism (IHH)
(b) Genetic defects of the gonadotropin subunits	(b) Kallmann syndrome
(c) Obesity-associated	
Laurence-Moon-Biedl-Bardet syndrome	
Prader-Willi syndrome	
(d) Associated with other pituitary hormone deficiencies	
II. Acquired	II. Acquired
(a) Tumors including craniopharyngiomas	(a) Hypothalamic amenorrhea ("functional")
(b) Autoimmune hypophysitis	(b) Eating disorders
(c) Infiltrative diseases (hemochromatosis)	(c) Excessive exercise
(d) Infarction	(d) Stress or trauma
(e) Medications(e.g., opiates, anabolic steroids)	
(f) Chronic medical illness	
(g) Radiation, trauma, surgery	
(h) Obesity	
(i) Chronic medical illness	
(j) Destructive processes tumor	
(k) Radiation	
(l) Infection	
(m) Infiltrative disease	

chromosomes exist but are rare. KS is not uncommon and occurs in from 1/600 to 1/1,000 live births. Upward of 70% of KS cases, however, go undiagnosed; furthermore only 10% of cases are diagnosed before puberty [2, 10]. The most common symptom leading to diagnosis is infertility. Occasionally the syndrome is discovered based on a set of clinical findings: small testes, androgen deficiency, narrow shoulders, broad hips, increased height, sparse hair, gynecomastia, and low verbal intelligence. Recently a form of the syndrome was described with the phenotype of central obesity, glucose intolerance, and dysfunctional lipid metabolism [2, 10].

3.8.3 Bone Health in KS

Numerous studies have demonstrated a decrease in bone mineral density (BMD) in individuals with KS [10]. Bojesen et al. demonstrated that individuals with KS had a relative risk of 2.40 (95% CI 1.98–2.91) for musculoskeletal disease [11]. Swerdlow et al. demonstrated an increase in death from fractures, such as femoral fracture, in individuals with KS [100]. Decreased BMD has been found in 25–48% of men with KS, and 6–15% of this population has been found to develop osteoporosis [13, 14, 27].

The pathophysiology of the bone disease component of KS is not well understood. The remodeling defect of bone in KS is thought to be due to both reduced bone formation and increased bone resorption [27]. Initially it seemed that hypogonadism leading to reduced androgen levels was the source of this defect. This hypothesis was supported by evidence that KS individuals have normal BMD until they reach puberty. Furthermore, endogenous testosterone levels appear to correlate with BMD. Testosterone deficiency during puberty is a critical factor in low bone mass in KS. Loss of cancellous bone, decreased osteoblastic activity, decreased apposition rate, and decreased osteoid seam width all have been found in hypogonadal KS individuals [27]. A number of recent studies, however, appear to challenge the simplistic view that all the bone pathology of KS is due solely to hypogonadism. Seo et al. [92] found that KS individuals with normal testosterone levels still had reduced BMD. While some studies demonstrated the ability of testosterone therapy to produce normal BMD if given before the age of 20 [56], a number of other studies have shown an inability of testosterone therapy to improve BMD [27]. A recent study by Bojesen et al. demonstrated that KS individuals who were receiving hormone replacement, compared with those who had/were not, had no difference in markers of bone metabolism [10].

Several reasons have been put forth to explain this seeming failure of testosterone to correct bone health in KS patients. A number of authors suggest that current testosterone replacement regimens are insufficient, as noted by the often continued elevation in LH despite treatment [10, 27]. Bojesen et al. suggest that muscle strength is a more direct determinant of BMD and bone health in this population [10]. With low testosterone, KS individuals have reduced muscle strength, which leads to less stress on bones and thus less bone growth. When given testosterone, KS individuals may need to engage in resistance exercise to build muscle strength and thus improve bone health indirectly.

Other recent studies suggest that sex hormones are not the only hormones that influence bone health in individuals with KS. Zitzmann et al. [108] described a nonrandom inactivation of X chromosomes in men with multiple X chromosomes; those X chromosomes with androgen receptors that had fewer CAG repeats were more likely to be inactivated. This inactivation selects androgen receptors that are less functional, which may lead to a different clinical outcome and response to androgen replacement or to a decreased bone mass even when androgen levels are normal [28].

Another hormone that may influence bone health in KS individuals is insulin-like factor 3(INSL3). This hormone is produced pre- and postnatally by differentiated Leydig cells and likely reflects the differentiation status of Leydig cells [27]. Levels of INSL3 follow those of serum testosterone and have been shown in KS to abnormally level off in puberty in a manner similar to testosterone. Receptors for INSL3 have been demonstrated on osteoblasts; thus, ISL3 may impair osteoblast function and thus explain why testosterone replacement alone does not totally reverse the diminished bone health of patients with KS.

3.8.4 Treatment of KS

Testosterone replacement in KS or primary testicular failure from other etiologies will generally depend on the age of diagnosis. If the diagnosis is made in childhood, treatment is recommended at the prepubertal stage in young men and adolescents. Testosterone replacement is started at low doses and gradually increased with the development of secondary sexual characteristics. Generally this is achieved by intramuscular testosterone administration but may also be accomplished with transdermal testosterone, which may have a benefit of mimicking a more physiologic and pharmacokinetic profile. Therapy is generally lifelong beginning at puberty to ensure secondary sexual characteristics development, normal sexual function and maintenance of normal muscle, bone and red blood cell count. However, the optimal testosterone regimen for patients with KS remains to be established. Human chorionic gonadotropin or HCG injections also can be used and will promote growth of testes, but may also give rise to gynecomastia. This therapy also may have the benefit of improving sufficient sperm counts to achieve fertility and conception. Pulsatile GnRH stimulation via subcutaneous pump administration every 2 h is optimal for testicular growth and achievement of sperm counts adequate for fertility [79]; however, it is currently not approved by the FDA for treatment of infertility and only available at specialized research centers.

3.8.5 Treatment for Bone Health

As with any patient at higher risk for osteoporosis, treatment of bone health in KS starts with encouraging calcium and vitamin D supplementation. Calcium intake should be set at about 1,200 mg/day. Vitamin D should be given to maintain 25-hydroxy vitamin D levels in the serum at or slightly above 30 ng/mL. Furthermore, weight-bearing exercise should be encouraged. Muscle strengthening or resistance training is important, as individuals with KS often have less muscle strength, which may by extension lead to less bone accrual. Thus, resistance training and low-impact exercise are preferable [27].

DEXA scans are recommended every 2–5 years after diagnosis. In patients with low testosterone and low BMD, testosterone supplementation is recommended as described above. Some physicians recommend that testosterone should be supplemented until LH is in the mid-normal range; however, optimal dosing and levels are not well established and may depend on which end points are being considered. In patients with normal testosterone level but low BMD, bisphosphonates can be given as primary therapy [27]. Studies on bisphosphonate early usage in KS individuals to improve BMD have not yielded conclusive results [99]. While providing promising new information about the pathophysiology of KS, no therapies for androgen insensitivity or INSL3 deficiency are currently in use.

3.8.6 Primary Hypogonadism in Women

Primary gonadal failure in women, also known as primary ovarian insufficiency (POI), may be severe, associated with absent pubertal development and primary amenorrhea, or may have post-pubertal onset characterized by disappearance of menstrual cycles (secondary amenorrhea) associated with defective folliculogenesis. POI is generally characterized by low levels of gonadal hormones (estrogens and inhibins) and high levels of gonadotropins (LH and FSH) (hypergonadotropic amenorrhea). POI affects approximately 1 in 10,000 women by age 20; 1 in 1,000 women by age 30; 1 in 100 women by age 40 [19]. Most common inherited causes seen in younger women include Turner syndrome (gonadal dysgenesis), a relatively common disorder, discussed in detail below. Turner syndrome may cause primary or secondary amenorrhea. Other genetic conditions associated with anomalies of the X chromosome also may be associated with POI.

3.8.7 Turner Syndrome

Turner syndrome is a disease of women in which one of the X chromosomes is affected. Approximately 50% of individuals with Turner syndrome have a 45X karyotype, 20% have a 45X/46XX mosaicism, and the remainder have structural abnormalities of the X chromosome. The prevalence of Turner syndrome is significant as it is the most common sex chromosome abnormality in female conceptions and affects ~1 in 2,500 live female births [2].

3.8.8 Bone Health

Skeletal abnormalities have been noted in Turner syndrome since its initial description in 1938 [1]. Early observational studies showed hypomineralization on radiograms. Furthermore, physical characteristics of Turner syndrome such as scoliosis, genu valgum, Madelung deformity, a high arched palate, and short stature all suggest abnormalities in skeletal function. In fact, the most common abnormality of Turner syndrome is not gonadal dysgenesis, but rather growth failure and short statue [87].

Beyond physical abnormalities, the structural integrity of the skeletal system in Turner syndrome patients is compromised. A number of epidemiological studies have demonstrated an increased risk of fractures in these patients. Gravholt et al., in a retrospective analysis of the Danish Cytogenetic Central Register and Danish National Registry, found a 2.16 relative risk at 10 years (95% CI: 1.5–3.0) of fracture in women with Turner syndrome vs. normal karyotype females. This study was, however, performed prior to the widespread use of hormone replacement therapy (HRT) to improve bone health in patients with Turner syndrome [6, 33].

Other smaller studies have suggested a much more modest increase in fracture risk. Bakalov et al. found a nonsignificant increase in fracture rate in women with Turner syndrome vs. those with a normal karyotype [7]. Ross et al. found a significant increase in forearm fractures in women with Turner syndrome [85]. Furthermore, Landin-Wilhelmsen et al. found a significant increase in fractures in women with Turner syndrome, with a particular increase in fractures after the age of 45 [57]. A recent review by Bakalov and Bondy indicated that there was a small increase risk of fracture in patients with Turner syndrome, particularly in the forearm region [6].

3.8.9 Sex Hormone Deficiency

Initial focus on bone disease in Turner syndrome was on the lack of sex hormones due to gonadal dysgenesis. Low estrogen levels are common in individuals with Turner syndrome as their ovaries fail at an early age, often before menarche [68, 86]. As estrogen is essential for proper bone mineralization, the assumption was that low estrogen levels in these individuals contributed to osteopenia, osteoporosis, and other skeletal pathologies. Furthermore, recent evidence has suggested that estrogen has an anabolic effect on bone. Therefore decreased estrogen in adolescence could contribute to these individuals' short stature and delayed bone formation and may impact peak bone mass [22, 58]. The skeletal abnormalities common to Turner syndrome patients were, therefore, thought not to be intrinsic to the disorder, but rather secondary to estrogen deficiency [22].

As a result of these investigations and theories, early HRT in patients with Turner syndrome was recommended. Such treatment brought significant results. A study by G. Khastgir et al. [49] demonstrated that treatment with subcutaneous estrogen leads to increased bone mineralization. Over 3 years, subcutaneous estrogen implants in 21 women aged 20–40 with Turner syndrome increased the DXA T-score of the lumbar spine and femur from −1.4 and −1.1 to −0.2 and −0.4, respectively. Furthermore, BMD was normalized in 19 women, and bone biopsy showed an increase in trabecular bone density.

HRT also has been demonstrated to be essential in preventing the development of osteoporosis in women with Turner syndrome. Hanton et al. [37] performed a comparative study of 50 women, 34 of whom had received and continued HRT (with at least 75% adherence to therapy) and 16 who had not. Of those in the HRT nonadherent group, 38% met criteria for osteoporosis and 19% had lumber compression fractures; however, 0% of the HRT adherent individuals had either condition [37].

3.8.10 DEXA Scans in Turner Syndrome Patients

Some studies have suggested that even with HRT, Turner syndrome individuals still have low BMD [58]. A possible explanation for this finding is that DEXA scans underestimate BMD in individuals with short stature [34]. DEXA measures areal bone density; thus, the larger bones of larger individuals project more density on the surface measured than seen in the smaller bones of smaller individuals. This is particularly true of individuals less than 150 cm in height, a condition quite common in individuals with Turner syndrome.

Physicians can take steps to ensure the proper analysis of BMD in Turner syndrome patients. First quantitative computer-assisted tomography (QCT) can be utilized to measure volumetric bone density, which is independent of bone size. Unfortunately QCT is expensive, involves more radiation, and has not been scientifically validated to predict fractures. Another option is converting DEXA scans into volumetric measures of bone density such as bone mineral apparent density and/or width-adjusted BMD. In pediatric patients, it is often necessary to determine DEXA scan Z-scores based on height-adjusted age or bone age, instead of calendar age [6].

3.8.11 SHOX Gene Haploid Insufficiency

While clearly an important component of the bone disease found in individuals with Turner syndrome, estrogen deficiency does not completely explain the observed bone pathology. For one, despite estrogen replacement therapy, individuals with Turner syndrome continue to have short stature. Also, estrogen deficiency does not explain the congenital structural skeletal abnormalities seen with Turner syndrome. Studies also have shown disproportionality in the skeletal size of different skeletal regions of individuals with Turner syndrome [34]. Finally, HRT does not completely reverse the fracture risk in Turner syndrome patients. Gravholt et al. demonstrated through a questionnaire issued to women in Denmark with Turner syndrome that even with 70% of Turner syndrome subjects adherent to HRT, the relative risk of fractures was 1.35 (95% CI 1.04–1.75). While this relative risk was reduced from the previous Gravholt study, it does not appear that HRT eliminates the fracture risk in Turner syndrome individuals [33].

Some studies have found increased fracture rates in Turner syndrome individuals, despite relatively normal BMD [85]. Other studies have found no difference in the BMD of those Turner syndrome individuals with fractures and those without [7]. This observation further suggests that estrogen deficiency alone is not the cause of diminished bone health in Turner syndrome individuals because BMD, the factor estrogen corrects or stabilizes, does not appear to be the only factor involved in the increased risk of fractures.

Further supporting a process of diminished bone health other than estrogen deficiency, Zuckerman-Levin et al. found that Turner syndrome individuals often had normal DEXA BMD, but also had low speed of sound on quantitative ultrasound measurement of the tibia and radius. These results suggested a defect in cortical bone, and not in the trabecular bone that estrogen is known to target [110]. Bechtold et al. supported this finding, as they used OCT to demonstrate decreased cortical bone thickness at the radial metaphysic and diaphysis. Furthermore, Bakalov et al. used dual x-ray absorptiometry to demonstrate decreased cortical BMD independent of hormone deficiency [9].

Therefore, another process, other than sex hormone deficiency, appears to be affecting bone health in individuals with Turner syndrome. The likely cause is haploinsufficiency of the SHOX gene. The SHOX gene is located in the p11.2–p22.1 region of the X chromosome [107]. This region is missing in almost all karyotypes consistent with Turner syndrome [6]. The lack of both copies of the gene leads to a decrease in homeobox regulatory protein, translating to improper chondrocyte development in the growth plates. The lack of SHOX gene is common in other genetic syndromes, such as Leri-Weill dyschondrosteosis (LWD). A comparison of individuals with LWD to individuals with Turner syndrome shows that both populations have very similar skeletal abnormalities [84]. It thus appears likely that some of the skeletal abnormalities and diminished bone health seen in Turner syndrome are the results of haploinsufficiency of the SHOX gene of the X chromosome.

3.8.12 Treatment

Maintaining bone health is an essential aspect of the treatment of Turner syndrome. As the syndrome is congenital, measures to ensure the best possible bone health should be initiated at a very young age. To start, calcium supplementation of 1,200–1,500 mg/day and age-appropriate vitamin D are recommended for all individuals with Turner syndrome. As muscle tone is helpful in maintaining bone density, low-impact and weight-bearing exercise is recommended to begin at a young age. If possible, exercises should focus on the long bones and hips – that is, exercises such as walking with weights [6].

Early HRT is essential to prevent osteoporosis. To prevent growth-plate fusion and ensure maximum height, starting therapy at about 14 years of age is often recommended. Most oral contraceptives contain enough estrogen for young adults. A full adult dose would be 100 mcg transdermal patch, 2 mg oral estradiol, or 1.25 mg conjugated estrogen [6]. Education about the need for continued HRT beyond puberty for bone health is essential to ensure adherence to the treatment plan [37]. HRT should be tapered to be discontinued in an age-appropriate manner in the late 30s to early 40s – that is, similar to the time of menopause.

A bone density scan should be performed at the time an individual with Turner syndrome is transitioned to adult care. The results of such scans must be read in the context of the height of the individual as described above. If the scan is normal, it does not need to be repeated until the patient is 40–45 years old. If the patient has further risk factors for osteoporosis, scans may need to be repeated more frequently, particularly once the patient has reached the age of 45. An abnormal scan may indicate the need to start bisphosphonates or change HRT regimens.

Currently there is no known effective treatment to increase the thickness of cortical bone in individuals with Turner syndrome [6]. An alternative therapy is growth hormone replacement. While such therapy has been shown to increase the final height of affected individuals, there is little evidence that the growth hormone replacement has any effect on bone health [4, 5]. Furthermore, a recent randomized clinical trial of 14 patients with Turner syndrome assessed the use of androgen replacement therapy (oral testosterone) for 1 year to improve the morbidity associated with Turner syndrome. The study found an increase in BMD, but further longitudinal prospective studies need to be performed to assess the effectiveness of androgen replacement [109].

3.9 Secondary Hypogonadism in Men and Women

Hypothalamic and pituitary disorders may result in secondary gonadal failure in men and women and are associated with low levels of sex steroids and inappropriately low levels of FSH and LH. These can be congenital or acquired, hypothalamic or pituitary, or may be related to radiation, chronic medical and inflammatory disorders, anorexia, obesity (male), opiates, and illicit use of anabolic steroids. Head trauma or encephalitis also can contribute to gonadotropin deficiency. In women, secondary hypogonadism resulting in amenorrhea also may be caused by constitutional delay of adolescence, organic illness, vigorous exercise (e.g., ballet dancing, running), stressful life events, dieting, or anorexia nervosa; however, these conditions should not be assumed to account for amenorrhea without a full physical and endocrinologic evaluation. Hypothalamic and pituitary etiologies for secondary hypogonadism include genetic deficiency of GnRH and/or gonadotropins, which may be isolated or associated with other pituitary deficiencies or diminished olfaction as in Kallmann syndrome. The approach to idiopathic hypogonadotropic hypogonadism (IHH) including the congenital disorder, Kallmann syndrome, will be discussed in further detail.

3.9.1 Hypogonadotropic Hypogonadism: Kallmann Syndrome in Men and Women

Hypogonadotropic hypogonadism (HH) refers to a group of disorders, which may be congenital or acquired, in which low sex hormone levels are associated with low levels of gonadotropins (FSH, LH). Failure of the episodic GnRH secretion or action or disruption of the axis results in the clinical syndrome of HH. Congenital abnormalities are rare but well described and can occur in an isolated manner (IHH) and more recently also called isolated GnRH deficiency (IGD). When they occur with anosmia (inability to detect odors), the condition is known as Kallmann syndrome. IGD is caused by impaired gonadotropin release in the setting of otherwise normal anterior pituitary anatomy and function and in the absence of secondary causes of HH. Mutations have been described in the GnRH receptor as well as in both LH-β and FSH-β subunits. IHH is a rare disorder with an estimated occurrence between 1/10,000 and 1/86,000 individuals. Isolated GnRH deficiency occurs more commonly in men than in women in a ratio of 4:1.

Acquired causes of HH are not uncommon and are due to underlying conditions that affect the hypothalamic-pituitary axis. The clinical features of HH typically first appear at puberty. Normally, a marked increase in the GnRH pulse generator occurs and is required for the initiation of puberty and the normal reproductive axis in humans. The phenotypic presentation of HH varies with age of onset (congenital vs. acquired), duration (functional vs. permanent), and severity (complete vs. partial). The presentation is one of lack of development of secondary sexual characteristics, tall stature with eunuchoid body habitus, delayed bone age and prepubertal sized testes, and mild anemia. The diagnosis of IHH or Kallmann syndrome can also be made in infant boys who present with micropenis and cryptorchidism. At puberty, most individuals with IGD have abnormal sexual maturation, usually with incomplete development of secondary sexual characteristics. However, the degree to which sexual maturation is impaired can vary. Less frequently, the diagnosis is made in adult males who demonstrate incomplete sexual maturation and secondary sexual characteristics on physical exam as they have prepubertal testicular volume of less than 4 mL, absence of facial and axillary hair growth, and absence of voice deepening. In addition, they may have muscle mass decrease, low bone density, and erectile dysfunction with decreased libido and infertility. Affected adult females can have primary amenorrhea or lack of breast development. Rates of linear growth are normal; however, absence of pubertal growth spurt is typical. Anosmia is present and individuals may or may not be aware of it. Other findings can include unilateral renal agenesis, sensory neural hearing loss, cleft lip or palate, agenesis of teeth, brachydactyly, syndactyly, synkinesia of the digits, and agenesis of the corpus callosum. In individuals with IHH with a normal sense of smell, about two-thirds of cases are sporadic and one-third are inherited [76]. Cases can be either autosomal dominant or autosomal recessive. Discussion of detailed genetics of these disorders is complex and beyond the scope of this chapter.

In order to meet the diagnostic criteria, an isolated defect in GnRH secretion is evidenced by (1) complete or partial absence of GnRH-induced LH pulsations; (2) normalization of pituitary-gonadal axis function in response to physiological regimens of exogenous GnRH replacement; (3) otherwise normal hormonal testing of the anterior pituitary including a normal ferritin level; and (4) normal hypothalamic-pituitary region as demonstrated by imaging.

3.9.2 Treatment of IHH or HH

Treatment options for the hypogonadism of IGD include sex steroids, gonadotropins, and pulsatile GnRH administration. Choice of therapy is determined by the goal(s) of treatment, that is, to induce and maintain secondary sex characteristics and/or to restore fertility or maintain bone health. A baseline bone density should be obtained. Clearly that potential for low bone density in individuals with IHH or HH is evident. Factors to consider include timing of puberty, duration of hypogonadism, and whether other osteoporotic risk factors coexist. In a study of 11 congenital hypogonadal men, bone density values were obtained to assess the effects of testosterone replacement on skeletal integrity [44]. In this small study, 11 men were compared to 10 healthy young men who served as controls. The population of IHH consisted of men receiving intramuscular testosterone enanthate 250 mg every 4 weeks for a mean duration of 21 years (7–43 years). The authors measured distal BMD at the radius by peripheral quantitative computerized tomography (QCT). The researchers found significantly lower bone density in the patient group than in the healthy men at the whole radial bone density as well as the trabecular bone density. In addition, the authors found that whole radial bone density correlated negatively with the patient's age at the initiation of the testosterone, such that the later the age of replacement, the lower the BMD. The patient group had significant osteopenia, which persisted long after testosterone replacement. It should be noted that this study was limited by its small number of subjects and cross-sectional design.

In another study, a retrospective analysis, stature and bone age before and during androgen replacement, was evaluated in 25 men with isolated IHH. Before initiation of androgen therapy, stature was lower for chronological age but normal for bone age in this group of 25 men. Bone mass was within normal limits of published controls either before initiation or after androgen treatment. However, BMD was below the 50th percentile of controls prior to androgen treatment and only increased slightly during treatment. These authors concluded that deficiency of androgen prior to puberty may cause permanent defects in bone density, which may not be adequately corrected by androgen replacement if instituted after this critical window [103].

In women, initial treatment for congenital IGD should consist of unopposed estrogen replacement via one of several modes of treatment to allow optimal breast development. After a period of approximately 6 months, when breast development has been optimized, a progestin should be added for endometrial protection. Many formulations of estrogens and progestins are available, and these can be given in either cyclical or continuous fashion. Preference of the individual plays an important role in choosing the right treatment plan, although low estrogen formulations should be considered in individuals with clotting abnormalities. Pulsatile GnRH stimulation is also an approved therapy for folliculogenesis in women with IGD. Intravenous administration of GnRH at various frequencies throughout the menstrual cycle closely mimics normal cycle dynamics with the resulting ovulation of a single follicle [89]. This therapy offers a clear advantage over the traditional treatment with exogenous gonadotropins, which involves higher rates of both multiple gestation and ovarian hyperstimulation syndrome. For either approach, however, the rate of conception is approximately 30% per ovulatory cycle [62]. Specific treatment for decreased bone mass should be considered depending on the degree of bone mineralization.

There are few studies evaluating the effect of IHH on bone health in women, although HH has been evaluated extensively in women in the context of functional hypothalamic amenorrhea (HA) seen in the "female athlete triad," which results from the interaction among energy availability, menstrual function, and bone metabolism that may lead to amenorrhea and osteopenia or osteoporosis. Functional HA has been described as a reversible form of GnRH deficiency commonly triggered by stressors such as excessive exercise, nutritional deficits, or psychological distress that result in the absence of menses, low or normal gonadotropin levels, and hypoestrogenemia without organic abnormality [81]. HA is associated with a spectrum of abnormal GnRH-secretion patterns, and administration of exogenous pulsatile GnRH can restore functionality of the hypothalamic-pituitary-gonadal axis [89]. Caronia et al. have reported on an increased incidence of the rare variants of genes associated with idiopathic hypogonadotropic hypogonadism in women with HA, suggesting that these mutations may contribute to the variable susceptibility of women to the functional changes in GnRH secretion that characterize HA [16].

Typically, high-impact weight-bearing exercise is associated with a 5–15% higher BMD in athletes compared to nonathletes [29]. Weight-bearing activity optimizes mineral accrual in the bone in the premenarchal years and in adolescent girls [80]. In a study examining the prevalence of female athlete triad among high school girls, Nichols et al. [70] found that eumenorrheic high school athletes participating in high-/odd-impact loading sports had consistently higher hip BMD values compared to eumenorrheic athletes participating in low/repetitive-impact sports. In addition, higher spine BMD was recorded in eumenorrheic high/odd-impact athletes compared to oligo/amenorrheic repetitive/nonimpact athletes [69]. The type of impact loading seems to affect BMD at the hip contrary to gonadal steroids that influence mostly spine BMD. Lumbar spine is considered estrogen sensitive and is more severely affected in the presence of amenorrhea [17]. In another 4-year prospective study, Sowińska-Przepiera et al. evaluated the effects of 4-year estrogen progestin therapy (EP) on the BMD of 16–17-year-old girls with functional HA in 78 women and found a progressive increase in BMD with the treatment, although it still remained below the control group after 4 years [97].

Functional HA with estrogen deficiency also has been described in the setting of anorexia nervosa (AN). AN is associated with bone loss during adulthood, but also may delay skeletal growth and mineral accrual during growth related to estrogen deficiency, malnutrition, and low body weight. In a study comparing bone densities in HA women with amenorrhea and women with AN, Grinspoon et al. found that the bone densities were significantly lower in women with AN suggesting that the estrogen status and lean body mass both were determinants of BMD [36]. In a study evaluating bone density in women with AN, Seeman et al. [91] evaluated the effect of estrogen containing oral contraceptives (OCPs) and exercise in women with AN, and found that OCPs had a positive effect on spine bone density while exercise helped with the hip bone density although the BMD stayed below the control group. Karlsson et al. [47] compared vertebral and femoral neck BMC in untreated women with AN and compared them to women on estrogen containing OCP and women who had recovered from AN. They found that vertebral and femoral neck BMC and volumetric BMD were lower in untreated women and very similar in HRT-treated women and in recovered women after adjusting for changes in body composition. These findings led them to conclude that a substantial proportion of the deficit in bone mass in women with AN relative to controls is due to their smaller bone size; that HRT is associated with higher volumetric BMD (vBMD) and bone size relative to untreated women; recovery from illness is associated with a near-normal bone size and vBMD; and that incomplete recovery of lean and fat mass may account for part of the remaining deficits in bone size, not vBMD. In a study evaluating women with AN and functional HA to healthy controls, Lawson et al. [59] described normal-weight women with HA as an intermediate phenotype between healthy menstruating women and those with AN in terms of severity of bone loss, hypercortisolemia, and mood disturbances. They evaluated the cortisol levels in this group and its relationship to bone loss and found that cortisol levels negatively correlated with BMD. Similarly, Grinspoon et al. [36] showed in a study of 49 amenorrheic women (30 with AN and 19 with HA) matched for age of menarche and duration of amenorrhea, and 30 healthy controls, T-scores at the AP spine and hip were lower in HA compared with healthy controls and lowest in those with AN.

3.10 Measurement of Testosterone

The most optimal methodology for measurement of testosterone is not clearly agreed upon by experts in endocrine disorders. Testosterone circulates bound to plasma proteins including sex hormone–binding globulin (SHBG) and to albumin. Free testosterone, which is unbound, is often the component considered to have most access to body cells. Additionally, bioavailable testosterone, defined as the concentration of testosterone that is free or unbound *plus* that which is bound to albumin to which it is weakly bound, can be measured in some laboratories. Bioavailable testosterone may be the best assay to determine the most accurate amount of testosterone available to the tissues; however, variations in assay methodology make it difficult to compare among laboratories. Bioavailable testosterone has been reported to correlate well with free testosterone by equilibrium dialysis. Recently, the Endocrine Society released their position statement regarding measurement of testosterone, as many nonstandardized methodologies in use have made for difficulties in this field [83]. The key findings are that although current methodologies often are unsatisfactory, establishing a clinical standard should be sought. In the interim, the recommendations are to know the type of quality of assay that is being used in the clinical laboratory of choice, as well as the reference intervals that are used. When screening for hypogonadism, the serum total testosterone should be obtained on more than one morning sample. If hypogonadism treatment is required, then most clinicians will follow the measurement of testosterone that is available in one's local clinical laboratory.

3.11 Obesity and Hypogonadism in Older Men

Obesity is defined as a body mass index (BMI) of >30 kg/m^2, and low testosterone levels commonly occur in the same individuals [106]. Low SHBG with low total testosterone levels with normal free testosterone levels is commonly seen; thus, these men are not truly hypogonadal. However, as obesity increases, free or bioavailable testosterone decreases as well, and FSH and LH remain inappropriately normal, resulting in secondary hypogonadism.

Testosterone treatment can prevent bone loss in men who are hypogonadal even in those who are of older age [8]. However, studies of testosterone replacement in older men with low or low normal levels have yielded conflicting results, and there are no studies to date regarding testosterone benefits on fracture risk reduction. MrOS, Osteoporotic Fractures in Men Study, a longitudinal cohort study of older men, showed that only 12% of osteoporotic men are below the testosterone threshold of 200 ng/dL where it is believed that replacement therapy is indicated. This may potentially explain why testosterone concentrations do not have significant effects on skeletal outcomes, although results should be interpreted with caution. Androgens also can impact muscle maintenance; therefore, testosterone therapy in older men may be beneficial for muscle strength, and this can indirectly affect the risk of fracture and falls independent of bone density. In fact, the MrOS study did report that men with lower bioavailable testosterone levels had a higher incidence of falls [72]. A recent study [71] suggests that testosterone therapy in frail older men with low levels demonstrated an increased lean body mass and muscle strength; however, the effect does not last after discontinuation of hormone therapy.

The role of SHBG has been elucidated somewhat more recently. A number of recent studies show that SHBG is inversely and independently related to bone density, although it is unclear to what extent the association of SHBG with male skeletal health outcomes including osteoporotic fractures can be explained by the decreasing bioavailability of sex steroids with aging. Thus, the MrOS study has suggested that free estradiol and sex hormone–binding globulin (SHGB), but not free testosterone, were similarly associated with fracture risk [60]. This also has been reported in other studies. Thus, SHGB appears to have a bone mass effect in older men, but further research is needed to clarify its exact role.

Conclusion

The discussion in this chapter focused on the role of gonadal steroids in early bone development through the later stages of the life cycle. Further studies are needed to better define the exact role of androgens and estrogens in men and women, respectively, as recent evidence suggests the complexity of these relationships and their influence on bone health in both the male and female skeleton.

References

1. Classic pages in obstetrics and gynecology by Henry H. Turner. A syndrome of infantilism, congenital webbed neck, and cubitus valgus. Endocrinology. 1938;23: 566–74. Am J Obstet Gynecol 113: 279, 1972.

2. Achermann JC, Jameson J. Disorders of sex development. In: Fauci AS, Braunwald E, Kasper DL, Kauser SL, Longo DL, Jameson JL, Loscalzo J, editors. Harrison's principles of internal medicine. New York: McGraw-Hill; 2008. Access medicine.
3. Ammann P, Rizzoli R, Bonjour JP, Bourrin S, Meyer JM, Vassalli P, Garcia I. Transgenic mice expressing soluble tumor necrosis factor-receptor are protected against bone loss caused by estrogen deficiency. J Clin Invest. 1997;99:1699–703.
4. Amundson E, Boman UW, Barrenas ML, Bryman I, Landin-Wilhelmsen K. Impact of growth hormone therapy on quality of life in adults with turner syndrome. J Clin Endocrinol Metab. 2010;95:1355–9.
5. Andrade AC, Baron J, Manolagas SC, Shaw NJ, Rappold GA, Donaldson MD, Gault EJ, Savendahl L. Hormones and genes of importance in bone physiology and their influence on bone mineralization and growth in Turner syndrome. Horm Res Paediatr. 2010;73:161–5.
6. Bakalov VK, Bondy CA. Fracture risk and bone mineral density in Turner syndrome. Rev Endocr Metab Disord. 2008;9:145–51.
7. Bakalov VK, Chen ML, Baron J, Hanton LB, Reynolds JC, Stratakis CA, Axelrod LE, Bondy CA. Bone mineral density and fractures in Turner syndrome. Am J Med. 2003;115:259–64.
8. Bassil N. Late-onset hypogonadism. Med Clin North Am. 2011;95:507–23.
9. Bechtold S, Rauch F, Noelle V, Donhauser S, Neu CM, Schoenau E, Schwarz HP. Musculoskeletal analyses of the forearm in young women with Turner syndrome: a study using peripheral quantitative computed tomography. J Clin Endocrinol Metab. 2001;86: 5819–23.
10. Bojesen A, Birkebaek N, Kristensen K, Heickendorff L, Mosekilde L, Christiansen JS, Gravholt CH. Bone mineral density in Klinefelter syndrome is reduced and primarily determined by muscle strength and resorptive markers, but not directly by testosterone. Osteoporos Int. 2011;22(5):1441–50.
11. Bojesen A, Juul S, Birkebaek NH, Gravholt CH. Morbidity in Klinefelter syndrome: a Danish register study based on hospital discharge diagnoses. J Clin Endocrinol Metab. 2006;91:1254–60.
12. Borjesson AE, Lagerquist MK, Liu C, Shao R, Windahl SH, Karlsson C, Sjogren K, Moverare-Skrtic S, Antal MC, Krust A, Mohan S, Chambon P, Savendahl L, Ohlsson C. The role of estrogen receptor alpha in growth plate cartilage for longitudinal bone growth. J Bone Miner Res. 2010;25:2690–700.
13. Breuil V, Euller-Ziegler L. Gonadal dysgenesis and bone metabolism. Joint Bone Spine. 2001;68:26–33.
14. Callewaert F, Venken K, Ophoff J, De Gendt K, Torcasio A, van Lenthe GH, Van Oosterwyck H, Boonen S, Bouillon R, Verhoeven G, Vanderschueren D. Differential regulation of bone and body composition in male mice with combined inactivation of androgen and estrogen receptor-alpha. FASEB J. 2009;23:232–40.
15. Carani C, Qin K, Simoni M, Faustini-Fustini M, Serpente S, Boyd J, Korach KS, Simpson ER. Effect of testosterone and estradiol in a man with aromatase deficiency. N Engl J Med. 1997;337:91–5.
16. Caronia LM, Martin C, Welt CK, Sykiotis GP, Quinton R, Thambundit A, Avbelj M, Dhruvakumar S, Plummer L, Hughes VA, Seminara SB, Boepple PA, Sidis Y, Crowley Jr WF, Martin KA, Hall JE, Pitteloud N. A genetic basis for functional hypothalamic amenorrhea. N Engl J Med. 2011;364:215–25.
17. Christo K, Prabhakaran R, Lamparello B, Cord J, Miller KK, Goldstein MA, Gupta N, Herzog DB, Klibanski A, Misra M. Bone metabolism in adolescent athletes with amenorrhea, athletes with eumenorrhea, and control subjects. Pediatrics. 2008;121:1127–36.
18. Clarke BL, Khosla S. Female reproductive system and bone. Arch Biochem Biophys. 2010;503:118–28.
19. Coulam CB, Adamson SC, Annegers JF. Incidence of premature ovarian failure. Obstet Gynecol. 1986;67: 604–6.
20. Couse JF, Korach KS. Estrogen receptor null mice: what have we learned and where will they lead us? Endocr Rev. 1999;20:358–417.
21. Dang ZC, van Bezooijen RL, Karperien M, Papapoulos SE, Lowik CW. Exposure of KS483 cells to estrogen enhances osteogenesis and inhibits adipogenesis. J Bone Miner Res. 2002;17:394–405.
22. Davies MC, Gulekli B, Jacobs HS. Osteoporosis in Turner's syndrome and other forms of primary amenorrhoea. Clin Endocrinol (Oxf). 1995;43:741–6.
23. Bremner WJ, Matsumoto AM, Sussman AM, Paulsen CA. Follicle stimulating hormone and spermatogenesis. J Clin Invest. 1981;68:1044–1052.
24. DiVasta AD, Gordon CM. Bone health in adolescents. Adolesc Med Clin. 2006;17:639–52; abstract xi.
25. Dufau ML, Catt KJ. Gonadotropin receptors and regulation of steroidogenesis in the testis and ovary. Vitam Horm. 1978;36:461–592.
26. Eghbali-Fatourechi G, Khosla S, Sanyal A, Boyle WJ, Lacey DL, Riggs BL. Role of RANK ligand in mediating increased bone resorption in early postmenopausal women. J Clin Invest. 2003;111:1221–30.
27. Ferlin A, Schipilliti M, Di Mambro A, Vinanzi C, Foresta C. Osteoporosis in Klinefelter's syndrome. Mol Hum Reprod. 2010;16:402–10.
28. Ferlin A, Schipilliti M, Foresta C. Bone density and risk of osteoporosis in Klinefelter syndrome. Acta Paediatr. 2011;100:878–84.
29. Ferretti JL, Cointry GR, Capozza RF, Frost HM. Bone mass, bone strength, muscle-bone interactions, osteopenias and osteoporoses. Mech Ageing Dev. 2003;124:269–79.
30. Gibson JH, Mitchell A, Harries MG, Reeve J. Nutritional and exercise-related determinants of bone density in elite female runners. Osteoporos Int. 2004;15:611–8.
31. Girasole G, Jilka RL, Passeri G, Boswell S, Boder G, Williams DC, Manolagas SC. 17 beta-estradiol inhibits interleukin-6 production by bone marrow-derived stromal cells and osteoblasts in vitro: a potential

mechanism for the antiosteoporotic effect of estrogens. J Clin Invest. 1992;89:883–91.
32. Gordon CM. Bone density issues in the adolescent gynecology patient. J Pediatr Adolesc Gynecol. 2000;13:157–61.
33. Gravholt CH, Juul S, Naeraa RW, Hansen J. Morbidity in Turner syndrome. J Clin Epidemiol. 1998;51: 147–58.
34. Gravholt CH, Lauridsen AL, Brixen K, Mosekilde L, Heickendorff L, Christiansen JS. Marked disproportionality in bone size and mineral, and distinct abnormalities in bone markers and calcitropic hormones in adult turner syndrome: a cross-sectional study. J Clin Endocrinol Metab. 2002;87:2798–808.
35. Andersson AM. Inhibin B in the assessment of seminiferous tubular function. Baillieres Best Pract Res Clin Endocrinol Metab. 2000;14:389 /contents/evaluation-of-male-infertility/abstract/78.
36. Grinspoon S, Miller K, Coyle C, Krempin J, Armstrong C, Pitts S, Herzog D, Klibanski A. Severity of osteopenia in estrogen-deficient women with anorexia nervosa and hypothalamic amenorrhea. J Clin Endocrinol Metab. 1999;84:2049–55.
37. Hanton L, Axelrod L, Bakalov V, Bondy CA. The importance of estrogen replacement in young women with Turner syndrome. J Womens Health (Larchmt). 2003;12:971–7.
38. Hayes FJ, DeCruz S, Seminara SB, Boepple PA, Crowley Jr WF. Differential regulation of gonadotropin secretion by testosterone in the human male: absence of a negative feedback effect of testosterone on follicle-stimulating hormone secretion. J Clin Endocrinol Metab. 2001;86:53–8.
39. Ho AY, Kung AW. Determinants of peak bone mineral density and bone area in young women. J Bone Miner Metab. 2005;23:470–5.
40. Hofbauer LC, Khosla S, Dunstan CR, Lacey DL, Spelsberg TC, Riggs BL. Estrogen stimulates gene expression and protein production of osteoprotegerin in human osteoblastic cells. Endocrinology. 1999;140: 4367–70.
41. Huber DM, Bendixen AC, Pathrose P, Srivastava S, Dienger KM, Shevde NK, Pike JW. Androgens suppress osteoclast formation induced by RANKL and macrophage-colony stimulating factor. Endocrinology. 2001;142:3800–8.
42. Hughes DE, Dai A, Tiffee JC, Li HH, Mundy GR, Boyce BF. Estrogen promotes apoptosis of murine osteoclasts mediated by TGF-beta. Nat Med. 1996;2: 1132–6.
43. Imai Y, Youn MY, Kondoh S, Nakamura T, Kouzmenko A, Matsumoto T, Takada I, Takaoka K, Kato S. Estrogens maintain bone mass by regulating expression of genes controlling function and life span in mature osteoclasts. Ann N Y Acad Sci. 2009; 1173 Suppl 1:E31–9.
44. Ishizaka K, Suzuki M, Kageyama Y, Kihara K, Yoshida K. Bone mineral density in hypogonadal men remains low after long-term testosterone replacement. Asian J Androl. 2002;4:117–21.
45. Jilka RL, Hangoc G, Girasole G, Passeri G, Williams DC, Abrams JS, Boyce B, Broxmeyer H, Manolagas SC. Increased osteoclast development after estrogen loss: mediation by interleukin-6. Science. 1992; 257:88–91.
46. Johnston Jr CC, Slemenda CW. Determinants of peak bone mass. Osteoporos Int. 1993;3 Suppl 1:54–5.
47. Karlsson MK, Weigall SJ, Duan Y, Seeman E. Bone size and volumetric density in women with anorexia nervosa receiving estrogen replacement therapy and in women recovered from anorexia nervosa. J Clin Endocrinol Metab. 2000;85:3177–82.
48. Khalid O, Baniwal SK, Purcell DJ, Leclerc N, Gabet Y, Stallcup MR, Coetzee GA, Frenkel B. Modulation of Runx2 activity by estrogen receptor-alpha: implications for osteoporosis and breast cancer. Endocrinology. 2008;149:5984–95.
49. Khastgir G, Studd JW, Fox SW, Jones J, Alaghband-Zadeh J, Chow JW. A longitudinal study of the effect of subcutaneous estrogen replacement on bone in young women with Turner's syndrome. J Bone Miner Res. 2003;18:925–32.
50. Khosla S. Estrogen and bone: insights from estrogen-resistant, aromatase-deficient, and normal men. Bone. 2008;43:414–7.
51. Kimble RB, Srivastava S, Ross FP, Matayoshi A, Pacifici R. Estrogen deficiency increases the ability of stromal cells to support murine osteoclastogenesis via an interleukin-1and tumor necrosis factor-mediated stimulation of macrophage colony-stimulating factor production. J Biol Chem. 1996;271:28890–7.
52. Kimble RB, Vannice JL, Bloedow DC, Thompson RC, Hopfer W, Kung VT, Brownfield C, Pacifici R. Interleukin-1 receptor antagonist decreases bone loss and bone resorption in ovariectomized rats. J Clin Invest. 1994;93:1959–67.
53. Kitazawa R, Kimble RB, Vannice JL, Kung VT, Pacifici R. Interleukin-1 receptor antagonist and tumor necrosis factor binding protein decrease osteoclast formation and bone resorption in ovariectomized mice. J Clin Invest. 1994;94:2397–406.
54. Kousteni S, Bellido T, Plotkin LI, O'Brien CA, Bodenner DL, Han L, Han K, DiGregorio GB, Katzenellenbogen JA, Katzenellenbogen BS, Roberson PK, Weinstein RS, Jilka RL, Manolagas SC. Nongenotropic, sex-nonspecific signaling through the estrogen or androgen receptors: dissociation from transcriptional activity. Cell. 2001;104:719–30.
55. Kousteni S, Han L, Chen JR, Almeida M, Plotkin LI, Bellido T, Manolagas SC. Kinase-mediated regulation of common transcription factors accounts for the bone-protective effects of sex steroids. J Clin Invest. 2003;111:1651–64.
56. Kubler A, Schulz G, Cordes U, Beyer J, Krause U. The influence of testosterone substitution on bone mineral density in patients with Klinefelter's syndrome. Exp Clin Endocrinol. 1992;100:129–32.
57. Landin-Wilhelmsen K, Bryman I, Windh M, Wilhelmsen L. Osteoporosis and fractures in Turner syndrome-importance of growth promoting and

oestrogen therapy. Clin Endocrinol (Oxf). 1999;51: 497–502.
58. Lanes R, Gunczler P, Esaa S, Martinis R, Villaroel O, Weisinger JR. Decreased bone mass despite long-term estrogen replacement therapy in young women with Turner's syndrome and previously normal bone density. Fertil Steril. 1999;72:896–9.
59. Lawson EA, Donoho D, Miller KK, Misra M, Meenaghan E, Lydecker J, Wexler T, Herzog DB, Klibanski A. Hypercortisolemia is associated with severity of bone loss and depression in hypothalamic amenorrhea and anorexia nervosa. J Clin Endocrinol Metab. 2009;94:4710–6.
60. LeBlanc ES, Nielson CM, Marshall LM, Lapidus JA, Barrett-Connor E, Ensrud KE, Hoffman AR, Laughlin G, Ohlsson C, Orwoll ES. The effects of serum testosterone, estradiol, and sex hormone binding globulin levels on fracture risk in older men. J Clin Endocrinol Metab. 2009;94:3337–46.
61. Manolagas SC, Jilka RL. Bone marrow, cytokines, and bone remodeling. Emerging insights into the pathophysiology of osteoporosis. N Engl J Med. 1995;332:305–11.
62. Martin K, Santoro N, Hall J, Filicori M, Wierman M, Crowley Jr WF. Clinical review 15: management of ovulatory disorders with pulsatile gonadotropin-releasing hormone. J Clin Endocrinol Metab. 1990;71:1081A–G.
63. Migliaccio S, Newbold RR, Bullock BC, Jefferson WJ, Sutton Jr FG, McLachlan JA, Korach KS. Alterations of maternal estrogen levels during gestation affect the skeleton of female offspring. Endocrinology. 1996;137:2118–25.
64. Mircea CN, Lujan ME, Pierson RA. Metabolic fuel and clinical implications for female reproduction. J Obstet Gynaecol Can. 2007;29:887–902.
65. Modder UI, Clowes JA, Hoey K, Peterson JM, McCready L, Oursler MJ, Riggs BL, Khosla S. Regulation of circulating sclerostin levels by sex steroids in women and in men. J Bone Miner Res. 2011;26:27–34.
66. Molina P. Chapter9: Female reproductive system. In: Molina PE, editor. Endocrine physiology. 3rd ed. New York: McGraw-Hill; 2009.
67. Morishima A, Grumbach MM, Simpson ER, Fisher C, Qin K. Aromatase deficiency in male and female siblings caused by a novel mutation and the physiological role of estrogens. J Clin Endocrinol Metab. 1995;80:3689–98.
68. Neely EK, Marcus R, Rosenfeld RG, Bachrach LK. Turner syndrome adolescents receiving growth hormone are not osteopenic. J Clin Endocrinol Metab. 1993;76:861–6.
69. Nichols JF, Rauh MJ, Barrack MT, Barkai HS. Bone mineral density in female high school athletes: interactions of menstrual function and type of mechanical loading. Bone. 2007;41:371–7.
70. Nichols JF, Rauh MJ, Lawson MJ, Ji M, Barkai HS. Prevalence of the female athlete triad syndrome among high school athletes. Arch Pediatr Adolesc Med. 2006;160:137–42.
71. O'Connell MD, Roberts SA, Srinivas-Shankar U, Tajar A, Connolly MJ, Adams JE, Oldham JA, Wu FC. Do the effects of testosterone on muscle strength, physical function, body composition, and quality of life persist six months after treatment in intermediate-frail and frail elderly men? J Clin Endocrinol Metab. 2011;96:454–8.
72. Orwoll E, Lambert LC, Marshall LM, Blank J, Barrett-Connor E, Cauley J, Ensrud K, Cummings SR. Endogenous testosterone levels, physical performance, and fall risk in older men. Arch Intern Med. 2006;166:2124–31.
73. Oursler MJ, Cortese C, Keeting P, Anderson MA, Bonde SK, Riggs BL, Spelsberg TC. Modulation of transforming growth factor-beta production in normal human osteoblast-like cells by 17 beta-estradiol and parathyroid hormone. Endocrinology. 1991;129: 3313–20.
74. Oursler MJ, Pederson L, Fitzpatrick L, Riggs BL, Spelsberg T. Human giant cell tumors of the bone (osteoclastomas) are estrogen target cells. Proc Natl Acad Sci USA. 1994;91:5227–31.
75. Pacifici R, Brown C, Puscheck E, Friedrich E, Slatopolsky E, Maggio D, McCracken R, Avioli LV. Effect of surgical menopause and estrogen replacement on cytokine release from human blood mononuclear cells. Proc Natl Acad Sci USA. 1991;88:5134–8.
76. Pallais JC, Au M, Au M, Seminara S, Crowley Jr WF. Kallmann syndrome. Seattle: University of Washington; 2007.
77. Pederson L, Kremer M, Judd J, Pascoe D, Spelsberg TC, Riggs BL, Oursler MJ. Androgens regulate bone resorption activity of isolated osteoclasts in vitro. Proc Natl Acad Sci USA. 1999;96:505–10.
78. Pitsillides AA, Rawlinson SC, Suswillo RF, Bourrin S, Zaman G, Lanyon LE. Mechanical strain-induced NO production by bone cells: a possible role in adaptive bone (re)modeling? FASEB J. 1995;9:1614–22.
79. Pitteloud N, Hayes FJ, Dwyer A, Boepple PA, Lee H, Crowley Jr WF. Predictors of outcome of long-term GnRH therapy in men with idiopathic hypogonadotropic hypogonadism. J Clin Endocrinol Metab. 2002; 87:4128–36.
80. Rautava E, Lehtonen-Veromaa M, Kautiainen H, Kajander S, Heinonen OJ, Viikari J, Mottonen T. The reduction of physical activity reflects on the bone mass among young females: a follow-up study of 142 adolescent girls. Osteoporos Int. 2007;18:915–22.
81. Reindollar RH, Novak M, Tho SP, McDonough PG. Adult-onset amenorrhea: a study of 262 patients. Am J Obstet Gynecol. 1986;155:531–43.
82. Rigotti NA, Neer RM, Skates SJ, Herzog DB, Nussbaum SR. The clinical course of osteoporosis in anorexia nervosa. A longitudinal study of cortical bone mass. JAMA. 1991;265:1133–8.
83. Rosner W, Auchus RJ, Azziz R, Sluss PM, Raff H. Position statement: utility, limitations, and pitfalls in measuring testosterone: an endocrine society position statement. J Clin Endocrinol Metab. 2007;92: 405–13.

84. Ross JL, Kowal K, Quigley CA, Blum WF, Cutler Jr GB, Crowe B, Hovanes K, Elder FF, Zinn AR. The phenotype of short stature homeobox gene (SHOX) deficiency in childhood: contrasting children with Leri-Weill dyschondrosteosis and Turner syndrome. J Pediatr. 2005;147:499–507.
85. Ross JL, Long LM, Feuillan P, Cassorla F, Cutler Jr GB. Normal bone density of the wrist and spine and increased wrist fractures in girls with Turner's syndrome. J Clin Endocrinol Metab. 1991;73:355–9.
86. Ross JL, Long LM, Loriaux DL, Cutler Jr GB. Growth hormone secretory dynamics in Turner syndrome. J Pediatr. 1985;106:202–6.
87. Saenger P. Turner's syndrome. N Engl J Med. 1996;335:1749–54.
88. Santen RJ. Is aromatization of testosterone to estradiol required for inhibition of luteinizing hormone secretion in men? J Clin Invest. 1975;56:1555–63.
89. Santoro N, Filicori M, Crowley Jr WF. Hypogonadotropic disorders in men and women: diagnosis and therapy with pulsatile gonadotropin-releasing hormone. Endocr Rev. 1986;7:11–23.
90. Seeman E. Pathogenesis of bone fragility in women and men. Lancet. 2002;359:1841–50.
91. Seeman E, Szmukler GI, Formica C, Tsalamandris C, Mestrovic R. Osteoporosis in anorexia nervosa: the influence of peak bone density, bone loss, oral contraceptive use, and exercise. J Bone Miner Res. 1992;7:1467–74.
92. Seo JT, Lee JS, Oh TH, Joo KJ. The clinical significance of bone mineral density and testosterone levels in Korean men with non-mosaic Klinefelter's syndrome. BJU Int. 2007;99:141–6.
93. Shevde NK, Bendixen AC, Dienger KM, Pike JW. Estrogens suppress RANK ligand-induced osteoclast differentiation via a stromal cell independent mechanism involving c-Jun repression. Proc Natl Acad Sci USA. 2000;97:7829–34.
94. Simonet WS, Lacey DL, Dunstan CR, Kelley M, Chang MS, Luthy R, Nguyen HQ, Wooden S, Bennett L, Boone T, Shimamoto G, DeRose M, Elliott R, Colombero A, Tan HL, Trail G, Sullivan J, Davy E, Bucay N, Renshaw-Gegg L, Hughes TM, Hill D, Pattison W, Campbell P, Sander S, Van G, Tarpley J, Derby P, Lee R, Boyle WJ. Osteoprotegerin: a novel secreted protein involved in the regulation of bone density. Cell. 1997;89:309–19.
95. Smith EP, Boyd J, Frank GR, Takahashi H, Cohen RM, Specker B, Williams TC, Lubahn DB, Korach KS. Estrogen resistance caused by a mutation in the estrogen-receptor gene in a man. N Engl J Med. 1994;331:1056–61.
96. Sowers MF. Lower peak bone mass and its decline. Baillieres Best Pract Res Clin Endocrinol Metab. 2000;14:317–29.
97. Sowinska-Przepiera E, Chelstowski K, Friebe Z, Syrenicz A. Bone mineral density in girls with functional hypothalamic amenorrhea subjected to estroprogestagen treatment – a 4-year prospective study. Gynecol Endocrinol. 2011;27(11):966–70.
98. Srivastava S, Toraldo G, Weitzmann MN, Cenci S, Ross FP, Pacifici R. Estrogen decreases osteoclast formation by down-regulating receptor activator of NF-kappa B ligand (RANKL)-induced JNK activation. J Biol Chem. 2001;276:8836–40.
99. Stepan JJ, Burckhardt P, Hana V. The effects of three-month intravenous ibandronate on bone mineral density and bone remodeling in Klinefelter's syndrome: the influence of vitamin D deficiency and hormonal status. Bone. 2003;33:589–96.
100. Swerdlow AJ, Higgins CD, Schoemaker MJ, Wright AF, Jacobs PA. Mortality in patients with Klinefelter syndrome in Britain: a cohort study. J Clin Endocrinol Metab. 2005;90:6516–22.
101. Tanaka S, Takahashi N, Udagawa N, Tamura T, Akatsu T, Stanley ER, Kurokawa T, Suda T. Macrophage colony-stimulating factor is indispensable for both proliferation and differentiation of osteoclast progenitors. J Clin Invest. 1993;91:257–63.
102. Tomkinson A, Reeve J, Shaw RW, Noble BS. The death of osteocytes via apoptosis accompanies estrogen withdrawal in human bone. J Clin Endocrinol Metab. 1997;82:3128–35.
103. Van der Werff ten Bosch JJ, Bot A. Some skeletal dimensions of males with isolated gonadotrophin deficiency. Neth J Med. 1992;41:259–63.
104. Wahlstrom T, Huhtaniemi I, Hovatta O, Seppala M. Localization of luteinizing hormone, follicle-stimulating hormone, prolactin, and their receptors in human and rat testis using immunohistochemistry and radioreceptor assay. J Clin Endocrinol Metab. 1983;57:825–30.
105. Warren MP, Brooks-Gunn J, Fox RP, Holderness CC, Hyle EP, Hamilton WG. Osteopenia in exercise-associated amenorrhea using ballet dancers as a model: a longitudinal study. J Clin Endocrinol Metab. 2002;87:3162–8.
106. Wu FC, Tajar A, Beynon JM, Pye SR, Silman AJ, Finn JD, O'Neill TW, Bartfai G, Casanueva FF, Forti G, Giwercman A, Han TS, Kula K, Lean ME, Pendleton N, Punab M, Boonen S, Vanderschueren D, Labrie F, Huhtaniemi IT. Identification of late-onset hypogonadism in middle-aged and elderly men. N Engl J Med. 2010;363:123–35.
107. Zinn AR, Tonk VS, Chen Z, Flejter WL, Gardner HA, Guerra R, Kushner H, Schwartz S, Sybert VP, Van Dyke DL, Ross JL. Evidence for a Turner syndrome locus or loci at Xp11.2-p22.1. Am J Hum Genet. 1998;63:1757–66.
108. Zitzmann M, Nieschlag E. The CAG repeat polymorphism within the androgen receptor gene and maleness. Int J Androl. 2003;26:76–83.
109. Zuckerman-Levin N, Frolova-Bishara T, Militianu D, Levin M, Aharon-Peretz J, Hochberg Z. Androgen replacement therapy in Turner syndrome: a pilot study. J Clin Endocrinol Metab. 2009;94:4820–7.
110. Zuckerman-Levin N, Yaniv I, Schwartz T, Guttmann H, Hochberg Z. Normal bone mineral density but frail cortical bone in Turner's syndrome. Clin Endocrinol (Oxf). 2007;67:60–4.

Thyroid and Thyroid Hormone: Normal Function, Diseases, Disorders, Emerging Therapeutics

4

Paula H. Stern

Keywords
Thyroid • Thyroid hormone • Thyroxin • Triiodothyronine • Deiodinase • Thyroid-stimulating hormone • Hypothyroidism • Hyperthyroidism

4.1 Introduction

Throughout life, thyroid hormones exert important effects on bone. From the fetal period on, thyroid hormones are critical to ensure normal growth and development of the skeleton. In the adult, thyroid hormones stimulate both anabolic and resorptive activity, with an age-dependent increase in resorption over formation. Both systemic and local environment factors influence how thyroid hormones affect the quantity and nature of bone responses. Finally, it is now recognized that thyroid hormones are a component of a tightly regulated feedback system that makes it difficult to determine the immediate cause of a given effect.

Thyroid hormones are synthesized and secreted via a feedback-regulated mechanism involving the hypothalamus and pituitary gland [113]. The thyroid hormones, thyroxin (T4) and triiodothyronine (T3), are biosynthesized in the thyroid gland from the amino acid tyrosine. The gland accumulates iodide through a sodium/iodide symporter located at the basolateral membrane of the thyroid follicular cells. Thyroperoxidase at the apical membrane of the gland cells oxidizes the iodide and catalyzes iodination of tyrosyl residues on the protein thyroglobulin. Coupling of the iodinated tyrosines by the peroxidase generates T3 and T4, and stimulation of the gland by thyroid-stimulating hormone (TSH) results in the hydrolysis of thyroglobulin and the release of T3 and T4. In the circulation, T3 and T4 are tightly bound to thyroxine-binding globulin, transthyretin, and albumin. Free T3 and T4 interact with receptors in the hypothalamus and pituitary gland. This suppresses secretion of thyrotropin-releasing hormone (TRH) and TSH. TRH production is also regulated by neuronal inputs from brain stem and hypothalamic arcuate and dorsomedial nuclei through leptin, neuropeptide Y, α-melanocyte-stimulating hormone, agouti-related peptide, and norepinephrine [47, 144]. TRH acts through G-protein-coupled transmembrane receptors of the Gαq family and a calcium signal transduction system that stimulates the synthesis and secretion of the glycoprotein TSH in the pituitary. The TSH receptor in the thyroid gland is a G-protein-coupled transmembrane receptor that couples primarily to Gαs and

P.H. Stern, Ph.D.
Department of Molecular Pharmacology and Biological Chemistry,
Northwestern University Feinberg School of Medicine,
303 E. Chicago Ave., Chicago, IL 60611, USA
e-mail: p-stern@northwestern.edu

F. Bronner et al. (eds.), *Bone-Metabolic Functions and Modulators*, Topics in Bone Biology,
DOI 10.1007/978-1-4471-2745-1_4, © Springer-Verlag London 2012

activates adenylate cyclase. Recent studies have found that TSH has direct effects on bone cells (see below).

4.2 Thyroid Hormone Uptake and Metabolism in Bone

Tissue uptake and thyroid hormone release are mediated by several transporters. The mRNAs for three transporters, L-type amino acid transporter 1 (LAT1), L-type amino acid transporter 2 (LAT2), and the monocarboxylate transporter 8 (MCT8), are expressed in MC3T3-E1 calvarial and femur-derived osteoblastic cells of fetal and postnatal mice [28]. LAT1 and LAT2 expressions do not change with cell differentiation, age, or thyroid hormone status. MCT8 expression, on the other hand, increases with differentiation of the MC3T3-E1 preosteoblastic cells and decreases in the course of days 4–35 of postnatal development. MCT8 is upregulated in hypothyroid mice and downregulated when the mice are treated with T3. Other studies have shown that MCT8 transcripts are present in chondrocytes, osteoblasts, and osteoclasts in both primary cells and cell lines, and are maintained in the cells as they differentiate [211]. The significance of skeletal MCT8 is yet to be established. MCT8 mutations in humans result in skeletal disorders; however, these may be secondary to neurologic impairment [88].

Much of the T3 in peripheral target tissues derives from the peripheral conversion of the weaker prohormone T4 by type 1 and type 2 5′-deiodinases, selenoenzymes that remove the iodine from the 5 position of the outer ring. A type 3 deiodinase inactivates both thyroid hormones by removing iodine from the inner ring. Recent studies have determined the functional significance and consequences of deletion of these deiodinases in skeletal tissue. Type 3 deiodinase is found in primary chondrocytes, osteoblasts, and osteoclasts [211]. Type 3 deiodinase expression during mouse fetal development negatively correlates with the sensitivity of the growth plate to thyroid hormone. This suggests that the enzyme is an important regulator of thyroid hormone signaling during development [29]. Type 2 5′-deiodinase mRNA increases during later stages of fetal development and later in postnatal life. Type 2 deiodinase is restricted to mature osteoblasts [211]. Type 2 deiodinase knockout mice have normal serum levels of T3, but their bones are brittle and highly susceptible to fracture, with signs of excessive mineralization [15]. In these mice, bone formation is decreased, but resorption and microarchitecture are normal. It has been proposed that type 2 deiodinase acts as a local regulator to maintain thyroid hormone function in osteoblasts [15]. Patients with a Thr92Ala polymorphism in type 2 deiodinase have an enzyme with a lower V_{max}. Their femoral neck BMD is decreased and their bone turnover is elevated, independent of serum thyroid hormone levels. This indicates the importance of local type 2 deiodinase in normal bone physiology [78].

4.3 Mechanism of Thyroid Hormone Action in Bone

The action of thyroid hormones is mediated largely through nuclear receptors that interact with the thyroid response element (TRE) on target genes (Fig. 4.1), although there is also evidence of other mechanisms. In the absence of thyroid hormone, nuclear receptors repress gene transcription. Under these conditions, the receptor interacts with a corepressor complex that includes a nuclear receptor corepressor NCoR, the silencing mediator for retinoic acid receptor (SMRT), the repressor Sin3, and histone deacetylases [195, 216]. The repressor complex undergoes dissociation when T3 binds to the receptor. This allows the receptor to associate with one of several coactivator complexes. One of these, the HAT coactivator complex, involves the steroid receptor coactivator (SRC), CREB-binding protein (CBP), p300 protein, and a p300/CBP-associated factor (PCAF) that confers histone acetyltransferase activity [131, 195]. Another coactivator complex, the vitamin D receptor interacting protein/TR-associated protein (DRIP/TRAP) complex, recruits and stabilizes the RNA polymerase [25, 86, 158, 181]. Activation of

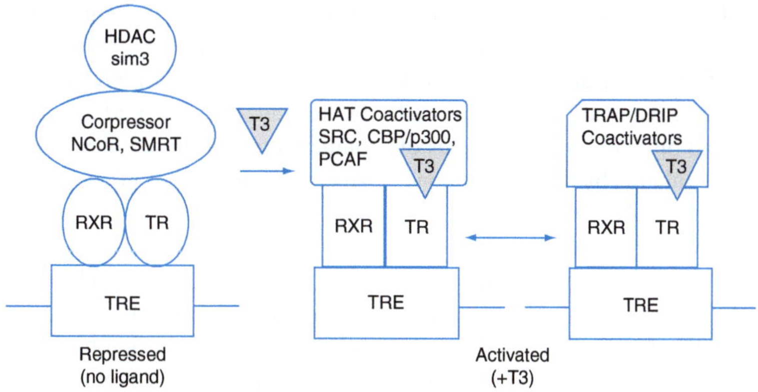

Fig. 4.1 Thyroid hormone receptor complexes in the absence (no ligand) and presence (+ T3) of thyroid hormone. *HDAC* histone deacetylase, *NCoR* nuclear receptor corepressor, *SMRT* silencing mediator for retinoic acid receptor, *RXR* retinoid X receptor, *TR* thyroid hormone receptor, *TRE* thyroid response element, *HAT* histone acetyltransferase, *SRC* steroid receptor coactivator, *CBP* CREB-binding protein, *PCAF* p300/CBP-associated factor, *DRIP/TRAP* vitamin D receptor interacting protein/TR-associated protein

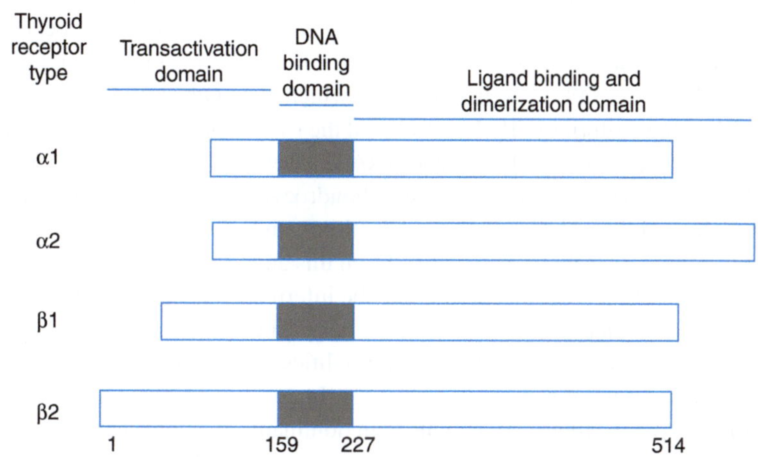

Fig. 4.2 Thyroid hormone receptors

various genes can require differential recruitment of coactivators and histone acetylation [120].

Thyroid hormone receptors are members of the steroid receptor superfamily and have a carboxy-terminal ligand binding domain that binds to the coactivators or corepressors and a centrally located zinc finger DNA-binding domain [44]. The DNA-binding sites for thyroid hormone receptors on target genes include monomeric, palindromic, inverted repeat, and direct repeat response elements, derived from a common AGGT(C/A)A motif. Thyroid hormone receptors bind to DNA in multiple forms, including monomers, homodimers, and heterodimers between isoforms of thyroid hormone receptors and heterodimers with retinoid and vitamin D receptors. DNA binding and transcriptional activation are enhanced when the thyroid receptor isoforms interact as heterodimers with the retinoid or vitamin D receptors [23, 62, 212, 213].

Several thyroid hormone receptors have been identified (Fig. 4.2). Thyroid receptor α (TRα) is encoded by a gene on chromosome 17. Four carboxy-terminal products are generated by alternative splicing [30, 87]. TRα1 is the commonly expressed active TRα isoform, whereas TRα2, which is homologous to the v-erb A oncogene, is a nonbinding isoform that may act as a dominant negative repressor [101, 169]. There are also two truncated isoforms that have dominant negative activity [18]. Thyroid receptor β (TRβ) is encoded by a gene on chromosome 3. TRβ1 and the amino-terminal splice variant TRβ2 are both active. TRβ2, however, is most highly expressed in hypothalamus and pituitary [115], the sites of negative feedback regulation by thyroid hormone. In various studies, mRNAs for TRα1, TRα2, and TRβ1 and TRβ2 have been found in osteoblasts, osteoblast cell lines, chondrocytes, and osteoclastic cells [2, 3, 10, 212]. Transcripts encoding TRα1, TRα2, and TRαβ1 are expressed in vivo [2, 135, 150], particularly at bone-modeling sites. TRα1 mRNA levels are 12-fold higher than TRβ1 mRNA levels in tibia and femurs of 7-week-old male mice [150]. In contrast to the findings regarding mRNA expression, TRα1 protein is limited to osteoblasts at sites of remodeling and to undifferentiated chondrocytes [3].

TR-deficient mouse strains have revealed the importance of the various isoforms [16, 17, 49, 59, 64, 90, 91, 148, 150]. In a model in which all of the TRα isoforms (TRα1, TRα2, and the truncated splice variants TRΔα1 and TRΔα2) were deleted, growth was retarded, and chondrocyte development, endochondral ossification, and mineralization were impaired [17]. From this and other models of TRα deletion, it may be inferred that TRα mediates the effects of T3 on bone. The knockout animals do not have abnormalities in circulating thyroid hormones or in TSH. In contrast, TRβ knockouts and animals with dominant negative mutations designed to mimic the mutations found in syndromes of resistance to thyroid hormone exhibit enhanced endochondral and intramembranous ossification and bone mineral deposition, and their cortical bone has increased thickness [17, 148, 150]. The animals are short because the growth plate matures early. The animals have elevated T3, T4, and TSH levels with a bone phenotype that is consistent with thyrotoxicosis. The findings support the inference that TRα is a principal receptor for thyroid hormone effects on bone, and that TRβ is the predominant regulator of hypothalamic and pituitary feedback regulation in response to thyroid hormone.

There is evidence for rapid nongenomic effects of thyroid hormones on bone. The integrin $\alpha_v\beta_3$ is a target for thyroid hormone action [173]. A neutralizing antibody to $\alpha_v\beta_3$ inhibits the effects of 10-min treatment with T3 and T4 to activate ERK, a component of the MAP kinase pathway, and prevents the subsequent ERK-dependent stimulation by T3 and T4 on thymidine incorporation in the human osteoblastic cell lines MG-63 and SaOS-2. Another nongenomic effect of T3 in bone is the suppression of Src in primary mouse calvarial osteoblasts [12]. This rapid effect, seen within 5 min of treatment, leads to a later increase in osteocalcin expression, demonstrated by the attenuation of osteocalcin expression by constitutively active Src (Y527F). Treatment of fetal rat limb bones for 30 s with thyroid hormones stimulated prostaglandin-dependent production of inositol phosphates, an effect not produced by inactive analogues [109]. Nongenomic effects of T3 on inositol phosphate metabolism have been implicated in effects on mitochondrial oxidative phosphorylation and gating of the mitochondrial permeability transition pore in vivo and in cultured Jurkat cells [215]. Other nongenomic effects of thyroid hormones and their significance for the maintenance of steady-state cell function have been reviewed [32, 172]. Differences in tissue distribution of the receptor isoforms and the presence of nongenomic effects have suggested the possibility of generating selective thyroid hormone analogues that have the cholesterol-lowering properties of T3 without the deleterious effects on the cardiovascular system or bone. The TRβ-selective analogue GC-1 has greater effects on lipids and less on the heart [20]. GC-1 mimicked T3 in reducing serum TSH. GC-1 could offer an advantage over the naturally occurring thyroid hormones based on the finding that, in contrast with T3, it does not reduce bone mineral density in vertebrae and limb bones.

4.4 Thyroid Hormone Effects on Bone Tissues and Cells

4.4.1 Chondrocytes and the Growth Plate

Thyroid hormones inhibit chondrocyte proliferation and promote chondrocyte maturation, leading to a hypertrophic phenotype and endochondral mineralization. Treatment with thyroid hormones decreases expression of type II collagen and increases expression of alkaline phosphatase and type X collagen, a protein unique to hypertrophic chondrocytes [13, 21, 22, 26, 60, 85, 132, 145]. Chondrocytes express TRα and TRβ isoforms [114, 156]. The effects of T3 on chondrocytes isolated from mouse rib are mediated by the TRβ receptor isoform, but not by the TRα isoform [156]. Vascular endothelial cell factors act synergistically with thyroid hormones to promote the expression of type X collagen and alkaline phosphatase and the acquisition of the hypertrophic phenotype that leads to mineralization [21]. Work from several laboratories has produced a model of how thyroid hormones promote chondrocyte maturation, with bone morphogenetic protein 4 (BMP4) playing a central role [114]. In a chick sternum chondrocyte cell culture, T3 has been found to stimulate collagen X gene transcription, but with a time delay of 1 day. Thyroid hormone treatment of the chondrocytes results within 1 day in a progressive decrease in mRNA encoding the BMP4 inhibitor noggin and an increase in BMP4 mRNA levels. As noggin decreased and BMP4 increased, collagen X mRNA levels increased dramatically. Exogenous noggin prevented the effect of T3 on the collagen X promoter. A similar temporal pattern of noggin, BMP4, and collagen X occurs during normal development; Wnt signaling appears to be involved. BMPs increased Wnt8c in sternal chondrocytes [37], and Wnt and β-catenin stimulate gene expression of collagen X in the cells [38]. T3 increases Wnt4 expression and stabilizes β-catenin in rat growth plate chondrocytes [209]. Further studies implicate the induction of carboxypeptidase Z by thyroid hormone in the activation of and terminal differentiation of the chondrocytes [210]. Interactions with fibroblast growth factors (FGFs) also may be involved in the actions of thyroid hormones on the growth plate. The effects are complicated, and their significance has not yet been established. T3 enhances FGF2 expression and FGF18 activation of MAP kinase in chondrocytes but inhibits FGF activation of STAT-1 [14]. There is also evidence that thyroid hormones regulate hypertrophic chondrocyte differentiation at the growth plate through expression of parathyroid hormone-related peptide [187].

4.4.2 Osteoblasts and Bone Anabolic Factors

Thyroid hormones elicit anabolic effects on bone. T3 has variable effects on the proliferation of osteoblasts, influenced in complex ways by dose, duration of incubation, cell type, passage number, and degree of confluence. Stimulatory effects on proliferation have been reported in human and rodent osteoblasts [42, 84, 94, 151], but effects are inhibitory in murine MC3T3-E1 cells [93]. T3 has no significant effects on proliferation in rat ROS 25/1, UMR-106, and ROS 17/2.8 cultures [116, 171, 212]. In neonatal mouse calvaria, a dose-dependent effect of T3 on thymidine incorporation has been reported [95]. Prostaglandin production antagonizes this effect; this suggests that local production of the eicosanoid may be the factor that produces varying responses in other models.

Thyroid hormone promotes the differentiation of osteoblasts, stimulating osteoblast phenotypic markers. Thyroid hormones increase alkaline phosphatase in many osteoblast cell models [41, 42, 93, 94, 99, 171]. The effect is not seen in other models, possibly due to high basal levels of alkaline phosphatase in those cell lines [82, 116, 177]. Alkaline phosphatase expression is stimulated by thyroid hormones in isolated tibiae [188]. Osteocalcin expression is increased by T3 in some osteoblast models [162, 171], although T3 does not increase osteocalcin mRNA levels in bone marrow stromal-derived ST2 cells [204]. Also, the site from which cells are derived determines their response to T3. When cells derived from femoral bone marrow were cultured under conditions that lead to osteogenic differentiation, T3 prevented the time-dependent decrease in osteocalcin mRNA levels, whereas in similarly treated cultures from vertebral marrow, osteocalcin mRNA levels did not decline and the response was unaffected by T3 [135]. Site-dependent effects also have been observed in T3 effects on type I collagen [135]. T3 exerted stimulation in femoral bones, but not in vertebral bones [135]. T3 inhibited type I carboxy terminal propeptide production in cells from human trabecular bone explants [94]. Collagen and noncollagenous protein synthesis was inhibited when rat osteoblast-like cells were treated with T3 [42]. However, in MC3T3-E1 cells, T3 increased the mRNA expression of genes for two enzymes that are involved in posttranslational modification of collagen, and mRNA for the processing enzyme of the lysyl oxidase precursor and of procollagen [203]. In mouse calvaria precultured with indomethacin, collagen and noncollagenous protein synthesis was stimulated by T3. This again suggests that anabolic effects of T3 are antagonized by prostaglandin production [95]. A series of studies from a team of investigators in Vienna demonstrated other effects of T3 in MC3T3-E1 cells [54, 55, 121–123, 199, 201, 202, 204] and have shown that the treatment also increased c-fos, c-jun, osteoprotegerin (OPG), osteocalcin, and matrix metalloproteinase-13 (MMP-13). Osteocalcin attenuated the effect of T3 on MMP-13. T3 elicited marked changes in cytoskeletal proteins and in the cell structure.

The growth factors insulin-like growth factor-I (IGF-I) and FGF have been implicated in the bone anabolic effects of thyroid hormones. IGF-I mRNA was increased by T3 treatment in MC3T3-E1 cells [99, 200]. Thyroid hormones increased IGF-I in fetal rat bones, rat calvarial osteoblasts, and UMR-106 cells [99, 106, 177, 200]. In contrast to some of the other phenotypic effects described above, T3 had greater effects on IGF-I in vertebral marrow cultures than in femoral cultures [135]. IGF-I is likely to be a mediator of anabolic effects of thyroid hormones on bone. Antisense oligonucleotides, antibodies, and antagonist peptides to IGF-I decreased the stimulatory effects of T3 on alkaline phosphatase, osteocalcin, and collagen synthesis in primary mouse calvarial osteoblasts and MC3T3-E1 cells [82]. The IGF binding proteins IGFBP-2, IGFBP-3, and IGFBP-4 are increased by T3 in various osteoblast models [61, 177]. IGF binding proteins have complex physiological roles, and their importance in the anabolic effects of T3 is unclear. In bone, IGFBP-2 and IGFBP-4 can inhibit IGF-I actions [48, 138], and IGFBP-3 has both enhancing and inhibitory effects [43, 176, 178]. FGF receptor mRNA and protein were stimulated by T3, and TRα knockout mice had decreased expression of FGF receptor I [186]. A thyroid hormone response element was demonstrated in the fgfr1 gene [149]. Thyroid hormone effects on mineralization have been studied in calvarial cells in a bone nodule model [84]. The observed effects were biphasic, with lower concentrations promoting the stimulatory effect of dexamethasone on bone nodule formation and higher concentrations inhibiting bone nodule formation and attenuating the effect of dexamethasone.

4.4.3 Osteoclasts and Resorption

Thyroid hormones stimulate bone resorption in vivo and in organ culture [81, 96, 98, 103, 110, 141]. The responses to thyroid hormones are slower and maximum responses smaller than those elicited by parathyroid hormone [96, 98, 110, 141]. T3 stimulates the degradation of collagen in bone organ culture [74] and increases mRNA expression of collagenase-3 and gelatinase B in cultures of osteoblastic cells [155]. Addition of thyroid hormone to osteoclast precursor cells fails to stimulate their differentiation into mature osteoclasts [8], supporting the conclusion that the stimulation of resorption is indirectly mediated [8, 24]. There are both positive [136] and negative [170] findings as to whether thyroid hormone stimulate expression of receptor activator of NFκB ligand (RANKL) in osteoblastic cells. The findings suggest that thyroid hormones stimulate osteoclastogenesis by interacting with receptors in osteoblasts but that the effect is weak, possibly involving a mediators other than RANKL. Thyroid hormone effects on resorption in organ cultures are inhibited by immunosuppressive cyclosporines [110], interferon-β [98], and a neutralizing antibody to transforming growth factor β (TGFβ) [99]. Thyroid hormones increase expression of interleukin-6 in osteoblasts [183, 194], bone marrow stromal cells [97, 183], and organ culture models [192]. T3 promotes calcitriol-induced osteoclast formation through an interleukin-6 (IL-6)-dependent pathway [174].

In addition, T3 potentiates the bone-resorbing effects of interleukin-1 (IL-1) [192]. There is mutual upregulation of thyroid hormone and parathyroid hormone receptors in osteoblastic osteosarcoma cells [71]. Possibly, these types of interactions mediate and modulate the in vivo thyroid hormone stimulation of resorption. The absence of a potent effect of thyroid hormones in in vitro models is consistent with the variable effects of thyroid hormones on bone loss when the hormones are used therapeutically; see Sect. 4.6.3.

4.5 Skeletal Effects of Thyroid Hormone in Animal Studies

Animal studies have provided substantial information on the impact of the thyroid on the skeleton in both young and older animals. Findings in younger animals are consistent with cell studies that have shown that thyroid hormones promote differentiation of chondrocytes and osteoblasts. Treatment of neonatal rats with T3 has led to narrowing of the sagittal suture of the skull and increased mineral apposition rates at the osseous edges of the sutures [7]. This was accompanied by intense immunohistochemical staining for IGF-I along the suture margins, possibly reflecting the involvement of IGF-I. Age-dependent effects of thyroid hormone on bone growth have been demonstrated in hypophysectomized rats [63]. T4 restored bone growth without affecting weight in infant rats, but had no effect in older rats [63]. In transgenic mouse pups of the TG66-19 strain in which thyrocytes are decreased and T3 and T4 are undetectable, growth is markedly delayed [208]. Treatment of young rats with the thyroid hormone synthesis inhibitor methimazole for 7 weeks resulted in a marked increase in the trabecular bone volume of the subchondral spongiosa of the mandibular condyles [119]. IGF-I was present in the condyles from the control animals, but not in the condyles from the methimazole-treated. Studies in older animals provide further evidence of the in vivo bone-resorbing effects of thyroid hormones. A model using orthodontic procedures revealed that T3 treatment enhanced orthodontic tooth movement [182]. Thyroid and gonadal hormones interact in rats in their effects on bone. Ovariectomized rats are more sensitive to T4, with 12-week treatment causing greater bone turnover and lower bone density [214]. T4 also enhances the anabolic effects of estradiol in ovariectomized rats. Animals receiving both estradiol and T4 have greater bone mass and a higher mineral apposition rate than animals receiving only one hormone treatment [214]. In another study, bone turnover, evaluated by serum osteocalcin and urinary pyridinolines and the loss of bone mineral, was greater in ovariectomized rats when the animals were treated with T4 [218]. In ovariectomized thyroidectomized rats, estradiol prevented the decrease in bone mineral density elicited by T3 treatment, but had no effect without T3 [36]. This could suggest cross talk between the receptors at the target sites. Most of the studies demonstrating effects on resorption have utilized high doses of thyroid hormones. With lower doses, T4 administration to ovariectomized rats caused bone mineral density of both lumbar and vertebral bones to increase, as opposed to the bone mineral loss elicited by the higher doses [65]. Thyroid hormones have been reported to promote cortical bone healing around titanium implants [46]. A histomorphometric study that compared 12-week treatment with T4 or with propylthiouracil, to inhibit thyroid hormone synthesis, has shown that T4 increases bone mineral apposition and mineral deposition rates and causes bone surfaces to erode more. Bone volume was increased in the propylthiouracil-treated rats. This is consistent with thyroid hormone increasing bone remodeling [9]. In vivo studies have demonstrated differences in the sensitivity of bones at different sites, a difference also noted in in vitro studies (see above). In hyperthyroid animals, the femur, which has more cortical bone, is more sensitive to thyroid hormone–induced bone loss than the spine at which the bone is more trabecular [65, 152, 189, 190, 218].

4.6 Effects of Thyroid Hormones in Human Physiology and Pathophysiology

4.6.1 Hypothyroidism

Childhood hypothyroidism delays skeletal maturation, and dysgenesis occurs at the epiphyses. In children with congenital hypothyroidism treated with T4, serum T4 and bone age positively correlated with the treatment dose [80]. Individuals with resistance to T4 (RTH) have a characteristic short stature and exhibit delayed skeletal maturation and stippled epiphyses [159]. Bone turnover is decreased in hypothyroidism [140]. The decrease in bone resorption is also reflected in a reduction of urinary pyridinium cross-links [143]. Serum IGF-I is lower, again consistent with a role of IGF-I in thyroid hormone action [107].

4.6.2 Hyperthyroidism

In 1981, von Recklinghausen described the bone loss resulting from thyrotoxicosis [207]. Histomorphometric analyses showed increased osteoclast numbers and resorbing surfaces, with loss of trabecular bone volume [133, 140]. Bone turnover is increased, with elevation of pyridinoline and hydroxypyridinoline excretion, urinary N-terminal telopeptide of type I collagen (NTX), serum carboxy-terminal 1-telopeptide (ICTP), alkaline phosphatase, osteocalcin, and carboxy-terminal propeptide of type I procollagen (PICP) [6]. Although bone resorption and formation are both increased, formation and resorption are not in balance, with a disproportionately greater increase in resorption and net bone loss in each remodeling cycle. Bone mineral content is decreased, and the risk of fracture is increased. In healthy postmenopausal women having T3 and T4 in the high normal range, bone mineral density is reduced and the risk of vertebral fracture in increased [142]. Estrogen deficiency potentiates the effects of thyroid hormone and, when combined with mild hyperthyroidism, increases bone loss in postmenopausal women [108]. In children, the disease generally has different characteristics, with the anabolic effects of the hormone accelerating skeletal development and growth [166, 175]. Thyroid stimulation of IGF-I production may be greater in children than adults. This could explain why Graves disease or thyroid hormone treatment does not have the same deleterious skeletal effects in children as seen in adults [35, 102, 117, 196, 198, 205]. The receptor activator of NFκB ligand (RANKL) decoy receptor OPG is increased in patients with Graves disease [11, 137] and decreased by antithyroid treatment [137]. Amato et al. [11] have proposed that OPG production may constitute a mechanism to protect against excessive bone turnover due to thyroid hormone stimulation.

4.6.3 T4 Therapy

Patients who have undergone thyroidectomy or who have autoimmune thyroiditis are typically treated with replacement T4. T4 treatment is used for suppression in cases of toxic nodular goiter and thyroid cancer. Thyroid hormone therapy had no adverse effects in some studies [33, 51, 57, 67, 72, 75, 77, 100, 112, 127, 134, 146, 157, 160, 161, 167, 180, 193] but, in others, has led to accelerated bone turnover, decreased bone density, and increased risk of fracture [4, 5, 27, 31, 34, 40, 45, 56, 58, 66, 69, 73, 89, 118, 128, 130, 154, 165, 184, 191]. Dose and duration of treatment are probably the major determinants of the occurrence of bone loss [5, 27, 68, 126, 197]. However, a previous history of hyperthyroidism, increased age, menopausal status, and low dietary calcium also increase risk [5, 39, 50, 58, 66, 69, 89, 104, 105, 185]. The apparent lack of effects in some studies may be because the patients with hypothyroidism had higher bone density at the time of treatment, and that the normal bone density may reflect a loss [164]. It also has been postulated that the bone loss could be transient, and the point at which the study was carried out could affect the conclusions [31, 147, 206]. Following cessation of suppressive therapy, there is variability in the recovery of bone, although younger individuals appear to recover more readily [53, 166].

The bone loss due to thyroid hormone treatment is responsive to estrogen, estrogen/progestin, androgen, and bisphosphonates [52, 111, 124, 125, 163, 179] alone or in conjunction with antithyroid therapy. Long-term suppressive therapy with high doses of T4 was reported to decrease the effectiveness of alendronate treatment for postmenopausal osteoporosis [153].

4.7 TSH

TSH may function as an additional independent regulator of the skeleton [83, 217]. In a mouse model in which the TSH receptor was knocked out through homologous recombination in embryonic stem cells, the animal exhibited a decrease in femur length, decreased trabecular bone area, and an increase in the tartrate-resistant acid phosphatase (TRAP) labeled surface and in focal sclerosis [1]. These findings suggest that TSH is a regulator of bone, and that the bone loss in the hyperthyroid state may be due to the suppression of TSH. Treatment of hematopoietic stem cells or RAW-C3 bone cells with recombinant human TSH has decreased osteoclast markers and stimulated apoptosis of osteoclasts and precursor cells, possibly mediated by tumor necrosis factor α (TNFα), C-Jun N-terminal kinase (JNK), and nuclear factor κB (NFkB) [76]. Normal human osteoblasts and SaOS-2 osteosarcoma cells have TSH receptors, with TSH stimulating cAMP production in SaOS-2 cells [139]. TSH also stimulates the type 2 deiodinase [139]. Additionally, TSH increases alkaline phosphatase and osteocalcin and stimulates mineralization in osteoblasts [168], with low-density-lipoprotein-receptor-related protein 5 (LRP5) and the vascular endothelial growth factor receptor Flk-1 implicated in this response [1]. A finding inconsistent with the functional significance of TSH is that in TRβ knockout animals in which TSH is elevated due to deficient feedback inhibition at the pituitary gland, there was decreased trabecular bone and increased osteoclast activity [17].

Clinical studies have also come to contradictory conclusions regarding TSH and bone. A relationship of serum TSH and remodeling, independent of thyroid hormone, was found in a study of cured patients with differentiated thyroid carcinoma [79]. In another study, administration of TSH to a group of postmenopausal women with papillary thyroid carcinoma and near-total thyroidectomy produced a transient decrease in serum calcium and urinary excretion of C- and N-telopeptides of type I collagen [92]. In women with normal thyroid function, low serum TSH was correlated with vertebral fractures. This was independent of T4 levels, age, and bone mineral density [129]. Other clinical data, however, are not in accord with a dominant regulatory role of TSH in normal bone function. In the Tromsø study, serum TSH was not associated with bone mineral density in women and men who have TSH values within the normal range [19, 70]. The tight regulation of the system along with local regulation by tissue deiodinases makes it difficult to reach definitive conclusions on the regulatory role of TSH.

4.8 Summary

In summary, thyroid hormones play a significant role in the normal development of the skeleton. Thyroid hormones stimulate remodeling throughout life. Thyroid hormones can produce bone loss and increased susceptibility to fractures at high doses or in the presence of other factors that promote bone loss or when protective growth factors are deficient. Thyroid hormone function is largely mediated through nuclear receptors, and there may be modulation by nongenomic signals. Greater understanding of the mechanisms critical for local regulation of thyroid hormones, such as the transporters and deiodinases, and further understanding of the role of TSH will provide a more complete picture and may point to novel therapies in the future.

References

1. Abe E, Marians RC, Yu W, Wu XB, Ando T, Li Y, Iqbal J, Eldeiry L, Rajendren G, Blair HC, Davies TF, Zaidi M. TSH is a negative regulator of skeletal remodeling. Cell. 2003;115(2):151–62.

2. Abu EO, Bord S, Horner A, Chatterjee VK, Compston JE. The expression of thyroid hormone receptors in human bone. Bone. 1997;21(2):137–42.
3. Abu EO, Horner A, Teti A, Chatterjee VK, Compston JE. The localization of thyroid hormone receptor mRNAs in human bone. Thyroid. 2000;10(4):287–93.
4. Adlin EV, Maurer AH, Marks AD, Channick BJ. Bone mineral density in postmenopausal women treated with L-thyroxine. Am J Med. 1991;90(3):360–6.
5. Affinito P, Sorrentino C, Farace MJ, di Carlo C, Moccia G, Canciello P, Palomba S, Nappi C. Effects of thyroxine therapy on bone metabolism in postmenopausal women with hypothyroidism. Acta Obstet Gynecol Scand. 1996;75(9):843–8.
6. Ahn KH, Lee SH, Park HT, Kim T, Hur JY, Kim YT, Kim SH. Effect of adiponectin and sex steroid hormones on bone mineral density and bone formation markers in postmenopausal women with subclinical hyperthyroidism. J Obstet Gynaecol Res. 2010;36(2):370–6.
7. Akita S, Nakamura T, Hirano A, Fujii T, Yamashita S. Thyroid hormone action on rat calvarial sutures. Thyroid. 1994;4(1):99–106.
8. Allain TJ, Chambers TJ, Flanagan AM, McGregor AM. Tri-iodothyronine stimulates rat osteoclastic bone resorption by an indirect effect. J Endocrinol. 1992;133(3):327–31.
9. Allain TJ, Thomas MR, McGregor AM, Salisbury JR. A histomorphometric study of bone changes in thyroid dysfunction in rats. Bone. 1995;16(5):505–9.
10. Allain TJ, Yen PM, Flanagan AM, McGregor AM. The isoform-specific expression of the tri-iodothyronine receptor in osteoblasts and osteoclasts. Eur J Clin Invest. 1996;26(5):418–25.
11. Amato G, Mazziotti G, Sorvillo F, Piscopo M, Lalli E, Biondi B, Iorio S, Molinari A, Giustina A, Carella C. High serum osteoprotegerin levels in patients with hyperthyroidism: effect of medical treatment. Bone. 2004;35(3):785–91.
12. Asai S, Cao X, Yamauchi M, Funahashi K, Ishiguro N, Kambe F. Thyroid hormone non-genomically suppresses Src thereby stimulating osteocalcin expression in primary mouse calvarial osteoblasts. Biochem Biophys Res Commun. 2009;387(1):92–6.
13. Ballock RT, Reddi AH. Thyroxine is the serum factor that regulates morphogenesis of columnar cartilage from isolated chondrocytes in chemically defined medium. J Cell Biol. 1994;126(5):1311–8.
14. Barnard JC, Williams AJ, Rabier B, Chassande O, Samarut J, Cheng SY, Bassett JH, Williams GR. Thyroid hormones regulate fibroblast growth factor receptor signaling during chondrogenesis. Endocrinology. 2005;146(12):5568–80.
15. Bassett JH, Boyde A, Howell PG, Bassett RH, Galliford TM, Archanco M, Evans H, Lawson MA, Croucher P, St Germain DL, Galton VA, Williams GR. Optimal bone strength and mineralization requires the type 2 iodothyronine deiodinase in osteoblasts. Proc Natl Acad Sci USA. 2010;107(16):7604–9.
16. Bassett JH, Nordstrom K, Boyde A, Howell PG, Kelly S, Vennstrom B, Williams GR. Thyroid status during skeletal development determines adult bone structure and mineralization. Mol Endocrinol. 2007;21(8):1893–904.
17. Bassett JH, O'Shea PJ, Sriskantharajah S, Rabier B, Boyde A, Howell PG, Weiss RE, Roux JP, Malaval L, Clement-Lacroix P, Samarut J, Chassande O, Williams GR. Thyroid hormone excess rather than thyrotropin deficiency induces osteoporosis in hyperthyroidism. Mol Endocrinol. 2007;21(5):1095–107.
18. Bassett JH, Williams GR. The skeletal phenotypes of TRalpha and TRbeta mutant mice. J Mol Endocrinol. 2009;42(4):269–82.
19. Bauer DC. Bone: does TSH concentration influence skeletal health? Nat Rev Endocrinol. 2009;5(5):245–6.
20. Beber EH, Capelo LP, Fonseca TL, Costa CC, Lotfi CF, Scanlan TS, Gouveia CH. The thyroid hormone receptor (TR) beta-selective agonist GC-1 inhibits proliferation but induces differentiation and TR beta mRNA expression in mouse and rat osteoblast-like cells. Calcif Tissue Int. 2009;84(4):324–33.
21. Bittner K, Vischer P, Bartholmes P, Bruckner P. Role of the subchondral vascular system in endochondral ossification: endothelial cells specifically derepress late differentiation in resting chondrocytes in vitro. Exp Cell Res. 1998;238(2):491–7.
22. Bohme K, Conscience-Egli M, Tschan T, Winterhalter KH, Bruckner P. Induction of proliferation or hypertrophy of chondrocytes in serum-free culture: the role of insulin-like growth factor-I, insulin, or thyroxine. J Cell Biol. 1992;116(4):1035–42.
23. Brent GA, Moore DD, Larsen PR. Thyroid hormone regulation of gene expression. Annu Rev Physiol. 1991;53:17–35.
24. Britto JM, Fenton AJ, Holloway WR, Nicholson GC. Osteoblasts mediate thyroid hormone stimulation of osteoclastic bone resorption. Endocrinology. 1994;134(1):169–76.
25. Burakov D, Crofts LA, Chang CP, Freedman LP. Reciprocal recruitment of DRIP/mediator and p160 coactivator complexes in vivo by estrogen receptor. J Biol Chem. 2002;277(17):14359–62.
26. Burch WM, Van Wyk JJ. Triiodothyronine stimulates cartilage growth and maturation by different mechanisms. Am J Physiol. 1987;252(2 Pt 1):E176–82.
27. Campbell J, Day P, Diamond T. Fine adjustments in thyroxine replacement and its effect on bone metabolism. Thyroid. 1996;6(2):75–8.
28. Capelo LP, Beber EH, Fonseca TL, Gouveia CH. The monocarboxylate transporter 8 and L-type amino acid transporters 1 and 2 are expressed in mouse skeletons and in osteoblastic MC3T3-E1 cells. Thyroid. 2009;19(2):171–80.
29. Capelo LP, Beber EH, Huang SA, Zorn TM, Bianco AC, Gouveia CH. Deiodinase-mediated thyroid hormone inactivation minimizes thyroid hormone signaling in the early development of fetal skeleton. Bone. 2008;43(5):921–30.

30. Chassande O, Fraichard A, Gauthier K, Flamant F, Legrand C, Savatier P, Laudet V, Samarut J. Identification of transcripts initiated from an internal promoter in the c-erbA alpha locus that encode inhibitors of retinoic acid receptor-alpha and triiodothyronine receptor activities. Mol Endocrinol. 1997;11(9):1278–90.
31. Coindre JM, David JP, Riviere L, Goussot JF, Roger P, de Mascarel A, Meunier PJ. Bone loss in hypothyroidism with hormone replacement. A histomorphometric study. Arch Intern Med. 1986;146(1):48–53.
32. Davis PJ, Davis FB, Lin HY, Mousa SA, Zhou M, Luidens MK. Translational implications of nongenomic actions of thyroid hormone initiated at its integrin receptor. Am J Physiol Endocrinol Metab. 2009;297(6):E1238–46.
33. De Rosa G, Testa A, Maussier ML, Calla C, Astazi P, Albanese C. A slightly suppressive dose of L-thyroxine does not affect bone turnover and bone mineral density in pre- and postmenopausal women with nontoxic goitre. Horm Metab Res. 1995;27(11):503–7.
34. Diamond T, Nery L, Hales I. A therapeutic dilemma: suppressive doses of thyroxine significantly reduce bone mineral measurements in both premenopausal and postmenopausal women with thyroid carcinoma. J Clin Endocrinol Metab. 1991;72(6):1184–8.
35. Dickerman Z, De Vries L. Prepubertal and pubertal growth, timing and duration of puberty and attained adult height in patients with congenital hypothyroidism (CH) detected by the neonatal screening programme for CH – a longitudinal study. Clin Endocrinol (Oxf). 1997;47(6):649–54.
36. DiPippo VA, Lindsay R, Powers CA. Estradiol and tamoxifen interactions with thyroid hormone in the ovariectomized-thyroidectomized rat. Endocrinology. 1995;136(3):1020–33.
37. Dong Y, Drissi H, Chen M, Chen D, Zuscik MJ, Schwarz EM, O'Keefe RJ. Wnt-mediated regulation of chondrocyte maturation: modulation by TGF-beta. J Cell Biochem. 2005;95(5):1057–68.
38. Dong YF, Soung do Y, Schwarz EM, O'Keefe RJ, Drissi H. Wnt induction of chondrocyte hypertrophy through the Runx2 transcription factor. J Cell Physiol. 2006;208(1):77–86.
39. Duncan WE, Chang A, Solomon B, Wartofsky L. Influence of clinical characteristics and parameters associated with thyroid hormone therapy on the bone mineral density of women treated with thyroid hormone. Thyroid. 1994;4(2):183–90.
40. Eftekhari M, Asadollahi A, Beiki D, Izadyar S, Gholamrezanezhad A, Assadi M, Fard-Esfahani A, Fallahi B, Takavar A, Saghari M. The long term effect of levothyroxine on bone mineral density in patients with well differentiated thyroid carcinoma after treatment. Hell J Nucl Med. 2008;11(3):160–3.
41. Egrise D, Martin D, Neve P, Verhas M, Schoutens A. Effects and interactions of 17 beta-estradiol, T3 and 1,25(OH)2D3 on cultured osteoblasts from mature rats. Bone Miner. 1990;11(3):273–83.
42. Ernst M, Froesch ER. Triiodothyronine stimulates proliferation of osteoblast-like cells in serum-free culture. FEBS Lett. 1987;220(1):163–6.
43. Ernst M, Rodan GA. Increased activity of insulin-like growth factor (IGF) in osteoblastic cells in the presence of growth hormone (GH): positive correlation with the presence of the GH-induced IGF-binding protein BP-3. Endocrinology. 1990;127(2):807–14.
44. Evans RM. The steroid and thyroid hormone receptor superfamily. Science. 1988;240(4854):889–95.
45. Fallon MD, Perry HM, Bergfeld M, Droke D, Teitelbaum SL, Avioli LV. Exogenous hyperthyroidism with osteoporosis. Arch Intern Med. 1983;143(3):442–4.
46. Feitosa Dda S, Bezerra Bde B, Ambrosano GM, Nociti FH, Casati MZ, Sallum EA, de Toledo S. Thyroid hormones may influence cortical bone healing around titanium implants: a histometric study in rats. J Periodontol. 2008;79(5):881–7.
47. Fekete C, Lechan RM. Negative feedback regulation of hypophysiotropic thyrotropin-releasing hormone (TRH) synthesizing neurons: role of neuronal afferents and type 2 deiodinase. Front Neuroendocrinol. 2007;28(2–3):97–114.
48. Feyen JH, Evans DB, Binkert C, Heinrich GF, Geisse S, Kocher HP. Recombinant human [Cys281] insulin-like growth factor-binding protein 2 inhibits both basal and insulin-like growth factor I-stimulated proliferation and collagen synthesis in fetal rat calvariae. J Biol Chem. 1991;266(29):19469–74.
49. Fraichard A, Chassande O, Plateroti M, Roux JP, Trouillas J, Dehay C, Legrand C, Gauthier K, Kedinger M, Malaval L, Rousset B, Samarut J. The T3R alpha gene encoding a thyroid hormone receptor is essential for post-natal development and thyroid hormone production. EMBO J. 1997;16(14):4412–20.
50. Franklyn J, Betteridge J, Holder R, Daykin J, Lilley J, Sheppard M. Bone mineral density in thyroxine treated females with or without a previous history of thyrotoxicosis. Clin Endocrinol (Oxf). 1994;41(4):425–32.
51. Franklyn JA, Betteridge J, Daykin J, Holder R, Oates GD, Parle JV, Lilley J, Heath DA, Sheppard MC. Long-term thyroxine treatment and bone mineral density. Lancet. 1992;340(8810):9–13.
52. Franklyn JA, Betteridge J, Holder R, Sheppard MC. Effect of estrogen replacement therapy upon bone mineral density in thyroxine-treated postmenopausal women with a past history of thyrotoxicosis. Thyroid. 1995;5(5):359–63.
53. Fraser SA, Anderson JB, Smith DA, Wilson GM. Osteoporosis and fractures following thyrotoxicosis. Lancet. 1971;1(7707):981–3.
54. Fratzl-Zelman N, Glantschnig H, Rumpler M, Nader A, Ellinger A, Varga F. The expression of matrix metalloproteinase-13 and osteocalcin in mouse osteoblasts is related to osteoblastic differentiation and is modulated by 1,25-dihydroxyvitamin D3 and thyroid hormones. Cell Biol Int. 2003;27(6):459–68.

55. Fratzl-Zelman N, Horandner H, Luegmayr E, Varga F, Ellinger A, Erlee MP, Klaushofer K. Effects of triiodothyronine on the morphology of cells and matrix, the localization of alkaline phosphatase, and the frequency of apoptosis in long-term cultures of MC3T3-E1 cells. Bone. 1997;20(3):225–36.
56. Frevert EU, Biester A, Muller MJ, Schmidt-Gayk H, von zur Muhlen A, Brabant G. Markers of bone metabolism during short-term administration of thyroxine in healthy volunteers. Eur J Endocrinol. 1994; 131(2):145–9.
57. Fujiyama K, Kiriyama T, Ito M, Kimura H, Ashizawa K, Tsuruta M, Nagayama Y, Villadolid MC, Yokoyama N, Nagataki S. Suppressive doses of thyroxine do not accelerate age-related bone loss in late postmenopausal women. Thyroid. 1995;5(1):13–7.
58. Garton M, Reid I, Loveridge N, Robins S, Murchison L, Beckett G, Reid D. Bone mineral density and metabolism in premenopausal women taking L-thyroxine replacement therapy. Clin Endocrinol (Oxf). 1994; 41(6):747–55.
59. Gauthier K, Chassande O, Plateroti M, Roux JP, Legrand C, Pain B, Rousset B, Weiss R, Trouillas J, Samarut J. Different functions for the thyroid hormone receptors TRalpha and TRbeta in the control of thyroid hormone production and post-natal development. EMBO J. 1999;18(3):623–31.
60. Glade MJ, Kanwar YS, Stern PH. Insulin and thyroid hormones stimulate matrix metabolism in primary cultures of articular chondrocytes from young rabbits independently and in combination. Connect Tissue Res. 1994;31(1):37–44.
61. Glantschnig H, Varga F, Klaushofer K. Thyroid hormone and retinoic acid induce the synthesis of insulin-like growth factor-binding protein-4 in mouse osteoblastic cells. Endocrinology. 1996;137(1): 281–6.
62. Glass CK. Differential recognition of target genes by nuclear receptor monomers, dimers, and heterodimers. Endocr Rev. 1994;15(3):391–407.
63. Glasscock GF, Nicoll CS. Hormonal control of growth in the infant rat. Endocrinology. 1981;109(1): 176–84.
64. Gothe S, Wang Z, Ng L, Kindblom JM, Barros AC, Ohlsson C, Vennstrom B, Forrest D. Mice devoid of all known thyroid hormone receptors are viable but exhibit disorders of the pituitary-thyroid axis, growth, and bone maturation. Genes Dev. 1999;13(10): 1329–41.
65. Gouveia CH, Jorgetti V, Bianco AC. Effects of thyroid hormone administration and estrogen deficiency on bone mass of female rats. J Bone Miner Res. 1997; 12(12):2098–107.
66. Grant DJ, McMurdo ME, Mole PA, Paterson CR. Is previous hyperthyroidism still a risk factor for osteoporosis in post-menopausal women? Clin Endocrinol (Oxf). 1995;43(3):339–45.
67. Grant DJ, McMurdo ME, Mole PA, Paterson CR, Davies RR. Suppressed TSH levels secondary to thyroxine replacement therapy are not associated with osteoporosis. Clin Endocrinol (Oxf). 1993;39(5): 529–33.
68. Greenspan SL, Greenspan FS. The effect of thyroid hormone on skeletal integrity. Ann Intern Med. 1999;130(9):750–8.
69. Greenspan SL, Greenspan FS, Resnick NM, Block JE, Friedlander AL, Genant HK. Skeletal integrity in premenopausal and postmenopausal women receiving long-term L-thyroxine therapy. Am J Med. 1991;91(1): 5–14.
70. Grimnes G, Emaus N, Joakimsen RM, Figenschau Y, Jorde R. The relationship between serum TSH and bone mineral density in men and postmenopausal women: the Tromso study. Thyroid. 2008;18(11): 1147–55.
71. Gu WX, Stern PH, Madison LD, Du GG. Mutual upregulation of thyroid hormone and parathyroid hormone receptors in rat osteoblastic osteosarcoma 17/2.8 cells. Endocrinology. 2001;142(1):157–64.
72. Gurlek A, Gedik O. Effect of endogenous subclinical hyperthyroidism on bone metabolism and bone mineral density in premenopausal women. Thyroid. 1999;9(6):539–43.
73. Hadji P, Hars O, Sturm G, Bauer T, Emons G, Schulz KD. The effect of long-term, non-suppressive levothyroxine treatment on quantitative ultrasonometry of bone in women. Eur J Endocrinol. 2000; 142(5):445–50.
74. Halme J, Uitto J, Kivirikko KI, Saxen L. Effect of triiodothyronine in the metabolism of collagen in cultured embryonic bones. Endocrinology. 1972; 90(6):1476–82.
75. Hanna FW, Pettit RJ, Ammari F, Evans WD, Sandeman D, Lazarus JH. Effect of replacement doses of thyroxine on bone mineral density. Clin Endocrinol (Oxf). 1998;48(2):229–34.
76. Hase H, Ando T, Eldeiry L, Brebene A, Peng Y, Liu L, Amano H, Davies TF, Sun L, Zaidi M, Abe E. TNFalpha mediates the skeletal effects of thyroid-stimulating hormone. Proc Natl Acad Sci USA. 2006; 103(34):12849–54.
77. Hawkins F, Rigopoulou D, Papapietro K, Lopez MB. Spinal bone mass after long-term treatment with L-thyroxine in postmenopausal women with thyroid cancer and chronic lymphocytic thyroiditis. Calcif Tissue Int. 1994;54(1):16–9.
78. Heemstra KA, Hoftijzer H, van der Deure WM, Peeters RP, Hamdy NA, Pereira A, Corssmit EP, Romijn JA, Visser TJ, Smit JW. The type 2 deiodinase Thr92Ala polymorphism is associated with increased bone turnover and decreased femoral neck bone mineral density. J Bone Miner Res. 2010;25(6):1385–91.
79. Heemstra KA, van der Deure WM, Peeters RP, Hamdy NA, Stokkel MP, Corssmit EP, Romijn JA, Visser TJ, Smit JW. Thyroid hormone independent associations between serum TSH levels and indicators of bone turnover in cured patients with differentiated thyroid carcinoma. Eur J Endocrinol. 2008;159(1):69–76.

80. Heyerdahl S, Kase BF, Stake G. Skeletal maturation during thyroxine treatment in children with congenital hypothyroidism. Acta Paediatr. 1994;83(6):618–22.
81. Hoffmann O, Klaushofer K, Koller K, Peterlik M, Mavreas T, Stern P. Indomethacin inhibits thrombin-, but not thyroxin-stimulated resorption of fetal rat limb bones. Prostaglandins. 1986;31(4):601–8.
82. Huang BK, Golden LA, Tarjan G, Madison LD, Stern PH. Insulin-like growth factor I production is essential for anabolic effects of thyroid hormone in osteoblasts. J Bone Miner Res. 2000;15(2):188–97.
83. Imam A, Iqbal J, Blair HC, Davies TF, Huang CL, Zallone A, Zaidi M, Sun L. Role of the pituitary-bone axis in skeletal pathophysiology. Curr Opin Endocrinol Diabetes Obes. 2009;16(6):423–9.
84. Ishida H, Bellows CG, Aubin JE, Heersche JN. Triiodothyronine (T3) and dexamethasone interact to modulate osteoprogenitor cell differentiation in fetal rat calvaria cell cultures. Bone. 1995;16(5):545–9.
85. Ishikawa Y, Genge BR, Wuthier RE, Wu LN. Thyroid hormone inhibits growth and stimulates terminal differentiation of epiphyseal growth plate chondrocytes. J Bone Miner Res. 1998;13(9):1398–411.
86. Ito M, Roeder RG. The TRAP/SMCC/Mediator complex and thyroid hormone receptor function. Trends Endocrinol Metab. 2001;12(3):127–34.
87. Izumo S, Mahdavi V. Thyroid hormone receptor alpha isoforms generated by alternative splicing differentially activate myosin HC gene transcription. Nature. 1988;334(6182):539–42.
88. Jansen J, Friesema EC, Kester MH, Schwartz CE, Visser TJ. Genotype-phenotype relationship in patients with mutations in thyroid hormone transporter MCT8. Endocrinology. 2008;149(5):2184–90.
89. Jodar E, Begona Lopez M, Garcia L, Rigopoulou D, Martinez G, Hawkins F. Bone changes in pre- and postmenopausal women with thyroid cancer on levothyroxine therapy: evolution of axial and appendicular bone mass. Osteoporos Int. 1998;8(4):311–6.
90. Kaneshige M, Kaneshige K, Zhu X, Dace A, Garrett L, Carter TA, Kazlauskaite R, Pankratz DG, Wynshaw-Boris A, Refetoff S, Weintraub B, Willingham MC, Barlow C, Cheng S. Mice with a targeted mutation in the thyroid hormone beta receptor gene exhibit impaired growth and resistance to thyroid hormone. Proc Natl Acad Sci USA. 2000;97(24):13209–14.
91. Kaneshige M, Suzuki H, Kaneshige K, Cheng J, Wimbrow H, Barlow C, Willingham MC, Cheng S. A targeted dominant negative mutation of the thyroid hormone alpha 1 receptor causes increased mortality, infertility, and dwarfism in mice. Proc Natl Acad Sci USA. 2001;98(26):15095–100.
92. Karga H, Papaioannou G, Polymeris A, Papamichael K, Karpouza A, Samouilidou E, Papaioannou P. The effects of recombinant human TSH on bone turnover in patients after thyroidectomy. J Bone Miner Metab. 2010;28(1):35–41.
93. Kasono K, Sato K, Han DC, Fujii Y, Tsushima T, Shizume K. Stimulation of alkaline phosphatase activity by thyroid hormone in mouse osteoblast-like cells (MC3T3-E1): a possible mechanism of hyperalkaline phosphatasia in hyperthyroidism. Bone Miner. 1988;4(4):355–63.
94. Kassem M, Mosekilde L, Eriksen EF. Effects of triiodothyronine on DNA synthesis and differentiation markers of normal human osteoblast-like cells in vitro. Biochem Mol Biol Int. 1993;30(4):779 88.
95. Kawaguchi H, Pilbeam CC, Raisz LG. Anabolic effects of 3,3″,5-triiodothyronine and triiodothyroacetic acid in cultured neonatal mouse parietal bones. Endocrinology. 1994;135(3):971–6.
96. Kawaguchi H, Pilbeam CC, Woodiel FN, Raisz LG. Comparison of the effects of 3,5,3″-triiodothyroacetic acid and triiodothyronine on bone resorption in cultured fetal rat long bones and neonatal mouse calvariae. J Bone Miner Res. 1994;9(2):247–53.
97. Kim CH, Kim HK, Shong YK, Lee KU, Kim GS. Thyroid hormone stimulates basal and interleukin (IL)-1-induced IL-6 production in human bone marrow stromal cells: a possible mediator of thyroid hormone-induced bone loss. J Endocrinol. 1999;160(1):97–102.
98. Klaushofer K, Hoffmann O, Gleispach H, Leis HJ, Czerwenka E, Koller K, Peterlik M. Bone-resorbing activity of thyroid hormones is related to prostaglandin production in cultured neonatal mouse calvaria. J Bone Miner Res. 1989;4(3):305–12.
99. Klaushofer K, Varga F, Glantschnig H, Fratzl-Zelman N, Czerwenka E, Leis HJ, Koller K, Peterlik M. The regulatory role of thyroid hormones in bone cell growth and differentiation. J Nutr. 1995;125(7 Suppl):1996S–2003.
100. Knudsen N, Faber J, Sierbaek-Nielsen A, Vadstrup S, Sorensen HA, Hegedus L. Thyroid hormone treatment aiming at reduced, but not suppressed, serum thyroid-stimulating hormone levels in nontoxic goitre: effects on bone metabolism amongst premenopausal women. J Intern Med. 1998;243(2):149–54.
101. Koenig RJ, Lazar MA, Hodin RA, Brent GA, Larsen PR, Chin WW, Moore DD. Inhibition of thyroid hormone action by a non-hormone binding c-erbA protein generated by alternative mRNA splicing. Nature. 1989;337(6208):659–61.
102. Kooh SW, Brnjac L, Ehrlich RM, Qureshi R, Krishnan S. Bone mass in children with congenital hypothyroidism treated with thyroxine since birth. J Pediatr Endocrinol Metab. 1996;9(1):59–62.
103. Krieger NS, Stappenbeck TS, Stern PH. Characterization of specific thyroid hormone receptors in bone. J Bone Miner Res. 1988;3(4):473–8.
104. Kung AW, Lorentz T, Tam SC. Thyroxine suppressive therapy decreases bone mineral density in postmenopausal women. Clin Endocrinol (Oxf). 1993;39(5):535–40.
105. La Vignera S, Vicari E, Tumino S, Ciotta L, Condorelli R, Vicari LO, Calogero AE. L-thyroxin

treatment and post-menopausal osteoporosis: relevance of the risk profile present in clinical history. Minerva Ginecol. 2008;60(6):475–84.
106. Lakatos P, Caplice MD, Khanna V, Stern PH. Thyroid hormones increase insulin-like growth factor I content in the medium of rat bone tissue. J Bone Miner Res. 1993;8(12):1475–81.
107. Lakatos P, Foldes J, Nagy Z, Takacs I, Speer G, Horvath C, Mohan S, Baylink DJ, Stern PH. Serum insulin-like growth factor-I, insulin-like growth factor binding proteins, and bone mineral content in hyperthyroidism. Thyroid. 2000;10(5):417–23.
108. Lakatos P, Hollo I, Horvath C. Severe postmenopausal osteoporosis and thyroid hormones. Arch Intern Med. 1986;146(9):1859.
109. Lakatos P, Stern PH. Evidence for direct nongenomic effects of triiodothyronine on bone rudiments in rats: stimulation of the inositol phosphate second messenger system. Acta Endocrinol (Copenhagen). 1991;125(5):603–8.
110. Lakatos P, Stern PH. Effects of cyclosporins and transforming growth factor beta 1 on thyroid hormone action in cultured fetal rat limb bones. Calcif Tissue Int. 1992;50(2):123–8.
111. Lakatos P, Tarjan G, Merei J, Foldes J, Hollo I. Androgens and bone mineral content in patients with subtotal thyroidectomy for benign nodular disease. Acta Med Hung. 1989;46(4):297–305.
112. Langdahl BL, Loft AG, Eriksen EF, Mosekilde L, Charles P. Bone mass, bone turnover and body composition in former hypothyroid patients receiving replacement therapy. Eur J Endocrinol. 1996;134(6):702–9.
113. Larsen P, Davies TF, Schlumberber M-J, Hay ID. In: Kronenberg H, Shlomo M, Polonsky KS, Larsen PR, editors. Williams textbook of endocrinology. Philadelphia: Saunders Elsevier; 2008.
114. Lassova L, Niu Z, Golden EB, Cohen AJ, Adams SL. Thyroid hormone treatment of cultured chondrocytes mimics in vivo stimulation of collagen X mRNA by increasing BMP 4 expression. J Cell Physiol. 2009;219(3):595–605.
115. Lazar MA. Thyroid hormone receptors: multiple forms, multiple possibilities. Endocr Rev. 1993;14(2):184–93.
116. LeBron BA, Pekary AE, Mirell C, Hahn TJ, Hershman JM. Thyroid hormone 5′-deiodinase activity, nuclear binding, and effects on mitogenesis in UMR-106 osteoblastic osteosarcoma cells. J Bone Miner Res. 1989;4(2):173–8.
117. Leger J, Ruiz JC, Guibourdenche J, Kindermans C, Garabedian M, Czernichow P. Bone mineral density and metabolism in children with congenital hypothyroidism after prolonged L-thyroxine therapy. Acta Paediatr. 1997;86(7):704–10.
118. Lehmke J, Bogner U, Felsenberg D, Peters H, Schleusener H. Determination of bone mineral density by quantitative computed tomography and single photon absorptiometry in subclinical hyperthyroidism: a risk of early osteopaenia in postmenopausal women. Clin Endocrinol (Oxf). 1992;36(5):511–7.
119. Lewinson D, Bialik GM, Hochberg Z. Differential effects of hypothyroidism on the cartilage and the osteogenic process in the mandibular condyle: recovery by growth hormone and thyroxine. Endocrinology. 1994;135(4):1504–10.
120. Liu Y, Xia X, Fondell JD, Yen PM. Thyroid hormone-regulated target genes have distinct patterns of coactivator recruitment and histone acetylation. Mol Endocrinol. 2006;20(3):483–90.
121. Luegmayr E, Glantschnig H, Varga F, Klaushofer K. The organization of adherens junctions in mouse osteoblast-like cells (MC3T3-E1) and their modulation by triiodothyronine and 1,25-dihydroxyvitamin D3. Histochem Cell Biol. 2000;113(6):467–78.
122. Luegmayr E, Varga F, Frank T, Roschger P, Klaushofer K. Effects of triiodothyronine on morphology, growth behavior, and the actin cytoskeleton in mouse osteoblastic cells (MC3T3-E1). Bone. 1996;18(6):591–9.
123. Luegmayr E, Varga F, Glantschnig H, Fratzl-Zelman N, Rumpler M, Ellinger A, Klaushofer K. 1,25-Dihydroxy vitamin D3 and tri-iodothyronine stimulate the expression of a protein immunologically related to osteocalcin. J Histochem Cytochem. 1998;46(4):477–86.
124. Lupoli G, Nuzzo V, Di Carlo C, Affinito P, Vollery M, Vitale G, Cascone E, Arlotta F, Nappi C. Effects of alendronate on bone loss in pre- and postmenopausal hyperthyroid women treated with methimazole. Gynecol Endocrinol. 1996;10(5):343–8.
125. Majima T, Komatsu Y, Doi K, Takagi C, Shigemoto M, Fukao A, Morimoto T, Corners J, Nakao K. Clinical significance of risedronate for osteoporosis in the initial treatment of male patients with Graves' disease. J Bone Miner Metab. 2006;24(2):105–13.
126. Marcocci C, Golia F, Bruno-Bossio G, Vignali E, Pinchera A. Carefully monitored levothyroxine suppressive therapy is not associated with bone loss in premenopausal women. J Clin Endocrinol Metab. 1994;78(4):818–23.
127. Marcocci C, Golia F, Vignali E, Pinchera A. Skeletal integrity in men chronically treated with suppressive doses of L-thyroxine. J Bone Miner Res. 1997;12(1):72–7.
128. Matusik P, Malecka-Tendera E, Franek E, Januszek-Trzciakowska A. Bone mineral density and metabolism in levothyroxine-treated adolescent girls with euthyroid diffuse goiter. Endokrynol Pol. 2010;61(1):14–9.
129. Mazziotti G, Porcelli T, Patelli I, Vescovi PP, Giustina A. Serum TSH values and risk of vertebral fractures in euthyroid post-menopausal women with low bone mineral density. Bone. 2010;46(3):747–51.
130. McDermott MT, Perloff JJ, Kidd GS. A longitudinal assessment of bone loss in women with

levothyroxine-suppressed benign thyroid disease and thyroid cancer. Calcif Tissue Int. 1995;56(6): 521–5.
131. McKenna NJ, O'Malley BW. Combinatorial control of gene expression by nuclear receptors and coregulators. Cell. 2002;108(4):465–74.
132. Mello MA, Tuan RS. Effects of TGF-beta1 and triiodothyronine on cartilage maturation: in vitro analysis using long-term high-density micromass cultures of chick embryonic limb mesenchymal cells. J Orthop Res. 2006;24(11):2095–105.
133. Meunier P, Bianchi GGS, Edouard CM. Bone manifestations of thyrotoxicosis. Orthop Clin North Am. 1972;3:745–74.
134. Mikosch P, Jauk B, Gallowitsch HJ, Pipam W, Kresnik E, Lind P. Suppressive levothyroxine therapy has no significant influence on bone degradation in women with thyroid carcinoma: a comparison with other disorders affecting bone metabolism. Thyroid. 2001;11(3):257–63.
135. Milne M, Kang MI, Cardona G, Quail JM, Braverman LE, Chin WW, Baran DT. Expression of multiple thyroid hormone receptor isoforms in rat femoral and vertebral bone and in bone marrow osteogenic cultures. J Cell Biochem. 1999;74(4):684–93.
136. Miura M, Tanaka K, Komatsu Y, Suda M, Yasoda A, Sakuma Y, Ozasa A, Nakao K. A novel interaction between thyroid hormones and 1,25(OH)(2)D(3) in osteoclast formation. Biochem Biophys Res Commun. 2002;291(4):987–94.
137. Mochizuki Y, Banba N, Hattori Y, Monden T. Correlation between serum osteoprotegerin and biomarkers of bone metabolism during anti-thyroid treatment in patients with Graves' disease. Horm Res. 2006;66(5):236–9.
138. Mohan S, Bautista CM, Wergedal J, Baylink DJ. Isolation of an inhibitory insulin-like growth factor (IGF) binding protein from bone cell-conditioned medium: a potential local regulator of IGF action. Proc Natl Acad Sci USA. 1989;86(21):8338–42.
139. Morimura T, Tsunekawa K, Kasahara T, Seki K, Ogiwara T, Mori M, Murakami M. Expression of type 2 iodothyronine deiodinase in human osteoblast is stimulated by thyrotropin. Endocrinology. 2005;146(4):2077–84.
140. Mosekilde L, Melsen F. A tetracycline-based histomorphometric evaluation of bone resorption and bone turnover in hyperthyroidism and hyperparathyroidism. Acta Med Scand. 1978;204(1–2):97–102.
141. Mundy GR, Shapiro JL, Bandelin JG, Canalis EM, Raisz LG. Direct stimulation of bone resorption by thyroid hormones. J Clin Invest. 1976;58(3):529–34.
142. Murphy E, Gluer CC, Reid DM, Felsenberg D, Roux C, Eastell R, Williams GR. Thyroid function within the upper normal range is associated with reduced bone mineral density and an increased risk of nonvertebral fractures in healthy euthyroid postmenopausal women. J Clin Endocrinol Metab. 2010;95(7):3173–81.
143. Nakamura H, Mori T, Genma R, Suzuki Y, Natsume H, Andoh S, Kitahara R, Nagasawa S, Nishiyama K, Yoshimi T. Urinary excretion of pyridinoline and deoxypyridinoline measured by immunoassay in hypothyroidism. Clin Endocrinol (Oxf). 1996;44(4):447–51.
144. Nillni EA. Regulation of the hypothalamic thyrotropin releasing hormone (TRH) neuron by neuronal and peripheral inputs. Front Neuroendocrinol. 2010; 31(2):134–56.
145. Nilsson A, Ohlsson C, Isaksson OG, Lindahl A, Isgaard J. Hormonal regulation of longitudinal bone growth. Eur J Clin Nutr. 1994;48 Suppl 1:S150–8; discussion S158–160.
146. Nuzzo V, Lupoli G, Esposito Del Puente A, Rampone E, Carpinelli A, Del Puente AE, Oriente P. Bone mineral density in premenopausal women receiving levothyroxine suppressive therapy. Gynecol Endocrinol. 1998;12(5):333–7.
147. Nystrom E, Lundberg PA, Petersen K, Bengtsson C, Lindstedt G. Evidence for a slow tissue adaptation to circulating thyroxine in patients with chronic L-thyroxine treatment. Clin Endocrinol (Oxf). 1989; 31(2):143–50.
148. O'Shea PJ, Bassett JH, Sriskantharajah S, Ying H, Cheng SY, Williams GR. Contrasting skeletal phenotypes in mice with an identical mutation targeted to thyroid hormone receptor alpha1 or beta. Mol Endocrinol. 2005;19(12):3045–59.
149. O'Shea PJ, Guigon CJ, Williams GR, Cheng SY. Regulation of fibroblast growth factor receptor-1 (FGFR1) by thyroid hormone: identification of a thyroid hormone response element in the murine Fgfr1 promoter. Endocrinology. 2007;148(12):5966–76.
150. O'Shea PJ, Harvey CB, Suzuki H, Kaneshige M, Kaneshige K, Cheng SY, Williams GR. A thyrotoxic skeletal phenotype of advanced bone formation in mice with resistance to thyroid hormone. Mol Endocrinol. 2003;17(7):1410–24.
151. Ohishi K, Ishida H, Nagata T, Yamauchi N, Tsurumi C, Nishikawa S, Wakano Y. Thyroid hormone suppresses the differentiation of osteoprogenitor cells to osteoblasts, but enhances functional activities of mature osteoblasts in cultured rat calvaria cells. J Cell Physiol. 1994;161(3):544–52.
152. Ongphiphadhanakul B, Jenis LG, Braverman LE, Alex S, Stein GS, Lian JB, Baran DT. Etidronate inhibits the thyroid hormone-induced bone loss in rats assessed by bone mineral density and messenger ribonucleic acid markers of osteoblast and osteoclast function. Endocrinology. 1993;133(6):2502–7.
153. Panico A, Lupoli GA, Fonderico F, Marciello F, Martinelli A, Assante R, Lupoli G. Osteoporosis and thyrotropin-suppressive therapy: reduced effectiveness of alendronate. Thyroid. 2009;19(5):437–42.
154. Paul TL, Kerrigan J, Kelly AM, Braverman LE, Baran DT. Long-term L-thyroxine therapy is associated with decreased hip bone density in premenopausal women. JAMA. 1988;259(21):3137–41.

155. Pereira RC, Jorgetti V, Canalis E. Triiodothyronine induces collagenase-3 and gelatinase B expression in murine osteoblasts. Am J Physiol. 1999;277(3 Pt 1):E496–504.
156. Rabier B, Williams AJ, Mallein-Gerin F, Williams GR, Chassande O. Thyroid hormone-stimulated differentiation of primary rib chondrocytes in vitro requires thyroid hormone receptor beta. J Endocrinol. 2006;191(1):221–8.
157. Rachedi F, Rohmer V, Six P, Duquenne M, Wion Barbot N, Minebois A, Bigorgne JC, Audran M. Prolonged suppressive L-thyroxine therapy. Longitudinal study of the effect of LT4 on bone mineral density and bone metabolism markers in 71 patients. Presse Med. 1999;28(7):323–9.
158. Rachez C, Freedman LP. Mediator complexes and transcription. Curr Opin Cell Biol. 2001;13(3):274–80.
159. Refetoff S, Weiss RE, Usala SJ. The syndromes of resistance to thyroid hormone. Endocr Rev. 1993; 14(3):348–99.
160. Reverter JL, Holgado S, Alonso N, Salinas I, Granada ML, Sanmarti A. Lack of deleterious effect on bone mineral density of long-term thyroxine suppressive therapy for differentiated thyroid carcinoma. Endocr Relat Cancer. 2005;12(4):973–81.
161. Ribot C, Tremollieres F, Pouilles JM, Louvet JP. Bone mineral density and thyroid hormone therapy. Clin Endocrinol (Oxf). 1990;33(2):143–53.
162. Rizzoli R, Poser J, Burgi U. Nuclear thyroid hormone receptors in cultured bone cells. Metabolism. 1986;35(1):71–4.
163. Rosen HN, Moses AC, Gundberg C, Kung VT, Seyedin SM, Chen T, Holick M, Greenspan SL. Therapy with parenteral pamidronate prevents thyroid hormone-induced bone turnover in humans. J Clin Endocrinol Metab. 1993;77(3):664–9.
164. Ross DS. Worm-eaten bones. Thyroid. 2000;10(4): 331–3.
165. Ross DS, Neer RM, Ridgway EC, Daniels GH. Subclinical hyperthyroidism and reduced bone density as a possible result of prolonged suppression of the pituitary-thyroid axis with L-thyroxine. Am J Med. 1987;82(6):1167–70.
166. Saggese G, Bertelloni S, Baroncelli GI. Bone mineralization and calciotropic hormones in children with hyperthyroidism. Effects of methimazole therapy. J Endocrinol Invest. 1990;13(7):587–92.
167. Saggese G, Bertelloni S, Baroncelli GI, Costa S, Ceccarelli C. Bone mineral density in adolescent females treated with L-thyroxine: a longitudinal study. Eur J Pediatr. 1996;155(6):452–7.
168. Sampath TK, Simic P, Sendak R, Draca N, Bowe AE, O'Brien S, Schiavi SC, McPherson JM, Vukicevic S. Thyroid-stimulating hormone restores bone volume, microarchitecture, and strength in aged ovariectomized rats. J Bone Miner Res. 2007; 22(6):849–59.
169. Sap J, Munoz A, Damm K, Goldberg Y, Ghysdael J, Leutz A, Beug H, Vennstrom B. The c-erb-A protein is a high-affinity receptor for thyroid hormone. Nature. 1986;324(6098):635–40.
170. Saraiva PP, Teixeira SS, Padovani CR, Nogueira CR. Triiodothyronine (T3) does not induce Rankl expression in rat Ros 17/2.8 cells. Arq Bras Endocrinol Metabol. 2008;52(1):109–13.
171. Sato K, Han DC, Fujii Y, Tsushima T, Shizume K. Thyroid hormone stimulates alkaline phosphatase activity in cultured rat osteoblastic cells (ROS 17/2.8) through 3,5,3″-triiodo-L-thyronine nuclear receptors. Endocrinology. 1987;120(5):1873–81.
172. Scapin S, Leoni S, Spagnuolo S, Gnocchi D, De Vito P, Luly P, Pedersen JZ, Incerpi S. Short-term effects of thyroid hormones during development: focus on signal transduction. Steroids. 2010;75(8–9):576–84.
173. Scarlett A, Parsons MP, Hanson PL, Sidhu KK, Milligan TP, Burrin JM. Thyroid hormone stimulation of extracellular signal-regulated kinase and cell proliferation in human osteoblast-like cells is initiated at integrin alphaVbeta3. J Endocrinol. 2008; 196(3):509–17.
174. Schiller C, Gruber R, Ho GM, Redlich K, Gober HJ, Katzgraber F, Willheim M, Hoffmann O, Pietschmann P, Peterlik M. Interaction of triiodothyronine with 1alpha,25-dihydroxyvitamin D3 on interleukin-6-dependent osteoclast-like cell formation in mouse bone marrow cell cultures. Bone. 1998;22(4):341–6.
175. Schlesinger B, Fisher OD. Accelerated skeletal development from thyrotoxicosis and thyroid overdosage in childhood. Lancet. 1951;2(6677):289–90.
176. Schmid C, Rutishauser J, Schlapfer I, Froesch ER, Zapf J. Intact but not truncated insulin-like growth factor binding protein-3 (IGFBP-3) blocks IGF I-induced stimulation of osteoblasts: control of IGF signalling to bone cells by IGFBP-3-specific proteolysis? Biochem Biophys Res Commun. 1991; 179(1):579–85.
177. Schmid C, Schlapfer I, Futo E, Waldvogel M, Schwander J, Zapf J, Froesch ER. Triiodothyronine (T3) stimulates insulin-like growth factor (IGF)-1 and IGF binding protein (IGFBP)-2 production by rat osteoblasts in vitro. Acta Endocrinol. 1992;126(5):467–73.
178. Schmid C, Schlapfer I, Keller A, Waldvogel M, Froesch ER, Zapf J. Effects of insulin-like growth factor (IGF) binding proteins (BPs) -3 and −6 on DNA synthesis of rat osteoblasts: further evidence for a role of auto-/paracrine IGF I but not IGF II in stimulating osteoblast growth. Biochem Biophys Res Commun. 1995;212(1):242–8.
179. Schneider DL, Barrett-Connor EL, Morton DJ. Thyroid hormone use and bone mineral density in elderly women. Effects of estrogen. J Am Med Assoc. 1994;271(16):1245–9.
180. Schneider DL, Barrett-Connor EL, Morton DJ. Thyroid hormone use and bone mineral density in elderly men. Arch Intern Med. 1995;155(18): 2005–7.

181. Sharma D, Fondell JD. Ordered recruitment of histone acetyltransferases and the TRAP/mediator complex to thyroid hormone-responsive promoters in vivo. Proc Natl Acad Sci USA. 2002;99(12):7934–9.
182. Shirazi M, Dehpour AR, Jafari F. The effect of thyroid hormone on orthodontic tooth movement in rats. J Clin Pediatr Dent. 1999;23(3):259–64.
183. Siddiqi A, Monson JP, Wood DF, Besser GM, Burrin JM. Serum cytokines in thyrotoxicosis. J Clin Endocrinol Metab. 1999;84(2):435–9.
184. Stall GM, Harris S, Sokoll LJ, Dawson-Hughes B. Accelerated bone loss in hypothyroid patients overtreated with L-thyroxine. Ann Intern Med. 1990;113(4):265–9.
185. Stepan JJ, Limanova Z. Biochemical assessment of bone loss in patients on long-term thyroid hormone treatment. Bone Miner. 1992;17(3):377–88.
186. Stevens DA, Harvey CB, Scott AJ, O'Shea PJ, Barnard JC, Williams AJ, Brady G, Samarut J, Chassande O, Williams GR. Thyroid hormone activates fibroblast growth factor receptor-1 in bone. Mol Endocrinol. 2003;17(9):1751–66.
187. Stevens DA, Hasserjian RP, Robson H, Siebler T, Shalet SM, Williams GR. Thyroid hormones regulate hypertrophic chondrocyte differentiation and expression of parathyroid hormone-related peptide and its receptor during endochondral bone formation. J Bone Miner Res. 2000;15(12):2431–42.
188. Stracke H, Rossol S, Schatz H. Alkaline phosphatase and insulin-like growth factor in fetal rat bone under the influence of thyroid hormones. Horm Metab Res. 1986;18(11):794.
189. Suwanwalaikorn S, Ongphiphadhanakul B, Braverman LE, Baran DT. Differential responses of femoral and vertebral bones to long-term excessive L-thyroxine administration in adult rats. Eur J Endocrinol. 1996;134(5):655–9.
190. Suwanwalaikorn S, Van Auken M, Kang MI, Alex S, Braverman LE, Baran DT. Site selectivity of osteoblast gene expression response to thyroid hormone localized by in situ hybridization. Am J Physiol. 1997;272(2 Pt 1):E212–7.
191. Taelman P, Kaufman JM, Janssens X, Vandecauter H, Vermeulen A. Reduced forearm bone mineral content and biochemical evidence of increased bone turnover in women with euthyroid goitre treated with thyroid hormone. Clin Endocrinol (Oxf). 1990;33(1):107–17.
192. Tarjan G, Stern PH. Triiodothyronine potentiates the stimulatory effects of interleukin-1 beta on bone resorption and medium interleukin-6 content in fetal rat limb bone cultures. J Bone Miner Res. 1995;10(9):1321–6.
193. Toh SH, Brown PH. Bone mineral content in hypothyroid male patients with hormone replacement: a 3-year study. J Bone Miner Res. 1990;5(5):463–7.
194. Tokuda H, Kozawa O, Harada A, Isobe KI, Uematsu T. Triiodothyronine modulates interleukin-6 synthesis in osteoblasts: inhibitions in protein kinase A and C pathways. Endocrinology. 1998;139(3):1300–5.
195. Torchia J, Glass C, Rosenfeld MG. Co-activators and co-repressors in the integration of transcriptional responses. Curr Opin Cell Biol. 1998;10(3):373–83.
196. Tumer L, Hasanoglu A, Cinaz P, Bideci A. Bone mineral density and metabolism in children treated with L-thyroxine. J Pediatr Endocrinol Metab. 1999;12(4):519–23.
197. Uzzan B, Campos J, Cucherat M, Nony P, Boissel JP, Perret GY. Effects on bone mass of long term treatment with thyroid hormones: a meta-analysis. J Clin Endocrinol Metab. 1996;81(12):4278–89.
198. Van Vliet G. Neonatal hypothyroidism: treatment and outcome. Thyroid. 1999;9(1):79–84.
199. Varga F, Luegmayr E, Fratzl-Zelman N, Glantschnig H, Ellinger A, Prinz D, Rumpler M, Klaushofer K. Tri-iodothyronine inhibits multilayer formation of the osteoblastic cell line, MC3T3-E1, by promoting apoptosis. J Endocrinol. 1999;160(1):57–65.
200. Varga F, Rumpler M, Klaushofer K. Thyroid hormones increase insulin-like growth factor mRNA levels in the clonal osteoblastic cell line MC3T3-E1. FEBS Lett. 1994;345(1):67–70.
201. Varga F, Rumpler M, Luegmayr E, Fratzl-Zelman N, Glantschnig H, Klaushofer K. Triiodothyronine, a regulator of osteoblastic differentiation: depression of histone H4, attenuation of c-fos/c-jun, and induction of osteocalcin expression. Calcif Tissue Int. 1997;61(5):404–11.
202. Varga F, Rumpler M, Spitzer S, Karlic H, Klaushofer K. Osteocalcin attenuates T3- and increases vitamin D3-induced expression of MMP-13 in mouse osteoblasts. Endocr J. 2009;56(3):441–50.
203. Varga F, Rumpler M, Zoehrer R, Turecek C, Spitzer S, Thaler R, Paschalis EP, Klaushofer K. T3 affects expression of collagen I and collagen cross-linking in bone cell cultures. Biochem Biophys Res Commun. 2010;402(2):180–5.
204. Varga F, Spitzer S, Klaushofer K. Triiodothyronine (T3) and 1,25-dihydroxyvitamin D3 (1,25D3) inversely regulate OPG gene expression in dependence of the osteoblastic phenotype. Calcif Tissue Int. 2004;74(4):382–7.
205. Verrotti A, Greco R, Altobelli E, Morgese G, Chiarelli F. Bone metabolism in children with congenital hypothyroidism – a longitudinal study. J Pediatr Endocrinol Metab. 1998;11(6):699–705.
206. Vestergaard P, Rejnmark L, Weeke J, Mosekilde L. Fracture risk in patients treated for hyperthyroidism. Thyroid. 2000;10(4):341–8.
207. Von Recklinghausen F. Die Fibrose oder deformierende Ostitis, die Osteomalazie und die osteoplasticsche Karcinose in ihre gegenseitigen Bezeihungen. Festschrift Rundolf Virchow. Berlin: G Reimer; 1891;1–89.
208. Wallace H, Pate A, Bishop JO. Effects of perinatal thyroid hormone deprivation on the growth and behaviour of newborn mice. J Endocrinol. 1995;145(2):251–62.

209. Wang L, Shao YY, Ballock RT. Thyroid hormone interacts with the Wnt/beta-catenin signaling pathway in the terminal differentiation of growth plate chondrocytes. J Bone Miner Res. 2007;22(12):1988–95.
210. Wang L, Shao YY, Ballock RT. Carboxypeptidase Z (CPZ) links thyroid hormone and Wnt signaling pathways in growth plate chondrocytes. J Bone Miner Res. 2009;24(2):265–73.
211. Williams AJ, Robson H, Kester MH, van Leeuwen JP, Shalet SM, Visser TJ, Williams GR. Iodothyronine deiodinase enzyme activities in bone. Bone. 2008;43(1):126–34.
212. Williams GR, Bland R, Sheppard MC. Characterization of thyroid hormone (T3) receptors in three osteosarcoma cell lines of distinct osteoblast phenotype: interactions among T3, vitamin D3, and retinoid signaling. Endocrinology. 1994;135(6):2375–85.
213. Williams GR, Bland R, Sheppard MC. Retinoids modify regulation of endogenous gene expression by vitamin D3 and thyroid hormone in three osteosarcoma cell lines. Endocrinology. 1995;136(10):4304–14.
214. Yamaura M, Nakamura T, Kanou A, Miura T, Ohara H, Suzuki K. The effect of 17 beta-estradiol treatment on the mass and the turnover of bone in ovariectomized rats taking a mild dose of thyroxin. Bone Miner. 1994;24(1):33–42.
215. Yehuda-Shnaidman E, Kalderon B, Azazmeh N, Bar-Tana J. Gating of the mitochondrial permeability transition pore by thyroid hormone. FASEB J. 2010;24(1):93–104.
216. Yen PM, Ando S, Feng X, Liu Y, Maruvada P, Xia X. Thyroid hormone action at the cellular, genomic and target gene levels. Mol Cell Endocrinol. 2006;246(1–2):121–7.
217. Zaidi M, Iqbal J, Blair HC, Zallone A, Davies T, Sun L. Paradigm shift in the pathophysiology of postmenopausal and thyrotoxic osteoporosis. Mt Sinai J Med. 2009;76(5):474–83.
218. Zeni S, Gomez-Acotto C, Di Gregorio S, Mautalen C. Differences in bone turnover and skeletal response to thyroid hormone treatment between estrogen-depleted and repleted rats. Calcif Tissue Int. 2000;67(2):173–7.

Pituitary Hormones and the Pathophysiology of Osteoporosis

5

Manasi Agrawal, Shitij Arora, Graziana Colaianni, Li Sun, Jameel Z. Iqbal, and Mone Zaidi

Keywords
Growth hormone • Insulin-like growth factors • Follicle-stimulating hormone • Thyroid-stimulating hormone • Oxytocin • Prolactin • Bone

M. Agrawal, M.B.B.S.
Internal Medicine, Maimonides Medical Center, 4802, 10th Avenue, Brooklyn, NY 11201, USA

S. Arora, M.D.
Internal Medicine, Wyckoff Heights Medical Center, 374 Stockholm Street, Brooklyn, NY 11237, USA
e-mail: drshitij@yahoo.com

G. Colaianni, Ph.D.
The Mount Sinai Bone Program, Mount Sinai School of Medicine, One Gustave Levy Place, New York, NY 10029, USA

L. Sun, M.D., Ph.D.
The Mount Sinai Bone Program, Mount Sinai School of Medicine, One Gustave L. Levy Place, New York, NY 10029, USA

J.Z. Iqbal, M.D., Ph.D.
Department of Pathology and Lab Medicine, University of Pennsylvania, 3400 Spruce Street, Philadelphia, PA 19104, USA

M. Zaidi, M.D., Ph.D., F.RC.P. (✉)
The Mount Sinai Bone Program, Department of Medicine, Mount Sinai School of Medicine, One Gustave L. Levy Place, New York, NY 10029, USA
e-mail: mone.zaidi@mountsinai.org

5.1 Introduction

Pituitary hormones orchestrate the structure and function of various organ systems in the body. A specific, limited function is ascribed to each pituitary hormone. We have come to appreciate that pituitary hormones have profound effects on bone, so much so that the "pituitary-bone axis" is now understood to be integral to skeletal biology. All pituitary hormones play a part in bone regulation, including growth hormone (GH), follicle-stimulating hormone (FSH), thyroid-stimulating hormone (TSH), adrenocorticotropic hormone (ACTH), prolactin and oxytocin. In mice, reduction in hormone levels due to haploinsufficiency for any one of several pituitary hormones or their receptors alters bone dynamics, while the "primary" target organ remains unaffected. This finding indicates that bone is the more sensitive organ. An in-depth insight into the mechanism of action of each hormone gives us a better understanding of bone pathophysiology and opens up new avenues for treatment of osteoporosis. In this chapter, we discuss the interaction of each pituitary hormone with bone and the potential that targeting these interactions holds in management of osteoporosis.

F. Bronner et al. (eds.), *Bone-Metabolic Functions and Modulators*, Topics in Bone Biology,
DOI 10.1007/978-1-4471-2745-1_5,

5.2 Growth Hormone Action on Bone Occurs Primarily Through IGFs

Growth hormone (GH), a single-chain polypeptide of 191 amino acids in humans, secreted by the anterior pituitary, plays a vital role in skeletal homeostasis. The direct effects of GH on bone are mediated through the GH receptor, a member of the G-protein-coupled receptor family. Importantly, GH acts in close collaboration with insulin-like growth factors (IGFs) and other modulators. IGFs are a group of growth-promoting polypeptides with endocrine, paracrine, and autocrine actions. The IGFs, including IGF1 and IGF2, are single-chain polypeptides, which, despite sharing a similar secondary structure, have independent and different signaling outcomes. The predominant IGF, IGF-1, is synthesized mainly in the liver, and the majority of it (70–80%) circulates bound to IGF binding protein-3 (IGFBP3) and acid labile subunit (ALS) into a ternary structure, which prevents its degradation, prolongs its half-life, and modulates its endocrine actions. IGF-1 is also expressed by skeletal and other tissues where it has an autocrine function [101].

Most of GH-mediated effects on the skeleton are thought to occur indirectly through IGF-1. A study on bitransgenic mice with both GHR deletion and overexpression of IGF-1 demonstrated that the growth retardation and loss of skeletal strength seen in GHR null mice are restored with IGF-1 overexpression [19]. Similarly, the effects of GH on increasing the bone mineralizing perimeter (an index of osteoblastic activity) appear to be mediated through the IGF-1 pathway via parathyroid hormone (PTH) [78]; locally acting IGF-1 uses PTH to mediate its anabolic effects [95]. Nonetheless, GH does have effects on bone that are exclusive of IGF-1. GH replacement can reverse the increased adiposity in hypophysectomized rats, while IGF-1 replacement cannot. These findings suggest that this effect is probably a direct function of GH that is mediated through the GHR [60].

A relevant consideration in GH treatment is protein intake. Rats with a low protein intake show decreases in bone mass, density, and strength on GH treatment, in contrast to rats with a normal protein intake that display increases in bone mass, with both groups having an intact IGF-1 response [6]. This observation calls for caution in using GH therapy, especially in the malnourished and the elderly who may have low protein in their diets.

5.3 Circulating IGF-1 Is Needed for Bone Growth, While Autocrine IGF-1 Regulates Bone Homeostasis

The genetic deletion of IGF-1 complex components has helped assign specific roles to these factors. Liver IGF-1-deficient (LID) mice show a 75% reduction in IGF-1, but display normal growth and development [100]. ALS knockout (ALSKO) mice show a reduction in serum IGF-1 and IGFBP levels due to increased degradation; these mice, however, have only a slight reduction in body weight [92]. In a combined knockout (KO) mouse model (LID+ALSKO), serum IGF-1 is significantly reduced, while GH is markedly elevated because of the absence of negative feedback. In this model, linear growth and bone strength both are dramatically retarded [101]. In all three mouse models, skeletal IGF-1 levels were comparable, suggesting that it is the circulating IGF-1 that plays a vital role in the acquisition of peak bone mass. Also, it appears that a threshold level of serum IGF-1 is required for adequate bone formation, and only when it is lower than this level does peak bone density become affected, as occurs in the double KO mice [101].

Various inbred strains of mice that have variable allelic expression in the quantitative trait loci (QTL) on chromosome 6 exhibit differences in IGF-1 expression and femoral bone mineral density (BMD) [74]. Human studies further corroborate the evidence; lower circulating IGF-1 is associated with lower BMD [45] and higher fracture risk [30]. A cross-sectional study has demonstrated recently that once skeletal maturity is reached, an association between declining serum IGF-1 and increased levels of bone turnover markers becomes evident, even in premenopausal women [2]. Whether this association is causal or not has yet to be determined.

It appears that circulating liver IGF-1 is a major determinant of skeletal growth during puberty, while autocrine and paracrine IGF-1 regulates skeletal growth during the prenatal and postnatal periods [33]. Mice with overexpression of liver IGF-1 have an increase in body size and skeletal strength [24]. Conversely, mice with genetic deletion of skeletal IGF-1 and overexpression of liver IGF-1 demonstrate early retardation of skeletal expansion. These mice catch up growth during puberty, with restoration of both skeletal morphology and strength, mediated by liver IGF-1. These effects are mediated independently of GH levels, as they remained unaffected in all of these mice models. The observations underscore the distinctive roles of local and circulating IGF-1 in accelerating skeletal growth during both early and pubertal periods, respectively. Elevated levels of circulating IGF-1 can compensate for early growth deficit.

Global deletion of IGF-1 leads to marked osteopenia [86], while overexpression of the same factor in mouse osteoblasts accelerates bone formation [104]. Also, serum IGF-1 regulates subperiosteal expansion and mineralized cortical tissue deposition through its dual effects on osteoblasts and osteoclasts [99]. Based on these findings, it appears that IGF-1 is integral in mediating the continuous remodeling in the skeleton in response to mechanical load and stress.

Interestingly, in ovariectomized LID mice, the sensitivity to GH increases, and administration of GH can reverse osteopenia [27]. In older women with depleted levels of estrogen and IGF-1, GH rescues the skeleton from osteoporotic bone loss. Pregnancy-associated plasma protein-A (PAPP-A) is anabolic and promotes fetal skeleton growth and strength during pregnancy [91]. PAPP-A's effects are mediated indirectly through IGFs, as PAPP-A increases their bioavailability [70].

GH also increases osteoclastic activity by stimulating local IGF-1 production by bone marrow stromal cells [35]. IGF-1, in turn, acts to promote bone resorption. Osteoclasts possess IGF-1 receptors, as has been seen in rabbit models [38]; these receptors mediate the direct effects of IGF-1. Receptor activator for NF-κB ligand (RANKL) and osteoprotegerin (OPG) are secreted by stromal osteoblasts. RANKL stimulates osteoclastogenesis by binding with RANK, while OPG prevents this action [65]. IGF-1 alters the RANKL/OPG ratio [76] in favor of osteoclastogenesis. IGF-1 decreases the synthesis of OPG in a dose- and time-dependent manner, a regulation that occurs at the transcriptional level; in contrast, IGF-1 increases the expression of RANKL [76]. Similar results have been noted in vivo [76]; OPG decreases on rhIGF-1 treatment and remains unaffected with rhGH treatment.

Both GH and IGF-1 thus stimulate bone formation and resorption, thereby increasing bone turnover [93]. Short-term treatment with GH in postmenopausal women and in the elderly elevates IGF-1 along with bone resorption markers [13]. Treatment with IGF-1 in normal women results in both bone formation and resorption, with the effect on bone formation being predominant [22].

5.4 Elevations in FSH Cause Bone Loss

Follicle-stimulating hormone (FSH) has traditionally been identified with ovarian folliculogenesis and estrogen production. However, we now believe that the late perimenopausal and early postmenopausal spike in FSH stimulates osteoclastogenesis and bone resorption. During the late perimenopause, even before estrogen has declined, FSH levels rise. Accompanying this rise, there occur a sharp elevation in the markers of bone resorption [83] and an increase in trabecular perforation [3] that weakens bone and increases fracture risk. Approximately half of the bone loss in woman's lifetime occurs within the first five years of menopause. Interestingly, much of this loss occurs before significant estrogen decline [71].

Independent of the species studied, mouse or human, FSH stimulates osteoclast formation from its precursors in the presence of RANKL through the $G_{i2\alpha}$-coupled FSH receptor (FSHR),

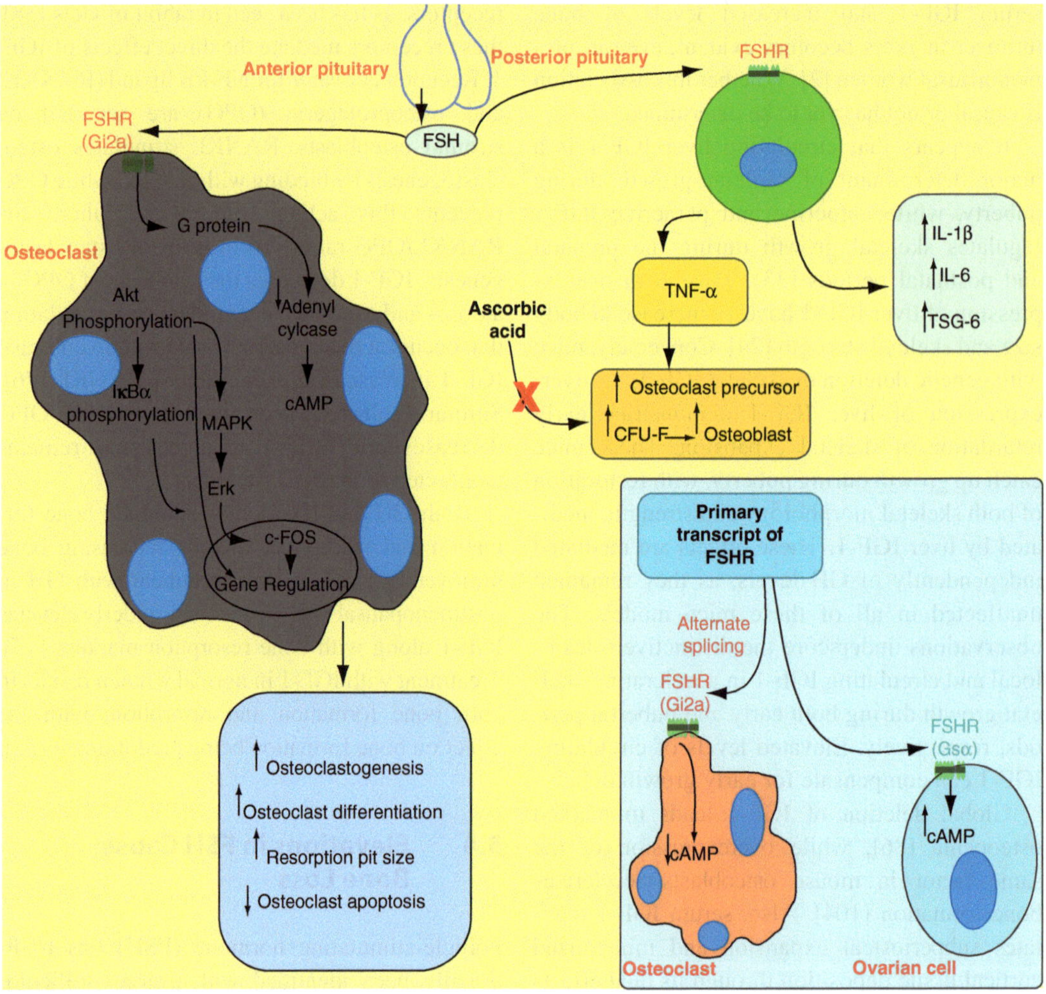

Fig. 5.1 The action of follicle-stimulating hormone (FSH) on bone. *FSHR* follicle-stimulating hormone receptor, *cAMP* cyclic adenosine monophosphate, *MAPK* mitogen-activated protein kinase, *ERK* extracellular signal regulated kinase, *IκBα* nuclear factor of kappa light polypeptide gene enhancer in B cells inhibitor alpha, *TNF-α* tumor necrosis factor α, *IL-1β* interleukin-1β, *TSG-6* tumor necrosis factor-inducible gene 6 protein, *CFU-F* colony-forming unit-fibroblast

present on both osteoclast precursors and osteoclasts [87, 97]. FSHR activation enhances the phosphorylation of downstream RANKL sensitive kinases, Erk (extracellular signal-regulated kinases) and Akt, as well as IκBα, an inhibitor of NF-κB; all these pathways are known to transduce the proresorptive actions of RANKL [87]. Figure 5.1 illustrates the actions of FSH on bone metabolism.

Haploinsufficiency in FSHβ heterozygotic mice reduces FSH levels and results in a high bone mass; this is true even though these heterozygotic animals have normal gonadal function and estrogen levels. The high bone mass phenotype is due to a decrease in bone resorption, evident by histomorphometric features of tissues and activity measurements in ex vivo cultures of bone marrow cells. FSHβ$^{-/-}$ and FSHR$^{-/-}$ mice do not show bone loss despite being severely hypogonadal [87]. Part of this protective effect is exerted through mild hyperandrogenemia [29]. However, aromatase null mice that display equivalent hyperandrogenemia lose bone profusely and have high FSH levels; this suggests that it is the absence of FSH that is, at least in part, protective against bone loss.

FSH also stimulates monocytes to produce interleukin (IL)-1β, which, in turn, mobilizes osteoclasts for bone resorption [14]. Furthermore, FSH stimulates the production of TNF-α from the bone marrow precursor macrophages [40]. Polymorphisms in the FSHR gene in humans are associated with bone loss. Women with the single nucleotide polymorphism (SNP) AA rs6166 have a significantly higher incidence of osteoporosis than those with the GG rs6166 allele, even with comparable circulating levels of FSH and estrogen [72].

There is a strong positive correlation between basal FSH and markers of bone remodeling [83]. Changes in FSH levels over four years can predict changes in bone mass [84]. Women with amenorrhea having a higher serum FSH have more significant bone loss compared to those with lower serum FSH, even when estrogen levels are similar [20]. Also, bone loss is highest during 2–3 years before and after the final menstrual period when with serum FSH > 34 mIU/mL [85]. The above evidence suggests causality between FSH and bone resorption.

Besides the spine and long bones, a connection between FSH and other diseases involving bone loss has been noted. For example, FSH aggravates periodontitis-associated alveolar bone loss in ovariectomized rats [47], and treatment with leuprolide, an inhibitor of FSH release, is protective [48]. Another cross-sectional analysis suggests that long-term cadmium exposure is associated with elevated FSH and lower BMD in perimenopausal women [28]. Although this study does not determine causality, it does strengthen the negative correlation between FSH and BMD.

5.5 Clinical Relevance of the FSH-Bone Axis

Knowing that a significant amount of bone loss occurs during late perimenopause, we can prevent and treat menopausal osteoporosis more effectively. Women can be screened earlier for bone loss, and those requiring more aggressive treatment can be identified. The diagnosis of osteoporosis is traditionally made through the measurement of T-scores, which compare the patient's BMD, a measure of bone mineral content across a given area, against a database of young, 30-year-old Caucasian women [62]. The microarchitectural deterioration caused likely in part, by FSH during late perimenopause, in the form of trabecular perforations [3], may not decrease the T-score significantly enough to fall into the osteoporotic range. However, it does decrease the bone strength [50]. Hence, although the BMD may be normal, bone fragility increases and mostly escapes detection. This discrepancy points toward the need to develop and use other screening methods besides BMD that have higher accuracy for detecting skeletal deterioration.

Markers of bone resorption, such as urinary N-telopeptide and serum C-telopeptide, are measures of osteoclastic activity. Both markers can be used to detect bone loss. These markers assume even greater clinical relevance during perimenopause and early menopause when BMD is normal or near normal. In one study, urinary N-telopeptide levels were found to be 19% higher in perimenopausal than in postmenopausal women [21]. Similarly, high osteocalcin levels (a marker of bone formation that rises in tandem with resorption) predicted severe and diffuse bone loss across the perimenopause [15]. An increase of one standard deviation (SD) in N-telopeptide and in osteocalcin levels increases the probability by 2.1% of losing spinal BMD, the most commonly affected site during early menopause [73]. The Study of Women's Health Across the Nation (SWAN) also showed cross-sectional positive correlations between N-telopeptide and serum FSH levels [83, 84].

The final menstrual period is determined retrospectively, after a year of amenorrhea, by which time, substantial and largely irreversible bone resorption has already occurred. Sowers et al. have categorized the lifetime pattern of FSH variation into four distinct stages; by their criteria, maximal bone resorption occurs during stage 3, a time when FSH levels shoot up [85]. In an endeavor to improve early diagnosis and more timely management, measuring serum FSH over time can predict the transition into stage 3 and the onset of significant bone loss in transmenopausal women.

An important issue concerns the time that is right to start treatment for osteoporosis. Is it when significant bone loss has occurred or earlier? Is it before bone loss becomes significant? Should the therapy be aimed at prevention? Further studies are needed to elucidate the possible benefits of new diagnostic and therapeutic protocols for preventative osteoporosis management.

5.6 TSH: The Bone-Suppressing Hormone

Thyroid-stimulating hormone (TSH) has been thought to solely regulate thyroid follicular growth and thyroid hormone secretion [64]. In vitro and organ culture studies have shown that thyroid hormones are proresorptive due to an imbalance between bone formation and resorption, in part, mediated by TNF-α and IL-6 [42]. The high-turnover osteoporosis and hip fractures in hyperthyroidism and Graves' disease have been attributed solely to elevated thyroid hormones [75, 96]. Interestingly, however, the therapeutic suppression of TSH or subclinical hyperthyroidism, in which TSH is low and thyroid hormones are normal, are both associated with equally profound osteoporosis and a high fracture risk, prominently at the hip, suggesting an bone protective action of TSH [9].

On the other hand, thyroid hormones stimulate osteoblasts directly and play an important role in bone formation during growth and development [41] probably mediated through IGF-1. Both mice and humans, when hypothyroid, show a common phenotype characterized by skeletal runting. Thyrotoxicosis can increase intrauterine skeletal growth and premature ossification postnatally in mice bearing a knock-in thyroid hormone receptor β gene (TRβPV), simulating juvenile human hyperthyroidism [10]. Thyroid hormones thus have a dual action on the skeleton: they are a necessary anabolic stimulus during growth and development, but promote bone resorption in the mature skeleton [5].

Some of the skeletal morphology in thyroid dysfunction cannot, however, be explained by thyroid hormones alone. First, mice deficient in both α1 and β thyroid receptors have skeletal runting, rather than defects in bone remodeling [32]. Second, patients with subclinical hyperthyroidism with normal thyroid hormones and elevated TSH display high-turnover osteoporosis. Third, fracture risk and BMD have a strong correlation with serum levels of TSH, but not particularly with thyroid hormones [11, 63].

TSH appears to be a direct inhibitor of osteoblast and osteoclast activity [1]. Haploinsufficiency of TSHR in heterozygotic mice results in a high-turnover osteoporosis phenotype, while the thyroid hormone profile remains unaffected [69]. $TSHR^{-/-}$ mice are osteoporotic. This bone loss cannot be explained by the proosteoclastic action of thyroid hormones; on the contrary, they are deficient. On thyroid hormone replacement, skeletal runting is reversed, but not the osteoporotic changes. This suggests that TSH acts on bone independently of thyroid hormones and that the osteoporosis of hyperthyroidism may, at least in part, be due to low TSH [105].

$TSHR^{-/-}$ mice show evidence of increased osteoclastic activity, as do hyt/hyt mice, which have defective TSHR signaling [12, 88]. Studies also show that recombinant TSH attenuates the genesis, function, and survival of osteoclasts in vitro [1]. Likewise, overexpression of constitutively activated TSHR in osteoclast precursor RAW-C3 cells [62] or transgenically in mouse precursors [88] inhibits osteoclastogenesis.

The antiosteoclastogenic action of TSH is mediated by a reduction in NF-κB and JNK signaling and in TNF-α production [1, 36]. It has been demonstrated that the effect of TSH on TNF-α synthesis is mediated transcriptionally by binding of two high mobility group box proteins, HMGB1 and HMGB2, to the promoter of the TNF-α gene [102].

As expected, TNF-α production is upregulated in $TSHR^{-/-}$ mice, which increases osteoclastic activity and contributes to the osteopenic phenotype [1]. To further corroborate these findings, the genetic deletion of TNF-α in $TSHR^{-/-}$ mice was studied, and bone resorption was found to be reversed [36]. Recently, it was demonstrated that TSH inhibits osteoclastogenesis in murine stem cells, suggesting it plays a role early in bone [53].

The role of TSH is osteoblast regulation is less explicit, except that TSHR deficiency is associated with increased osteoblastogenesis and expression of low-density lipoprotein receptor-like protein-5 and Flk-1 proteins. Although administration of recombinant TSH inhibits the expression of these receptors, it does not alter that of Osterix or Runx-2, two key osteoblastic transcription factors [1]. On the whole, there is data suggesting that TSH inhibits both osteoblast and osteoclast function, and that its deficiency contributes to high-turnover osteoporosis irrespective of the thyroid hormone status.

As opposed to its catabolic effects likely exerted at a constant high level, intermittently administered TSH appears to be anabolic [77]. In rats, TSH injected thrice a week inhibits and reverses ovariectomy-induced bone loss. These effects are mediated by a direct anabolic action of intermittent TSH, as demonstrated by calcein-labeled bone apposition rates [77].

In postmenopausal women, a single subcutaneous injection of recombinant human TSH lowers serum C-telopeptide to premenopausal levels within two days, with recovery at day 7 [58]. In none of the studies with TSH replacement did thyroid hormone levels increase, exemplifying the notion that the pituitary-bone axis is more primitive than the pituitary-thyroid axis.

Recombinant TSH in clinical studies shows a reduction in serum C-telopeptide levels [58], although the effect on serum RANKL and OPG is less clear. In a study by Giusti et al. [31], there was no alteration in these cytokines in response to recombinant TSH in patients receiving L-thyroxine for differentiated thyroid carcinoma. Martini et al. [56], however, demonstrated an increase in RANKL levels following an increase in type 1 procollagen N-terminal propeptide (PINP), a marker of bone formation. This validates the conclusion drawn from previous studies that a bolus dose of TSH is anabolic [77].

5.7 Clinical Relevance of the TSH-Bone Axis

A decline in serum TSH levels predisposes to increased bone resorption, an association fortified by clinical data. There is a 4.5-fold increase in the risk of vertebral fractures and 3.2-fold increase in the risk of nonvertebral fractures when serum TSH falls below 0.1 IU/L [11]. Another study showed a strong negative correlation between serum TSH and C-telopeptide in postmenopausal women; there was no correlation between thyroid hormone levels and markers of bone resorption [106]. In patients receiving L-thyroxine treatment for thyroid disease, there is a significantly greater bone loss in those with suppressed TSH than those with no suppression [8]. The Tromso study reported that participants with serum TSH levels below 2 SD had a significantly lower BMD, those with TSH levels above 2 SD had a significantly increased BMD, while there was no association between TSH levels and BMD at normal TSH levels [34]. In patients taking suppressive doses of L-thyroxine for thyroid cancer, the serum level of cathepsin K, a surrogate but yet unvalidated marker for bone resorption, was elevated [61]. The second Nord-Trøndelag Health Study (HUNT) assessed the association between TSH and BMD and found a positive correlation, stronger at the distal than at the ultradistal forearm. This is expected as the distal site has predominantly cortical bone, compared to the ultradistal site, which is more sensitive to a low TSH [89].

In an elaborate epidemiologic study using data from the third US National Health and Nutrition Examination Survey, the odds ratio for correlations between serum TSH and bone mass was in the range of 2–3.4. The correlation was especially strong between increasing serum TSH within the reference range and increasing bone mass in both Caucasian and African-American women [63]. In patients receiving L-thyroxine therapy, serum TSH and bone microarchitecture (using heel ultrasound measurements) showed no statistically significant association [66].

Another prospective study showed that euthyroid women with serum TSH in the lower tertile of the normal range had a higher incidence of vertebral fractures, independent of age, BMD, and thyroid hormones [57]. The strongest evidence in support of a causal association between TSH and bone mass regulation comes from studying TSH receptor polymorphisms. Patients with the TSHR-D727E polymorphism have a high bone mass, demonstrated after correcting for body weight [37]. The same allelic association is reported in postmenopausal women from the United Kingdom and in the Rotterdam study [4]. Another polymorphism, T + 140974TC, seen in the Korean population, is associated with increased BMD at the lumbar vertebrae and femoral necks, more so in patient groups with elevated TSH, substantiating the role of TSH in protecting against bone loss [94].

5.8 Oxytocin Is a Bone Anabolic Hormone

Oxytocin (OT) is a nine amino acids peptide synthesized in the hypothalamus, released into circulation by the posterior pituitary [103]. Its primary function is to mediate the milk ejection reflex in nursing mammals. It also stimulates uterine contraction during parturition; however, it is not absolutely required for this to occur. OT null mice deliver pups normally, but are unable to nurse. This phenotype is completely reversed upon subcutaneous OT administration, attesting to this being a peripheral, as opposed to a central action [68].

OT also regulates social behavior, including both sexual and maternal behavior, affiliation, social memory, and penile erection and ejaculation in males [7]. OT controls food, predominantly carbohydrate, intake [79]. These actions appear to be centrally mediated as social amnesia, aggressive behavior, and overfeeding observed in $OT^{-/-}$, and $Oxtr^{-/-}$ mice are reversed on intracerebroventricular OT injection [25]. Hence, OT has both central and hormonally mediated peripheral actions.

There has been considerable interest in the role of OT in bone regulation, and it has been determined that OT is anabolic in both sexes in basal physiological conditions and contributes to skeletal homeostasis [90], to maternal bone remodeling during pregnancy [68], and to fetal trabecular growth and maturation [49]. It has a potential role in osteoporosis management.

The oxytocin receptor (Oxtr), a G-protein-coupled receptor, is present on osteoblasts [17], osteoclasts, and their precursors [16]. These receptors are present in large loci on the mature multinucleate osteoclasts and homogenously in smaller numbers on preosteoclasts, suggesting that the expression of the receptor depends on the level of osteoclast maturation. Furthermore, the Oxtr is functional and its activation causes a rise in intracellular Ca^{2+} in presence of OT [16].

In vivo, OT stimulates osteoblast proliferation and bone formation with no discernable effect on osteoclasts. $OT^{-/-}$ or $Oxtr^{-/-}$ mice demonstrate severe osteoporosis. Mice haploinsufficient for OT also display bone loss, while lactation and weight remain unaffected [90]. This phenotype indicates the exquisite sensitivity of bone to OT, again emphasizing the more primitive pituitary-bone axis. Ex vivo, OT has a dual action on osteoclasts, increasing their number while decreasing the activity of mature osteoclasts.

That the skeletal actions of OT are mediated peripherally is proven by reversal of bone loss upon intraperitoneal injection, whereupon there is a significant increase in BMD and osteoblast formation [90]. Another study demonstrated that OT injections in wild-type rats altered the RANKL/OPG ratio in favor of bone formation, attesting to the anabolic action of OT in this scenario [23].

OT appears to have an indispensible role in bone homeostasis during pregnancy and lactation. Accelerated bone resorption occurs during pregnancy and lactation, with the loss of up to 80 g of calcium displaced toward fetal bone growth [98]. This bone loss is completely reversed on weaning by a yet unidentified mechanism [82]. OT peaks in blood during late pregnancy and lactation, coinciding with the period of maximum fetal skeletogenesis and maternal bone loss. OT seems to assist in intergenerational calcium transfer, enhancing maternal bone resorption to mobilize calcium toward fetal bone growth. At the same time, it appears to prevent excessive bone loss in the mother postlactation and helps recovery of bone mass.

Bone marrow cultures from pregnant wild-type mice demonstrated accelerated osteoclastogenesis and a near doubling of plasma C-telopeptide, a marker of bone resorption, with a strong temporal association [49]. These changes have been reproduced by addition of OT to bone marrow

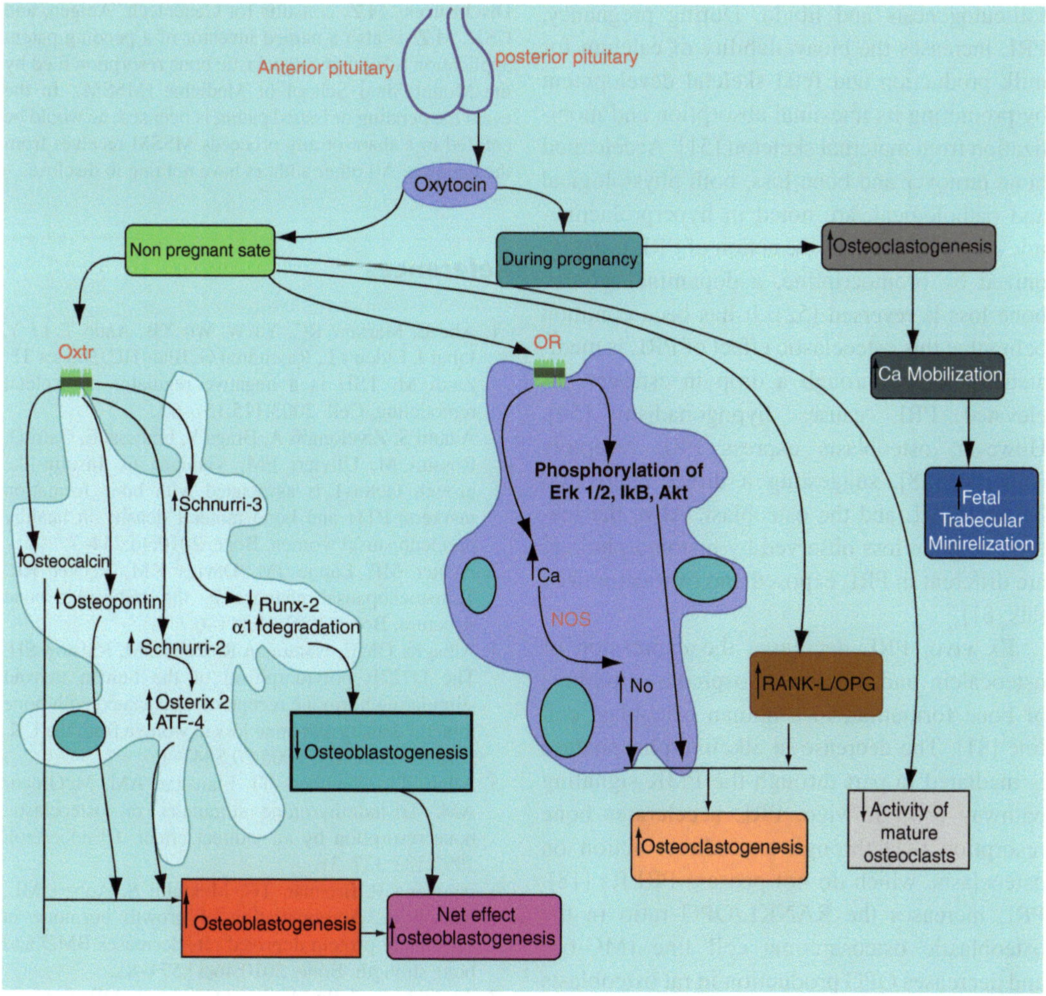

Fig. 5.2 The action of oxytocin on bone. *OXTR* oxytocin receptor, *ATF-4* activating transcription factor-4, *ERK* extracellular signal regulated kinase, *IκB* nuclear factor of kappa light polypeptide gene enhancer in B cells inhibitor, *Ca* calcium, *NOS* nitric oxide synthase, *NO* nitric oxide, *RANKL* receptor activator for nuclear factor kappa B cells ligand, *OPG* osteoprotegerin

cultures and intraperitoneal OT injection to mice. $OT^{-/-}$ and $OT^{+/-}$ mice have a drastic reduction in osteoclastogenesis, by up to 80% in homozygous OT null mice. This observation strongly suggests that bone homeostasis is dependent, at least in part, on an intact pituitary-bone axis, mediated by OT. The bone actions of OT are graphically demonstrated in Fig. 5.2.

OT null pups have increased trabecular numbers with hypomineralization, but no gross differences [49]. We thus conclude that OT is an integral, although not the only, stimulus for regulating maternal and fetal bone growth and can reverse pregnancy-and lactation-induced osteoporosis, at least in part. The safety of OT in humans is already documented.

5.9 Prolactin Has Contrasting Effects on Bone Depending on Age

Prolactin (PRL) is a peptide hormone secreted by the anterior pituitary. It primarily acts in females to induce and maintain lactation and prevent the occurrence of another pregnancy by suppressing folliculogenesis and libido. During pregnancy, PRL increases the bioavailability of calcium for milk production and fetal skeletal development by promoting its intestinal absorption and mobilization from maternal skeleton [51]. Accelerated bone turnover and bone loss, both physiological and pathological, are noted in hyperprolactinemic adults [67]. When the action of PRL is antagonized by bromocriptine, a dopamine agonist, bone loss is reversed [52]. It has been common belief that this osteoclastic effect of PRL is mediated indirectly through a drop in estrogen, as elevated PRL causes hypogonadism [59]. However, osteoblasts express PRL receptors (PRLRs) [18], suggesting a direct interaction between PRL and the osteoblast. Also, the features of bone loss observed by histomorphology are different in PRL exposed and ovariectomized rats [81].

Ex vivo, PRL decreases the expression of osteocalcin and alkaline phosphatase, markers of bone formation, in a human osteoblast cell line [81]. The decrease in alkaline phosphatase is mediated in part through the PI3K signaling pathway [80]. In vivo, PRL accelerates bone resorption [81] through an indirect action on osteoclasts, which do not possess PRLRs [18]. PRL increases the RANKL/OPG ratio in the osteoblastic osteosarcoma cell line (MG-63) and decreases OPG production in rat osteoblasts [81], hence constituting a putative mechanism of increased bone resorption. On the other hand, PRL causes net bone gain in infant rat [44] and increased osteocalcin expression and decreased RANKL/OPG ratio in human fetal osteoblast cells ex vivo [80].

It appears that the net effect of PLR on bone depends on the biological maturity of the organism. In the fetal stage, it promotes bone growth and mineralization while accelerating bone resorption in the mother to make available nutrients. Further insight is needed to clarify the role of PRL in bone metabolism and determine the cellular pathways.

Acknowledgments M.Z. is supported by grants from the National Institutes of Health. J.I. acknowledges the support of the American Federation for Aging Research.

Disclosures M.Z. consults for Genentech, Amgen, and GSK. M.Z. is also a named inventor of a pending patent application related to osteoclastic bone resorption filed by the Mount Sinai School of Medicine (MSSM). In the event the pending or issued patent is licensed, he would be entitled to a share of any proceeds MSSM receives from the licensee. All other authors have nothing to disclose.

References

1. Abe E, Marians RC, Yu W, Wu XB, Ando T, Li Y, Iqbal J, Eldeiry L, Rajendren G, Blair HC, Davies TF, Zaidi M. TSH is a negative regulator of skeletal remodeling. Cell. 2003;115:151–62.
2. Adami S, Zivelonghi A, Braga V, Fracassi E, Gatti D, Rossini M, Ulivieri FM, Viapiana O. Insulin-like growth factor-1 is associated with bone formation markers, PTH and bone mineral density in healthy premenopausal women. Bone. 2010;46:244–7.
3. Akhter MP, Lappe JM, Davies KM, Recker RR. Transmenopausal changes in the trabecular bone structure. Bone. 2007;41:111–6.
4. Albagha OME, Natarajan R, Reid DM, Ralston SH. The D727E polymorphism of the human thyroid stimulating hormone receptor is associated with bone mineral density and bone loss in women from the UK. J Bone Miner Res. 2005;20:S341–1.
5. Allain TJ, Chambers TJ, Flanagan AM, McGregor AM. Tri-iodothyronine stimulates rat osteoclastic bone resorption by an indirect effect. J Endocrinol. 1992;133:327–31.
6. Ammann P, Brennan TC, Mekraldi S, Aubert ML, Rizzoli R. Administration of growth hormone in selectively protein-deprived rats decreases BMD and bone strength. Bone. 2010;46(1):574–81.
7. Argiolas A, Collu M, Gessa GL, Melis MR, Serra G. The oxytocin antagonist d(CH2)5Tyr(Me)-Orn8-vasotocin inhibits male copulatory behaviour in rats. Eur J Pharmacol. 1988;149:389–92.
8. Baqi L, Payer J, Killinger Z, Susienkova K, Jackuliak P, Cierny D, Langer P. The level of TSH appeared favourable in maintaining bone mineral density in postmenopausal women. Endocr Regul. 2010;44:9–15.
9. Baran DT. Thyroid hormone and bone mass: the clinician's dilemma. Thyroid. 1994;4:143–4.
10. Bassett JH, Nordstrom K, Boyde A, Howell PG, Kelly S, Vennstrom B, Williams GR. Thyroid status during skeletal development determines adult bone structure and mineralization. Mol Endocrinol. 2007; 21:1893–904.
11. Bauer DC, Ettinger B, Nevitt MC, Stone KL. Risk for fracture in women with low serum levels of thyroid-stimulating hormone. Ann Intern Med. 2001;134:561–8.
12. Britto JM, Fenton AJ, Holloway WR, Nicholson GC. Osteoblasts mediate thyroid hormone stimulation of osteoclastic bone resorption. Endocrinology. 1994; 134:169–76.

13. Brixen K, Kassem M, Nielsen HK, Loft AG, Flyvbjerg A, Mosekilde L. Short-term treatment with growth hormone stimulates osteoblastic and osteoclastic activity in osteopenic postmenopausal women: a dose response study. J Bone Miner Res. 1995;10(1):865–74.
14. Cannon JG, Cortez-Cooper M, Meaders E, Stallings J, Haddow S, Kraj B, Sloan G, Mulloy A. Follicle-stimulating hormone, interleukin-1, and bone density in adult women. Am J Physiol Regul Integr Comp Physiol. 2010;298:R790–8.
15. Chapurlat RD, Garnero P, Sornay-Rendu E, Arlot ME, Claustrat B, Delmas PD. Longitudinal study of bone loss in pre- and perimenopausal women: evidence for bone loss in perimenopausal women. Osteoporos Int. 2000;11:493–8.
16. Colucci S, Colaianni G, Mori G, Grano M, Zallone A. Human osteoclasts express oxytocin receptor. Biochem Biophys Res Commun. 2002;297:442–5.
17. Copland JA, Ives KL, Simmons DJ, Soloff MS. Functional oxytocin receptors discovered in human osteoblasts. Endocrinology. 1999;140(4):371–4.
18. Coss D, Yang L, Kuo CB, Xu X, Luben RA, Walker AM. Effects of prolactin on osteoblast alkaline phosphatase and bone formation in the developing rat. Am J Physiol Endocrinol Metab. 2000;279:E1216–25.
19. De Jesus K, Wang X, Liu JL. A general IGF-I overexpression effectively rescued somatic growth and bone deficiency in mice caused by growth hormone receptor knockout. Growth Factors. 2009;27:438–47.
20. Devleta B, Adem B, Senada S. Hypergonadotropic amenorrhea and bone density: new approach to an old problem. J Bone Miner Metab. 2004;22:360–4.
21. Ebeling PR, Atley LM, Guthrie JR, Burger HG, Dennerstein L, Hopper JL, Wark JD. Bone turnover markers and bone density across the menopausal transition. J Clin Endocrinol Metab. 1996;81(3):366–71.
22. Ebeling PR, Jones JD, O'Fallon WM, Janes CH, Riggs BL. Short-term effects of recombinant human insulin-like growth factor I on bone turnover in normal women. J Clin Endocrinol Metab. 1993;77(1):384–7.
23. Elabd SK, Sabry I, Hassan WB, Nour H, Zaky K. Possible neuroendocrine role for oxytocin in bone remodeling. Endocr Regul. 2007;41:131–41.
24. Elis S, Courtland HW, Wu Y, Rosen CJ, Sun H, Jepsen KJ, Majeska RJ, Yakar S. Elevated serum levels of IGF-1 are sufficient to establish normal body size and skeletal properties even in the absence of tissue IGF-1. J Bone Miner Res. 2010;25(1):257–66.
25. Ferguson JN, Young LJ, Hearn EF, Matzuk MM, Insel TR, Winslow JT. Social amnesia in mice lacking the oxytocin gene. Nat Genet. 2000;25:284–8.
26. Flynn RW, Bonellie SR, Jung RT, MacDonald TM, Morris AD, Leese GP. Serum thyroid-stimulating hormone concentration and morbidity from cardiovascular disease and fractures in patients on long-term thyroxine therapy. J Clin Endocrinol Metab. 2010; 95:186–93.
27. Fritton JC, Emerton KB, Sun H, Kawashima Y, Mejia W, Wu Y, Rosen CJ, Panus D, Bouxsein M, Majeska RJ, Schaffler MB, Yakar S. Growth hormone protects against ovariectomy-induced bone loss in states of low circulating insulin-like growth factor (IGF-1). J Bone Miner Res. 2010;25:235–46.
28. Gallagher CM, Moonga BS, Kovach JS. Cadmium, follicle-stimulating hormone, and effects on bone in women age 42–60 years, NHANES III. Environ Res. 2010;110:105–11.
29. Gao J, Tiwari-Pandey R, Samadfam R, Yang Y, Miao D, Karaplis AC, Sairam MR, Goltzman D. Altered ovarian function affects skeletal homeostasis independent of the action of follicle-stimulating hormone. Endocrinology. 2007;148(2):613–21.
30. Garnero P, Sornay-Rendu E, Delmas PD. Low serum IGF-1 and occurrence of osteoporotic fractures in postmenopausal women. Lancet. 2000;355:898–9.
31. Giusti M, Cecoli F, Ghiara C, Rubinacci A, Villa I, Cavallero D, Mazzuoli L, Mussap M, Lanzi R, Minuto F. Recombinant human thyroid stimulating hormone does not acutely change serum osteoprotegerin and soluble receptor activator of nuclear factor-kappaBeta ligand in patients under evaluation for differentiated thyroid carcinoma. Hormones (Athens). 2007;6:304–13.
32. Gothe S, Wang Z, Ng L, Kindblom JM, Barros AC, Ohlsson C, Vennstrom B, Forrest D. Mice devoid of all known thyroid hormone receptors are viable but exhibit disorders of the pituitary-thyroid axis, growth, and bone maturation. Genes Dev. 1999;13(1):329–41.
33. Govoni KE, Wergedal JE, Florin L, Angel P, Baylink DJ, Mohan S. Conditional deletion of insulin-like growth factor-I in collagen type 1alpha2-expressing cells results in postnatal lethality and a dramatic reduction in bone accretion. Endocrinology. 2007;148(5):706–15.
34. Grimnes G, Emaus N, Joakimsen RM, Figenschau Y, Jorde R. The relationship between serum TSH and bone mineral density in men and postmenopausal women: the Tromso study. Thyroid. 2008;18(1):147–55.
35. Guicheux J, Heymann D, Rousselle AV, Gouin F, Pilet P, Yamada S, Daculsi G. Growth hormone stimulatory effects on osteoclastic resorption are partly mediated by insulin-like growth factor I: an in vitro study. Bone. 1998;22:25–31.
36. Hase H, Ando T, Eldeiry L, Brebene A, Peng Y, Liu L, Amano H, Davies TF, Sun L, Zaidi M, Abe E. TNFalpha mediates the skeletal effects of thyroid-stimulating hormone. Proc Natl Acad Sci USA. 2006;103:12849–54.
37. Heemstra KA, van der Deure WM, Peeters RP, Hamdy NA, Stokkel MP, Corssmit EP, Romijn JA, Visser TJ, Smit JW. Thyroid hormone independent associations between serum TSH levels and indicators of bone turnover in cured patients with differentiated thyroid carcinoma. Eur J Endocrinol. 2008;159:69–76.
38. Hou P, Sato T, Hofstetter W, Foged NT. Identification and characterization of the insulin-like growth factor I receptor in mature rabbit osteoclasts. J Bone Miner Res. 1997;12:534–40.

39. Insel TR, Harbaugh CR. Lesions of the hypothalamic paraventricular nucleus disrupt the initiation of maternal behavior. Physiol Behav. 1989;45(1):033–41.
40. Iqbal J, Sun L, Kumar TR, Blair HC, Zaidi M. Follicle-stimulating hormone stimulates TNF production from immune cells to enhance osteoblast and osteoclast formation. Proc Natl Acad Sci USA. 2006;103: 14925–30.
41. Ishikawa Y, Genge BR, Wuthier RE, Wu LN. Thyroid hormone inhibits growth and stimulates terminal differentiation of epiphyseal growth plate chondrocytes. J Bone Miner Res. 1998;13(1):398–411.
42. Kim CH, Kim HK, Shong YK, Lee KU, Kim GS. Thyroid hormone stimulates basal and interleukin (IL)-1-induced IL-6 production in human bone marrow stromal cells: a possible mediator of thyroid hormone-induced bone loss. J Endocrinol. 1999;160: 97–102.
43. Kindblom JM, Gevers EF, Skrtic SM, Lindberg MK, Gothe S, Tornell J, Vennstrom B, Ohlsson C. Increased adipogenesis in bone marrow but decreased bone mineral density in mice devoid of thyroid hormone receptors. Bone. 2005;36:607–16.
44. Krishnamra N, Seemoung J. Effects of acute and long-term administration of prolactin on bone 45Ca uptake, calcium deposit, and calcium resorption in weaned, young, and mature rats. Can J Physiol Pharmacol. 1996;74(1):157–65.
45. Langlois JA, Rosen CJ, Visser M, Hannan MT, Harris T, Wilson PW, Kiel DP. Association between insulin-like growth factor I and bone mineral density in older women and men: the Framingham Heart Study. J Clin Endocrinol Metab. 1998;83(4):257–62.
46. La Vignera S, Vicari E, Tumino S, Ciotta L, Condorelli R, Vicari LO, Calogero AE. L-thyroxin treatment and post-menopausal osteoporosis: relevance of the risk profile present in clinical history. Minerva Ginecol. 2008;60:475–84.
47. Liu S, Cheng Y, Fan M, Chen D, Bian Z. FSH aggravates periodontitis-related bone loss in ovariectomized rats. J Dent Res. 2010;89:366–71.
48. Liu S, Cheng Y, Xu W, Bian Z. Protective effects of follicle-stimulating hormone inhibitor on alveolar bone loss resulting from experimental periapical lesions in ovariectomized rats. J Endod. 2010;36:658–63.
49. Liu X, Shimono K, Zhu LL, Li J, Peng Y, Imam A, Iqbal J, Moonga S, Colaianni G, Su C, Lu Z, Iwamoto M, Pacifici M, Zallone A, Sun L, Zaidi M. Oxytocin deficiency impairs maternal skeletal remodeling. Biochem Biophys Res Commun. 2009;388:161–6.
50. Liu XS, Sajda P, Saha PK, Wehrli FW, Guo XE. Quantification of the roles of trabecular microarchitecture and trabecular type in determining the elastic modulus of human trabecular bone. J Bone Miner Res. 2006;21(1):608–17.
51. Lotinun S, Limlomwongse L, Krishnamra N. The study of a physiological significance of prolactin in the regulation of calcium metabolism during pregnancy and lactation in rats. Can J Physiol Pharmacol. 1998;76:218–28.
52. Lotinun S, Limlomwongse L, Sirikulchayanonta V, Krishnamra N. Bone calcium turnover, formation, and resorption in bromocriptine- and prolactin-treated lactating rats. Endocrine. 2003;20:163–70.
53. Ma R, Latif R, Zaidi M, Davies T. Thyroid and bone: TSH inhibits osteoclastogenesis from embryonic stem cells. In: Presented at the 91st annual meeting of the Endocrine Society, Washington D.C.; 2009.
54. Mantella RC, Vollmer RR, Li X, Amico JA. Female oxytocin-deficient mice display enhanced anxiety-related behavior. Endocrinology. 2003;144(2):291–6.
55. Marcus R, Butterfield G, Holloway L, Gilliland L, Baylink DJ, Hintz RL, Sherman BM. Effects of short term administration of recombinant human growth hormone to elderly people. J Clin Endocrinol Metab. 1990;70:519–27.
56. Martini G, Gennari L, De Paola V, Pilli T, Salvadori S, Merlotti D, Valleggi F, Campagna S, Franci B, Avanzati A, Nuti R, Pacini F. The effects of recombinant TSH on bone turnover markers and serum osteoprotegerin and RANKL levels. Thyroid. 2008;18: 455–60.
57. Mazziotti G, Porcelli T, Patelli I, Vescovi PP, Giustina A. Serum TSH values and risk of vertebral fractures in euthyroid post-menopausal women with low bone mineral density. Bone. 2010;46:747–51.
58. Mazziotti G, Sorvillo F, Piscopo M, Cioffi M, Pilla P, Biondi B, Iorio S, Giustina A, Amato G, Carella C. Recombinant human TSH modulates in vivo C-telopeptides of type-1 collagen and bone alkaline phosphatase, but not osteoprotegerin production in postmenopausal women monitored for differentiated thyroid carcinoma. J Bone Miner Res. 2005;20:480–6.
59. Meaney AM, Smith S, Howes OD, O'Brien M, Murray RM, O'Keane V. Effects of long-term prolactin-raising antipsychotic medication on bone mineral density in patients with schizophrenia. Br J Psychiatry. 2004;184:503–8.
60. Menagh PJ, Turner RT, Jump DB, Wong CP, Lowry MB, Yakar S, Rosen CJ, Iwaniec UT. Growth hormone regulates the balance between bone formation and bone marrow adiposity. J Bone Miner Res. 2010;25: 757–68.
61. Mikosch P, Kerschan-Schindl K, Woloszczuk W, Stettner H, Kudlacek S, Kresnik E, Gallowitsch HJ, Lind P, Pietschmann P. High cathepsin K levels in men with differentiated thyroid cancer on suppressive L-thyroxine therapy. Thyroid. 2008;18:27–33.
62. Miller PD. Guidelines for the diagnosis of osteoporosis: T-scores vs fractures. Rev Endocr Metab Disord. 2006;7:75–89.
63. Morris MS. The association between serum thyroid-stimulating hormone in its reference range and bone status in postmenopausal American women. Bone. 2007;40(1):128–34.
64. Murphy E, Williams GR. The thyroid and the skeleton. Clin Endocrinol (Oxf). 2004;61:285–98.
65. Murthy RK, Morrow PK, Theriault RL. Bone biology and the role of the RANK ligand pathway. Oncology (Williston Park). 2009;23:9–15.

66. Nagata M, Suzuki A, Sekiguchi S, Ono Y, Nishiwaki-Yasuda K, Itoi T, Yamamoto S, Imamura S, Katoh T, Hayakawa N, Oda N, Hashimoto S, Itoh M. Subclinical hypothyroidism is related to lower heel QUS in post-menopausal women. Endocr J. 2007;54:625–30.
67. Naylor KE, Iqbal P, Fledelius C, Fraser RB, Eastell R. The effect of pregnancy on bone density and bone turnover. J Bone Miner Res. 2000;15:129–37.
68. Nishimori K, Young LJ, Guo Q, Wang Z, Insel TR, Matzuk MM. Oxytocin is required for nursing but is not essential for parturition or reproductive behavior. Proc Natl Acad Sci USA. 1996;93:11699–704.
69. Novack DV. TSH, the bone suppressing hormone. Cell. 2003;115:129–30.
70. Phang D, Rehage M, Bonafede B, Hou D, Xing W, Mohan S, Wergedal JE, Qin X. Inactivation of insulin-like-growth factors diminished the anabolic effects of pregnancy-associated plasma protein-A (PAPP-A) on bone in mice. Growth Horm IGF Res. 2010;20: 192–200.
71. Recker R, Lappe J, Davies KM, Heaney R. Bone remodeling increases substantially in the years after menopause and remains increased in older osteoporosis patients. J Bone Miner Res. 2004;19(1):628–33.
72. Rendina D, Gianfrancesco F, De Filippo G, Merlotti D, Esposito T, Mingione A, Nuti R, Strazzullo P, Mossetti G, Gennari L. FSHR gene polymorphisms influence bone mineral density and bone turnover in postmenopausal women. Eur J Endocrinol. 2010;163:165–72.
73. Rosen CJ, Chesnut 3rd CH, Mallinak NJ. The predictive value of biochemical markers of bone turnover for bone mineral density in early postmenopausal women treated with hormone replacement or calcium supplementation. J Clin Endocrinol Metab. 1997;82(1): 904–10.
74. Rosen CJ, Dimai HP, Vereault D, Donahue LR, Beamer WG, Farley J, Linkhart S, Linkhart T, Mohan S, Baylink DJ. Circulating and skeletal insulin-like growth factor-I (IGF-I) concentrations in two inbred strains of mice with different bone mineral densities. Bone. 1997;21:217–23.
75. Ross DS. Hyperthyroidism, thyroid hormone therapy, and bone. Thyroid. 1994;4:319–26.
76. Rubin J, Ackert-Bicknell CL, Zhu L, Fan X, Murphy TC, Nanes MS, Marcus R, Holloway L, Beamer WG, Rosen CJ. IGF-I regulates osteoprotegerin (OPG) and receptor activator of nuclear factor-kappaB ligand in vitro and OPG in vivo. J Clin Endocrinol Metab. 2002;87(4):273–9.
77. Sampath TK, Simic P, Sendak R, Draca N, Bowe AE, O'Brien S, Schiavi SC, McPherson JM, Vukicevic S. Thyroid-stimulating hormone restores bone volume, microarchitecture, and strength in aged ovariectomized rats. J Bone Miner Res. 2007;22:849–59.
78. Schmidt IU, Dobnig H, Turner RT. Intermittent parathyroid hormone treatment increases osteoblast number, steady state messenger ribonucleic acid levels for osteocalcin, and bone formation in tibial metaphysis of hypophysectomized female rats. Endocrinology. 1995;136(5):127–34.
79. Sclafani A, Rinaman L, Vollmer RR, Amico JA. Oxytocin knockout mice demonstrate enhanced intake of sweet and nonsweet carbohydrate solutions. Am J Physiol Regul Integr Comp Physiol. 2007;292: R1828–33.
80. Seriwatanachai D, Charoenphandhu N, Suthiphongchai T, Krishnamra N. Prolactin decreases the expression ratio of receptor activator of nuclear factor kappaB ligand/osteoprotegerin in human fetal osteoblast cells. Cell Biol Int. 2008;32(1):126–35.
81. Seriwatanachai D, Thongchote K, Charoenphandhu N, Pandaranandaka J, Tudpor K, Teerapornpuntakit J, Suthiphongchai T, Krishnamra N. Prolactin directly enhances bone turnover by raising osteoblast-expressed receptor activator of nuclear factor kappaB ligand/osteoprotegerin ratio. Bone. 2008;42: 535–46.
82. Sowers M, Eyre D, Hollis BW, Randolph JF, Shapiro B, Jannausch ML, Crutchfield M. Biochemical markers of bone turnover in lactating and nonlactating postpartum women. J Clin Endocrinol Metab. 1995; 80(2):210–6.
83. Sowers MR, Greendale GA, Bondarenko I, Finkelstein JS, Cauley JA, Neer RM, Ettinger B. Endogenous hormones and bone turnover markers in pre- and perimenopausal women: SWAN. Osteoporos Int. 2003;14: 191–7.
84. Sowers MR, Jannausch M, McConnell D, Little R, Greendale GA, Finkelstein JS, Neer RM, Johnston J, Ettinger B. Hormone predictors of bone mineral density changes during the menopausal transition. J Clin Endocrinol Metab. 2006;91(1):261–7.
85. Sowers MR, Zheng H, Jannausch ML, McConnell D, Nan B, Harlow S, Randolph Jr JF. Amount of bone loss in relation to time around the final menstrual period and follicle-stimulating hormone staging of the transmenopause. J Clin Endocrinol Metab. 2010; 95(2):155–62.
86. Stabnov L, Kasukawa Y, Guo R, Amaar Y, Wergedal JE, Baylink DJ, Mohan S. Effect of insulin-like growth factor-1 (IGF-1) plus alendronate on bone density during puberty in IGF-1-deficient MIDI mice. Bone. 2002;30:909–16.
87. Sun L, Peng Y, Sharrow AC, Iqbal J, Zhang Z, Papachristou DJ, Zaidi S, Zhu LL, Yaroslavskiy BB, Zhou H, Zallone A, Sairam MR, Kumar TR, Bo W, Braun J, Cardoso-Landa L, Schaffler MB, Moonga BS, Blair HC, Zaidi M. FSH directly regulates bone mass. Cell. 2006;125:247–60.
88. Sun L, Vukicevic S, Baliram R, Yang G, Sendak R, McPherson J, Zhu LL, Iqbal J, Latif R, Natrajan A, Arabi A, Yamoah K, Moonga BS, Gabet Y, Davies TF, Bab I, Abe E, Sampath K, Zaidi M. Intermittent recombinant TSH injections prevent ovariectomy-induced bone loss. Proc Natl Acad Sci USA. 2008;105: 4289–94.
89. Svare A, Nilsen TI, Bjoro T, Forsmo S, Schei B, Langhammer A. Hyperthyroid levels of TSH correlate with low bone mineral density: the HUNT 2 study. Eur J Endocrinol. 2009;161:779–86.

90. Tamma R, Colaianni G, Zhu LL, DiBenedetto A, Greco G, Montemurro G, Patano N, Strippoli M, Vergari R, Mancini L, Colucci S, Grano M, Faccio R, Liu X, Li JH, Usmani S, Bachar M, Bab I, Nishimori K, Younge LJ, Buettner C, Iqbal J, Sun L, Zaidi M, Zallone A. Oxytocin is an anabolic bone hormone. Proc Natl Acad Sci USA. 2009;106:7149–54.
91. Tanner SJ, Hefferan TE, Rosen CJ, Conover CA. Impact of pregnancy-associated plasma protein-a deletion on the adult murine skeleton. J Bone Miner Res. 2008;23:655–62.
92. Ueki I, Ooi GT, Tremblay ML, Hurst KR, Bach LA, Boisclair YR. Inactivation of the acid labile subunit gene in mice results in mild retardation of postnatal growth despite profound disruptions in the circulating insulin-like growth factor system. Proc Natl Acad Sci USA. 2000;97:6868–73.
93. Ueland T. GH/IGF-I and bone resorption in vivo and in vitro. Eur J Endocrinol. 2005;152:327–32.
94. van der Deure WM, Uitterlinden AG, Hofman A, Rivadeneira F, Pols HA, Peeters RP, Visser TJ. Effects of serum TSH and FT4 levels and the TSHR-Asp727Glu polymorphism on bone: the Rotterdam Study. Clin Endocrinol (Oxf). 2008;68:175–81.
95. Wang Y, Nishida S, Boudignon BM, Burghardt A, Elalieh HZ, Hamilton MM, Majumdar S, Halloran BP, Clemens TL, Bikle DD. IGF-I receptor is required for the anabolic actions of parathyroid hormone on bone. J Bone Miner Res. 2007;22(1):329–37.
96. Wenzel KW. Thyroid hormone and bone. Thyroid. 1994;4:508–9.
97. Wu Y, Torchia J, Yao W, Lane NE, Lanier LL, Nakamura MC, Humphrey MB. Bone microenvironment specific roles of ITAM adapter signaling during bone remodeling induced by acute estrogen-deficiency. PLoS One. 2007;2:e586.
98. Wysolmerski JJ. The evolutionary origins of maternal calcium and bone metabolism during lactation. J Mammary Gland Biol Neoplasia. 2002;7:267–76.
99. Yakar S, Canalis E, Sun H, Mejia W, Kawashima Y, Nasser P, Courtland HW, Williams V, Bouxsein M, Rosen C, Jepsen KJ. Serum IGF-1 determines skeletal strength by regulating subperiosteal expansion and trait interactions. J Bone Miner Res. 2009;24(1):481–92.
100. Yakar S, Liu JL, Stannard B, Butler A, Accili D, Sauer B, LeRoith D. Normal growth and development in the absence of hepatic insulin-like growth factor I. Proc Natl Acad Sci USA. 1999;96:7324–9.
101. Yakar S, Rosen CJ, Beamer WG, Ackert-Bicknell CL, Wu Y, Liu JL, Ooi GT, Setser J, Frystyk J, Boisclair YR, LeRoith D. Circulating levels of IGF-1 directly regulate bone growth and density. J Clin Invest. 2002;110:771–81.
102. Yamoah K, Brebene A, Baliram R, Inagaki K, Dolios G, Arabi A, Majeed R, Amano H, Wang R, Yanagisawa R, Abe E. High-mobility group box proteins modulate tumor necrosis factor-alpha expression in osteoclastogenesis via a novel deoxyribonucleic acid sequence. Mol Endocrinol. 2008;22(1):141–53.
103. Young 3rd WS, Shepard E, DeVries AC, Zimmer A, LaMarca ME, Ginns EI, Amico J, Nelson RJ, Hennighausen L, Wagner KU. Targeted reduction of oxytocin expression provides insights into its physiological roles. Adv Exp Med Biol. 1998;449:231–40.
104. Zhao G, Monier-Faugere MC, Langub MC, Geng Z, Nakayama T, Pike JW, Chernausek SD, Rosen CJ, Donahue LR, Malluche HH, Fagin JA, Clemens TL. Targeted overexpression of insulin-like growth factor I to osteoblasts of transgenic mice: increased trabecular bone volume without increased osteoblast proliferation. Endocrinology. 2000;141(2):674–82.
105. Zaidi M, Sun L, Davies TF, Abe E. Low TSH triggers bone loss: fact or fiction? Thyroid. 2006;16:1075–6.
106. Zofkova I, Hill M. Biochemical markers of bone remodeling correlate negatively with circulating TSH in postmenopausal women. Endocr Regul. 2008;42:121–7.

6 Calcitonin: Its Physiological Role and Emerging Therapeutics

Jillian Cornish, Dorit Naot, and T. John Martin

Keywords
Calcitonin • Calcitonin gene-related peptide (CGRP) • Calcitonin receptor Receptor activity modifying proteins (RAMP) • Calcium homeostasis

6.1 Introduction

Calcitonin was discovered more than 40 years ago as a hormone that lowers circulating calcium levels [14, 15]. In mammals, the major site of calcitonin synthesis is the parafollicular cells of the thyroid, which secrete calcitonin in response to an increase in plasma calcium concentration and in response to a number of gut hormones, including gastrin and glucagon. Calcitonin is metabolized in the kidneys and has a plasma half-life of approximately 5 min. Calcitonin has been identified in many species, and salmon calcitonin, which shares only 50% sequence identity with human calcitonin, shows much greater potency than human calcitonin in most biological assays [31]. Human calcitonin is a 32-amino-acid peptide with a disulfide bridge between the cysteine residues at positions 1 and 7 and a proline-amide group at the C-terminus [6]. Both the bridge and the amide group along with the full amino acid sequence are necessary for calcitonin's biological activity.

A group of peptide hormones that share structural and functional similarities with calcitonin includes α-calcitonin gene-related peptide (αCGRP), βCGRP, amylin, adrenomedullin, and adrenomedullin 2 (intermedin) (Fig. 6.1). Calcitonin and αCGRP are produced by tissue-specific alternative RNA splicing of the gene *CALCA*, with αCGRP being predominantly produced in neural tissue [58]. A second form of CGRP, βCGRP, which differs from αCGRP by one amino acid in the rat and three amino acids in the human, is produced by a separate gene. The receptors for the calcitonin family peptides are also related to each other. The calcitonin receptor (CTR) is a seven-transmembrane domain G-protein-coupled receptor that can bind calcitonin with high affinity. Receptors for the other peptides of the calcitonin family are formed by heterodimerization of the calcitonin receptor or the closely related calcitonin receptor-like receptor (CLR) with one of three receptor activity modifying proteins (RAMPs) [54]. Although the different combinations of these proteins create receptors with distinct ligand specificities, there is a degree of cross-reactivity, and the receptors

J. Cornish, Ph.D. (✉) • D. Naot, Ph.D.
Department of Medicine, University of Auckland, Private Bag 92019, Auckland 1142, New Zealand
e-mail: j.cornish@auckland.ac.nz

T.J. Martin, M.D., D.Sc.
Bone Cell Biology and Disease, St. Vincent's Institute of Medical Research, 9 Princes St., Fitzroy, VIC 3065, Australia

F. Bronner et al. (eds.), *Bone-Metabolic Functions and Modulators*, Topics in Bone Biology, DOI 10.1007/978-1-4471-2745-1_6, © Springer-Verlag London 2012

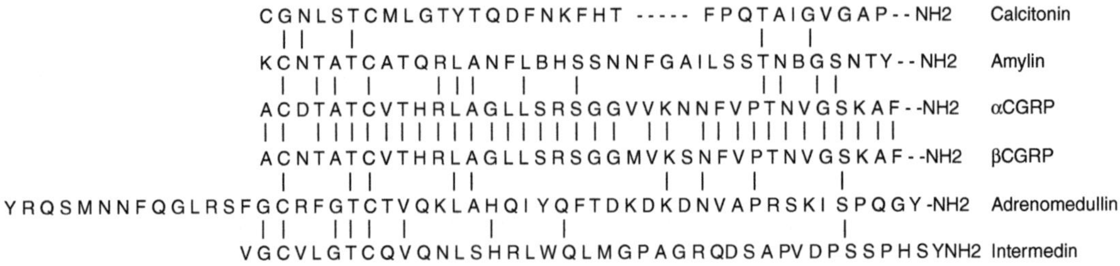

Fig. 6.1 Peptides of the calcitonin family (Reprinted from Naot and Cornish [48], Copyright 2008, with permission from Elsevier)

can bind other ligands from the family, usually with lower affinity.

Bone and kidney are the two primary targets of calcitonin, and both are important for the activity of calcitonin to acutely decrease circulating levels of calcium. In bone, calcitonin acts directly on osteoclasts, reducing calcium release into the plasma through inhibition of bone resorption, whereas in the kidneys calcitonin decreases renal tubular resorption of calcium and phosphate. In vitro and in several experimental animal models, amylin, and CGRP are also effective in inhibiting osteoclast activity and bone resorption.

Despite the large number of studies investigating calcitonin activity and although its effect to acutely reduce circulating calcium levels is well established, the physiological role of calcitonin is still uncertain and is much debated. Chronic calcitonin deficiency as seen in thyroidectomized patients or the excess of calcitonin produced in patients with medullary carcinoma of the thyroid do not appear to significantly affect calcium or bone metabolism. This chapter will review the activity of calcitonin in bone and present the current understanding of calcitonin's physiological role and its use as a therapeutic agent.

6.2 Effects of Calcitonin in Bone

6.2.1 Osteoclasts and Bone Resorption

Injection of calcitonin leads to a powerful lowering of plasma calcium levels in experimental animals, which results mainly from inhibition of bone resorption [7]. Studies of the mechanisms of action of calcitonin in osteoclasts showed that binding of calcitonin to CTR has two major effects: (1) inhibition of osteoclast motility and induction of a quiescent state through a cAMP-dependent mechanism and (2) osteoclast pseudopodial retraction, which is mediated through intracellular calcium signaling [1, 74]. Both changes decrease the area of the osteoclast contact with the bone surface. The inhibition of osteoclast activity by calcitonin is well established; however its effect on fusion of osteoclast precursors and the formation of multinucleated tartrate-resistant acid phosphatase (TRAP)-positive cells remains controversial and varies in different experimental systems. In murine bone marrow cultures stimulated to generate osteoclasts by 1,25 Vitamin D_3, calcitonin dose-dependently decreased the numbers of TRAP-positive multinucleated cells [18], but in other studies, short treatment with calcitonin had no effect on the number of multinucleated TRAP-positive cells [55, 70].

A number of studies showed that the effects of calcitonin in osteoclasts are transient, and prolonged exposure results in desensitization of the treated cells. Early studies showed that stimulation of bone resorption in organ cultures by parathyroid hormone (PTH) could be inhibited by the addition of calcitonin, but over time the cells manage to "escape" this inhibitory effect [72]. This "escape phenomenon" was later found to be due to ligand-induced internalization of the receptor, as well as inhibition of de novo synthesis of the calcitonin receptor [64, 69].

The other members of the calcitonin family vary in their abilities to regulate osteoclast activity and bone resorption. Similar to calcitonin, injection of amylin or CGRP to animals also reduces circulating calcium levels, but amylin and CGRP are less potent than calcitonin in inducing hypocalcemia by several orders of magnitude [41, 65]. CGRP and amylin inhibit osteoclast motility and decrease the numbers of TRAP-positive multinucleated cells in murine bone marrow cultures, although with much lower potency than calcitonin. Adrenomedullin does not induce hypocalcemia and does not appear to have an inhibitory effect on osteoclasts [19].

Following its discovery, calcitonin was thought to account for the tight control of serum calcium, but this has now been questioned. Concepts of the role of bone in maintaining extracellular fluid calcium had relied upon observations made in young animals in which rapid bone resorption and formation are required for development of the skeleton. Clearly, if bone accretion continued at the same rate and bone resorption were inhibited in these animals, the result would be a lowering of plasma calcium. It would therefore be expected that the calcium-lowering effect of calcitonin should be greater in younger than in older animals, and this consistently was found to be the case. In normal adult human subjects, even quite large doses of calcitonin have little effect on serum calcium levels.

The antiresorptive activity of calcitonin led to its therapeutic use in patients with increased bone turnover (e.g., cancer hypercalcemia, Paget's disease).

6.2.2 Osteoblasts and Bone Formation

Although several early pharmacological studies reported that calcitonin stimulated osteoblast proliferation and differentiation [24, 71], followed later by in vitro and even in vivo studies showing that calcitonin increased indices of bone formation, these osteoblast effects do not appear to be of physiological relevance. The effects were only seen when very high concentrations of calcitonin were used [17, 19, 20, 67, 68]. In comparison, in a local injection model, with the peptides administered by daily subcutaneous injection over one of the hemicalvaria of adult mice, calcitonin significantly inhibited eroded surfaces, indicating inhibition of bone resorption, but did not significantly alter any bone formation indices [16, 17]. There are no obvious explanations for any direct effects of calcitonin on osteoblasts as no evidence has been produced on the existence of genuine receptors in osteoblasts, for example, by CTR autoradiography [51]. Thus, studies overall have indicated that the osteoblast is not a primary target of calcitonin.

6.3 Receptors of the Calcitonin Family of Peptides

CTR belongs to the seven-transmembrane domain class II G-protein-coupled receptors, a group that includes other receptors that bind regulatory peptides such as PTH-/PTH-related peptide and secretin [39]. CLR was cloned independently by two groups, as a novel receptor that showed high homology to the CTR [8, 52]. For several years, CTR was only recognized as a calcitonin receptor and CLR was an "orphan receptor" with no known ligands. A breakthrough in the understanding of these receptors came with the discovery of RAMPs, as described above. In a study that was designed to identify the CGRP receptor, McLatchie et al. screened pools of clones of a cDNA library from the human neuroblastoma cell line SK-N-MC by expressing them in *Xenopus* oocytes and measuring cAMP response to CGRP treatment [45]. All three known RAMPs were discovered in this study [45]. CGRP receptor was found to be a heterodimer, and only coexpression of RAMP1 with CLR could reconstitute a CGRP receptor with identical pharmacology to the one expressed in SK-N-MC cells. A sequence database search for expressed sequences similar to RAMP1 identified RAMP2 and RAMP3 [45]. Although the three RAMPs show only about 30% amino acid sequence identity, they share a similar basic structure – a large extracellular domain containing four conserved cysteine residues, a single transmembrane domain, and a short intracellular domain. The combinations of the receptors CTR, CLR, and RAMP1–3 were subsequently identified as the receptors for all the peptides of the calcitonin family, as summarized in Fig. 6.2

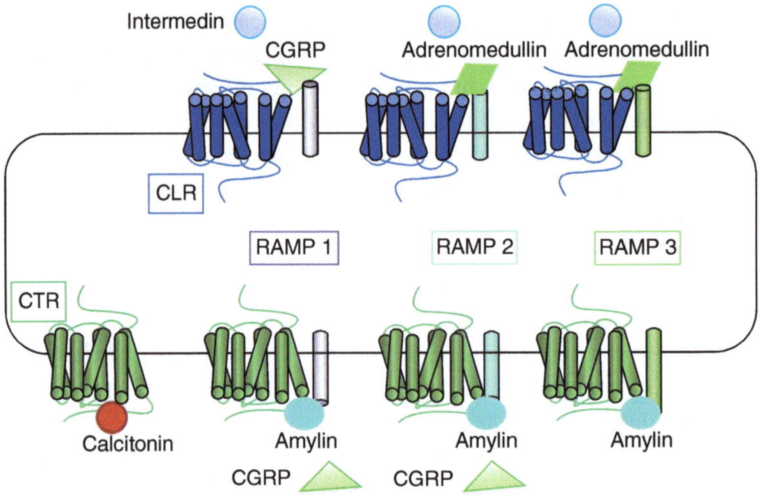

Fig. 6.2 Receptors for peptides of the calcitonin family and their ligand specificities. CTR is a high-affinity, specific calcitonin receptor that can form dimers with each of the RAMPs to produce amylin receptors. The combinations CTR/RAMP1 and CTR/RAMP2 can also bind CGRP. CLR can only bind ligands when coexpressed with one of the RAMPs. CLR/RAMP1 forms a specific, high-affinity receptor for CGRP, while CLR/RAMP2 and CLR/RAMP3 are adrenomedullin receptors. Intermedin binds nonselectively to all three CLR/RAMP receptors

[13, 46, 54]. Detailed analysis of the interactions between the receptors of the calcitonin family and their ligands demonstrated a degree of cross-reactivity with some of the receptor combinations, and the specific affinities were also dependent on the experimental system [46]. Although CTR and CLR share >50% amino acid identity, CTR itself acts as a specific calcitonin receptor, whereas CLR does not function as an independent receptor. Transport of CLR to the plasma membrane and its ability to bind ligands depend on its heterodimerization with one of the RAMPs [12, 13]. RAMPs do not interact exclusively with CTR and CLR, but also can form dimers with other class II as well as some of class III G-protein-coupled receptors [5, 12].

6.4 Expression of Receptors for the Calcitonin Family in Bone

In the osteoclast linage, CTR expression is induced during osteoclastogenesis, and it is highly expressed before cell fusion and the formation of multinucleated osteoclasts [26]. CTR, CLR, and RAMP2, but not RAMP1 and RAMP3, were detectable in a pure population of osteoclast-like cells prepared by laser capture microdissection from cocultures of mouse bone marrow and spleen cells [47].

We used quantitative PCR to investigate the expression of mRNA-encoding CTR, CLR, and RAMP1–3 in 32 samples from human bone that had been collected from patients undergoing orthopedic surgery [48]. Sixteen of the samples were explant cultures of human osteoblast-like cells that were grown from bone fragments and showed characteristics of osteoblasts including staining with alkaline phosphatase, expression of type 1 collagenα1, and osteocalcin. The other 16 samples were cells grown from bone marrow, containing a mixed cell population of stromal cells and cells of hematopoietic origin. The details of the protocols have been described previously in a study that used these samples as controls [50]. As shown in Fig. 6.3, CTR was absent from all the osteoblast samples and showed low levels of expression in the bone marrow samples, most likely indicating the presence of a small number of differentiated osteoclasts. RAMP3 was not expressed in any of the samples we tested. CLR and RAMP1 had very high levels of expression whereas RAMP2 showed higher expression in bone marrow than in primary osteoblasts. In primary rat osteoblasts, expression of CTR could not be detected by RT-PCR and

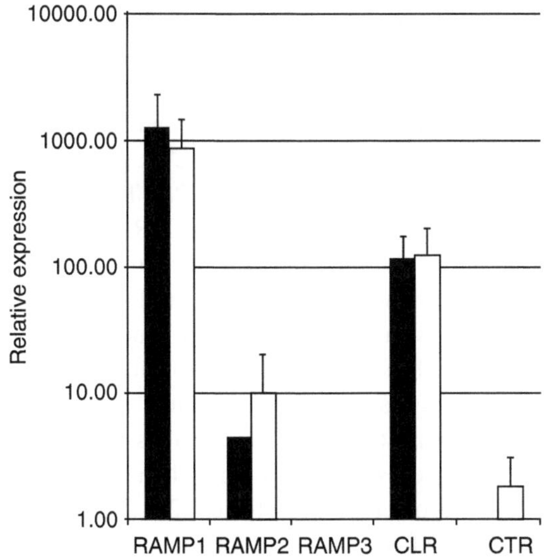

Fig. 6.3 Relative mRNA expression of receptors for the calcitonin peptide family in human osteoblasts and bone marrow cells. The relative levels of expression of RAMP1–3, CLR, and CTR were determined by quantitative PCR in 16 samples of cultured human osteoblasts (*black bars*) and 16 samples of bone marrow cells (*clear bars*). The data are presented as means + standard deviations (Reprinted from Naot and Cornish [48], Copyright 2008, with permission from Elsevier)

northern blot analysis, whereas CLR was detected in these cells [49]. RAMP2 showed high levels of expression in the primary rat osteoblasts, and RAMP1 and RAMP3 had lower levels of expression [49]. In a recent study, CTR mRNA and protein were identified in osteocytes, and once again, immunohistochemistry and quantitative PCR in this study confirmed that primary osteoblasts do not express CTR [25]. The significance of these findings will be discussed further, in relation to newer findings regarding the physiological role of calcitonin.

The relative expression levels of CTR, CLR, and RAMP1–3 determine which of the calcitonin family peptides a cell is more likely to bind with high affinity, and the expression of the receptor components can be regulated by extracellular factors. For example, PTH treatment in mouse primary osteoblasts has been shown to upregulate the expression of RAMP3 [53], whereas dexamethasone increases the expression of RAMP1 and RAMP2 mRNA, leaving RAMP3 levels unchanged and decreasing CLR expression [66].

6.5 Physiological Role of Calcitonin in Bone

Ideas of the physiological role of calcitonin have included that it is an inhibitor of bone resorption; however, argument about the physiological function has continued over the decades. Debate culminated in the suggestion by one of the codiscoverers of calcitonin that calcitonin is *not* involved in calcium homeostasis or in any other important physiological function, except possibly in protection of the skeleton under calcium stress [29]. It was thought that the role of calcitonin in its effect on bone throughout life might be that of a regulator of the bone resorptive process, whatever the overall rate of the latter. In the young or in pathological states of increased bone resorption in maturity (e.g., Paget's disease, thyrotoxicosis), calcitonin inhibition of bone resorption can lower the serum calcium level and may even have a calcium homeostatic role for endogenous calcitonin in those circumstances. The physiological function of calcitonin in maturity may nevertheless be to regulate the bone resorptive process in either a continuous or intermittent manner. It follows that calcitonin should *not* necessarily be regarded as a "calcium-regulating hormone" in maturity, but may yet be shown to be such in stages of rapid growth (e.g., in the young or in states of increased bone turnover).

It is nevertheless important that bone resorption be regulated, and calcitonin is the only hormone known to be capable of carrying out this function by a direct action on bone. Such a role might become more important in circumstances in which skeletal loss particularly needs to be prevented (e.g., in pregnancy and lactation). Evidence in support of such an important physiological role for endogenous calcitonin in protecting against bone loss is provided by experiments showing that trabecular bone loss in thyroparathyroidectomized rats treated with PTH was greater than that in similarly treated sham-operated controls [27]. Other clinical evidence has shown that small doses of calcium in men suppress PTH but do not increase bone density, suggesting that PTH is not the only factor involved in the effect of calcium supplements on bone [57]. Calcitonin is a candidate for mediating the rapid suppression of bone resorption with these supplements [56].

In the last few years though, further interesting possibilities on the physiological role of calcitonin have been raised through studies carried out initially in genetically manipulated mice. A knockout mouse deficient of the *Calca* gene, which encodes both calcitonin and CGRP, compared to wild-type mice were much less able to overcome hypercalcemia induced by a calcium load [30] and lost excessive bone during lactation [73]. Surprisingly, these *Calca–/–* mice had an unexpected phenotype [30]. The animals did not have the predicted osteoporotic phenotype due to accelerated bone resorption, but rather had higher bone volume and trabecular number resulting from a significant increase in bone formation, implying an inhibitory effect of calcitonin or αCGRP on bone formation. A subsequent long-term study of the bone phenotype of these animals showed that in the *Calca*-deficient mice, the bone phenotype developed with age, so that at 12 and 18 months, the increased bone formation was accompanied by evidence for increased bone resorption [32]. This high bone turnover state resulted in hyperostotic lesions in 20% of the *Calca*-deficient mice. However, it is difficult to interpret the physiological role of calcitonin in the regulation of bone metabolism from the phenotype of the *Calca*-deficient mice, given the complex genotype of these animals, which lack both calcitonin and αCGRP. Following these studies, mice deficient for CGRPα alone were studied, and the increased bone formation phenotype was *not* found, leaving calcitonin deficiency likely responsible for the increased bone formation in *Calca–/–* mice [60].

The next observations consistent with these results were receptor-deficient mice. CTR–/– mice were found to be not viable, thus two alternative knockout animal models were developed to study the physiological role of CTR. CTR haploinsufficiency was produced in heterozygous CTR+/– mice, where the expression of CTR in osteoclasts was half that of the wild type [22]. These animals had high bone mass due to increased bone formation without changes in bone resorption, similar to the phenotype described initially for the *Calca*-deficient mice [30]. A second animal model for the study of the physiological role of CTR in bone metabolism is a viable global CTR knockout mouse with deletion of more than 94% but less than 100% of the CTR gene developed using the Cre/*lox*P system [23]. The study of these animals demonstrated that CTR has a modest role in the physiological regulation of bone and calcium homeostasis in the basal state, yielding mice with a mild increase in bone formation rate, but plays a major role in conditions of calcium stress, such as hypocalcemia induced by 1,25 vitamin D_3. These observations indicate an inhibitory effect of calcitonin on bone formation, as in the other genetic studies [22, 23, 30, 33]. How the effect on bone formation comes about remains to be determined. The lack of evidence for specific calcitonin receptors and responses in osteoblasts is compelling, so it seems that the physiological roles of calcitonin in bone might be brought about through two possible pathways: (1) a direct effect on osteoclasts to inhibit resorption and (2) an indirect one resulting in the elaboration of a critical, locally active factor that is necessary for bone formation. This could result from signals through receptors either in the osteoclast or in the hypothalamus in each of which CTR is abundantly expressed [51, 59]. It could also be explained by an effect of calcitonin to promote sclerostin production, as discussed below.

One interpretation of these findings might have come from the hypothesized role of active osteoclasts in the coupling process since the best-documented action of calcitonin is its acute inhibition of osteoclast function. If the initiation of bone formation at sites of activation of bone multicellular units requires osteoclasts to be transiently activated to enable them to produce coupling activity, then the lack of calcitonin could result in osteoclasts remaining active, enabling them to continue contributing to bone formation, giving rise to the phenotype expressed in *calcitonin–/–* mice and in *CTR–/–* mice [44]. This would have revealed calcitonin as a short-term regulator of osteoclast activity which, through its action on the osteoclast, also regulates bone formation by limiting the duration of osteoclast activation in response to the anabolic stimulus.

In pursuing this possibility, we administered a low dose of salmon calcitonin to young rats receiving an anabolic PTH regimen (discussed in Chap. 1). Coadministration of salmon calcitonin significantly blunted the anabolic effect of PTH, and remarkably, sclerostin mRNA was significantly enhanced in bone by calcitonin treatment, whereas the expression of two other osteocyte gene products, MEPE and DMP1, were downregulated. Immunohistochemistry confirmed that calcitonin administration increased the percentage of osteocytes expressing sclerostin, suggesting a mechanism by which calcitonin reduced the anabolic effect of PTH [25].

Neither mRNA-encoding calcitonin receptor nor labeled calcitonin binding could be detected in sclerostin-enriched cells differentiated from primary calvarial osteoblasts. In contrast, immunohistochemistry revealed colocalization of CTR and sclerostin in osteocytes in calvarial sections. Furthermore, osteocytes freshly isolated from calvariae expressed a high level of CTR mRNA, the authenticity of which was established by sequencing of the cDNA and showing that the CTR was of the 1a isoform [25]. Thus, the impaired PTH anabolic effect in response to calcitonin in the young rats might be explained by direct stimulation of sclerostin production in osteocytes by calcitonin. Thus, the findings directly implicate calcitonin as a negative regulator of bone formation through a previously unsuspected mechanism and could explain the bone formation phenotypes exhibited in the genetically manipulated mice. Importantly though, as mice lacking calcitonin aged, they developed high turnover bone loss [32, 37], consistent with the predicted role for calcitonin as an inhibitor of bone remodeling. Taking the data further, this might imply that the physiological roles of calcitonin differ between younger and old animals. This possibility clearly needs to be resolved in further work.

In summary, there exists a large body of evidence showing that administration of calcitonin inhibits bone resorption, and in addition, the increased bone formation identified in the *Calca*-deficient mice suggests an unexpected physiological role for calcitonin as an inhibitor of bone formation (Fig. 6.4). The use of different experimental systems and different species in the study of calcitonin peptides and their receptors in bone produced many interesting results that are not always congruent. The fact that animals deficient in calcitonin, CGRP, or amylin have a bone phenotype different than the wild type suggests that these peptides are physiological regulators of bone metabolism. However, understanding of the physiological roles of the calcitonin peptides in bone will require more rigorous investigation of existing animal models as well as the development of conditional knockout animals in which inactivation of the genes of interest could be regulated in a time- and tissue-specific manner. In addition, the significance of peptides of the calcitonin family in regulation of bone and calcium metabolism in these animal models could be determined under various conditions of calcium stress, such as pregnancy, lactation, and low-calcium diet. Cellular and molecular biology approaches together with studies in whole animal models are likely to find the missing components that will elucidate the mechanism of action of calcitonin peptides in bone.

6.6 Emerging Therapeutics

The discovery of calcitonin as an inhibitor of bone resorption identified it as a potential therapeutic, and indeed it has been used as such for the treatment of osteoporosis, Paget's disease of bone, and hypercalcemia of malignancy. It has been approved as a resorption inhibitor in several countries.

Calcitonin given by subcutaneous injection was long recognized to be effective in the treatment of Paget's disease, with relief of pain, return of biochemical indices of disease activity toward normal, formation of normal lamellar bone, and filling in of osteolytic lesions [38]. In chronic treatment of Paget's disease with calcitonin, the number of osteoclasts declines progressively, either because of a direct effect on osteoclast precursors or as an indirect consequence of the acute inhibition of osteoclast function by calcitonin. The use of calcitonin in Paget's disease has been overtaken by the success of bisphosphonates

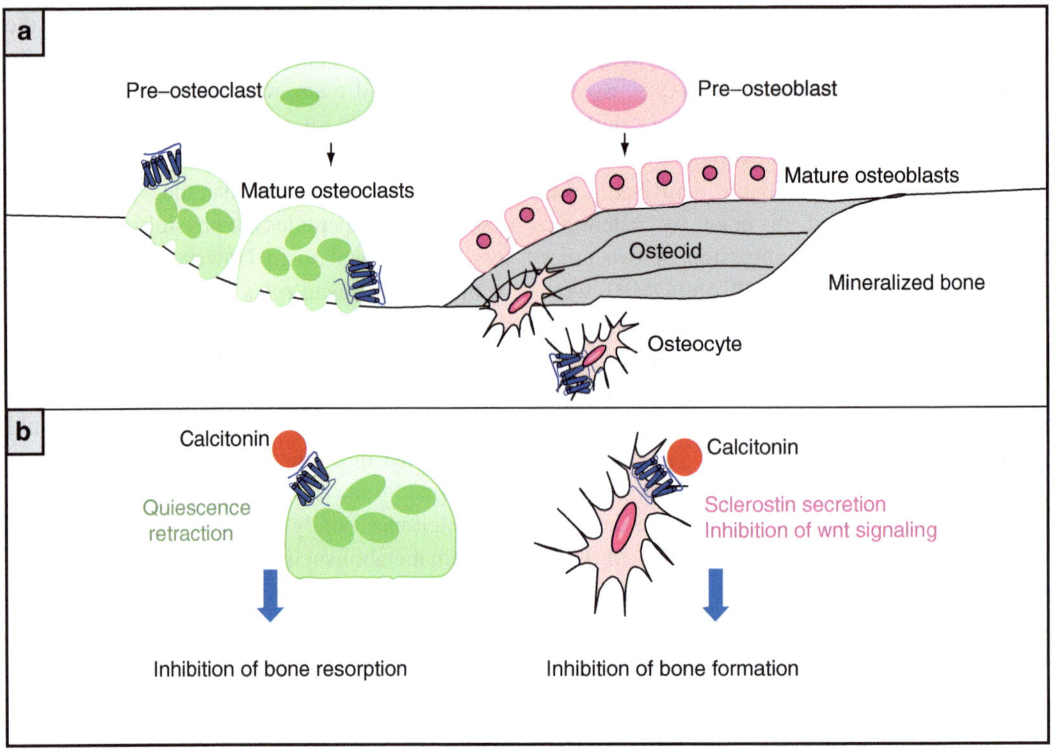

Fig. 6.4 Calcitonin receptor expression and calcitonin activity in bone cells. (**a**) A schematic representation of the bone-remodeling unit. Preosteoclasts that develop from mononuclear hematopoietic cells fuse to form multinucleated cells that resorb bone. Preosteoblasts that originate from mesenchymal stem cells differentiate into mature osteoblasts that initially lay down unmineralized extracellular matrix (osteoid) and subsequently calcify it to form mineralized bone. Osteocytes are terminally differentiated osteoblasts that are embedded in the bone matrix and play important regulatory roles. A large number of local and systemic signals are involved in coupling of bone resorption and formation, ensuring that at the end of the process, the amount of old bone removed has been accurately replaced with new bone. Expression of calcitonin receptor has been identified in differentiated osteoclasts and in osteocytes. (**b**) Mechanisms of action of calcitonin in bone cells. Binding of calcitonin to osteoclasts inhibits bone resorption by inducing a quiescent state and retraction of osteoclast pseudopodia. The first evidence for calcitonin's inhibitory effect on bone formation came from studies in transgenic mice deficient of calcitonin or CTR. Recent findings suggest a possible mechanism for this activity (see text). The osteocyte has been discovered as a target cell of calcitonin, where calcitonin induces secretion of the wnt-signaling inhibitor, sclerostin, which could explain the inhibition of osteoblast activity

producing long-term reductions in disease activity. In the case of the hypercalcemia in cancer, it was expected that calcitonin, as a powerful inhibitor of bone resorption, would provide effective treatment, but it has been fairly disappointing in this respect. It is effective in some patients with hypercalcemia of cancer or primary hyperparathyroidism, but more often it has little benefit. The phenomenon of calcitonin-induced resistance to its own action might contribute to this; glucocorticoids have been used together with calcitonin in an attempt to overcome this [4].

Salmon calcitonin, administered either by injection or by nasal spray, has been found to decrease vertebral fracture risk in postmenopausal osteoporotic women [9]. The PROOF trial of intranasal salmon calcitonin in the prevention of fractures [11] suffered from a high dropout rate, and in addition, a 200-IU per day dose appeared to be effective, but a higher dose ineffective [21]. A reported advantage of calcitonin is its analgesic effect on bone pain, which is probably mediated centrally [9]; calcitonin treatment has at best modest effects on bone density or bone turnover markers. The results of the QUEST study in which effects of calcitonin on bone structure were assessed by high-resolution MRI suggest therapeutic benefit of calcitonin nasal spray compared with placebo in maintaining trabecular microarchitecture at multiple skeletal sites [10]. Similar protection by calcitonin of bone structure was obtained in ovariectomized sheep, again using MRI to assess bone changes [34].

A number of recent studies have suggested the potential benefit of calcitonin in osteoarthritis. Both in vitro and in vivo [3, 62], calcitonin was found to attenuate the indices of progression of osteoarthritis, including degradation of collagen type II, a hallmark of articular cartilage damage. In humans, treatment with an orally deliverable form of salmon calcitonin reduced circulating carboxy-terminal collagen cross-links (CTX)-II [2] and improved functional disability in patients, albeit in a small test group, selected for active disease [43]. The mechanism of action of calcitonin in this putative chondroprotection is not clear, but there is evidence that calcitonin has direct effects on bovine articular chondrocytes *via* the CTR [63]. In contrast, a recent study was unable to find either CTR expression or responsiveness to calcitonin in human chondrocytes [40]. The findings are nonetheless intriguing, and benefits could result from effects of calcitonin on subchondral bone, as have been described for bisphosphonate treatment of animal models of osteoarthritis [28]. Potential benefits of calcitonin have also been suggested for inflammatory arthritis since it was found to preserve bone morphology in a rat model of rheumatoid arthritis, particularly when used with prednisolone [42].

The promising data in development of an orally deliverable form of calcitonin has reawakened interest in calcitonin as a therapeutic, both in osteoarthritis and in osteoporosis. An initial study showed in an osteoporosis trial of postmenopausal women that 1 mg of orally delivered salmon calcitonin maintained an acute reduction of serum and urinary CTX and bone-specific alkaline phosphatase through 3 months of treatment. A pharmacokinetic comparison of 0.8-mg calcitonin with 200-IU intranasal calcitonin showed similar pharmacokinetic profiles, but the oral form resulted in more than ten times higher peak plasma concentrations [35]. A detailed account of the development of the tablet form is provided in a review, including discussion of the optimal conditions for reproducible absorption of the peptide [36].

Oral salmon calcitonin was used in a model of osteoporotic bone loss in ovariectomized rats, where the peptide was as effective as 17β-estradiol in reducing serum levels of CTX-II [62]. In a 3-month dose-ranging study in postmenopausal women, orally delivered salmon calcitonin produced dose-dependent decreases in urinary CTX-I and CTX-II [2]. The early data with the oral preparation looks sufficiently interesting to warrant its thorough investigation as a resorption inhibitor, likely using an approach based on the known nocturnal increase in bone resorption [61].

6.7 Summary

Peptides of the calcitonin family have been the focus of many studies that investigated their mechanisms of action and physiological roles as well as their potential clinical use. In the years following its initial discovery, it has been well established that calcitonin lowers calcium blood levels and that it directly inhibits osteoclast function. These activities suggested that the physiological roles of calcitonin might include regulation of calcium homeostasis and bone resorption. However, no direct pathology is associated with calcitonin excess or deficiency, and the current understanding is that calcitonin is only important in protecting the skeleton under conditions of rapid bone growth and calcium stress. Another skeletal effect of calcitonin was discovered in studies of the bone phenotype of a number of transgenic mice strains, which determined that calcitonin can inhibit bone formation. This activity is likely to be mediated either systemically or locally through the osteoclasts and osteocytes, as calcitonin has no direct effect on osteoblasts. Salmon calcitonin has been in clinical use for a number of years for the treatment of diseases of increased bone turnover, including Paget's disease and osteoporosis.

However, calcitonin is no longer in wide use as bisphosphonates proved to be more effective in producing long-term reductions in disease activity. Recent development of a salmon calcitonin preparation that can be delivered orally and studies showing potential benefit of calcitonin use in osteoarthritis suggest that calcitonin might return to a wider clinical use in the future.

References

1. Alam AS, Bax CM, Shankar VS, Bax BE, Bevis PJ, Huang CL, Moonga BS, Pazianas M, Zaidi M. Further studies on the mode of action of calcitonin on isolated rat osteoclasts: pharmacological evidence for a second site mediating intracellular Ca^{2+} mobilization and cell retraction. J Endocrinol. 1993;136:7–15.
2. Bagger YZ, Tanko LB, Alexandersen P, Karsdal MA, Olson M, Mindeholm L, Azria M, Christiansen C. Oral salmon calcitonin induced suppression of urinary collagen type II degradation in postmenopausal women: a new potential treatment of osteoarthritis. Bone. 2005;37:425–30.
3. Behets C, Williams JM, Chappard D, Devogelaer JP, Manicourt DH. Effects of calcitonin on subchondral trabecular bone changes and on osteoarthritic cartilage lesions after acute anterior cruciate ligament deficiency. J Bone Miner Res. 2004;19:1821–6.
4. Binstock ML, Mundy GR. Effect of calcitonin and glutocorticoids in combination on the hypercalcemia of malignancy. Ann Intern Med. 1980;93:269–72.
5. Bouschet T, Martin S, Henley JM. Receptor-activity-modifying proteins are required for forward trafficking of the calcium-sensing receptor to the plasma membrane. J Cell Sci. 2005;118:4709–20.
6. Breimer LH, MacIntyre I, Zaidi M. Peptides from the calcitonin genes: molecular genetics, structure and function. Biochem J. 1988;255:377–90.
7. Chambers TJ, Magnus CJ. Calcitonin alters behaviour of isolated osteoclasts. J Pathol. 1982;136:27–39.
8. Chang CP, Pearse 2nd RV, O'Connell S, Rosenfeld MG. Identification of a seven transmembrane helix receptor for corticotropin-releasing factor and sauvagine in mammalian brain. Neuron. 1993;11: 1187–95.
9. Chesnut 3rd CH, Azria M, Silverman S, Engelhardt M, Olson M, Mindeholm L. Salmon calcitonin: a review of current and future therapeutic indications. Osteoporos Int. 2008;19:479–91.
10. Chesnut 3rd CH, Majumdar S, Newitt DC, Shields A, Van Pelt J, Laschansky E, Azria M, Kriegman A, Olson M, Eriksen EF, Mindeholm L. Effects of salmon calcitonin on trabecular microarchitecture as determined by magnetic resonance imaging: results from the QUEST study. J Bone Miner Res. 2005;20: 1548–61.
11. Chesnut 3rd CH, Silverman S, Andriano K, Genant H, Gimona A, Harris S, Kiel D, LeBoff M, Maricic M, Miller P, Moniz C, Peacock M, Richardson P, Watts N, Baylink D. A randomized trial of nasal spray salmon calcitonin in postmenopausal women with established osteoporosis: the prevent recurrence of osteoporotic fractures study. PROOF study group. Am J Med. 2000;109:267–76.
12. Christopoulos A, Christopoulos G, Morfis M, Udawela M, Laburthe M, Couvineau A, Kuwasako K, Tilakaratne N, Sexton PM. Novel receptor partners and function of receptor activity-modifying proteins. J Biol Chem. 2003;278:3293–7.
13. Christopoulos G, Perry KJ, Morfis M, Tilakaratne N, Gao Y, Fraser NJ, Main MJ, Foord SM, Sexton PM. Multiple amylin receptors arise from receptor activity-modifying protein interaction with the calcitonin receptor gene product. Mol Pharmacol. 1999;56: 235–42.
14. Copp DH, Cheney B. Calcitonin-a hormone from the parathyroid which lowers the calcium-level of the blood. Nature. 1962;193:381–2.
15. Copp DH, Cameron EC, Cheney BA, Davidson AG, Henze KG. Evidence for calcitonin – a new hormone from the parathyroid that lowers blood calcium. Endocrinology. 1962;70:638–49.
16. Cornish J, Reid IR. Skeletal effects of amylin and related peptides. Endocrinologist. 1999;9:183–9.
17. Cornish J, Callon KE, Cooper GJ, Reid IR. Amylin stimulates osteoblast proliferation and increases mineralized bone volume in adult mice. Biochem Biophys Res Commun. 1995;207:133–9.
18. Cornish J, Callon KE, Bava U, Kamona SA, Cooper GJ, Reid IR. Effects of calcitonin, amylin, and calcitonin gene-related peptide on osteoclast development. Bone. 2001;29:162–8.
19. Cornish J, Callon KE, Coy DH, Jiang NY, Xiao L, Cooper GJ, Reid IR. Adrenomedullin is a potent stimulator of osteoblastic activity in vitro and in vivo. Am J Physiol. 1997;273:E1113–20.
20. Cornish J, Callon KE, Lin CQ, Xiao CL, Gamble GD, Cooper GJ, Reid IR. Comparison of the effects of calcitonin gene-related peptide and amylin on osteoblasts. J Bone Miner Res. 1999;14:1302–9.
21. Cummings SR, Chapurlat RD. What PROOF proves about calcitonin and clinical trials. Am J Med. 2000;109:330–1.
22. Dacquin R, Davey RA, Laplace C, Levasseur R, Morris HA, Goldring SR, Gebre-Medhin S, Galson DL, Zajac JD, Karsenty G. Amylin inhibits bone resorption while the calcitonin receptor controls bone formation in vivo. J Cell Biol. 2004;164: 509–14.
23. Davey RA, Turner AG, McManus JF, Chiu WS, Tjahyono F, Moore AJ, Atkins GJ, Anderson PH, Ma C, Glatt V, MacLean HE, Vincent C, Bouxsein M, Morris HA, Findlay DM, Zajac JD. Calcitonin receptor plays a physiological role to protect against hypercalcemia in mice. J Bone Miner Res. 2008;23: 1182–93.

24. Farley JR, Tarbaux NM, Hall SL, Linkhart TA, Baylink DJ. The anti-bone-resorptive agent calcitonin also acts in vitro to directly increase bone formation and bone cell proliferation. Endocrinology. 1988;123: 159–67.
25. Gooi JH, Pompolo S, Karsdal MA, Kulkarni NH, Kalajzic I, McAhren SH, Han B, Onyia JE, Ho PW, Gillespie MT, Walsh NC, Chia LY, Quinn JM, Martin TJ, Sims NA. Calcitonin impairs the anabolic effect of PTH in young rats and stimulates expression of sclerostin by osteocytes. Bone. 2010;46:1486–97.
26. Granholm S, Lundberg P, Lerner UH. Expression of the calcitonin receptor, calcitonin receptor-like receptor, and receptor activity modifying proteins during osteoclast differentiation. J Cell Biochem. 2008;104: 920–33.
27. Harper C, Toverud SU. Ability of thyrocalcitonin to protect against hypercalcemia in adult rats. Endocrinology. 1973;93:1354–9.
28. Hayami T, Pickarski M, Wesolowski GA, McLane J, Bone A, Destefano J, Rodan GA, le Duong T. The role of subchondral bone remodeling in osteoarthritis: reduction of cartilage degeneration and prevention of osteophyte formation by alendronate in the rat anterior cruciate ligament transection model. Arthritis Rheum. 2004;50:1193–206.
29. Hirsch PF, Baruch H. Is calcitonin an important physiological substance? Endocr J. 2003;21:201–8.
30. Hoff AO, Catala-Lehnen P, Thomas PM, Priemel M, Rueger JM, Nasonkin I, Bradley A, Hughes MR, Ordonez N, Cote GJ, Amling M, Gagel RF. Increased bone mass is an unexpected phenotype associated with deletion of the calcitonin gene. J Clin Invest. 2002;110:1849–57.
31. Houssami S, Findlay DM, Brady CL, Martin TJ, Epand RM, Moore EE, Murayama E, Tamura T, Orlowski RC, Sexton PM. Divergent structural requirements exist for calcitonin receptor binding specificity and adenylate cyclase activation. Mol Pharmacol. 1995;47:798–809.
32. Huebner AK, Schinke T, Priemel M, Schilling S, Schilling AF, Emeson RB, Rueger JM, Amling M. Calcitonin deficiency in mice progressively results in high bone turnover. J Bone Miner Res. 2006;21: 1924–34.
33. Huebner AK, Keller J, Catala-Lehnen P, Perkovic S, Streichert T, Emeson RB, Amling M, Schinke T. The role of calcitonin and alpha-calcitonin gene-related peptide in bone formation. Arch Biochem Biophys. 2008;473:210–7.
34. Jiang Y, Zhao J, Geusens P, Liao EY, Adriaensens P, Gelan J, Azria M, Boonen S, Caulin F, Lynch JA, Ouyang X, Genant HK. Femoral neck trabecular microstructure in ovariectomized ewes treated with calcitonin: MRI microscopic evaluation. J Bone Miner Res. 2005;20:125–30.
35. Karsdal MA, Byrjalsen I, Riis BJ, Christiansen C. Optimizing bioavailability of oral administration of small peptides through pharmacokinetic and pharmacodynamic parameters: the effect of water and timing of meal intake on oral delivery of Salmon calcitonin. BMC Clin Pharmacol. 2008;8:5.
36. Karsdal MA, Henriksen K, Bay-Jensen AC, Molloy B, Arnold M, John MR, Byrjalsen I, Azria M, Riis BJ, Qvist P, Christiansen C. Lessons learned from the development of oral calcitonin: the first tablet formulation of a protein in phase III clinical trials. J Clin Pharmacol. 2010. doi:10.1177/0091270010372625.
37. Keller JH, Huebner AK, Catala-Lehnen P, Schinke T, Amling M. High bone mass due to increased bone formation in mice lacking the calcitonin receptor. J Bone Miner Res. 2008;23S:S171.
38. Langston AL, Ralston SH. Management of Paget's disease of bone. Rheumatology (Oxford). 2004;43:955–9.
39. Lin HY, Harris TL, Flannery MS, Aruffo A, Kaji EH, Gorn A, Kolakowski Jr LF, Yamin M, Lodish HF, Goldring SR. Expression cloning and characterization of a porcine renal calcitonin receptor. Trans Assoc Am Physicians. 1991;104:265–72.
40. Lin Z, Pavlos NJ, Cake MA, Wood DJ, Xu J, Zheng MH. Evidence that human cartilage and chondrocytes do not express calcitonin receptor. Osteoarthritis Cartilage. 2008;16:450–7.
41. MacIntyre I. Amylinamide, bone conservation, and pancreatic beta cells. Lancet. 1989;2:1026–7.
42. Mancini L, Paul-Clark MJ, Rosignoli G, Hannon R, Martin JE, Macintyre I, Perretti M. Calcitonin and prednisolone display antagonistic actions on bone and have synergistic effects in experimental arthritis. Am J Pathol. 2007;170:1018–27.
43. Manicourt DH, Azria M, Mindeholm L, Thonar EJ, Devogelaer JP. Oral salmon calcitonin reduces Lequesne's algofunctional index scores and decreases urinary and serum levels of biomarkers of joint metabolism in knee osteoarthritis. Arthritis Rheum. 2006;54: 3205–11.
44. Martin TJ, Sims NA. Osteoclast-derived activity in the coupling of bone formation to resorption. Trends Mol Med. 2005;11:76–81.
45. McLatchie LM, Fraser NJ, Main MJ, Wise A, Brown J, Thompson N, Solari R, Lee MG, Foord SM. RAMPs regulate the transport and ligand specificity of the calcitonin-receptor-like receptor. Nature. 1998;393: 333–9.
46. Muff R, Buhlmann N, Fischer JA, Born W. An amylin receptor is revealed following co-transfection of a calcitonin receptor with receptor activity modifying proteins-1 or -3. Endocrinology. 1999;140:2924–7.
47. Nakamura M, Morimoto S, Yang Q, Hisamatsu T, Hanai N, Nakamura Y, Mori I, Kakudo K. Osteoclast-like cells express receptor activity modifying protein 2: application of laser capture microdissection. J Mol Endocrinol. 2005;34:257–61.
48. Naot D, Cornish J. The role of peptides and receptors of the calcitonin family in the regulation of bone metabolism. Bone. 2008;43:813–8.
49. Naot D, Callon KE, Grey A, Cooper GJ, Reid IR, Cornish J. A potential role for adrenomedullin as a local regulator of bone growth. Endocrinology. 2001;142:1849–57.

50. Naot D, Bava U, Matthews B, Callon KE, Gamble GD, Black M, Song S, Pitto RP, Cundy T, Cornish J, Reid IR. Differential gene expression in cultured osteoblasts and bone marrow stromal cells from patients with Paget's disease of bone. J Bone Miner Res. 2007;22:298–309.
51. Nicholson GC, Moseley JM, Sexton PM, Mendelsohn FA, Martin TJ. Abundant calcitonin receptors in isolated rat osteoclasts. Biochemical and autoradiographic characterization. J Clin Invest. 1986;78:355–60.
52. Njuki F, Nicholl CG, Howard A, Mak JC, Barnes PJ, Girgis SI, Legon S. A new calcitonin-receptor-like sequence in rat pulmonary blood vessels. Clin Sci. 1993;85:385–8.
53. Phelps E, Bezouglaia O, Tetradis S, Nervina JM. Parathyroid hormone induces receptor activity modifying protein-3 (RAMP3) expression primarily via 3′,5′-cyclic adenosine monophosphate signaling in osteoblasts. Calcif Tissue Int. 2005;77:96–103.
54. Poyner DR, Sexton PM, Marshall I, Smith DM, Quirion R, Born W, Muff R, Fischer JA, Foord SM. International union of pharmacology. XXXII. The mammalian calcitonin gene-related peptides, adrenomedullin, amylin, and calcitonin receptors. Pharmacol Rev. 2002;54:233–46.
55. Rakopoulos M, Ikegame M, Findlay DM, Martin TJ, Moseley JM. Short treatment of osteoclasts in bone marrow culture with calcitonin causes prolonged suppression of calcitonin receptor mRNA. Bone. 1995;17:447–53.
56. Reid IR, Schooler BA, Hannan SF, Ibbertson HK. The acute biochemical effects of four proprietary calcium preparations. Aust N Z J Med. 1986;16:193–7.
57. Reid IR, Ames R, Mason B, Reid HE, Bacon CJ, Bolland MJ, Gamble GD, Grey A, Horne A. Randomized controlled trial of calcium supplementation in healthy, nonosteoporotic, older men. Arch Intern Med. 2008;168:2276–82.
58. Rosenfeld MG, Mermod JJ, Amara SG, Swanson LW, Sawchenko PE, Rivier J, Vale WW, Evans RM. Production of a novel neuropeptide encoded by the calcitonin gene via tissue-specific RNA processing. Nature. 1983;304:129–35.
59. Rouleau MF, Warshawsky H, Goltzman D. Specific receptors for calcitonin in the subfornical organ of the brain. Brain. 1984;107(Pt 1):107–14.
60. Schinke T, Liese S, Priemel M, Haberland M, Schilling AF, Catala-Lehnen P, Blicharski D, Rueger JM, Gagel RF, Emeson RB, Amling M. Decreased bone formation and osteopenia in mice lacking alpha-calcitonin gene-related peptide. J Bone Miner Res. 2004; 19:2049–56.
61. Schlemmer A, Hassager C, Jensen SB, Christiansen C. Marked diurnal variation in urinary excretion of pyridinium cross-links in premenopausal women. J Clin Endocrinol Metab. 1992;74:476–80.
62. Sondergaard BC, Oestergaard S, Christiansen C, Tanko LB, Karsdal MA. The effect of oral calcitonin on cartilage turnover and surface erosion in an ovariectomized rat model. Arthritis Rheum. 2007;56: 2674–8.
63. Sondergaard BC, Wulf H, Henriksen K, Schaller S, Oestergaard S, Qvist P, Tanko LB, Bagger YZ, Christiansen C, Karsdal MA. Calcitonin directly attenuates collagen type II degradation by inhibition of matrix metalloproteinase expression and activity in articular chondrocytes. Osteoarthritis Cartilage. 2006; 14:759–68.
64. Takahashi S, Goldring S, Katz M, Hilsenbeck S, Williams R, Roodman GD. Downregulation of calcitonin receptor mRNA expression by calcitonin during human osteoclast-like cell differentiation. J Clin Invest. 1995;95:167–71.
65. Tippins JR, Morris HR, Panico M, Etienne T, Bevis P, Girgis S, MacIntyre I, Azria M, Attinger M. The myotropic and plasma-calcium modulating effects of calcitoningene-relatedpeptide(CGRP).Neuropeptides. 1984;4:425–34.
66. Uzan B, de Vernejoul MC, Cressent M. RAMPs and CRLR expressions in osteoblastic cells after dexamethasone treatment. Biochem Biophys Res Commun. 2004;321:802–8.
67. Villa I, Rubinacci A, Ravasi F, Ferrara AF, Guidobono F. Effects of amylin on human osteoblast-like cells. Peptides. 1997;18:537–40.
68. Villa I, Melzi R, Pagani F, Ravasi F, Rubinacci A, Guidobono F. Effects of calcitonin gene-related peptide and amylin on human osteoblast-like cells proliferation. Eur J Pharmacol. 2000;409:273–8.
69. Wada S, Martin TJ, Findlay DM. Homologous regulation of the calcitonin receptor in mouse osteoclast-like cells and human breast cancer T47D cells. Endocrinology. 1995;136:2611–21.
70. Wada S, Udagawa N, Nagata N, Martin TJ, Findlay DM. Calcitonin receptor down-regulation relates to calcitonin resistance in mature mouse osteoclasts. Endocrinology. 1996;137:1042–8.
71. Weiss RE, Singer FR, Gorn AH, Hofer DP, Nimni ME. Calcitonin stimulates bone formation when administered prior to initiation of osteogenesis. J Clin Invest. 1981;68:815–8.
72. Wener JA, Gorton SJ, Raisz LG. Escape from inhibition or resorption in cultures of fetal bone treated with calcitoninand parathyroid hromone. Endocrinology. 1972;90:752–9.
73. Woodrow JP, Sharpe CJ, Fudge NJ, Hoff AO, Gagel RF, Kovacs CS. Calcitonin plays a critical role in regulating skeletal mineral metabolism during lactation. Endocrinology. 2006;147:4010–21.
74. Zaidi M, Datta HK, Moonga BS, MacIntyre I. Evidence that the action of calcitonin on rat osteoclasts is mediated by two G proteins acting via separate post-receptor pathways. J Endocrinol. 1990;126:473–81.

Glucocorticoids, Inflammation, and Bone

7

Kong Wah Ng and T. John Martin

Keywords
Glucocorticoids • Bone loss • Inflammation • Cytokines
Glucocorticoid-induced osteoporosis • Rheumatoid arthritis

7.1 Introduction

7.1.1 Normal Function

Cortisol (hydrocortisone) is the principal glucocorticoid secreted from the adrenal cortex with a major role in the regulation of protein, carbohydrate, lipid, and nucleic acid metabolism. The production of glucocorticoids from the adrenal cortex is controlled by a classical negative feedback loop in which neurons in the hypothalamus detect circulating concentrations of glucocorticoids and in response stimulate or inhibit the release from the hypothalamus of corticotrophin-releasing hormone (CRH) and arginine vasopressin (AVP). CRH acts on corticotrophs in the anterior pituitary to stimulate the synthesis and release of adrenocorticotrophin (ACTH). The main action of ACTH on the adrenal cortex is to stimulate the synthesis and release of glucocorticoids and androgens.

Glucocorticoids readily cross cell membranes to combine with the glucocorticoid receptor (GR) in target tissues. There are two isoforms of the glucocorticoid receptor, GR alpha (GRα) and GR beta (GFβ). In bone cells, GRα is more abundantly expressed than GRβ [15]. Ligation of GRα leads to its dissociation from the protein complex that contains several heat shock proteins, mitogen-activated protein kinases (MAPKs), and chaperons, thus allowing GRα to translocate the nucleus and to form a homodimer. The zinc fingers in the DNA-binding domain of the dimerized receptors interact with the corresponding glucocorticoid response element of target genes to stimulate or repress gene transcription.

Prereceptor metabolism of glucocorticoids provides a way of modulating their action within a given tissue. The glucocorticoid metabolizing enzymes, 11beta-hydroxysteroid dehydrogenases (11βHSD), play a major role in modulating local cortisol levels [141]. The two isoenzymes, 11βHSD1 and 11βHSD2, act in opposing directions. 11βHSD2 acts as a dehydrogenase, converting active cortisol to the inactive cortisone, whereas 11βHSD1 acts as a reductase,

K.W. Ng, M.D.
Department of Endocrinology and Diabetes,
St. Vincent's Hospital, 41 Victoria Parade,
Fitzroy, VIC 3065, Australia

T.J. Martin, M.D., D.Sc. (✉)
Bone Cell Biology and Disease,
St. Vincent's Institute of Medical Research,
9 Princes Street, Fitzroy, VIC 3065, Australia
e-mail: jmartin@svi.edu.au

F. Bronner et al. (eds.), *Bone-Metabolic Functions and Modulators*, Topics in Bone Biology,
DOI 10.1007/978-1-4471-2745-1_7, © Springer-Verlag London 2012

regenerating active glucocorticoids in a tissue-specific manner [74]. Within specific cell types, the enzymes control glucocorticoid access to glucocorticoid receptors. Thus, cells that express 11βHSD2 are glucocorticoid resistant, whereas cells that express 11βHSD1 boost intracellular glucocorticoid levels. Intracellular glucocorticoid concentrations can, therefore, differ from plasma glucocorticoid levels depending on the 11βHSD isoenzyme expressed.

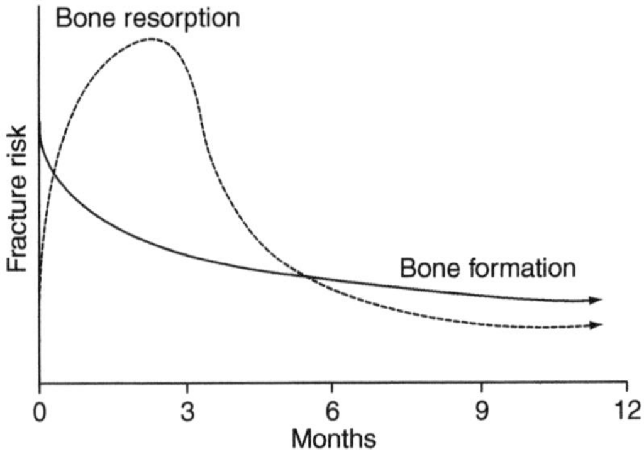

Fig. 7.1 Conceptual diagram for the time course of glucocorticoid-induced osteoporosis. There is an early phase of increased bone resorption when the risk of fracture is greatest, followed by a later phase of decreased bone formation and reduced bone turnover. Bone resorption is represented by *dotted line*, and bone formation by *solid line*

7.1.2 Glucocorticoids and Osteoporosis

The conclusion that physiological amounts of endogenous glucocorticoids are necessary for efficient osteoblast differentiation [53, 147, 148] was reached from studies of mice rendered null for the 11βHSD isoenzymes. On the other hand, excess amounts of glucocorticoids cause osteoporosis and other adverse effects such as glucose intolerance, dyslipidemia, central adiposity, hypertension, myopathy, and increased susceptibility to infections. Glucocorticoid-induced osteoporosis (GIO) is the most common form of secondary osteoporosis [108, 142]. Glucocorticoids are extensively used in the treatment of chronic inflammatory conditions such as rheumatoid arthritis (RA), asthma, inflammatory bowel disease, and multiple sclerosis. Glucocorticoids are well known to induce apoptosis of mononuclear cells, especially of lymphocytes and, to a lesser extent, of monocytes. It is these observations that have provided the rationale for using glucocorticoids to treat many lymphoid diseases and to prevent solid organ and stem cell transplant rejection [18, 158].

In GIO, bone loss occurs rapidly soon after initiation of therapy, with fracture risk increasing within 3 months of therapy. This occurs even before significant loss of BMD and is followed by a later phase of decreased bone formation [25, 39, 106] (Fig. 7.1). Within the first year, BMD is reduced by 6–12% and by about 3% in each subsequent year of additional treatment. The relative risk of fracture escalates by as much as 75% within the first 3 months after initiation of steroid therapy [163, 176]. Up to 50% of patients develop vertebral fractures if under prolonged treatment with systemic glucocorticoids [27, 41, 50, 115]. Some studies have shown that glucocorticoid-induced fractures tend to be multiple and occur at BMD values that are higher than in patients with other kinds of osteoporosis. The adverse effects on bone of excess glucocorticoid may, therefore, be partly due to abnormalities that are not related to the decline in bone mass [121, 176].

An increase in fracture risk occurs with daily doses of prednisolone as low as 2.5–7.5 mg. Although fractures can occur early in the course of glucocorticoid therapy, as pointed out above, fracture risk is also associated with the dose and duration of glucocorticoid exposure [33, 108, 164].

We shall now discuss the cellular aspects of glucocorticoid action in bone, highlighting the immunomodulatory roles of glucocorticoids in acute and chronic inflammation.

7.2 Acute Inflammation and Immunomodulatory Role of Glucocorticoids

Glucocorticoids were first used by Philip Hench in collaboration with Edward Kendall to treat inflammation in the late 1940s. For their successful use of cortisone to treat RA, they were awarded a Nobel Prize in 1950.

Glucocorticoids are a necessary component of a coordinated inflammatory response to injury and exert potent immunomodulatory rather than simply anti-inflammatory effects. Depending on concentration and timing, glucocorticoid treatment enhances and suppresses immune reactions. It, thus, shapes adaptive and innate immune responses [29, 30, 186].

Inflammation is a host defense mechanism activated in immediate response to injury or infection. It serves to control and eliminate invading pathogens and promote repair of damaged tissue [30]. The classic signs of inflammation, which include redness, swelling, heat, and pain, result from proinflammatory mediators such as tumor necrosis factor alpha (TNFα) and interleukin-1 (IL-1), released by resident mast cells and macrophages that cause increased vascular permeability and edema and promote migration of leukocytes into injured tissues. Macrophage differentiation is profoundly affected by the microenvironment: cytokines, microbial products, and hormones dictate their phenotype and responses. Thus, interferon gamma (IFNγ) and lipopolysaccharide (LPS) released early in the acute inflammatory response cause macrophages to differentiate to a phenotype that is strongly microbicidal [107].

Some stimulatory effects of glucocorticoids in the course of inflammation may be due to increased cellular expression of cytokine receptors. This enhances target T cell sensitivity to stimulation by cytokines. Glucocorticoids induce or enhance the expression of several cytokine receptors, including those for TNFα, IL-1, IL-2, and IL-6. Other receptors expressed are IFNγ and granulocyte-macrophage colony-stimulating factor (GM-CSF) in epithelial cells, lymphocytes, hepatocytes, monocytes, and neutrophils [6, 178]. The net effect may be to accelerate the onset and progression of an inflammatory response and a more rapid offset.

Glucocorticoids also play an important role in the resolution of inflammation because of their anti-inflammatory actions on mast cells, T lymphocytes, and monocytes. Glucocorticoids inhibit mast cell recruitment, proliferation, and survival, as well as mast cell degranulation and arachidonic acid metabolism [31]. They induce a shift in the cytokine response of stimulated CD4+ T cells with inhibition of the production of proinflammatory TNFα and IFNγ and by enhancing the anti-inflammatory actions of IL-4, IL-10, IL-1 receptor antagonist, and IL-13 and of the production of the transforming growth factor beta (TGFβ [7, 9, 13, 16, 126, 154]). Exposure of monocytes to glucocorticoids, IL-10, and TGFβ matures them into macrophages and reprograms their differentiation into a highly phagocytic "anti-inflammatory" phenotype with an enhanced ability to clear debris and ingest apoptotic cells [71, 102, 132, 167]. This process, thus, actively contributes to the resolution of inflammation.

Induction of 11βHSD1 to increase the availability of intracellular cortisol early in the course of an acute inflammation may play a significant role in its final resolution. This inference is supported by findings in the 11βHSD1 knockout mice, which have shown an exaggerated inflammatory response and altered resolution mechanisms. Compared to wild-type mice, $11\beta HSD^{-/-}$ mice show delayed acquisition of phagocytic competence following injection with thioglycollate [64]. Their weight loss is greater, and they have higher serum levels of TNFα, IL-6, and IL-12p40 following LPS administration [189]. 11βHSD1 is expressed in dendritic cells, T and B lymphocytes, as well as in macrophages [58, 188]. Increased 11βHSD1 activity and mRNA levels have been reported in synovial fibroblasts of patients with RA, where it is highly induced by IL-1 or TNFα [69], whereas 11βHSD2 is decreased. In general, 11βHSD1 expression is increased and 11βHSD2 decreased by proinflammatory stimuli or in the course of inflammation.

Glucocorticoid concentration within the systemic circulation is also increased during inflammation. TNFα, IL-1, and IL-6 released from a site of injury or following exposure to bacterial endotoxin activate the hypophyseal-pituitary-adrenal axis via a CRH-stimulated release of adrenocorticotropic hormone (ACTH) [32, 145]. This leads to an increase in production of glucocorticoids by the adrenal cortex.

The high concentrations of glucocorticoids commonly observed during major stresses are suppressive or anti-inflammatory and probably protect an animal from excessive inflammatory responses to injury [17, 54, 114]. In general, the inflammatory response is beneficial, with acute inflammation normally resolved quickly.

7.3 NFκB and the Anti-inflammatory Actions of Glucocorticoids

Nuclear factor kappa B (NFκB) proteins are a family of ubiquitously expressed transcription factors that play an essential role in most immune and inflammatory responses. In mammals, the NFκB family consists of five members: RelA (p65), RelB, c-Rel, NFκB1 (p50 and its precursor p105), and NFκB2 (p52 and its precursor p100). These compounds form a variety of homodimers and heterodimers, each of which activates its own set of genes that share a 300-amino acid domain, designated the Rel homology domain, which mediates their binding, dimerization, and nuclear translocation [19, 61, 135].

NFκB is present in the cytoplasm of almost all mammalian cells in an inactive form associated with the inhibitor kappaB (IκB) proteins, which include IκB alpha (IκBα), IκB beta (IκBβ), IκB epsilon (IκBε) and IκB gamma (IκBγ) [105]. The IκB proteins typically contain C-terminal ankyrin repeats that are crucial for their interaction with the NFκB proteins and an N-terminal leucine-rich nuclear export sequence that is important for the shuttling of IκB between the cytoplasm and nucleus. The shuttling is a mechanism important for the retention of the IκBα-p50-p65 complex in the cytoplasm. IκBα is also involved in the removal of NFκB proteins from the nucleus. Thus, IκB has both cytoplasmic and nuclear roles in regulating the NFκB pathway. In unstimulated cells, NFκB resides in the cytoplasm as an inactive NFκB–IκB complex. IκB binding hinders the recognition of the NFκB nuclear localization signal by nuclear import machinery so that NFκB is retained in the cytoplasm.

Many stimuli including the cytokines TNFα or IL-1, chemokines, bacterial and viral products, ultraviolet radiation, and free radicals activate the NFκB dimers by triggering a signaling pathway that leads to the degradation of IκB, occurring through consecutive steps of phosphorylation by IκB kinase (IKK), ubiquitination by $E3^{I\kappa B}$ ubiquitin ligase complex, and 26S proteasomal degradation. IKK is a complex composed of three subunits: IKKα, IKKβ, and IKKγ/NFκB, an essential modulator (NEMO). IKKα and IKKβ serve as the catalytic subunits, whereas IKKγ/NEMO is the regulatory subunit. IKKβ but not IKKα is essential for NFκB activation in response to proinflammatory and innate immune stimuli [187]. With few exceptions, release of NFκB is mediated by the degradation of IκB. The degradation of IκB exposes a nuclear localization signal on the NFκB proteins, which are then enabled to translocate into the nucleus and to stimulate transcription of specific genes [45].

NFκB regulates more than 150 genes, including those involved in immunity and inflammation, antiapoptosis, cell proliferation, and the negative feedback of the NFκB signal. NFκB regulates the expression of the cytokines IL-1 and TNFα, which are essential mediators of chronic inflammation and are implicated in leukocytosis, hyperplasia, and tissue breakdown. In turn, both TNFα and IL-1 are potent activators of NFκB activation, bringing about an interdependence of persistent NFκB activation and sustained levels of IL-1 and TNFα. Elevated levels of other NFκB-dependent gene products, including IL-6 and IL-15, the adhesion molecules E-selectin, VCAM-1 and ICAM-1, and the chemokines IL-8, MCP-1, and MIP-1α, promote recruitment and activation of inflammatory cells [135].

The NFκB signaling pathway has a number of built-in autoregulatory mechanisms that limit the duration and intensity of NFκB activation. NFκB rapidly induces the expression of its own inhibitor, IκB. The newly synthesized IκB enters the nucleus, where it dissociates NFκB from DNA and transports it to the cytoplasm. Another feedback mechanism acts on IKK. Activated IKKβ phosphorylates itself on its inhibitory loop, thereby limiting the duration of IKK activation. These feedback mechanisms ensure that NFκB-dependent transcription is only transiently activated in response to stimulation [105].

Glucocorticoids block the inflammatory action of TNFα by inducing the transcription of IκB. In the rat osteoblast-like cell line ROS 17/2.8, TNFα-dependent activation of NFκB was almost completely suppressed by treatment with the synthetic glucocorticoid, dexamethasone. Western blot and immunocytochemical analyses have shown that dexamethasone attenuates the TNFα-induced nuclear translocation of p65. Dexamethasone increases IκBα mRNA synergistically with TNFα, whereas it decreases p65 mRNA level. The increase in IκBα protein and concomitant decrease in p65 synthesis account for the dexamethasone-induced suppression of NFκB activation [93].

This action of glucocorticoid represses NFκB-mediated gene expression, decreasing proinflammatory cytokine production as well as inducing genes to inhibit cyclooxygenase-2 (COX-2) and adhesion molecules, as well as other inflammatory mediators [10]. This mechanism is strongly cell type and target gene dependent [45]. Whereas IκBα upregulation is predominantly and consistently observed in lymphocytes and monocytes, this is not so for endothelial or fibroblast cultures. Upregulation may begin as early as 30–60 min after drug administration and may take place even after a dose of prednisolone of 7.5 mg. This genomic effect may not occur until all the cytoplasmic glucocorticoid receptors are occupied, at prednisone doses of approximately 100 mg/day [21].

Apart from glucocorticoids, other anti-inflammatory drugs such as aspirin, sodium salicylate, sulfasalazine, and gold compounds also inhibit NFκB activity [55, 182] but are neither potent nor selective.

Even though NFκB plays an essential beneficial role in normal physiology, inappropriate regulation of NFκB activity has been implicated in the pathogenesis of several inflammatory and rheumatic diseases, such as RA, asthma, atherosclerosis, multiple sclerosis, inflammatory bowel disease, cancer, AIDs, and cachexia. The mechanisms that activate NFκB in chronic inflammation are unknown. Certain types of chronic inflammation are initiated by an autoimmune response that then progresses to a sustained, self-perpetuated inflammation. Experimental evidence suggests that NFκB is pivotal for initiation and perpetuation of chronic inflammation.

7.4 Chronic Inflammation and Bone Loss

When prolonged inflammation is not resolved, it ceases to be beneficial and contributes to the pathogenesis of many disease states. The hallmark of chronic inflammation is the sustained presence and accumulation of activated macrophages that continue to release proinflammatory mediators and that are responsible for much of the tissue damage. Chronic manifestations of these diseases typically represent a self-perpetuating hyperimmune, pathological phenomenon and cause progressive structural damage. It is likely that chronic inflammation such as occurs during RA or asthma results from an imbalance between the initial proinflammatory events needed to protect against infection and the mechanisms that terminate the inflammatory response, restoring homeostasis [70].

Inflammation per se is a risk factor for bone loss, independent of glucocorticoid therapy [94, 109]. A longitudinal study by van Staa and colleagues has demonstrated that disease activity and duration independently affect the risk of osteoporotic fracture in many skeletal sites, including the hip in patients with RA [165]. Virtually all forms of chronic inflammatory diseases besides RA, such as inflammatory bowel disease, systemic lupus erythematosus, and ankylosing spondylitis, are characterized by progressive bone loss [84, 85, 127]. Moreover, epidemiological studies have shown that the serum level of C-reactive protein predicts osteoporotic fracture independent of established risk factors [120, 143]. In contrast, when inflammation is treated aggressively and effectively, BMD can be preserved [68].

Rheumatoid arthritis is an autoimmune disease that is characterized by progressive destruction of periarticular and joint structures and loss of subchondral bone associated with generalized osteoporosis. The radiological hallmarks of RA are focal marginal joint erosions that are characteristically localized to the joint margins and subchondral bone adjacent to the bone marrow space into which the synovial inflammatory tissues have extended [67].

The involvement of the immune system is fundamental to the progression of RA. The molecular link between inflammation and bone resorption is not fully established, but it is widely acknowledged that cytokines such as TNFα, IL-1, and IL-6 play an essential role. These mediators link inflammation to bone loss by directly stimulating osteoclasts and by inducing the expression of factors essential for osteoclast formation [2, 3, 23]. There is solid evidence to support the idea that the vital link between chronic inflammation and bone function is provided by NFκB. Not only is it a central regulator of cellular responses to inflammation and to a broad range of diseases due to activation of the immune system, but it also plays a pivotal role in the formation and activation of osteoclasts [144, 159]. There is no question that osteoclasts are essential to the formation of focal joint erosions in inflammatory arthritis. RANKL knockout mice fail to develop functional osteoclasts and erosions [103, 122, 128].

7.4.1 RANKL/OPG/RANK and Osteoclast Formation

Under physiological conditions, mononuclear osteoclast precursor cells differentiate into multinucleate osteoclasts under the influence of the macrophage colony-stimulating factor (M-CSF) secreted by osteoblasts and the receptor activator of NFκB ligand (RANKL), an osteoblast protein that is regulated by osteotrophic hormones, i.e., parathyroid hormone and calcitriol, as well as by cytokines such as IL-1, IL-6, and IL-11. RANKL occurs in two forms: membrane bound and secreted. RANK, the receptor to which RANKL is bound, is expressed in mononuclear osteoclast precursors. The presence of M-CSF initiates the processes that lead to the formation of functional multinucleate osteoclasts. Osteoprotegerin (OPG), also produced by osteoblasts, functions as a decoy molecule to regulate and activate osteoclast differentiation by blocking the interaction of RANK and RANKL. It is relative RANKL and OPG levels that determine whether bone is formed or lost [95, 184, 185].

When RANK is bound to RANKL, signaling is initiated by the TNF receptor–associated factors (TRAFs) 1,2,3,5, and 6. TRAF-6 plays an important role in linking the interaction of RANK to the adaptor proteins downstream. Binding to TRAF adaptor proteins within the cytoplasmic domain of RANK is the initial step in the process of RANK signaling [116]. The downstream targets of TRAF-6 are the transcription factors, including NFκB, activator protein-1 (AP-1) and nuclear factor of activated T cells-1 (NFATc1), MAPKs such as p38 stress kinase, c-jun-terminal kinase (JNK), and the ERK and PI3K/AKT pathways [160]. NFATc1 is the master transcription factor for osteoclastogenesis [155, 156]. The pivotal role of NFκB in osteoclastogenesis is underscored by the fact that gene-specific deletion of both its p50 and p52 subunits leads to severe osteopetrosis, because osteoclastogenesis is suppressed [57, 79, 138].

7.4.2 RANKL/OPG/RANK System in Chronic Inflammation

RANKL is normally expressed by osteoblasts. However, in chronic inflammation, nonosteoblastic sources of RANKL assume greater importance. Both soluble and membrane-bound RANKL is produced by activated $CD4^+$ and $CD8^+$ T cells [75, 92]. RANKL is also expressed in lymph nodes, spleen, thymus, and intestinal lymphoid patches and by immature $CD4^-CD8^-$ thymocytes. Transgenic overexpression of RANKL in T cells restores osteoclastogenesis in a *rankl*$^{-/-}$ background and partially restores normal bone marrow cavities [87]. This demonstrates that T cells are crucial mediators of bone loss in vivo through their production of RANKL. RANKL may also be produced by other cells of the RA joint, such as synovial fibroblasts [150], chondrocytes [90], endothelial cells [36], activated macrophages [43], and neutrophils [123].

In inflammatory or autoimmune disease states, activated T cells produce RANKL and proinflammatory cytokines such as TNFα, IL-1, IL-6, or IL-11, all of which can induce RANKL expression in osteoblasts and bone marrow stromal cells. Thus, it seems that T cells promote bone resorption directly via RANKL expression and indirectly via expression of proinflammatory cytokines that mediate RANKL expression in non–T cells. TNFα also produced by activated macrophages as well as by synoviocytes, triggers bone erosion through induction of IL-1 [190]. TNFα also induces osteoclast formation independently of the RANKL/RANK interaction [88] by directly targeting macrophage precursors. This process requires constitutive amounts of RANKL which primes macrophages to commit to osteoclast phenotype in response to TNFα [97]. In a reciprocal fashion, TNFα "primes" these precursors to respond to relatively small amounts of RANKL. Another inflammatory mediator that has been implicated in destructive arthritis is the T cell product IL-17. IL-17 is abundant in active RA joints and constitutes a potent inducer of RANKL. It is produced by T-helper 17 (Th17) cells that also express RANKL and TNFα. Th17 cells are produced when naïve T cells are activated by TGFβ and IL-6 in the mouse, or by TGFβ and inflammatory stimuli in humans. IL-17 production is also promoted by IL-23 [5, 104, 119, 144].

Anti-inflammatory cytokines produced by T cells include IFNγ, GM-CSF, IL-3, OPG, IL-4, IL-10, IL-13, IL-12, osteoclast inhibitory lectin (OCIL), and secreted frizzled-related proteins (sFRPs) [63, 76, 125]. Even though IL-23 stimulates Th17 cells to secrete IL-17 and RANKL, it is also a potent stimulator of GM-CSF production. Some of these factors, such as GM-CSF, IL-3, and sFRPs, strongly block osteoclast formation when RANKL levels are high. IFNγ is generally considered to be a proinflammatory factor based on its strong activation of macrophage antimicrobial activity, antigen presentation, and synergy with TNFα and LPS in the activation of macrophage inflammatory functions [146]. There is solid evidence for the anti-inflammatory actions of IFNγ. IFNs suppress a broad range of proinflammatory and tissue-destructive activities of IL-1 through the modulation of IL-1 receptor expression. IFNγ-mediated downregulation of IL-1R type I expression is dependent on Stat1, a transcription factor considered to be a key mediator of macrophage activation by IFNs. Dual and opposing roles for Stat1 conform to a homeostatic paradigm in immune activation in which molecules that promote cell activation and effector function also play a role in limiting the response to avoid tissue damage and autoimmunity [77]. IFNγ also inhibits RANKL-mediated osteoclastogenesis, presumably via induction of TRAF6 ubiquitination and proteolytic TRAF6 degradation [8]. These counterregulatory measures control osteoclast activation and help limit, though not eliminate, structural bone damage in RA.

The anti-inflammatory and immunosuppressive actions of endogenous glucocorticoids may limit structural bone damage that arises from chronic inflammation. However, the beneficial action of glucocorticoids may be blunted when glucocorticoid-responsive tissues with an inflammatory response that is mediated by activated NFκB become resistant to glucocorticoid signaling because of a blocked GR function [46, 99]. Resistance is localized to the site of inflammation where cytokines are produced. This may explain why patients with glucocorticoid-resistant asthma respond to the endocrine and metabolic effects of glucocorticoids. Steroid resistance correlates with increased epithelial activation of stress-activated protein kinases such as MAPK and NFκB [60]. Enhanced JNK activation in steroid-resistant patients may contribute to steroid unresponsiveness, either by inhibiting GR activity or by blocking its phosphorylation or, indirectly, by increasing AP-1 activity, which transrepresses the glucocorticoid effects [56, 170]. Steroid resistance may be responsible for the need to initiate therapy of chronic inflammation with supraphysiological doses of glucocorticoids.

Bone loss in chronic inflammation is exacerbated by reduction in bone formation. Proinflammatory cytokines, particularly TNFα inhibit osteoblast differentiation [62] and bone-forming activity by downregulating the expression of Runx-2 and increasing the expression of Dickoff-1 (DKK-1), a potent Wnt antagonist found in inflamed joints [49]. The abundance of

DKK-1 in inflammatory arthritis reduces OPG expression and enhances RANKL sensitivity and osteoclast activity and subsequent bone loss [65].

7.5 Pathogenesis of Glucocorticoid-Induced Osteoporosis

7.5.1 Action of Glucocorticoids on Osteoblasts, Osteocytes, and Osteoclasts

Glucocorticoids act directly on bone cells. Osteoblasts, osteocytes, and osteoclasts express glucocorticoid receptors and glucocorticoid-modifying enzymes that determine the susceptibility to glucocorticoids [73].

Excess amounts of glucocorticoids reduce replication, alter differentiation, shorten life span, and impair osteoblast function. In the presence of excess glucocorticoids, the differentiation of bone marrow stroma is directed toward cells of the adipocytic lineage. Mechanisms involved in this redirection of stromal cells include induction of nuclear factors of the CCAAT enhancer binding protein family and induction of peroxisome proliferator–activated receptor gamma 2 (PPARγ 2) [169]. One mechanism involves repression of bone morphogenetic proteins, of the insulin-like growth factor-1 (IGF-1) and of TGFβ, which activate the osteoblastic transcription factors Runx2 and beta-catenin (β-catenin) [27, 171, 180]. Other effects of glucocorticoids on bone formation include inhibition of the Wnt signaling pathway and increased osteoblast and osteocyte apoptosis through activation by caspase 3 [89, 117, 149, 174]. Glucocorticoids suppress Wnt signaling by increasing the expression of DDK-1 and sFRP-1, as well as by stabilizing GSK3β [118, 152, 169]. The decrease in β-catenin inhibits LEF/TCF-mediated transcription. Reduced β-catenin levels downregulate OPG and upregulate RANKL [65, 66]. Glucocorticoids also impair bone matrix synthesis and composition. Gene expression of type I collagen is repressed by glucocorticoids through transcriptional and posttranscriptional mechanisms [48]. Following glucocorticoid treatment, bone strength is compromised due to increased expression of the mineralization inhibitors Dmp-1 and Phex [183].

The effect of excess glucocorticoids on osteocyte viability substantially contributes to impaired bone quality and strength, independent of bone loss, because osteocytes serve as mechanosensors and are involved in the repair of bone microdamage. Loss of osteocytes reduces the size of the vascular bed in bone and disrupts the osteocyte lacunar canalicular network. This leads to the failure to detect signals that stimulate processes that mediate the replacement of damaged bone [14]. Disruption of the osteocyte lacunar canalicular network disrupts fluid flow within the network and adversely affects the mechanical strength of bone, whether or not bone remodeling or mineral density has changed [98, 175, 176]. Age-dependent increases in endogenous glucocorticoids compromise bone strength in a manner similar to that of excess glucocorticoids [177]. In humans, endogenous glucocorticoids increase with age [124, 133] due to 11βHSD1 activity in osteoblasts [42] and because of the glucocorticoid feedback inhibition of ACTH that is blunted [179].

Low bone turnover and reduced bone formation are characteristic of long-term glucocorticoid therapy because of depletion of the osteoblastic cellular pool. This depletion is the result of the inhibition by glucocorticoids of osteoblast cell replication and differentiation and of the increase in apoptosis of mature osteoblasts.

The mechanisms that underlie the transient glucocorticoid-mediated increase in bone resorption have not been fully elucidated but include increased production by osteoblasts of M-CSF and RANKL [72, 137] and the downregulation of OPG, which brings about an increase in osteoclastogenesis and prolongs the osteoclast life span.

Glucocorticoid-mediated suppression of OPG production does not involve canonical Wnt signaling [65, 91]. An increase in the RANKL/OPG ratio has been observed in human osteoblast-like cells and in immortalized human bone marrow stromal cells, as well as in immortalized human fetal osteoblasts and in the osteoblastic cell line MG-63. The increase in the RANKL/OPG ratio may constitute a key mechanism of glucocorticoid-induced bone loss [20, 72, 78, 168]. Suppression of OPG may also contribute indirectly to osteoclast survival because of increased availability of RANKL [96].

Glucocorticoids induce or enhance the expression of several cytokine receptors, including those for TNFα, IL-1, IL-2, IL-6, IFNγ, and GM-CSF [6, 178]. Glucocorticoids suppress the expression of IFNβ, an inhibitor of osteoclastogenesis [51, 157], and cause a decrease in apoptosis of mature osteoclasts [81]. Swanson and colleagues have shown that the expression of mRNA encoding RANK in osteoclast progenitor cells is increased following treatment with dexamethasone [153]. The net result is an increase in osteoclasts with a prolonged life span even though this transient increase in osteoclast activity may be limited by a reduction in RANKL production due to the suppression of osteoblastogenesis by glucocorticoids [26].

Glucocorticoids, in addition to acting on bone target cells, mediate changes in the synthesis, receptor binding, or binding proteins of growth factors present in the bone microenvironment. Glucocorticoids suppress IGF-1 and IGFBP-5 gene transcription [59]. IGFBP-5 is a binding protein for IGF-1 with anabolic effects on skeletal cells. IGF-1 increases bone formation and synthesis of type I collagen; it also decreases bone collagen degradation and osteoblast apoptosis [24]. Glucocorticoids inhibit the release of gonadotropins, thereby affecting estrogen and testosterone production [166]. Hypogonadism reduced production of IGF-1, and increased losses of calcium from the kidney and intestine contribute indirectly to glucocorticoid-induced bone loss. In addition, decreased muscle strength and impaired musculoskeletal interactions increase fracture risk because of a higher propensity to falls. Nevertheless, of the effects of glucocorticoids on bone cells, the direct ones predominate [27].

7.5.2 Susceptibility to Glucocorticoid-Induced Osteoporosis

Because some individuals are more susceptible to develop GIO than others, glucocorticoid bioavailability may vary in individuals perhaps because of differences in local activity of glucocorticoid metabolizing enzymes or in expression levels of GR. Another possibility is that differences in the response are due to polymorphisms of the glucocorticoid receptor gene [181]. Exogenously administered glucocorticoids differ in affinity for the 11βHSD isoforms. For example, the oxidation of steroids by 11βHSD2 is lower in fluorinated or methylated glucocorticoid compounds, with the actual reduction by 11βHSD1 depending on the structure of the steroid in question. This is the reason why the metabolism of synthetic glucocorticoids needs to be taken into account. The target tissues (liver, fat tissue, bone, CNS) may express 11βHSD1 differentially, and this may help optimize systemic glucocorticoid therapy [162].

7.6 Emerging Therapies in Glucocorticoid-Induced Osteoporosis

In therapy, it is important to recognize that chronic inflammation per se can cause bone loss even before therapy is started. In any therapeutic approach, it is important to prevent or lessen the impact of glucocorticoid-induced osteoporosis [38, 52]. To achieve this may only require low doses of prednisolone in early treatment [40], inhibition of bone resorption, or stimulation of bone formation. Effective measures targeting specific pathways associated with inflammation reduce dependence on glucocorticoids as anti-inflammatory agents [28].

7.6.1 Inhibition of Bone Resorption

Oral and intravenous administration of antiresorptives like bisphosphonates inhibits osteoclast function and promotes osteoclast apoptosis [38]. The primary endpoint of bisphosphonate trials has been to stabilize or increase BMD, with the minimization of fracture risk a secondary endpoint [4, 34, 47, 130, 131, 139]. Notwithstanding the fact that most studies have been short term, bisphosphonate treatment has become the mainstay of GIO treatment.

Denosumab is a human monoclonal antibody that blocks binding to RANK and inhibits osteoclast development and activity. As a result, bone resorption is diminished and bone density is increased. In clinical trials, denosumab has reduced bone turnover and increased BMD in osteoporotic postmenopausal women with low BMD. Denosumab also reduces fracture risk and, when added to ongoing methotrexate treatment, inhibits structural damage in patients with RA [44, 100, 113]. It is currently under investigation for the treatment of GIO.

The early effect of high-dose glucocorticoid treatment needs to be kept in mind when used to reduce cerebral edema in patients with brain tumors. In those circumstances, antiresorptive treatment provides prophylaxis against rapid bone loss.

In animal models of arthritis, inhibition of bone resorption through the RANKL/OPG/RANK pathway prevents bone erosion but has no beneficial effect on inflammation [136, 151].

7.6.2 Stimulation of Bone Formation

Parathyroid hormone (PTH), given intermittently, constitutes an effective anabolic agent, causing trabecular number, bone thickness, and connectivity to increase [82]. PTH stimulates the MAPK pathway and, thus, modulates osteoblast differentiation, replication, and activity (see Chap. 1). It stimulates the differentiation and activation of quiescent lining cells, increasing the life span of osteoblasts and osteocytes by inhibiting apoptosis and regulating replication, differentiation, and survival of progenitors. It does so by modulating the synthesis and release of local mediators, including Wnt, bone morphogenetic proteins, TGFβ, IGF-1, fibroblast growth factor 2, and IL-6 [112, 173]. Several studies have shown that PTH is an effective treatment for patients with GIO [22, 129, 140] and it is the only anabolic agent that counteracts the deleterious effects of glucocorticoids on the skeleton.

7.6.3 Targeting the Inflammatory Pathway

The established anticytokine therapies in RA involve TNFα, IL-1 antagonists, and anti-TNFα agents, including adalimumab, etanercept, infliximab, golimumab, and certolizumab. These agents exhibit rapid action and reduce inflammation and joint destruction. Treatment with infliximab has also been successful in inflammatory bowel disease [1, 37]. Blockade of IL-1 action with an IL-1 receptor antagonist has been effective in treating RA and in suppressing joint damage [35]. Tocilizumab is a monoclonal antibody against the IL-6 receptor, but its cost and concern about infections that arise from immunosuppression have limited its clinical use in RA [12, 80].

7.6.4 Kinase Inhibitors

Spleen tyrosine kinase (SyK) is a tyrosine kinase present in synoviocytes of patients with RA. It is a component of the signal pathway to Fc receptors that bind to immunoglobulins and autoantibodies. Fc receptors are expressed on most immune cells and activate them when the receptors are occupied by immune complexes that originate from the binding of autoantibodies to their antigen. The activation of these cells promotes cytokine production. Other cell types, such as B cells, NK cells, and osteoclasts, also use SyK [134]. Weinblatt and colleagues have reported, on the basis of a 6-month phase 2 study with R788, an oral Syk inhibitor. It reduced disease activity in patients with RA [172].

7.6.5 NFκB as a Potential Therapeutic Target

The pivotal role occupied by NFκB in linking inflammation and bone destruction makes suppression of NFκB an attractive therapeutic intervention. Progress in understanding the mechanisms of NFκB signaling has led to novel therapeutic strategies aimed at the inhibition of key elements in the NFκB pathway. Proteasome function inhibitors, decoy oligonucleotides, RNA interference, and peptides that inhibit nuclear localization of NFκB have been utilized to inhibit NFκB signaling. Research in this area has so far been restricted to animal studies.

Bortezomib, an orally active proteasome function inhibitor used to treat multiple myeloma, significantly decreases NFκB activity and is associated with lower serum levels of IL-1, IL-16, and nitric oxide metabolites [86].

NFκB decoys are short double-stranded oligodeoxynucleotides that contain NFκB binding sites which compete for binding with native NFκB and its consensus sequences in the promoter region of target genes. It is administered by intra-articular injection into the hind joints of rats with collagen-induced arthritis to decrease inflammation and prevent joint destruction [161].

IKKβ is an appealing target because of its crucial role in NFκB activation. Gene therapy using an intra-articular delivery of a dominant-negative IKKβ adenovirus construct inhibits NFκB translocation [11]. An orally available IKKβ inhibitor, BMS-345541, has in a dose-dependent manner reduced the incidence of arthritis in murine type-II-collagen-induced arthritis [110]. A small synthetic peptide that disrupts the interaction between IKKβ and the IKKγ regulatory subunit and therefore prevents IKK from inhibiting inflammation-induced bone loss in a mouse model of arthritis also has been used [83]. Genetic constructs that overexpress IκB or express an engineered protein without the sites for phosphorylation (IκB super repressor) have also been used with some success [138].

RNA interference is initiated by a double-stranded RNA which, after being introduced into cells, is cleaved into 21 or 22nt dsRNA fragments. These fragments (siRNA) induce the formation of a ribonucleoprotein complex that mediates sequence-specific cleavage of the targeted transcript RNA by the antisense RNA strand. It thereby promotes mRNA degradation of a specific mRNA [111]. siRNA targeting of the NFκB p65 subunit has shown promising results in rat chondrocytes that are stimulated with IL-1β and TNFα [101, 111].

Inhibition of elements of the NFκB signaling pathway is not without its hazards. One common effect of the disruption of NFκB genes or signaling pathways impairs development of proper immune function. In animal models, inactivation of the RelA gene, *rela*, causes early embryonic death owing to massive liver apoptosis due to the increased sensitivity of $rela^{-/-}$ fetal hepatocytes to the toxicity brought about by the cytotoxicity of circulating TNFα. $Ikk\beta^{-/-}$ mice die at midgestation due to massive liver apoptosis. $Relb^{-/-}$ mice spontaneously develop a persistent multiorgan inflammation due to overexpression of inflammatory cytokines. Important issues that need to be addressed before specific NFκB inhibitors can even be considered for clinical trials involve the selection of optimal targets for therapeutic intervention and side effects that may result from the suppression of NFκB and raises the question of long-term safety [105].

Conclusion

Physicians treating patients with diseases associated with chronic inflammation still face many challenges notwithstanding the availability of effective anti-inflammatory treatments. Often, such treatment needs to be initiated early in the course of the disease to prevent major structural damage to joints and bone. Another major hurdle is the lack of understanding of the mechanisms that trigger the dysregulation of immune and inflammatory responses that underpin chronic inflammatory disease. The deleterious effects of excess glucocorticoids on bone structure are widely known. However, reliance on glucocorticoid as an effective anti-inflammatory agent can only be reduced if safe and effective alternative agents are available to target relevant points along the inflammatory signaling pathways. We need affordable small-molecule inhibitors that are specific, relatively short acting, and are delivered to trouble spots without causing unwanted systemic effects.

References

1. Abreu MT, Geller JL, Vasiliauskas EA, Kam LY, Vora P, Martyak LA, Yang H, Hu B, Lin YC, Keenan G, Price J, Landers CJ, Adams JS, Targan SR. Treatment with infliximab is associated with increased markers of bone formation in patients with Crohn's disease. J Clin Gastroenterol. 2006;40(1):55–63.

2. Abu-Amer Y, Ross FP, Edwards J, Teitelbaum SL. Lipopolysaccharide-stimulated osteoclastogenesis is mediated by tumor necrosis factor via its P55 receptor. J Clin Invest. 1997;100(6):1557–65.
3. Abu-Amer Y, Erdmann J, Alexopoulou L, Kollias G, Ross FP, Teitelbaum SL. Tumor necrosis factor receptors types 1 and 2 differentially regulate osteoclastogenesis. J Biol Chem. 2000;275(35):27307–10.
4. Adachi JD, Saag KG, Delmas PD, Liberman UA, Emkey RD, Seeman E, Lane NE, Kaufman JM, Poubelle PE, Hawkins F, Correa-Rotter R, Menkes CJ, Rodriguez-Portales JA, Schnitzer TJ, Block JA, Wing J, McIlwain HH, Westhovens R, Brown J, Melo-Gomes JA, Gruber BL, Yanover MJ, Leite MO, Siminoski KG, Nevitt MC, Sharp JT, Malice MP, Dumortier T, Czachur M, Carofano W, Daifotis A. Two-year effects of alendronate on bone mineral density and vertebral fracture in patients receiving glucocorticoids: a randomized, double-blind, placebo-controlled extension trial. Arthritis Rheum. 2001;44(1):202–11.
5. Adamopoulos IE, Bowman EP. Immune regulation of bone loss by Th17 cells. Arthritis Res Ther. 2008; 10(5):225.
6. Almawi WY, Beyhum HN, Rahme AA, Rieder MJ. Regulation of cytokine and cytokine receptor expression by glucocorticoids. J Leukoc Biol. 1996;60(5): 563–72.
7. Almawi WY, Irani-Hakime N. The antiproliferative effect of glucocorticoids: is it related to induction of TGF-beta? Nephrol Dial Transplant. 1998;13(10):2450–2.
8. Arron JR, Choi Y. Bone versus immune system. Nature. 2000;408(6812):535–6.
9. Asadullah K, Schacke H, Cato AC. Dichotomy of glucocorticoid action in the immune system. Trends Immunol. 2002;23(3):120–2.
10. Auphan N, DiDonato JA, Rosette C, Helmberg A, Karin M. Immunosuppression by glucocorticoids: inhibition of NF-kappa B activity through induction of I kappa B synthesis. Science. 1995;270(5234):286–90.
11. Aupperle K, Bennett B, Han Z, Boyle D, Manning A, Firestein G. NF-kappa B regulation by I kappa B kinase-2 in rheumatoid arthritis synoviocytes. J Immunol. 2001;166(4):2705–11.
12. Bansback NJ, Regier DA, Ara R, Brennan A, Shojania K, Esdaile JM, Anis AH, Marra CA. An overview of economic evaluations for drugs used in rheumatoid arthritis: focus on tumour necrosis factor-alpha antagonists. Drugs. 2005;65(4):473–96.
13. Barnes PJ. Anti-inflammatory actions of glucocorticoids: molecular mechanisms. Clin Sci (Lond). 1998; 94(6):557–72.
14. Baylink DJ, Wergedal JE. Bone formation by osteocytes. Am J Physiol. 1971;221(3):669–78.
15. Beavan S, Horner A, Bord S, Ireland D, Compston J. Colocalization of glucocorticoid and mineralocorticoid receptors in human bone. J Bone Miner Res. 2001;16(8):1496–504.
16. Berrebi D, Bruscoli S, Cohen N, Foussat A, Migliorati G, Bouchet-Delbos L, Maillot MC, Portier A, Couderc J, Galanaud P, Peuchmaur M, Riccardi C, Emilie D. Synthesis of glucocorticoid-induced leucine zipper (GILZ) by macrophages: an anti-inflammatory and immunosuppressive mechanism shared by glucocorticoids and IL-10. Blood. 2003;101(2):729–38.
17. Bertini R, Bianchi M, Ghezzi P. Adrenalectomy sensitizes mice to the lethal effects of interleukin 1 and tumor necrosis factor. J Exp Med. 1988;167(5):1708–12.
18. Boumpas DT, Chrousos GP, Wilder RL, Cupps TR, Balow JE. Glucocorticoid therapy for immune-mediated diseases: basic and clinical correlates. Ann Intern Med. 1993;119(12):1198–208.
19. Bouwmeester T, Bauch A, Ruffner H, Angrand PO, Bergamini G, Croughton K, Cruciat C, Eberhard D, Gagneur J, Ghidelli S, Hopf C, Huhse B, Mangano R, Michon AM, Schirle M, Schlegl J, Schwab M, Stein MA, Bauer A, Casari G, Drewes G, Gavin AC, Jackson DB, Joberty G, Neubauer G, Rick J, Kuster B, Superti-Furga G. A physical and functional map of the human TNF-alpha/NF-kappa B signal transduction pathway. Nat Cell Biol. 2004;6(2):97–105.
20. Brandstrom H, Bjorkman T, Ljunggren O. Regulation of osteoprotegerin secretion from primary cultures of human bone marrow stromal cells. Biochem Biophys Res Commun. 2001;280(3):831–5.
21. Buttgereit F, da Silva JA, Boers M, Burmester GR, Cutolo M, Jacobs J, Kirwan J, Kohler L, Van Riel P, Vischer T, Bijlsma JW. Standardised nomenclature for glucocorticoid dosages and glucocorticoid treatment regimens: current questions and tentative answers in rheumatology. Ann Rheum Dis. 2002;61(8): 718–22.
22. Buxton EC, Yao W, Lane NE. Changes in serum receptor activator of nuclear factor-kappaB ligand, osteoprotegerin, and interleukin-6 levels in patients with glucocorticoid-induced osteoporosis treated with human parathyroid hormone (1–34). J Clin Endocrinol Metab. 2004;89(7):3332–6.
23. Caetano-Lopes J, Canhao H, Fonseca JE. Osteoimmunology – the hidden immune regulation of bone. Autoimmun Rev. 2009;8(3):250–5.
24. Canalis E, Centrella M, Burch W, McCarthy TL. Insulin-like growth factor I mediates selective anabolic effects of parathyroid hormone in bone cultures. J Clin Invest. 1989;83(1):60–5.
25. Canalis E, Bilezikian JP, Angeli A, Giustina A. Perspectives on glucocorticoid-induced osteoporosis. Bone. 2004;34(4):593–8.
26. Canalis E. Mechanisms of glucocorticoid action in bone. Curr Osteoporos Rep. 2005;3(3):98–102.
27. Canalis E, Mazziotti G, Giustina A, Bilezikian JP. Glucocorticoid-induced osteoporosis: pathophysiology and therapy. Osteoporos Int. 2007;18(10): 1319–28.
28. Cantley MD, Smith MD, Haynes DR. Pathogenic bone loss in rheumatoid arthritis: mechanisms and therapeutic approaches. Int J Clin Rheumatol. 2009; 4(5):561–82.
29. Chapman KE, Coutinho A, Gray M, Gilmour JS, Savill JS, Seckl JR. Local amplification of glucocorticoids by 11beta-hydroxysteroid dehydroge-

nase type 1 and its role in the inflammatory response. Ann N Y Acad Sci. 2006;1088:265–73.
30. Chapman KE, Gilmour JS, Coutinho AE, Savill JS, Seckl JR. 11beta-hydroxysteroid dehydrogenase type 1 – a role in inflammation? Mol Cell Endocrinol. 2006;248(1–2):3–8.
31. Chapman KE, Coutinho AE, Gray M, Gilmour JS, Savill JS, Seckl JR. The role and regulation of 11beta-hydroxysteroid dehydrogenase type 1 in the inflammatory response. Mol Cell Endocrinol. 2009;301(1–2):123–31.
32. Chrousos GP. The hypothalamic-pituitary-adrenal axis and immune-mediated inflammation. N Engl J Med. 1995;332(20):1351–62.
33. Cohen A, Shane E. Osteoporosis after solid organ and bone marrow transplantation. Osteoporos Int. 2003;14(8):617–30.
34. Cohen S, Levy RM, Keller M, Boling E, Emkey RD, Greenwald M, Zizic TM, Wallach S, Sewell KL, Lukert BP, Axelrod DW, Chines AA. Risedronate therapy prevents corticosteroid-induced bone loss: a twelve-month, multicenter, randomized, double-blind, placebo-controlled, parallel-group study. Arthritis Rheum. 1999;42(11):2309–18.
35. Cohen S, Hurd E, Cush J, Schiff M, Weinblatt ME, Moreland LW, Kremer J, Bear MB, Rich WJ, McCabe D. Treatment of rheumatoid arthritis with anakinra, a recombinant human interleukin-1 receptor antagonist, in combination with methotrexate: results of a twenty-four-week, multicenter, randomized, double-blind, placebo-controlled trial. Arthritis Rheum. 2002;46(3):614–24.
36. Collin-Osdoby P, Rothe L, Anderson F, Nelson M, Maloney W, Osdoby P. Receptor activator of NF-kappa B and osteoprotegerin expression by human microvascular endothelial cells, regulation by inflammatory cytokines, and role in human osteoclastogenesis. J Biol Chem. 2001;276(23):20659–62.
37. Colombel JF, Sandborn WJ, Reinisch W, Mantzaris GJ, Kornbluth A, Rachmilewitz D, Lichtiger S, D'Haens G, Diamond RH, Broussard DL, Tang KL, van der Woude CJ, Rutgeerts P. Infliximab, azathioprine, or combination therapy for Crohn's disease. N Engl J Med. 2010;362(15):1383–95.
38. Compston J. Management of glucocorticoid-induced osteoporosis. Nat Rev Rheumatol. 2010;6(2):82–8.
39. Compston JE. Emerging consensus on prevention and treatment of glucocorticoid-induced osteoporosis. Curr Rheumatol Rep. 2007;9(1):78–84.
40. Conn DL, Lim SS. New role for an old friend: prednisone is a disease-modifying agent in early rheumatoid arthritis. Curr Opin Rheumatol. 2003;15(3):193–6.
41. Cooper C, Coupland C, Mitchell M. Rheumatoid arthritis, corticosteroid therapy and hip fracture. Ann Rheum Dis. 1995;54(1):49–52.
42. Cooper MS, Rabbitt EH, Goddard PE, Bartlett WA, Hewison M, Stewart PM. Osteoblastic 11beta-hydroxysteroid dehydrogenase type 1 activity increases with age and glucocorticoid exposure. J Bone Miner Res. 2002;17(6):979–86.
43. Crotti TN, Smith MD, Weedon H, Ahern MJ, Findlay DM, Kraan M, Tak PP, Haynes DR. Receptor activator NF-kappaB ligand (RANKL) expression in synovial tissue from patients with rheumatoid arthritis, spondyloarthropathy, osteoarthritis, and from normal patients: semiquantitative and quantitative analysis. Ann Rheum Dis. 2002;61(12):1047–54.
44. Cummings SR, San Martin J, McClung MR, Siris ES, Eastell R, Reid IR, Delmas P, Zoog HB, Austin M, Wang A, Kutilek S, Adami S, Zanchetta J, Libanati C, Siddhanti S, Christiansen C. Denosumab for prevention of fractures in postmenopausal women with osteoporosis. N Engl J Med. 2009;361(8):756–65.
45. De Bosscher K, Vanden Berghe W, Haegeman G. The interplay between the glucocorticoid receptor and nuclear factor-kappaB or activator protein-1: molecular mechanisms for gene repression. Endocr Rev. 2003;24(4):488–522.
46. de Haij S, Adcock IM, Bakker AC, Gobin SJ, Daha MR, van Kooten C. Steroid responsiveness of renal epithelial cells. Dissociation of transrepression and transactivation. J Biol Chem. 2003;278(7):5091–8.
47. de Nijs RN, Jacobs JW, Lems WF, Laan RF, Algra A, Huisman AM, Buskens E, de Laet CE, Oostveen AC, Geusens PP, Bruyn GA, Dijkmans BA, Bijlsma JW. Alendronate or alfacalcidol in glucocorticoid-induced osteoporosis. N Engl J Med. 2006;355(7):675–84.
48. Delany AM, Gabbitas BY, Canalis E. Cortisol downregulates osteoblast alpha 1 (I) procollagen mRNA by transcriptional and posttranscriptional mechanisms. J Cell Biochem. 1995;57(3):488–94.
49. Diarra D, Stolina M, Polzer K, Zwerina J, Ominsky MS, Dwyer D, Korb A, Smolen J, Hoffmann M, Scheinecker C, van der Heide D, Landewe R, Lacey D, Richards WG, Schett G. Dickkopf-1 is a master regulator of joint remodeling. Nat Med. 2007;13(2):156–63.
50. Doga M, Mazziotti G, Bonadonna S, Patelli I, Bilezikian JP, Canalis E, Giustina A. Prevention and treatment of glucocorticoid-induced osteoporosis. J Endocrinol Invest. 2008;31(7 Suppl):53–8.
51. Dovio A, Perazzolo L, Saba L, Termine A, Capobianco M, Bertolotto A, Angeli A. High-dose glucocorticoids increase serum levels of soluble IL-6 receptor alpha and its ratio to soluble gp130: an additional mechanism for early increased bone resorption. Eur J Endocrinol. 2006;154(5):745–51.
52. Ebeling PR. Approach to the patient with transplantation-related bone loss. J Clin Endocrinol Metab. 2009;94(5):1483–90.
53. Eijken M, Hewison M, Cooper MS, de Jong FH, Chiba H, Stewart PM, Uitterlinden AG, Pols HA, van Leeuwen JP. 11beta-hydroxysteroid dehydrogenase expression and glucocorticoid synthesis are directed by a molecular switch during osteoblast differentiation. Mol Endocrinol. 2005;19(3):621–31.
54. Elenkov IJ, Chrousos GP. Stress hormones, proinflammatory and antiinflammatory cytokines, and autoimmunity. Ann N Y Acad Sci. 2002;966:290–303.

55. Epinat JC, Gilmore TD. Diverse agents act at multiple levels to inhibit the Rel/NF-kappaB signal transduction pathway. Oncogene. 1999;18(49):6896–909.
56. Farrell RJ, Murphy A, Long A, Donnelly S, Cherikuri A, O'Toole D, Mahmud N, Keeling PW, Weir DG, Kelleher D. High multidrug resistance (P-glycoprotein 170) expression in inflammatory bowel disease patients who fail medical therapy. Gastroenterology. 2000;118(2):279–88.
57. Franzoso G, Carlson L, Xing L, Poljak L, Shores EW, Brown KD, Leonardi A, Tran T, Boyce BF, Siebenlist U. Requirement for NF-kappaB in osteoclast and B-cell development. Genes Dev. 1997;11(24): 3482–96.
58. Freeman L, Hewison M, Hughes SV, Evans KN, Hardie D, Means TK, Chakraverty R. Expression of 11beta-hydroxysteroid dehydrogenase type 1 permits regulation of glucocorticoid bioavailability by human dendritic cells. Blood. 2005;106(6):2042–9.
59. Gabbitas B, Pash JM, Delany AM, Canalis E. Cortisol inhibits the synthesis of insulin-like growth factor-binding protein-5 in bone cell cultures by transcriptional mechanisms. J Biol Chem. 1996;271(15): 9033–8.
60. Gallo KA, Johnson GL. Mixed-lineage kinase control of JNK and p38 MAPK pathways. Nat Rev Mol Cell Biol. 2002;3(9):663–72.
61. Ghosh S, Karin M. Missing pieces in the NF-kappaB puzzle. Cell. 2002;109(Suppl):S81–96.
62. Gilbert L, He X, Farmer P, Boden S, Kozlowski M, Rubin J, Nanes MS. Inhibition of osteoblast differentiation by tumor necrosis factor-alpha. Endocrinology. 2000;141(11):3956–64.
63. Gillespie MT. Impact of cytokines and T lymphocytes upon osteoclast differentiation and function. Arthritis Res Ther. 2007;9(2):103.
64. Gilmour JS, Coutinho AE, Cailhier JF, Man TY, Clay M, Thomas G, Harris HJ, Mullins JJ, Seckl JR, Savill JS, Chapman KE. Local amplification of glucocorticoids by 11 beta-hydroxysteroid dehydrogenase type 1 promotes macrophage phagocytosis of apoptotic leukocytes. J Immunol. 2006;176(12): 7605–11.
65. Glass 2nd DA, Bialek P, Ahn JD, Starbuck M, Patel MS, Clevers H, Taketo MM, Long F, McMahon AP, Lang RA, Karsenty G. Canonical Wnt signaling in differentiated osteoblasts controls osteoclast differentiation. Dev Cell. 2005;8(5):751–64.
66. Glass 2nd DA, Karsenty G. Canonical Wnt signaling in osteoblasts is required for osteoclast differentiation. Ann N Y Acad Sci. 2006;1068:117–30.
67. Goldring SR. Pathogenesis of bone erosions in rheumatoid arthritis. Curr Opin Rheumatol. 2002; 14(4):406–10.
68. Guler-Yuksel M, Bijsterbosch J, Goekoop-Ruiterman YP, de Vries-Bouwstra JK, Hulsmans HM, de Beus WM, Han KH, Breedveld FC, Dijkmans BA, Allaart CF, Lems WF. Changes in bone mineral density in patients with recent onset, active rheumatoid arthritis. Ann Rheum Dis. 2008;67(6):823–8.
69. Hardy R, Rabbitt EH, Filer A, Emery P, Hewison M, Stewart PM, Gittoes NJ, Buckley CD, Raza K, Cooper MS. Local and systemic glucocorticoid metabolism in inflammatory arthritis. Ann Rheum Dis. 2008;67(9): 1204–10.
70. Haslett C. Granulocyte apoptosis and its role in the resolution and control of lung inflammation. Am J Respir Crit Care Med. 1999;160(5 Pt 2):S5–11.
71. Heasman SJ, Giles KM, Ward C, Rossi AG, Haslett C, Dransfield I. Glucocorticoid-mediated regulation of granulocyte apoptosis and macrophage phagocytosis of apoptotic cells: implications for the resolution of inflammation. J Endocrinol. 2003;178(1):29–36.
72. Hofbauer LC, Gori F, Riggs BL, Lacey DL, Dunstan CR, Spelsberg TC, Khosla S. Stimulation of osteoprotegerin ligand and inhibition of osteoprotegerin production by glucocorticoids in human osteoblastic lineage cells: potential paracrine mechanisms of glucocorticoid-induced osteoporosis. Endocrinology. 1999;140(10):4382–9.
73. Hofbauer LC, Rauner M. Minireview: live and let die: molecular effects of glucocorticoids on bone cells. Mol Endocrinol. 2009;23(10):1525–31.
74. Holmes MC, Kotelevtsev Y, Mullins JJ, Seckl JR. Phenotypic analysis of mice bearing targeted deletions of 11beta-hydroxysteroid dehydrogenases 1 and 2 genes. Mol Cell Endocrinol. 2001;171(1–2):15–20.
75. Horwood NJ, Kartsogiannis V, Quinn JM, Romas E, Martin TJ, Gillespie MT. Activated T lymphocytes support osteoclast formation in vitro. Biochem Biophys Res Commun. 1999;265(1):144–50.
76. Horwood NJ, Elliott J, Martin TJ, Gillespie MT. IL-12 alone and in synergy with IL-18 inhibits osteoclast formation in vitro. J Immunol. 2001;166(8):4915–21.
77. Hu X, Ho HH, Lou O, Hidaka C, Ivashkiv LB. Homeostatic role of interferons conferred by inhibition of IL-1-mediated inflammation and tissue destruction. J Immunol. 2005;175(1):131–8.
78. Humphrey EL, Williams JH, Davie MW, Marshall MJ. Effects of dissociated glucocorticoids on OPG and RANKL in osteoblastic cells. Bone. 2006;38(5): 652–61.
79. Iotsova V, Caamano J, Loy J, Yang Y, Lewin A, Bravo R. Osteopetrosis in mice lacking NF-kappaB1 and NF-kappaB2. Nat Med. 1997;3(11):1285–9.
80. Irikura VM, Hirsch E, Hirsh D. Effects of interleukin-1 receptor antagonist overexpression on infection by *Listeria monocytogenes*. Infect Immun. 1999; 67(4):1901–9.
81. Jia D, O'Brien CA, Stewart SA, Manolagas SC, Weinstein RS. Glucocorticoids act directly on osteoclasts to increase their life span and reduce bone density. Endocrinology. 2006;147(12):5592–9.
82. Jiang Y, Zhao JJ, Mitlak BH, Wang O, Genant HK, Eriksen EF. Recombinant human parathyroid hormone (1–34) [teriparatide] improves both cortical and cancellous bone structure. J Bone Miner Res. 2003; 18(11):1932–41.
83. Jimi E, Aoki K, Saito H, D'Acquisto F, May MJ, Nakamura I, Sudo T, Kojima T, Okamoto F, Fukushima

H, Okabe K, Ohya K, Ghosh S. Selective inhibition of NF-kappa B blocks osteoclastogenesis and prevents inflammatory bone destruction in vivo. Nat Med. 2004;10(6):617–24.
84. Karberg K, Zochling J, Sieper J, Felsenberg D, Braun J. Bone loss is detected more frequently in patients with ankylosing spondylitis with syndesmophytes. J Rheumatol. 2005;32(7):1290–8.
85. Katz S. Osteoporosis in patients with inflammatory bowel disease: risk factors, prevention, and treatment. Rev Gastroenterol Disord. 2006;6(2):63–71.
86. Kawakami A, Nakashima T, Sakai H, Hida A, Urayama S, Yamasaki S, Nakamura H, Ida H, Ichinose Y, Aoyagi T, Furuichi I, Nakashima M, Migita K, Kawabe Y, Eguchi K. Regulation of synovial cell apoptosis by proteasome inhibitor. Arthritis Rheum. 1999;42(11):2440–8.
87. Kim N, Odgren PR, Kim DK, Marks Jr SC, Choi Y. Diverse roles of the tumor necrosis factor family member TRANCE in skeletal physiology revealed by TRANCE deficiency and partial rescue by a lymphocyte-expressed TRANCE transgene. Proc Natl Acad Sci USA. 2000;97(20):10905–10.
88. Kobayashi K, Takahashi N, Jimi E, Udagawa N, Takami M, Kotake S, Nakagawa N, Kinosaki M, Yamaguchi K, Shima N, Yasuda H, Morinaga T, Higashio K, Martin TJ, Suda T. Tumor necrosis factor alpha stimulates osteoclast differentiation by a mechanism independent of the ODF/RANKL-RANK interaction. J Exp Med. 2000;191(2): 275–86.
89. Kogianni G, Mann V, Ebetino F, Nuttall M, Nijweide P, Simpson H, Noble B. Fas/CD95 is associated with glucocorticoid-induced osteocyte apoptosis. Life Sci. 2004;75(24):2879–95.
90. Komuro H, Olee T, Kuhn K, Quach J, Brinson DC, Shikhman A, Valbracht J, Creighton-Achermann L, Lotz M. The osteoprotegerin/receptor activator of nuclear factor kappaB/receptor activator of nuclear factor kappaB ligand system in cartilage. Arthritis Rheum. 2001;44(12):2768–76.
91. Kondo T, Kitazawa R, Yamaguchi A, Kitazawa S. Dexamethasone promotes osteoclastogenesis by inhibiting osteoprotegerin through multiple levels. J Cell Biochem. 2008;103(1):335–45.
92. Kong YY, Feige U, Sarosi I, Bolon B, Tafuri A, Morony S, Capparelli C, Li J, Elliott R, McCabe S, Wong T, Campagnuolo G, Moran E, Bogoch ER, Van G, Nguyen LT, Ohashi PS, Lacey DL, Fish E, Boyle WJ, Penninger JM. Activated T cells regulate bone loss and joint destruction in adjuvant arthritis through osteoprotegerin ligand. Nature. 1999;402(6759): 304–9.
93. Kurokouchi K, Kambe F, Kikumori T, Sakai T, Sarkar D, Ishiguro N, Iwata H, Seo H. Effects of glucocorticoids on tumor necrosis factor alpha-dependent activation of nuclear factor kappaB and expression of the intercellular adhesion molecule 1 gene in osteoblast-like ROS17/2.8 cells. J Bone Miner Res. 2000;15(9): 1707–15.
94. Laan RF, Buijs WC, Verbeek AL, Draad MP, Corstens FH, van de Putte LB, van Riel PL. Bone mineral density in patients with recent onset rheumatoid arthritis: influence of disease activity and functional capacity. Ann Rheum Dis. 1993;52(1): 21–6.
95. Lacey DL, Timms E, Tan HL, Kelley MJ, Dunstan CR, Burgess T, Elliott R, Colombero A, Elliott G, Scully S, Hsu H, Sullivan J, Hawkins N, Davy E, Capparelli C, Eli A, Qian YX, Kaufman S, Sarosi I, Shalhoub V, Senaldi G, Guo J, Delaney J, Boyle WJ. Osteoprotegerin ligand is a cytokine that regulates osteoclast differentiation and activation. Cell. 1998;93(2):165–76.
96. Lacey DL, Tan HL, Lu J, Kaufman S, Van G, Qiu W, Rattan A, Scully S, Fletcher F, Juan T, Kelley M, Burgess TL, Boyle WJ, Polverino AJ. Osteoprotegerin ligand modulates murine osteoclast survival in vitro and in vivo. Am J Pathol. 2000;157(2):435–48.
97. Lam J, Takeshita S, Barker JE, Kanagawa O, Ross FP, Teitelbaum SL. TNF-alpha induces osteoclastogenesis by direct stimulation of macrophages exposed to permissive levels of RANK ligand. J Clin Invest. 2000;106(12):1481–8.
98. Lane NE, Yao W, Balooch M, Nalla RK, Balooch G, Habelitz S, Kinney JH, Bonewald LF. Glucocorticoid-treated mice have localized changes in trabecular bone material properties and osteocyte lacunar size that are not observed in placebo-treated or estrogen-deficient mice. J Bone Miner Res. 2006;21(3): 466–76.
99. Leung DY, de Castro M, Szefler SJ, Chrousos GP. Mechanisms of glucocorticoid-resistant asthma. Ann N Y Acad Sci. 1998;840:735–46.
100. Lewiecki EM. Denosumab update. Curr Opin Rheumatol. 2009;21(4):369–73.
101. Lianxu C, Hongti J, Changlong Y. NF-kappaBp65-specific siRNA inhibits expression of genes of COX-2, NOS-2 and MMP-9 in rat IL-1beta-induced and TNF-alpha-induced chondrocytes. Osteoarthritis Cartilage. 2006;14(4):367–76.
102. Liu Y, Cousin JM, Hughes J, Van Damme J, Seckl JR, Haslett C, Dransfield I, Savill J, Rossi AG. Glucocorticoids promote nonphlogistic phagocytosis of apoptotic leukocytes. J Immunol. 1999;162(6): 3639–46.
103. Lubberts E, Oppers-Walgreen B, Pettit AR, Van Den Bersselaar L, Joosten LA, Goldring SR, Gravallese EM, Van Den Berg WB. Increase in expression of receptor activator of nuclear factor kappaB at sites of bone erosion correlates with progression of inflammation in evolving collagen-induced arthritis. Arthritis Rheum. 2002;46(11):3055–64.
104. Lubberts E, Koenders MI, van den Berg WB. The role of T-cell interleukin-17 in conducting destructive arthritis: lessons from animal models. Arthritis Res Ther. 2005;7(1):29–37.
105. Makarov SS. NF-kappaB as a therapeutic target in chronic inflammation: recent advances. Mol Med Today. 2000;6(11):441–8.

106. Manolagas SC, Weinstein RS. New developments in the pathogenesis and treatment of steroid-induced osteoporosis. J Bone Miner Res. 1999;14(7): 1061–6.
107. Martinez FO, Gordon S, Locati M, Mantovani A. Transcriptional profiling of the human monocyte-to-macrophage differentiation and polarization: new molecules and patterns of gene expression. J Immunol. 2006;177(10):7303–11.
108. Mazziotti G, Angeli A, Bilezikian JP, Canalis E, Giustina A. Glucocorticoid-induced osteoporosis: an update. Trends Endocrinol Metab. 2006;17(4):144–9.
109. McInnes IB, Schett G. Cytokines in the pathogenesis of rheumatoid arthritis. Nat Rev Immunol. 2007;7(6):429–42.
110. McIntyre KW, Shuster DJ, Gillooly KM, Dambach DM, Pattoli MA, Lu P, Zhou XD, Qiu Y, Zusi FC, Burke JR. A highly selective inhibitor of I kappa B kinase, BMS-345541, blocks both joint inflammation and destruction in collagen-induced arthritis in mice. Arthritis Rheum. 2003;48(9):2652–9.
111. McManus MT, Sharp PA. Gene silencing in mammals by small interfering RNAs. Nat Rev Genet. 2002;3(10):737–47.
112. Migliaccio S, Brama M, Malavolta N. Management of glucocorticoids-induced osteoporosis: role of teriparatide. Ther Clin Risk Manag. 2009;5(2):305–10.
113. Miller PD. Denosumab: anti-RANKL antibody. Curr Osteoporos Rep. 2009;7(1):18–22.
114. Munck A, Naray-Fejes-Toth A. The ups and downs of glucocorticoid physiology. Permissive and suppressive effects revisited. Mol Cell Endocrinol. 1992;90(1):C1–4.
115. Naganathan V, Jones G, Nash P, Nicholson G, Eisman J, Sambrook PN. Vertebral fracture risk with long-term corticosteroid therapy: prevalence and relation to age, bone density, and corticosteroid use. Arch Intern Med. 2000;160(19):2917–22.
116. Naito A, Azuma S, Tanaka S, Miyazaki T, Takaki S, Takatsu K, Nakao K, Nakamura K, Katsuki M, Yamamoto T, Inoue J. Severe osteopetrosis, defective interleukin-1 signaling and lymph node organogenesis in TRAF6-deficient mice. Genes Cells. 1999;4(6):353–62.
117. O'Brien CA, Jia D, Plotkin LI, Bellido T, Powers CC, Stewart SA, Manolagas SC, Weinstein RS. Glucocorticoids act directly on osteoblasts and osteocytes to induce their apoptosis and reduce bone formation and strength. Endocrinology. 2004;145(4): 1835–41.
118. Ohnaka K, Tanabe M, Kawate H, Nawata H, Takayanagi R. Glucocorticoid suppresses the canonical Wnt signal in cultured human osteoblasts. Biochem Biophys Res Commun. 2005;329(1):177–81.
119. Pacifici R. T cells: critical bone regulators in health and disease. Bone. 2010;47(3):461–71.
120. Pasco JA, Kotowicz MA, Henry MJ, Nicholson GC, Spilsbury HJ, Box JD, Schneider HG. High-sensitivity C-reactive protein and fracture risk in elderly women. JAMA. 2006;296(11):1353–5.
121. Peel NF, Barrington NA, Blumsohn A, Colwell A, Hannon R, Eastell R. Bone mineral density and bone turnover in spinal osteoarthrosis. Ann Rheum Dis. 1995;54(11):867–71.
122. Pettit AR, Ji H, von Stechow D, Muller R, Goldring SR, Choi Y, Benoist C, Gravallese EM. TRANCE/RANKL knockout mice are protected from bone erosion in a serum transfer model of arthritis. Am J Pathol. 2001;159(5):1689–99.
123. Poubelle PE, Chakravarti A, Fernandes MJ, Doiron K, Marceau AA. Differential expression of RANK, RANK-L, and osteoprotegerin by synovial fluid neutrophils from patients with rheumatoid arthritis and by healthy human blood neutrophils. Arthritis Res Ther. 2007;9(2):R25.
124. Purnell JQ, Brandon DD, Isabelle LM, Loriaux DL, Samuels MH. Association of 24-hour cortisol production rates, cortisol-binding globulin, and plasma-free cortisol levels with body composition, leptin levels, and aging in adult men and women. J Clin Endocrinol Metab. 2004;89(1):281–7.
125. Quinn JM, Saleh H. Modulation of osteoclast function in bone by the immune system. Mol Cell Endocrinol. 2009;310(1–2):40–51.
126. Ramirez F, Fowell DJ, Puklavec M, Simmonds S, Mason D. Glucocorticoids promote a TH2 cytokine response by CD4+ T cells in vitro. J Immunol. 1996;156(7):2406–12.
127. Redlich K, Ziegler S, Kiener HP, Spitzauer S, Stohlawetz P, Bernecker P, Kainberger F, Grampp S, Kudlacek S, Woloszczuk W, Smolen JS, Pietschmann P. Bone mineral density and biochemical parameters of bone metabolism in female patients with systemic lupus erythematosus. Ann Rheum Dis. 2000;59(4): 308–10.
128. Redlich K, Hayer S, Ricci R, David JP, Tohidast-Akrad M, Kollias G, Steiner G, Smolen JS, Wagner EF, Schett G. Osteoclasts are essential for TNF-alpha-mediated joint destruction. J Clin Invest. 2002;110(10):1419–27.
129. Rehman Q, Lang TF, Arnaud CD, Modin GW, Lane NE. Daily treatment with parathyroid hormone is associated with an increase in vertebral cross-sectional area in postmenopausal women with glucocorticoid-induced osteoporosis. Osteoporos Int. 2003;14(1):77–81.
130. Reid DM, Adami S, Devogelaer JP, Chines AA. Risedronate increases bone density and reduces vertebral fracture risk within one year in men on corticosteroid therapy. Calcif Tissue Int. 2001;69(4):242–7.
131. Reid DM, Devogelaer JP, Saag K, Roux C, Lau CS, Reginster JY, Papanastasiou P, Ferreira A, Hartl F, Fashola T, Mesenbrink P, Sambrook PN. Zoledronic acid and risedronate in the prevention and treatment of glucocorticoid-induced osteoporosis (HORIZON): a multicentre, double-blind, double-dummy, randomised controlled trial. Lancet. 2009;373(9671):1253–63.
132. Ren Y, Stuart L, Lindberg FP, Rosenkranz AR, Chen Y, Mayadas TN, Savill J. Nonphlogistic clearance of

late apoptotic neutrophils by macrophages: efficient phagocytosis independent of beta 2 integrins. J Immunol. 2001;166(7):4743–50.
133. Reynolds RM, Dennison EM, Walker BR, Syddall HE, Wood PJ, Andrew R, Phillips DI, Cooper C. Cortisol secretion and rate of bone loss in a population-based cohort of elderly men and women. Calcif Tissue Int. 2005;77(3):134–8.
134. Rivera J, Colbert RA. Healing the Syk through kinase inhibitors. N Engl J Med. 2010;63(14): 1362–4.
135. Roman-Blas JA, Jimenez SA. NF-kappaB as a potential therapeutic target in osteoarthritis and rheumatoid arthritis. Osteoarthritis Cartilage. 2006; 14(9):839–48.
136. Romas E, Sims NA, Hards DK, Lindsay M, Quinn JW, Ryan PF, Dunstan CR, Martin TJ, Gillespie MT. Osteoprotegerin reduces osteoclast numbers and prevents bone erosion in collagen-induced arthritis. Am J Pathol. 2002;161(4):1419–27.
137. Rubin J, Biskobing DM, Jadhav L, Fan D, Nanes MS, Perkins S, Fan X. Dexamethasone promotes expression of membrane-bound macrophage colony-stimulating factor in murine osteoblast-like cells. Endocrinology. 1998;139(3):1006–12.
138. Ruocco MG, Karin M. IKK{beta} as a target for treatment of inflammation induced bone loss. Ann Rheum Dis. 2005;64 Suppl 4:vi81–5.
139. Saag KG, Emkey R, Schnitzer TJ, Brown JP, Hawkins F, Goemaere S, Thamsborg G, Liberman UA, Delmas PD, Malice MP, Czachur M, Daifotis AG. Alendronate for the prevention and treatment of glucocorticoid-inducedosteoporosis.Glucocorticoid-induced osteoporosis intervention study group. N Engl J Med. 1998;339(5):292–9.
140. Saag KG, Shane E, Boonen S, Marin F, Donley DW, Taylor KA, Dalsky GP, Marcus R. Teriparatide or alendronate in glucocorticoid-induced osteoporosis. N Engl J Med. 2007;357(20):2028–39.
141. Sandeep TC, Walker BR. Pathophysiology of modulation of local glucocorticoid levels by 11beta-hydroxysteroid dehydrogenases. Trends Endocrinol Metab. 2001;12(10):446–53.
142. Schacke H, Docke WD, Asadullah K. Mechanisms involved in the side effects of glucocorticoids. Pharmacol Ther. 2002;96(1):23–43.
143. Schett G, Kiechl S, Weger S, Pederiva A, Mayr A, Petrangeli M, Oberhollenzer F, Lorenzini R, Redlich K, Axmann R, Zwerina J, Willeit J. High-sensitivity C-reactive protein and risk of nontraumatic fractures in the Bruneck study. Arch Intern Med. 2006;166(22):2495–501.
144. Schett G, Teitelbaum SL. Osteoclasts and arthritis. J Bone Miner Res. 2009;24(7):1142–6.
145. Schreiber W, Pollmacher T, Fassbender K, Gudewill S, Vedder H, Wiedemann K, Galanos C, Holsboer F. Endotoxin- and corticotropin-releasing hormone-induced release of ACTH and cortisol. A comparative study in men. Neuroendocrinology. 1993;58(1):123–8.
146. Schroder K, Hertzog PJ, Ravasi T, Hume DA. Interferon-gamma: an overview of signals, mechanisms and functions. J Leukoc Biol. 2004;75(2): 163–89.
147. Sher LB, Woitge HW, Adams DJ, Gronowicz GA, Krozowski Z, Harrison JR, Kream BE. Transgenic expression of 11beta-hydroxysteroid dehydrogenase type 2 in osteoblasts reveals an anabolic role for endogenous glucocorticoids in bone. Endocrinology. 2004;145(2):922–9.
148. Sher LB, Harrison JR, Adams DJ, Kream BE. Impaired cortical bone acquisition and osteoblast differentiation in mice with osteoblast-targeted disruption of glucocorticoid signaling. Calcif Tissue Int. 2006;79(2):118–25.
149. Shi XM, Blair HC, Yang X, McDonald JM, Cao X. Tandem repeat of C/EBP binding sites mediates PPARgamma2 gene transcription in glucocorticoid-induced adipocyte differentiation. J Cell Biochem. 2000;76(3):518–27.
150. Shigeyama Y, Pap T, Kunzler P, Simmen BR, Gay RE, Gay S. Expression of osteoclast differentiation factor in rheumatoid arthritis. Arthritis Rheum. 2000;43(11):2523–30.
151. Sims NA, Green JR, Glatt M, Schlict S, Martin TJ, Gillespie MT, Romas E. Targeting osteoclasts with zoledronic acid prevents bone destruction in collagen-induced arthritis. Arthritis Rheum. 2004;50(7): 2338–46.
152. Smith E, Frenkel B. Glucocorticoids inhibit the transcriptional activity of LEF/TCF in differentiating osteoblasts in a glycogen synthase kinase-3beta-dependent and -independent manner. J Biol Chem. 2005;280(3):2388–94.
153. Swanson C, Lorentzon M, Conaway HH, Lerner UH. Glucocorticoid regulation of osteoclast differentiation and expression of receptor activator of nuclear factor-kappaB (NF-kappaB) ligand, osteoprotegerin, and receptor activator of NF-kappaB in mouse calvarial bones. Endocrinology. 2006;147(7): 3613–22.
154. Tabardel Y, Duchateau J, Schmartz D, Marecaux G, Shahla M, Barvais L, Leclerc JL, Vincent JL. Corticosteroids increase blood interleukin-10 levels during cardiopulmonary bypass in men. Surgery. 1996;119(1):76–80.
155. Takayanagi H, Kim S, Koga T, Nishina H, Isshiki M, Yoshida H, Saiura A, Isobe M, Yokochi T, Inoue J, Wagner EF, Mak TW, Kodama T, Taniguchi T. Induction and activation of the transcription factor NFATc1 (NFAT2) integrate RANKL signaling in terminal differentiation of osteoclasts. Dev Cell. 2002;3(6):889–901.
156. Takayanagi H. Mechanistic insight into osteoclast differentiation in osteoimmunology. J Mol Med. 2005;83(3):170–9.
157. Takuma A, Kaneda T, Sato T, Ninomiya S, Kumegawa M, Hakeda Y. Dexamethasone enhances osteoclast formation synergistically with transforming growth factor-beta by stimulating the priming of

osteoclast progenitors for differentiation into osteoclasts. J Biol Chem. 2003;278(45):44667–74.
158. Tauchmanova L, Colao A, Lombardi G, Rotoli B, Selleri C. Bone loss and its management in long-term survivors from allogeneic stem cell transplantation. J Clin Endocrinol Metab. 2007;92(12):4536–45.
159. Teitelbaum SL. Bone resorption by osteoclasts. Science. 2000;289(5484):1504–8.
160. Theoleyre S, Wittrant Y, Tat SK, Fortun Y, Redini F, Heymann D. The molecular triad OPG/RANK/RANKL: involvement in the orchestration of pathophysiological bone remodeling. Cytokine Growth Factor Rev. 2004;15(6):457–75.
161. Tomita T, Takeuchi E, Tomita N, Morishita R, Kaneko M, Yamamoto K, Nakase T, Seki H, Kato K, Kaneda Y, Ochi T. Suppressed severity of collagen-induced arthritis by in vivo transfection of nuclear factor kappaB decoy oligodeoxynucleotides as a gene therapy. Arthritis Rheum. 1999;42(12):2532–42.
162. Tomlinson JW, Walker EA, Bujalska IJ, Draper N, Lavery GG, Cooper MS, Hewison M, Stewart PM. 11beta-Hydroxysteroid dehydrogenase type 1: a tissue-specific regulator of glucocorticoid response. Endocr Rev. 2004;25(5):831–66.
163. Van Staa TP, Leufkens HG, Abenhaim L, Zhang B, Cooper C. Use of oral corticosteroids and risk of fractures. J Bone Miner Res. 2000;15(6):993–1000.
164. van Staa TP, Leufkens HG, Abenhaim L, Zhang B, Cooper C. Oral corticosteroids and fracture risk: relationship to daily and cumulative doses. Rheumatology (Oxford). 2000;39(12):1383–9.
165. van Staa TP, Geusens P, Bijlsma JW, Leufkens HG, Cooper C. Clinical assessment of the long-term risk of fracture in patients with rheumatoid arthritis. Arthritis Rheum. 2006;54(10):3104–12.
166. van Staa TP. The pathogenesis, epidemiology and management of glucocorticoid-induced osteoporosis. Calcif Tissue Int. 2006;79(3):129–37.
167. Varga G, Ehrchen J, Tsianakas A, Tenbrock K, Rattenholl A, Seeliger S, Mack M, Roth J, Sunderkoetter C. Glucocorticoids induce an activated, anti-inflammatory monocyte subset in mice that resembles myeloid-derived suppressor cells. J Leukoc Biol. 2008;84(3):644–50.
168. Vidal NO, Brandstrom H, Jonsson KB, Ohlsson C. Osteoprotegerin mRNA is expressed in primary human osteoblast-like cells: downregulation by glucocorticoids. J Endocrinol. 1998;159(1):191–5.
169. Wang FS, Ko JY, Yeh DW, Ke HC, Wu HL. Modulation of dickkopf-1 attenuates glucocorticoid induction of osteoblast apoptosis, adipocytic differentiation, and bone mass loss. Endocrinology. 2008;149(4):1793–801.
170. Webster JI, Carlstedt-Duke J. Involvement of multidrug resistance proteins (MDR) in the modulation of glucocorticoid response. J Steroid Biochem Mol Biol. 2002;82(4–5):277–88.
171. Wedel A, Ziegler-Heitbrock HW. The C/EBP family of transcription factors. Immunobiology. 1995;193(2–4):171–85.
172. Weinblatt ME, Kavanaugh A, Genovese MC, Musser TK, Grossbard EB, Magilavy DB. An oral spleen tyrosine kinase (Syk) inhibitor for rheumatoid arthritis. N Engl J Med. 2010;363(14):1303–12.
173. Weinstein RS, Jilka RL, Almeida M, Roberson PK, Manolagas SC. Intermittent parathyroid hormone administration counteracts the adverse effects of glucocorticoids on osteoblast and osteocyte viability, bone formation, and strength in mice. Endocrinology. 2010;151(6):2641–9.
174. Weinstein RS, Jilka RL, Parfitt AM, Manolagas SC. Inhibition of osteoblastogenesis and promotion of apoptosis of osteoblasts and osteocytes by glucocorticoids. Potential mechanisms of their deleterious effects on bone. J Clin Invest. 1998;102(2):274–82.
175. Weinstein RS. Glucocorticoids, osteocytes, and skeletal fragility: the role of bone vascularity. Bone. 2009;46(3):564–70.
176. Weinstein RS. Glucocorticoids, osteocytes, and skeletal fragility: the role of bone vascularity. Bone. 2010;46(3):564–70.
177. Weinstein RS, Wan C, Liu Q, Wang Y, Almeida M, O'Brien CA, Thostenson J, Roberson PK, Boskey AL, Clemens TL, Manolagas SC. Endogenous glucocorticoids decrease skeletal angiogenesis, vascularity, hydration, and strength in aged mice. Aging Cell. 2010;9(2):147–61.
178. Wiegers GJ, Reul JM. Induction of cytokine receptors by glucocorticoids: functional and pathological significance. Trends Pharmacol Sci. 1998;19(8):317–21.
179. Wilkinson CW, Petrie EC, Murray SR, Colasurdo EA, Raskind MA, Peskind ER. Human glucocorticoid feedback inhibition is reduced in older individuals: evening study. J Clin Endocrinol Metab. 2001;86(2):545–50.
180. Wu Z, Bucher NL, Farmer SR. Induction of peroxisome proliferator-activated receptor gamma during the conversion of 3 T3 fibroblasts into adipocytes is mediated by C/EBPbeta, C/EBPdelta, and glucocorticoids. Mol Cell Biol. 1996;16(8):4128–36.
181. Wust S, Van Rossum EF, Federenko IS, Koper JW, Kumsta R, Hellhammer DH. Common polymorphisms in the glucocorticoid receptor gene are associated with adrenocortical responses to psychosocial stress. J Clin Endocrinol Metab. 2004;89(2):565–73.
182. Yang JP, Merin JP, Nakano T, Kato T, Kitade Y, Okamoto T. Inhibition of the DNA-binding activity of NF-kappa B by gold compounds in vitro. FEBS Lett. 1995;361(1):89–96.
183. Yao W, Cheng Z, Pham A, Busse C, Zimmermann EA, Ritchie RO, Lane NE. Glucocorticoid-induced bone loss in mice can be reversed by the actions of parathyroid hormone and risedronate on different

pathways for bone formation and mineralization. Arthritis Rheum. 2008;58(11):3485–97.

184. Yasuda H, Shima N, Nakagawa N, Mochizuki SI, Yano K, Fujise N, Sato Y, Goto M, Yamaguchi K, Kuriyama M, Kanno T, Murakami A, Tsuda E, Morinaga T, Higashio K. Identity of osteoclastogenesis inhibitory factor (OCIF) and osteoprotegerin (OPG): a mechanism by which OPG/OCIF inhibits osteoclastogenesis in vitro. Endocrinology. 1998;139(3):1329–37.
185. Yasuda H, Shima N, Nakagawa N, Yamaguchi K, Kinosaki M, Mochizuki S, Tomoyasu A, Yano K, Goto M, Murakami A, Tsuda E, Morinaga T, Higashio K, Udagawa N, Takahashi N, Suda T. Osteoclast differentiation factor is a ligand for osteoprotegerin/osteoclastogenesis-inhibitory factor and is identical to TRANCE/RANKL. Proc Natl Acad Sci USA. 1998;95(7):3597–602.
186. Yeager MP, Guyre PM, Munck AU. Glucocorticoid regulation of the inflammatory response to injury. Acta Anaesthesiol Scand. 2004;48(7):799–813.
187. Zandi E, Rothwarf DM, Delhase M, Hayakawa M, Karin M. The IkappaB kinase complex (IKK) contains two kinase subunits, IKKalpha and IKKbeta, necessary for IkappaB phosphorylation and NF-kappaB activation. Cell. 1997;91(2):243–52.
188. Zhang TY, Ding X, Daynes RA. The expression of 11 beta-hydroxysteroid dehydrogenase type I by lymphocytes provides a novel means for intracrine regulation of glucocorticoid activities. J Immunol. 2005;174(2):879–89.
189. Zhang TY, Daynes RA. Macrophages from 11beta-hydroxysteroid dehydrogenase type 1-deficient mice exhibit an increased sensitivity to lipopolysaccharide stimulation due to TGF-beta-mediated up-regulation of SHIP1 expression. J Immunol. 2007;179(9):6325–35.
190. Zwerina J, Redlich K, Polzer K, Joosten L, Kronke G, Distler J, Hess A, Pundt N, Pap T, Hoffmann O, Gasser J, Scheinecker C, Smolen JS, van den Berg W, Schett G. TNF-induced structural joint damage is mediated by IL-1. Proc Natl Acad Sci USA. 2007;104(28):11742–7.

Diseases of Energy and Lipid Metabolism and Bone: Emerging Therapeutics

8

Sumithra K. Urs and Clifford J. Rosen

Keywords
Adipose tissue • Obesity • Osteoporosis • TDZ • Insulin • PPAR

8.1 Introduction

Lipids constitute a broad group of naturally occurring molecules that function as energy storage organs, as components of cell membranes, and as signaling molecules. Lipids and fatty acids are stored as triglycerides and are the most important source of energy for most organisms. When the body needs energy, lipolysis is initiated in adipocytes, and the triglycerides are hydrolyzed to glycerol and nonesterified fatty acids (NEFAs) [64]. The capacity to store triglycerides makes it possible to maintain energy homeostasis and prevent an abnormal toxic increase in plasma NEFAs. Under normal conditions, fat cells fine-tune the balance between lipogenesis and lipolysis of triglycerides in response to physiological needs. However, changes in lipid storage and metabolism, whether anabolic or catabolic, modulate whole body homeostasis. When fat mass is lacking as in lipoatrophy, there arise complications similar to those in type 2 diabetes, i.e., insulin resistance, dyslipidemia, hyperphagia, and liver steatosis. On the other hand, excessive lipid storage leads to obesity, along with a multitude of manifestations and clinical complications including altered insulin production. Fatty tissue accumulation is a major risk factor for chronic diseases, including the metabolic syndrome, also known as "syndrome X," a cluster of phenotypes that contribute to elevating the risk of disorders. Symptoms of the metabolic syndrome include insulin resistance, impaired glucose regulation, dyslipidemia, hypertension, central obesity, and microalbuminuria, with insulin resistance the major feature. Between 60% and 90% of type 2 diabetes cases are thought to be due to obesity. Altogether, adipose tissue is essential to maintaining health and in glucose and lipid homeostasis [64].

8.2 Relationship of Adipose Tissue to Bone

Our understanding of skeletal acquisition and maintenance has advanced considerably in the past decade, including a growing awareness that

S.K. Urs, Ph.D.
Center for Molecular Medicine,
Maine Medical Center Research Institute,
81 Research Drive, Scarborough, ME 04074, USA

C.J. Rosen, M.D. (✉)
Clinical and Translational Research,
Maine Medical Center Research Institute,
81 Research Drive, Scarborough, ME 04074, USA
e-mail: crofen@gmail.com

F. Bronner et al. (eds.), *Bone-Metabolic Functions and Modulators*, Topics in Bone Biology,
DOI 10.1007/978-1-4471-2745-1_8, © Springer-Verlag London 2012

bone remodeling requires a source of energy that is closely linked to other homeostatic pathways. Changes in glucose and fat metabolism, including diabetes mellitus, Cushing syndrome, and anorexia nervosa, severely impact skeletal health [52]. The link between energy and lipid metabolism and bone disorders is adipose tissue and factors associated with obesity. Adipose tissue is primarily responsible for dysregulation of lipid and energy metabolism and the effects on skeletal health of diabetes and osteoporosis.

8.3 Relationship Between Fat Mass, Bone Mass, and Skeletal Integrity

Obesity is simply the accumulation of fatty tissue. Worldwide, approximately 340 million people are obese. In the USA, 72.5 million adults can be categorized as obese. Obesity is a factor that contributes to several causes of death, including heart disease, stroke, diabetes, and some types of cancer [65]. Obesity has long been considered as protective of the skeletal system because adipose tissue can insulate the skeleton against trauma from falls and the severity of external forces that act on bone. Furthermore, gravitational forces are known to enhance periosteal bone formation and to strengthen bones, particularly during puberty. In postmenopausal women, an increase in adipose tissue enhances local aromatization of estradiol from testosterone. This causes bone resorption and menopausal bone loss to diminish. Men and women of low body weight tend to have less adipose tissue, low bone mass, and greater risk of fracture [31]. However, this tenet is highly questionable with observations and newer studies indicating a contrasting hypothesis.

The relationship between adiposity and bone in adults with obesity suggests the risk for fractures may be increased in obesity-associated disorders. In children, the relationship between body weight and fracture risk is complicated and confounded by puberty [12]. On the basis of studies like that from the Rancho Bernardo cohort of elderly men and women, the metabolic syndrome appears to be associated with a greater risk of fracture and lower areal bone mineral density (BMD) than is true for the individuals with normal body weight [63]. In Chinese men and women who have a low body mass index (BMI) (19–22 kg/m^2), body fat percentage, when corrected for body weight and mineral content, tend to be inversely related [25]. Osteoporosis and obesity coexist in syndromes of fat redistribution, such as Cushing's disease and drug-induced lipodystrophies [52]. Thus, notwithstanding abundant evidence that adipose tissue protects the skeleton, a number of studies also provide evidence to the contrary. Nevertheless, mechanistic explanations have been proposed to support the observed epidemiologic and functional associations between fat and bone. Because adipocytes and osteoblasts both differentiate from the same precursor cells, adipocyte-derived hormones modulate bone development [66]. These associations can to some degree be explained.

We will discuss the impact of lipid metabolism on specific conditions, i.e., diabetes, osteoporosis, and the role of adipokines and therapeutics.

8.4 Diabetes

8.4.1 Types of Diabetes

Diabetes belongs to the group of metabolic diseases that are characterized by insufficiency or absence of insulin, the principal hormone that regulates glucose uptake and determines how food is chemically transformed into energy. Diabetes affects more than 23.6 million or 7.8% of the US population. Fifty-seven million American adults have a prediabetic condition that raises the risk of developing type 2 diabetes as indicated by Centers for Diseases Control. Clinically, diabetes mellitus is classified as: type 1 insulin-dependent diabetes mellitus (IDDM) where the body produces little or no insulin. It is a condition that typically occurs in children and young adults, but can develop at any age; Type 2 diabetes is non insulin-dependent diabetes mellitus (NIDDM). In that condition, the body does not produce enough insulin or does not respond properly to insulin that is produced. Type 2 NIDDM is more common in people who are older, overweight, and inactive. It is characterized by high blood glucose which, because of insulin deficiency, has not gone down. Type 2 diabetes is due primarily to lifestyle factors and has a genetic basis. Individuals who do not smoke, consume alcohol in moderation, have high levels of physical activity, normal weight, a consumer diet (high in fiber, with a high ratio of polyunsaturated to saturated fat), and a relatively low mean glycemic index have an 82% lower rate of diabetes. Obesity has been found to account for approximately 55% of type 2 diabetes [48]. Environmental toxins contribute to increases in the rate of type 2 diabetes.

8.4.2 Diabetes and Bone

Dysregulation in blood glucose levels leads to complications and shifts in energy balance. Loss of cellular energy cells due to dysregulation of insulin, as in diabetes, results in disruption of the energy homeostasis. Prolonged exposure to such a state in humans leads to bone loss due to insufficient energy transport and distribution, along with a lack of cytokines and hormones required for normal bone metabolism [7, 8, 26]. In humans, type 1 diabetes is associated with a decrease in skeletal mass and a delay in the healing of fractures [38] as well as with an increased risk of osteopenia and osteoporosis [6, 42]. The Nord-Trondelag Health Survey from Norway showed that fracture rates had significantly increased among female type 1 diabetic patients compared with controls. Duration of diabetes appears to play a key role in bone health inasmuch as people who have had diabetes for >5 years had lower BMD [17]. In the Iowa Women's Health Study, women with type 1 diabetes were more than 12 times more likely to report a fracture than nondiabetic women. Diabetic patients exhibit reduced BMD as elevated at the lumbar spine and proximal femur by dual X-ray absorptiometry [55]. The bone formation rate is also reduced in diabetic people, perhaps because their osteoblast activity is lower than that of normal individuals. Type 1 diabetes develops in the young, when bone mass is accrued. Low bone mass is a predictable complication for type 1 diabetes (CDC-NIDDK).

Insight into the mechanisms of diabetes-associated bone disease has come largely from studies with animal models. In several models of type 1 diabetes, bone turnover is reduced, fracture is impaired, and mineralization is deficient. In streptozotocin-induced diabetic rats, abnormal bone repair is insulin dependent because the deficient osseous healing was reversed by insulin treatment [6]. This demonstrates the cause and effect relationship between insulin production and abnormal bone formation. The mechanism for the reduced bone turnover in type 1 diabetes therefore is likely multifactorial. Studies in uremic rats suggest that lack of insulin may diminish bone turnover [27]. However, insulin deficiency may also be important, inasmuch as decreased bone formation can be demonstrated in type 1 diabetics before the onset of clinical renal disease. The anabolic effects of insulin may be mediated through the insulin-like growth factor 1 (IGF-1) pathway. In type 1 diabetes, low levels of insulin and IGF-1 impair osteoblast function [14]. Bone histomorphometric studies in type 1 diabetes have generally, but not always, shown a low turnover of bone with bone formation reduced to a lesser degree than bone resorption. Reduced serum concentrations of osteocalcin, a marker of osteoblastic activity, are a sign of the decrease in bone formation. Resorption markers (such as serum tartrate-resistant acid phosphatase and urinary hydroxyproline) are increased in some patients, perhaps because of changes in renal function [24]. Children and adolescents with type 1 diabetes have reduced BMD at the forearm, but it is not clear whether this deficit is also present at the lumbar spine. Variable findings have been reported, from reductions in trabecular but not cortical BMD to no deficit when BMD is corrected for body weight. It is therefore assumed that any defect in BMD is due to a failure to acquire endosteal bone during growth [24]. In adults with type 1 diabetes, lumbar BMD is usually normal, whereas femoral BMD is reduced [41]. Most studies have failed to show a relationship between BMD and the duration of diabetes

Table 8.1 Effects of diabetes on bone

Features	Type 1 diabetes	Type 2 diabetes
Age of onset	Children	Older individuals
Body and bone morphology	Usually low BMI and low BMD	High BMI, overweight to obese, maybe increased BMD
Pathology and serum levels	Insulin deficiency, decreased bone formation, low bone turnover, increased bone fragility, increased fracture risk	Insulin resistance, hyperinsulinemia, decreased bone formation, low bone turnover, increased bone fragility, increased fracture risk

or glycemic control, but this is not uniformly true. One study of premenopausal women reported an increase in lumbar BMD and normal femoral BMD [21].

The majority of studies of type 2 diabetes have found that BMD in both women and men is normal or increased at the lumbar spine, femoral neck, and the mid and distal radius, and is correlated with BMI [44]. However, in studies that corrected for BMI, increase in BMD was found independent of obesity. A study of older well-functioning patients with type 2 diabetes showed higher hip, higher total body, and volumetric spine BMD in black and white men and women compared with controls. Yet, the spine bone volume was found to be lower in diabetic subjects, with bone strength possibly decreased. A recent report suggests that cortical porosity is increased in type 2 diabetics [54]. Bone loss or bone turnover in type 2 diabetes may also be due to treatment. Biguanide, a widely used drug used in type 2 diabetes, works primarily by reducing liver release of blood glucose from glycogen stores and secondarily by provoking an increase in cellular glucose uptake. Metformin also reduces insulin resistance and is preferred in obese patients, as it promotes weight loss. The most commonly used drugs in the past and currently belong to the sulfonylurea group, including glibenclamide and gliclazide. These increase glucose-stimulated insulin secretion by the pancreas and, thus, lowering blood glucose even in the face of insulin resistance. Their chief adverse effect is an increase in the chance of hypoglycemic episodes. Newer drugs include thiazolidinediones (TZDs) (rosiglitazone, pioglitazone, and troglitazone), all of which increase tissue insulin sensitivity by modulating gene expression. For further discussion of drugs in diabetes mellitus, see below. The effects of diabetes on bone are summarized in Table 8.1.

8.5 The Role of Insulin Signaling in Energy Metabolism

Insulin, by regulating energy and glucose metabolism in the body, provides a link between bone health and metabolic diseases. Research in recent years clarified the interaction of insulin signaling in bone and fat metabolism. Bone-derived osteocalcin, in its undercarboxylated, hormonal form, regulates fat deposition and induces insulin secretion which, in turn, regulates blood glucose [19]. Insulin signaling in osteoblasts activates transcriptional events that promote osteoblast differentiation and regulate the production and bioavailability of osteocalcin by activation of bone resorption. The undercarboxylated form of osteocalcin acts as a circulating hormone to regulate fat accumulation and insulin production and sensitivity. The mechanism of regulation has been explained as follows: first, insulin suppresses the (runt-related transcription factor 2) RUNX2 inhibitor Twist2, which promotes osteoblast differentiation necessary for normal bone formation. Second, insulin induces production of osteocalcin, which influences glucose utilization, perhaps by a regulatory loop wherein insulin, by signaling the osteoblast, modulates postnatal bone development and simultaneously regulates insulin sensitivity and pancreatic insulin secretion to regulate glucose homeostasis. As osteoblast signals the resorption process through cytokine release, the cell environment becomes more acidic. This, in turn, favors decarboxylation and activates more osteocalcin, which stimulates insulin production. Because insulin also favors

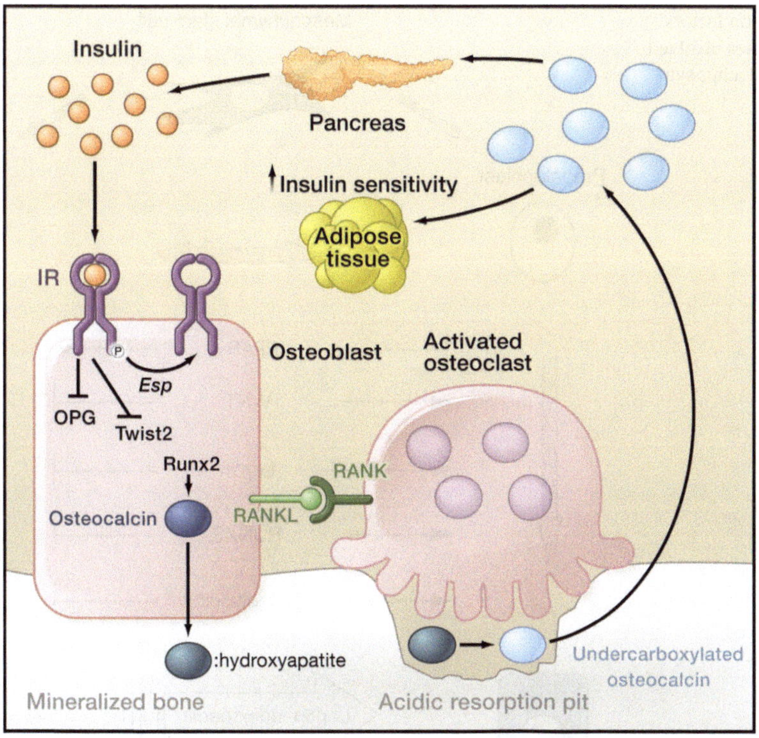

Fig. 8.1 Energy regulation and bone turnover by the insulin/osteocalcin axis. A putative feed-forward regulatory loop ties bone turnover to energy regulation as proposed by Ferron et al. [16] and Fulzele et al. [19]. Insulin activates skeletal remodeling (i.e., increases bone formation by osteoblasts and resorption by osteoclasts). This, in turn, releases uncarboxylated osteocalcin from the skeletal matrix into the circulation, enhances insulin secretion, and increases the insulin sensitivity of adipocytes. A tyrosine phosphatase OST-PTP, which is encoded by the *Esp* gene, binds the insulin receptor (IR) and suppresses its activation through dephosphorylation. The transcription factor Twist2 is a critical downstream suppressor of osteoblast differentiation. Osteoprotegerin (*OPG*) is an osteoblast-specific inhibitor of RANKL, acting as a decoy receptor to block bone resorption. Hydroxyapatite is the mineral component of bone (Adapted from Rosen and Motyl [53], Copyright 2010, with permission from Elsevier)

bone resorption, the process can be described as a "feed-forward" loop, whereby insulin signaling stimulates osteoblasts to start resorption [16, 22, 23]. As a result of this process, more osteocalcin is released, which then releases more insulin. Thus, insulin has been described as "a street-smart molecule" that takes advantage of the functional interplay between bone resorption and osteocalcin, to turn on the secretion and synthesis of more insulin. These findings strengthen the idea that diabetes can be treated by regulating levels of osteocalcin. This has implications for patients with diabetes and osteoporosis. The notion that hampering bone resorption has deleterious consequences on glucose homeostasis is medically important, inasmuch as most drugs used to treat osteoporosis target this aspect of bone remodeling. Fasting plasma glucose levels are elevated in women with osteoporosis who are treated with drugs that inhibit bone resorption and lower serum levels of undercarboxylated osteocalcin. Figure 8.1 illustrates energy regulation and bone turnover by insulin and the osteocalcin axis.

8.6 Osteoporosis

Osteoporosis is the most common metabolic bone disease and a major public health problem. The term osteoporosis literally means "porous bone." It can be defined as a skeletal disorder characterized by bone thinning that leads to low bone mass and bone fragility as a result of the disruption of

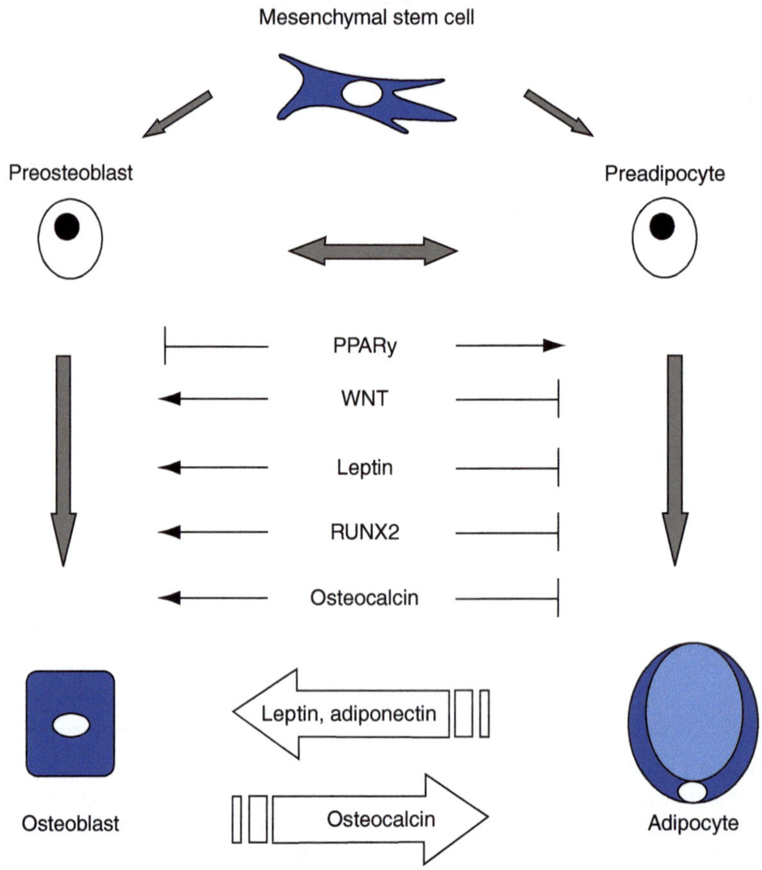

Fig. 8.2 Common factors shared in processes involved in osteoblast and adipocyte differentiation

bone microstructure, with an increase in the risk of fracture [46]. In the United States alone, some 10 million women and men have osteoporosis and 34 million people are at high risk for developing osteoporosis. In turn, this prevalence may result in over 1.5 million osteoporotic fractures per year [66, 67].

8.6.1 Obesity and Its Connection to Osteoporosis

Many similarities between obesity and osteoporosis have been identified. These include a pathophysiological linkage due to genetic and environmental factors that affect both diseases or their interaction.

- Normal aging is associated with both a high incidence of osteoporosis and bone marrow adiposity.
- Bone remodeling and adiposity are both regulated through the hypothalamus and the sympathetic nervous system [15, 51, 66].
- Adipocytes and osteoblasts arise from a common progenitor, the mesenchymal stem cell. These stem cells exhibit equal propensity for differentiation into adipocytes or osteoblasts, with the balance of the differentiation regulated by several interacting pathways that may contribute to the final effect of fat mass on bone. Figure 8.2 shows the possible function of common factors shared in osteoblast and adipocyte differentiation.

Adipocytes express and secrete a variety of biologically active molecules, such as estrogen, resistin, leptin, adiponectin, etc., that affect energy homeostasis and are involved in bone metabolism.

- Similarly, bone-secreted factors like osteocalcin, osteoprotegrin (OPG), and interleukin-6 respond to the antiapoptotic function of leptin, their serum levels increase, and they in turn modulate adipocytes [26].

These similarities indicate an interrelationship between bone and fat metabolism and their diseases, subject to genetic and environmental factors. The two cell types, adipocytes and osteoblasts, share a complicated inverse relationship. Mesenchymal stem cells arise in the bone marrow. Their differentiation depends on modulation of specific transcriptional factors that direct lineage specificity of the two cell types. For example, activation of the master regulatory transcription factor responsible for adipogenesis, PPARγ (peroxizome proliferator-activated receptor gamma), favors the differentiation of mesenchymal stem cells into adipocytes over that to osteoblasts [45]. In contrast, the Wnt-signaling pathway inhibits adipogenesis while promoting osteogenesis [3, 4, 20]. Based on these findings, an inverse relationship model, called the "see-saw paradigm" has been proposed to describe the relationship between fat mass and bone mass in bone marrow. Some potential effectors of osteoporosis are discussed below.

8.6.2 PPARgamma

PPARγ is a member of the nuclear receptor superfamily and is a critical transcription factor in adipogenesis. Activation of PPARγ requires the binding of a ligand and recruitment of specific coactivators to allow the PPARγ–RXRα heterodimer to induce gene transcription of insulin-sensitizing targets, such as adiponectin and lipoprotein lipase. Ligands for PPARγ include the naturally occurring prostaglandin compounds, as well as the TZD class of synthetic compounds. In 1999, two TZDs (rosiglitazone and pioglitazone) were approved by the US FDA for the treatment of type 2 diabetes mellitus because both enhance insulin sensitivity [32]. There are however differences within this class of agents, not only with respect to their lipid-lowering properties, but also with regard to their propensity to increase the risk of cardiovascular disease and, most intriguingly, their capacity to cause bone loss and marrow adipogenesis.

Regulation of PPARγ activity determines osteogenic recruitment, especially in the mesenchymal stem cell population in the bone marrow, as well as in adipose tissue derived from stromal cells. Molecules, like Sprouty and TAZ, also modulate PPARγ activity by directly or indirect binding to them [62]. PPARγ mediates the effects of fat cells on osteoblast function within the bone marrow, in part by regulating transcriptional activity of RUNX2. In addition, the adipocyte-secreted hormone adiponectin may modulate osteoblast function through adiponectin receptor-1-mediated changes in PPARγ expression. Cell apoptosis does not appear to play a role in the regulation by adipocytes of osteoblasts in bone marrow. Further research is needed to examine the molecular mechanisms through which PPARγ regulates RUNX2, in the hope of identifying possible therapeutic targets to modify age- and type 2 diabetes-related bone loss [37]. The effect of PPARγ on bone and obesity suggests that treatment with PPARγ antagonists might be therapeutically beneficial to intervene in age-related bone loss and marrow fat accumulation. In vitro treatment of cultured bone marrow-derived mesenchymal stem cells with PPARγ, cytokines (interleukin-1 (IL-1)), or TNF-α (tumor necrosis factor-alpha) inhibits adipogenesis and osteogenesis [66].

8.6.3 TZDs and Effect on Bone

There is now evidence that both TZDs, rosiglitazone and pioglitazone, have clinically important negative effects on the skeleton [9]. Fracture risk increased in women, but not men. In short-term clinical trials, both TZDs caused rapid bone loss in women [43]. Changes in bone turnover markers indicate a pattern of reduced bone formation without corresponding change in resorption. Although limited, these results give support to the hypothesis based on cultures of rodent models, that reduced bone formation resulting from activation of PPARγ is a central mechanism in the action of TZDs on bone. Research is needed to better understand the mechanisms of bone loss with TZDs and to identify and treat factors that affect susceptibility to TZD-induced osteoporosis. PPARγ activation with TZDs increases bone resorption and decreases bone formation. The PPARγ complex is activated by TZDs, which enhance insulin sensitivity, but also promote stromal cell entry into the fat lineage. TZD treatment improves glucose tolerance and results in modest weight gain and enhanced marrow adiposity. These effects are at the expense of the skeleton, but marrow fat cells can coexist with active osteoblasts. On the basis of experimental evidence, it may be possible to separate unwanted from beneficial effects of PPARγ by the use of selective PPARγ modulators [30]. Both rosiglitazone-mediated activation and overexpression of PPARγ have led to acceleration of osteoblast differentiation. However, in mice whose PPARγ was knocked out, osteoblast differentiation was diminished, but MSCs treated with rosiglitazone did not preferentially differentiate into adipocytes [8]. Yet the rosiglitazone-mediated acceleration of osteoblast differentiation was followed by accumulation of reactive oxygen species and apoptosis. In contrast to the osteogenic lineage, cells of the adipogenic lineage were protected. These findings suggest an explanation for why activated PPARγ suppresses bone and bone marrow adipogenesis. Implied in this explanation is that the osteogenic line is more susceptible than the adipogenic lineage to oxidative stress [2, 9, 11, 34, 56]. Rosiglitazone has also been found to decrease bone formation and to increase adipocyte and osteoclast numbers. The therapeutic potential effect of these events is under intense FDA consideration and review [1, 35, 49, 50].

8.6.4 Nonsteroidal Anti-inflammatory Drugs (NSAIDs)

Nonsteroidal anti-inflammatory drugs (NSAIDs) are widely used clinically as adjuncts to ameliorate postoperative pain. NSAIDs act through inhibition of cyclooxygenase (COX-2) enzymes and, therefore, diminish prostaglandin production. However, eicosanoids (prostaglandins) are intimately involved in the modulation of bone metabolism and favor bone anabolism. Inhibition of COX-2 downregulates osteoclast and osteoblast differentiation while favoring adipocyte differentiation [33]. Because insulin and/or glycemic status regulate osteogenesis, the consequences of diabetes and insulin treatment on bone formation and osteoblastogenesis lead to a decrease in new bone formation. Insulin treatment can restore bone formation to levels observed in nondiabetic controls; however, it does not significantly decrease adipogenesis. RUNX2 and several RUNX2 target genes, including matrix metalloproteinase-9, ALP (alkaline phosphatase), integrin-binding sialoprotein, Dmp1 (dentin matrix acidic phosphoprotein 1), Col1a2 (Collagen type 1, alpha 2), Phex (phosphate-regulating neutral endopeptidase), VDR (vitamin D receptor), osteocalcin, and osterix, are significantly downregulated during insulin-deficiency, hyperglycemia, and diabetic conditions, all of which contribute to diabetic bone diseases [18].

8.6.5 Hormone Therapy with Estrogen and Progesterone

Hormone therapy with estrogen and progesterone has been the most widely used treatment for osteoporosis because it raised hip and spine BMD by 5% and 2.5%, respectively. Combined hormone therapy has, however, come under question as a result of the findings in the NHLBI Women's Health Initiative (WHI) that indicated significant adverse events, including a greater risk of breast cancer. In type 2 diabetic women, combination hormone therapy is therefore limited to low-dose formulations, in part because glucose tolerance became impaired at higher estrogen doses. In men with gonadal insufficiency, androgen replacement improves BMD, but this approach cannot be used in men with a history of prostate cancer. It is not generally associated with impaired glucose tolerance. Raloxifene, a selective estrogen, is utilized to prevent and treat osteoporosis. Salmon calcitonin is a synthetic polypeptide with the molecular structure of calcitonin and is FDA approved for the treatment of postmenopausal osteoporosis (see Chap. 6). Current treatment has shifted to bisphosphonates (BPN), the use of which has been shown in several large-scale clinical trials to bring about a reduction of 40–50% in both spine and hip fractures. There are no large study reports that suggest an increased risk of diabetes in patients using BPNs. PTH (parathyroid hormone) is also approved for the treatment of osteoporosis. Treatment with this hormone is not associated with changes in body composition or diabetes mellitus.

8.7 Adipokines

Adipokines have been shown to participate in the complicated mechanisms that regulate bone metabolism. These findings not only reveal an added level of complexity but also provide molecular insight into the system of adipose–bone interactions [39].

8.7.1 Leptin

Leptin is a 16-kDa peptide adipokine that is synthesized by adipocytes that mediate energy homeostasis, appetite levels, and reproductive capacity. The signaling form of the leptin receptor is expressed in both osteoblasts and chondrocytes. Leptin increases proliferation and differentiation of osteoblasts and promotes bone nodule formation. It also increases chondrocyte growth. This accounts for the short limbs of animals with impaired leptin signaling. Leptin also regulates osteoclast development, at least in part through changes in production of receptor for nuclear factor-κB (RANK), RANK-ligand (RANKL), and osteoprotegerin. In obese individuals, leptin, by acting on bone formation and resorption, increases skeletal mass. The resulting skeleton has the greater strength needed to support the larger soft tissue mass [47].

Leptin regulates bone formation in mice through a complex neuroendocrine circuit that involves the hypothalamus, the sympathetic, and central nervous systems. Leptin also stimulates osteoblastic proliferation and differentiation in vitro and, when injected in high doses, leads to gain in bone mass, even though leptin's role on bone remodeling is limited [10, 29, 57]. Mouse models of lipodystrophy, as in A-ZIP transgenic and PPARγ hyp/hyp mice, also display a high bone mass phenotype. Low serum leptin levels induce an increase in bone mass regardless of body weight [60, 61]. Leptin deficiency is associated with reduced linear growth, reduced cortical bone mass, and an increase in the trabecular bone of the spine, but in the femora where huge adipocytes occupy much of the marrow space, trabecular bone is reduced. Systemic administration of leptin in intact or leptin-deficient animals usually enhances bone formation and skeletal mass and strength. In leptin replacement, leptin-deficient animals reverse the adipocyte phenotype and increase total body BMC by >30%. However, systemic administration of high doses of leptin may have negative effects that are similar when leptin is administered centrally [40], i.e., loss and decreases in serum IGF1 levels [47]. Deficiencies or resistance to leptin cause obesity, impaired fertility, and changes in appetite in humans and rodents. Surprisingly, leptin deficiency also results in high bone mass, even though in that situation estrogen concentrations are markedly suppressed.

The high bone mass of leptin deficiency is a result of a reduction in the sympathetic tone that innervates the two adrenergic receptors found in osteoblasts [52]. As for the indirect action of leptin, it has been demonstrated that intracerebroventricular infusion of the adipokine causes bone loss in leptin-deficient and wild-type mice, both by inhibiting bone formation [13] and stimulating bone resorption. Blockade of the sympathetic nervous system abrogates these effects, which appear to be mediated by the β-adrenoreceptor on the osteoblast [39]. It is therefore evident that leptin signaling regulates bone resorption via two antagonistic mechanisms [10, 29]. The first is a stimulation of bone resorption through the sympathetic nervous pathway. This increases RANKL expression in osteoblasts. The second is a reduction in bone resorption through upregulation of CART (cocaine- and amphetamine-regulated transcript). This decreases RANKL expression in osteoblasts through an as yet incompletely deciphered pathway. Leptin is, therefore, not only a hormone that modulates energy metabolism, but also constitutes an important determinant of bone remodeling.

Since the discovery of leptin 15 years ago, expectations have been widespread that targeting leptin might constitute an effective therapeutic approach to treat obesity and that leptin treatment would be an important adjunct to treating acquired lipodystrophic disorders, including chronic human immunodeficiency virus (HIV) infections and insulin-resistant diabetes mellitus. Leptin's role in skeletal function is complicated, but increasing the amount of circulating leptin could be therapeutically useful in bone diseases, particularly in states of disordered fat metabolism associated with bone marrow adiposity [30]. Therapeutic applications of leptin in human trials have been less successful. The role of leptin receptors and of agents that enhance leptin receptor sensitivity has been studied in obese mice models.

8.7.2 Adiponectin

Adiponectin, a 30-kDa adipocytokine, is highly expressed in visceral, subcutaneous, and bone marrow fat depots, as well as in bone [5]. It regulates energy homeostasis, glucose and lipid metabolism, and inflammatory pathways. Studies have shown that plasma concentrations of adiponectin relate inversely to visceral fat mass and BMI. Serum adiponectin levels correlate with insulin sensitivity. Low levels of adiponectin are found in subjects with coronary artery disease and type 2 diabetes mellitus. Both osteoblasts and osteoclasts have the receptors for adiponectin. They induce increased osteoblast proliferation and differentiation and mineralization of osteoblastic cells. Adiponectin may therefore also influence bone metabolism and be involved in the regulation of bone turnover and enhance the receptor activator of RANKL expression and in suppressing its decoy receptor, OPG. However, adiponectin does not act directly on osteoclasts. A rise in serum adiponectin improves not only osteoblastic dysfunction but also enhances low bone turnover, conditions typically seen in diabetic patients so far. However, only a few cross-sectional studies have been performed to study the association between serum adiponectin and bone markers in humans [28].

Adiponectin may increase bone mass in vivo, but studies in transgenic mice have been inconsistent. In 14-week old adiponectin-knockout mice, trabecular bone volume was 30% higher than in controls. This finding suggests that indirect of adipokine on bone are stronger than indirect effects. The latter may include modulation of insulin sensitivity and growth factor binding. The magnitude of the bone changes in the knockout mice indicates that adiponectin is likely to be a significant contributor to the fat–bone relationship. Clinical studies have shown the existence of inverse relationships between circulating adiponectin and BMD [47]. Adiponectin seems to function primarily to increase insulin sensitivity [36] via activation of PPARγ, another mechanism by which glucose and lipid metabolisms are regulated. Activation of the adiponectin receptors, AdipoR1 and AdipoR2, increases the activation of adenosine monophosphate protein kinase (AMPK), which results in insulin sensitivity. Patients with type 2 diabetes have lower adiponectin levels, and glycemic control in these patients may improve the impaired bone formation. In the clinic, serum adiponectin levels can help predict the beneficial bone reaction ahead of treatment. Further studies that have investigated the effects of current antidiabetic drugs including sulfonylurea, TZDs, and antihypertensive activation have shown that adiponectin levels increase regardless of activation of the PPARγ pathway [59]. TZDs increase adipocyte production of adiponectin by direct stimulation and also antagonize the effects of TNF-α, a known adiponectin antagonist. It has been proposed that adiponectin directly affects differentiating adipocytes that have not acquired insulin resistance. Recently, it has been hypothesized that adiponectin has at least three different actions on bone: (1) a positive one via the autocrine/paracrine pathway, (2) a negative direct endocrine one, and (3) a positive indirect endocrine action by enhancing insulin osteogenic signaling [58]. Discrepant findings may be due to the relative prevalence of positive and negative effects of adiponectin on bone formation. In humans, circulating adiponectin appears in general to diminish bone mass and constitute a predictor of lower bone mass.

The role of bone turnover in other adipokines, including resistin, visfatin, omentin, adipsin, is under current investigation. Resistin modestly increases proliferation of osteoblasts in both cell and organ culture systems and increases the formation and activity of osteoclasts. Visfatin/pre-B-cell-enhancing factor (PBEF)/nicotinamide phosphoribosyltranferase (Nampt) enhances the effect of IL-7 and stem cell factor on pre-B-cell colony formation. This indicates it exerts proinflammatory activities. Several independent studies have suggested that visfatin/PBEF/Nampt has insulin-like effects, although further elucidation of the signaling molecules used by visfatin/PBEF/Nampt is necessary to confirm its potential role as a novel insulin-mimetic adipokine. Plasma visfatin was not found to be associated with BMD in men. Vaspin (visceral adipose-tissue-derived serine protease inhibitor) is another recently identified adipokine, which shares some similarities with adiponectin in improving insulin sensitivity. Preliminary studies indicate that vaspin might also have anti-inflammatory effects, as it suppresses the production of TNF-α, leptin, and resistin, but no studies linking this molecule to bone metabolism have so far been published [39, 47, 59, 64]. Generally, adipokines are important local and systemic modulators of bone remodeling that involve direct and indirect mechanisms and a breadth of molecular signals. Additionally, cross talk is reciprocal, in that bone secretory products influence energy metabolism and adipokine release. Because adipocytes and osteoblasts arise from a common precursor cell in the bone marrow, their destiny is often connected and they share genetic, hormonal, and environmental dynamics.

8.8 Summary and Conclusion

What we have learned so far is that fat and bone by their reciprocal needs are tightly linked in mammalian physiology. Skeletal remodeling, as a finely tuned means of replenishing calcium and maintaining bone integrity, evolved over millions of year and demands a sustainable energy source from adipose tissue. Fat tissue, on the other hand, via signaling through the hypothalamus, regulates bone mass as a means of controlling energy use and modulating insulin secretion and sensitivity. The clinical correlates of this intimate relationship are profound and translatable to clinical practice. For example, the use of glucocorticoids or TZDs causes bone loss, principally by shifting the marrow equilibrium toward adipocyte differentiation [52]. This leads to the classical example of osteoporosis as a model disease that demonstrates the intrinsic interaction between fat and bone. Though obesity and osteoporosis were believed to be two unrelated diseases, current opinion holds that both diseases share common genetic and environmental factors.

Patients with diabetes typically have low bone turnover, with bone formation and, to a lesser degree, bone resorption both reduced. The mechanism for the reduction in bone turnover is likely multifactorial. In type 1 diabetes, low levels of insulin and IGF-1 may impair osteoblast function. In both type 1 and type 2 diabetes, the accumulation (as a result of hyperglycemia) of advanced glycation end products (AGE) in collagen may contribute to reduced bone formation. BMD is lower in patients with type-1 diabetes and normal or increased in patients with type 2 diabetes. Fracture risk is increased in both groups, possibly related to their diminished BMD, in turn due to the duration of the disease, to medical complications, to impaired bone quality, to medical treatment, and to the risk of falling. In the absence of studies specifically targeting osteoporosis in individuals with diabetes, treatment should follow for the recommended approach to treatment of osteoporosis in postmenopausal women and men.

In conclusion, patients with type 1 and 2 diabetes are at increased risk for developing an osteoporosis-related fracture. BMD measurements in this population may not be sufficient. All diabetes-related factors should be considered in assessing osteoporosis and fracture risk reduction. Diabetic patients with low-impact fractures or osteoporosis should be offered treatment that includes pharmacological and nonpharmacological therapies. The association of diabetes and osteoporosis is still not fully understood and investigation of additional treatment pathways continues to develop. Many of these pathways offer promising findings with respect to outcome, but clinical study and data are still in the early stages.

References

1. Ali AA, Weinstein RS, Stewart SA, Parfitt AM, Manolagas SC, Jilka RL. Rosiglitazone causes bone loss in mice by suppressing osteoblast differentiation and bone formation. Endocrinology. 2005;146:1226–35.
2. Aubert RE, Herrera V, Chen W, Haffner SM, Pendergrass M. Rosiglitazone and pioglitazone increase fracture risk in women and men with type 2 diabetes. Diabetes Obes Metab. 2010;12:716–21.
3. Bennett CN, Hodge CL, MacDougald OA, Schwartz J. Role of Wnt10b and C/EBPalpha in spontaneous adipogenesis of 243 cells. Biochem Biophys Res Commun. 2003;302:12–6.
4. Bennett CN, Ross SE, Longo KA, Bajnok L, Hemati N, Johnson KW, Harrison SD, MacDougald OA. Regulation of Wnt signaling during adipogenesis. J Biol Chem. 2002;277:30998–1004.
5. Berner HS, Lyngstadaas SP, Spahr A, Monjo M, Thommesen L, Drevon CA, Syversen U, Reseland JE. Adiponectin and its receptors are expressed in bone-forming cells. Bone. 2004;35:842–9.
6. Botolin S, McCabe LR. Bone loss and increased bone adiposity in spontaneous and pharmacologically induced diabetic mice. Endocrinology. 2007;148: 198–205.
7. Bouillon R. Diabetic bone disease. Calcif Tissue Int. 1991;49:155–60.
8. Bouillon R. Diabetic bone disease Low turnover osteoporosis related to decreased IGF-I production. Verh K Acad Geneeskd Belg. 1992;54:365–91; discussion 391–362.
9. Bruedigam C, Eijken M, Koedam M, van de Peppel J, Drabek K, Chiba H, van Leeuwen JP. A new concept underlying stem cell lineage skewing that explains the detrimental effects of thiazolidinediones on bone. Stem Cells. 2010;28:916–27.
10. Confavreux CB, Levine RL, Karsenty G. A paradigm of integrative physiology, the crosstalk between bone and energy metabolisms. Mol Cell Endocrinol. 2009;310:21–9.
11. Debiais F. Thiazolidinediones: antidiabetic agents with effects on bone. Joint Bone Spine. 2009;76: 221–3.
12. Dimitri P, Wales JK, Bishop N. Fat and bone in children: differential effects of obesity on bone size and mass according to fracture history. J Bone Miner Res. 2010;25:527–36.
13. Ducy P, Amling M, Takeda S, Priemel M, Schilling AF, Beil FT, Shen J, Vinson C, Rueger JM, Karsenty G. Leptin inhibits bone formation through a hypothalamic relay: a central control of bone mass. Cell. 2000;100:197–207.
14. Epstein S, Leroith D. Diabetes and fragility fractures – a burgeoning epidemic? Bone. 2008;43:3–6.
15. Felson DT, Zhang Y, Hannan MT, Anderson JJ. Effects of weight and body mass index on bone mineral density in men and women: the Framingham study. J Bone Miner Res. 1993;8:567–73.
16. Ferron M, Wei J, Yoshizawa T, Del Fattore A, DePinho RA, Teti A, Ducy P, Karsenty G. Insulin signaling in osteoblasts integrates bone remodeling and energy metabolism. Cell. 2010;142:296–308.
17. Forsen T, Eriksson J, Tuomilehto J, Reunanen A, Osmond C, Barker D. The fetal and childhood growth of persons who develop type 2 diabetes. Ann Intern Med. 2000;133:176–82.
18. Fowlkes JL, Bunn RC, Liu L, Wahl EC, Coleman HN, Cockrell GE, Perrien DS, Lumpkin Jr CK, Thrailkill KM. Runt-related transcription factor 2 (RUNX2) and RUNX2-related osteogenic genes are down-regulated throughout osteogenesis in type 1 diabetes mellitus. Endocrinology. 2008;149: 1697–704.
19. Fulzele K, Riddle RC, DiGirolamo DJ, Cao X, Wan C, Chen D, Faugere MC, Aja S, Hussain MA, Bruning JC, Clemens TL. Insulin receptor signaling in osteoblasts regulates postnatal bone acquisition and body composition. Cell. 2010;142:309–19.
20. Gimble JM, Zvonic S, Floyd ZE, Kassem M, Nuttall ME. Playing with bone and fat. J Cell Biochem. 2006;98:251–66.
21. Hadzibegovic I, Miskic B, Cosic V, Prvulovic D, Bistrovic D. Increased bone mineral density in postmenopausal women with type 2 diabetes mellitus. Ann Saudi Med. 2008;28:102–4.
22. Hinoi E, Gao N, Jung DY, Yadav V, Yoshizawa T, Kajimura D, Myers Jr MG, Chua Jr SC, Wang Q, Kim JK, Kaestner KH, Karsenty G. An osteoblast-dependent mechanism contributes to the leptin regulation of insulin secretion. Ann N Y Acad Sci. 2009;1173 Suppl 1:E20–3030.
23. Hinoi E, Gao N, Jung DY, Yadav V, Yoshizawa T, Myers Jr MG, Chua Jr SC, Kim JK, Kaestner KH, Karsenty G. The sympathetic tone mediates Leptin's inhibition of insulin secretion by modulating osteocalcin bioactivity. J Cell Biol. 2008;183:1235–42.
24. Hordon L. Bone disease in diabetes mellitus. In: uptodate; 2010. www.uptodate.com/contents/bone-disease-in-diabetes-mellitus.
25. Hsu YH, Venners SA, Terwedow HA, Feng Y, Niu T, Li Z, Laird N, Brain JD, Cummings SR, Bouxsein ML, Rosen CJ, Xu X. Relation of body composition, fat mass, and serum lipids to osteoporotic fractures and bone mineral density in Chinese men and women. Am J Clin Nutr. 2006;83:146–54.

26. Inzerillo AM, Epstein S. Osteoporosis and diabetes mellitus. Rev Endocr Metab Disord. 2004;5:261–8.
27. Jara A, Bover J, Felsenfeld AJ. Development of secondary hyperparathyroidism and bone disease in diabetic rats with renal failure. Kidney Int. 1995;47: 1746–51.
28. Kanazawa I, Yamaguchi T, Yamauchi M, Yamamoto M, Kurioka S, Yano S, Sugimoto T. Adiponectin is associated with changes in bone markers during glycemic control in type 2 diabetes mellitus. J Clin Endocrinol Metab. 2009;94:3031–7.
29. Karsenty G. Convergence between bone and energy homeostases: leptin regulation of bone mass. Cell Metab. 2006;4:341–8.
30. Kawai M, Devlin MJ, Rosen CJ. Fat targets for skeletal health. Nat Rev Rheumatol. 2009;5:365–72.
31. Kawai M, Rosen CJ. Bone: adiposity and bone accrual-still an established paradigm? Nat Rev Endocrinol. 2010;6:63–4.
32. Kawai M, Sousa KM, MacDougald OA, Rosen CJ. The many facets of PPARgamma: novel insights for the skeleton. Am J Physiol Endocrinol Metab. 2010;299:E3–99.
33. Kellinsalmi M, Parikka V, Risteli J, Hentunen T, Leskela HV, Lehtonen S, Selander K, Vaananen K, Lehenkari P. Inhibition of cyclooxygenase-2 down-regulates osteoclast and osteoblast differentiation and favours adipocyte formation in vitro. Eur J Pharmacol. 2007;572:102–10.
34. Lecka-Czernik B. Bone loss in diabetes: use of antidiabetic thiazolidinediones and secondary osteoporosis. Curr Osteoporos Rep. 2010;8(4):178–84.
35. Lecka-Czernik B, Ackert-Bicknell C, Adamo ML, Marmolejos V, Churchill GA, Shockley KR, Reid IR, Grey A, Rosen CJ. Activation of peroxisome proliferator-activated receptor gamma (PPARgamma) by rosiglitazone suppresses components of the insulin-like growth factor regulatory system in vitro and in vivo. Endocrinology. 2007;148:903–11.
36. Lee NK, Karsenty G. Reciprocal regulation of bone and energy metabolism. Trends Endocrinol Metab. 2008;19:161–6.
37. Liu LF, Shen WJ, Zhang ZH, Wang LJ, Kraemer FB. Adipocytes decrease Runx2 expression in osteoblastic cells: roles of PPARgamma and adiponectin. J Cell Physiol. 2010;225:837–45.
38. Lu H, Kraut D, Gerstenfeld LC, Graves DT. Diabetes interferes with the bone formation by affecting the expression of transcription factors that regulate osteoblast differentiation. Endocrinology. 2003;144:346–52.
39. Magni P, Dozio E, Galliera E, Ruscica M, Corsi MM. Molecular aspects of adipokine-bone interactions. Curr Mol Med. 2010;10:522–32.
40. Martin A, David V, Malaval L, Lafage-Proust MH, Vico L, Thomas T. Opposite effects of leptin on bone metabolism: a dose-dependent balance related to energy intake and insulin-like growth factor-I pathway. Endocrinology. 2007;148:3419–25.
41. Mastrandrea LD, Wactawski-Wende J, Donahue RP, Hovey KM, Clark A, Quattrin T. Young women with type 1 diabetes have lower bone mineral density that persists over time. Diabetes Care. 2008;31:1729–35.
42. McCabe LR. Understanding the pathology and mechanisms of type I diabetic bone loss. J Cell Biochem. 2007;102:1343–57.
43. McDonough AK, Rosenthal RS, Cao X, Saag KG. The effect of thiazolidinediones on BMD and osteoporosis. Nat Clin Pract Endocrinol Metab. 2008;4: 507–13.
44. Melton 3rd LJ, Riggs BL, Leibson CL, Achenbach SJ, Camp JJ, Bouxsein ML, Atkinson EJ, Robb RA, Khosla S. A bone structural basis for fracture risk in diabetes. J Clin Endocrinol Metab. 2008;93:4804–9.
45. Pei L, Tontonoz P. Fat's loss is bone's gain. J Clin Invest. 2004;113:805–6.
46. Raisz L. Pathogenesis of osteoporosis; 2010. www.mdconsult.com.
47. Reid IR. Fat and bone. Arch Biochem Biophys. 2010;503(1):20–7.
48. Riserus U, Willett WC, Hu FB. Dietary fats and prevention of type 2 diabetes. Prog Lipid Res. 2009;48: 44–51.
49. Rosen CJ. Revisiting the rosiglitazone story – lessons learned. N Engl J Med. 2010;363:803–6.
50. Rosen CJ. The rosiglitazone story – lessons from an FDA Advisory Committee meeting. N Engl J Med. 2007;357:844–6.
51. Rosen CJ, Bouxsein ML. Mechanisms of disease: is osteoporosis the obesity of bone? Nat Clin Pract Rheumatol. 2006;2:35–43.
52. Rosen CJ, Klibanski A. Bone, fat, and body composition: evolving concepts in the pathogenesis of osteoporosis. Am J Med. 2009;122:409–14.
53. Rosen CJ, Motyl KJ. No bones about it: insulin modulates skeletal remodeling. Cell. 2010;142:198–200.
54. Schafer AL, Vittinghoff E, Lang TF, Sellmeyer DE, Harris TB, Kanaya AM, Strotmeyer ES, Cawthon PM, Cummings SR, Tylavsky FA, Scherzinger AL, Schwartz AV. Fat infiltration of muscle, diabetes, and clinical fracture risk in older adults. J Clin Endocrinol Metab. 2010;95(11):E368–37272. Epub 2010 Jul 28.
55. Schwartz AV, Sellmeyer DE. Diabetes, fracture, and bone fragility. Curr Osteoporos Rep. 2007;5:105–11.
56. Schwartz AV, Sellmeyer DE. Effect of thiazolidinediones on skeletal health in women with Type 2 diabetes. Expert Opin Drug Saf. 2008;7:69–78.
57. Shi Y, Yadav VK, Suda N, Liu XS, Guo XE, Myers Jr MG, Karsenty G. Dissociation of the neuronal regulation of bone mass and energy metabolism by leptin in vivo. Proc Natl Acad Sci USA. 2008; 105:20529–33.
58. Shinoda Y, Yamaguchi M, Ogata N, Akune T, Kubota N, Yamauchi T, Terauchi Y, Kadowaki T, Takeuchi Y, Fukumoto S, Ikeda T, Hoshi K, Chung UI, Nakamura K, Kawaguchi H. Regulation of bone formation by adiponectin through autocrine/paracrine and endocrine pathways. J Cell Biochem. 2006;99:196–208.
59. Sonnett TE, Levien TL, Gates BJ, Robinson JD, Campbell RK. Diabetes mellitus, inflammation,

obesity: proposed treatment pathways for current and future therapies. Ann Pharmacother. 2010;44: 701–11.
60. Takeda S. Bone and development, topics in bone biology. London: Springer; 2010.
61. Takeda S, Elefteriou F, Levasseur R, Liu X, Zhao L, Parker KL, Armstrong D, Ducy P, Karsenty G. Leptin regulates bone formation via the sympathetic nervous system. Cell. 2002;111:305–17.
62. Urs S, Venkatesh D, Tang Y, Henderson T, Yang X, Friesel RE, Rosen CJ, Liaw L. Sprouty1 is a critical regulatory switch of mesenchymal stem cell lineage allocation. FASEB J. 2010;24:3264–73.
63. von Muhlen D, Safii S, Jassal SK, Svartberg J, Barrett-Connor E. Associations between the metabolic syndrome and bone health in older men and women: the Rancho Bernardo Study. Osteoporos Int. 2007; 18:1337–44.
64. Wang P, Mariman E, Renes J, Keijer J. The secretory function of adipocytes in the physiology of white adipose tissue. J Cell Physiol. 2008;216:3–13.
65. WHO. Diet and physical activity. www.who.int/dietphysicalactivity/en/.
66. Zhao LJ, Jiang H, Papasian CJ, Maulik D, Drees B, Hamilton J, Deng HW. Correlation of obesity and osteoporosis: effect of fat mass on the determination of osteoporosis. J Bone Miner Res. 2008;23:17–29.
67. Zhao LJ, Liu YJ, Liu PY, Hamilton J, Recker RR, Deng HW. Relationship of obesity with osteoporosis. J Clin Endocrinol Metab. 2007;92:1640–6.

Diseases of Mineral Metabolism and Bone: Emerging Therapeutics for Postmenopausal Osteoporosiss

9

Paul D. Miller

Keywords
Postmenopausal osteoporosis • Osteoporosis • Bisphosphonates • RANK ligand • Cathepsin K • Clinical trials

9.1 Introduction

The pharmacological management of postmenopausal osteoporosis (PMO) was heralded by the registration of injectable calcitonin, an antiresorptive agent that in the nasal formulation was shown to be effective to reduce the risk of incident vertebral fractures [14]. Other antiresorptive agents, with different mechanisms of action to inhibit bone resorption, then followed registration for management of PMO: estrogen, bisphosphonates, selective estrogen receptor modulators, and most recently, denosumab [6, 17, 20, 39, 40] Among these antiresorptive agents, the bisphosphonates became, and, to date, still are, the dominant pharmacological agent utilized to treat PMO [43, 47, 62, 66, 70]. Bisphosphonates this year celebrate their 40th anniversary since their introduction into clinical medicine [61].

Bisphosphonates have proven to be effective to reduce fracture risk in PMO, proven to be cost-effective when used in the higher risk population, and proven to be safe when used for the right duration of time. Bisphosphonates continue to have the lead among the registered pharmacological agents prescribed for the treatment of postmenopausal osteoporosis because evidence exists for the reduction of global (vertebral, nonvertebral, and hip) fracture risk. Bisphosphonates are not metabolized, ~40% are excreted into the urine unchanged, are retained in skeletal tissues, are recycled back into the circulation, and have the unique property of retaining effectiveness on bone mineral density, bone turnover markers, and perhaps fracture risk reduction for an uncertain, yet prolonged, period of time after discontinuation [61].

However, bisphosphonates have been impugned for inducing osteonecrosis of the jaw (ONJ) and atypical subtrochanteric femur fractures, without established causality [33, 64]. These rare associations (ONJ and atypical subtrochanteric femur fractures) and the media/legal attention that have accompanied these rare cases threaten to undermine the very good benefits that bisphosphonates have done for mankind. Bisphosphonates not only reduce fractures in PMO but also successfully manage male and glucocorticoid-induced osteoporosis as well as a whole different spectrum of metabolic bone diseases: male osteoporosis, glucocorticoid-induced osteoporosis, Paget's

P.D. Miller, M.D., FACP
Department of Medicine,
Colorado Center for Bone Research,
Lakewood, CO 80227, USA
e-mail: millerccbr@aol.com

F. Bronner et al. (eds.), *Bone-Metabolic Functions and Modulators*, Topics in Bone Biology,
DOI 10.1007/978-1-4471-2745-1_9, © Springer-Verlag London 2012

disease, osteogenesis imperfecta, metastatic cancer to the skeleton, and multiple myeloma [13, 15, 53, 59]. While bisphosphonates are still the established treatment for PMO, and we must continue to strive to understand their benefits and risk, science should continue to investigate and to understand various agents with different mechanisms of action for affecting bone remodeling, increasing bone strength, and reducing the risk for fracture.

In this regard, the anabolic agents emerged for the treatment of PMO [34, 51]. Anabolic agents increase bone formation [34, 52]. The first anabolic therapy for osteoporosis, teriparatide (rH 1–34 parathyroid hormone), is now registered for treatment of PMO, male, and glucocorticoid-induced osteoporosis [4, 5, 54, 63]. 1–84 PTH also is registered outside of the United States for PMO [25]. Strontium ranelate, whose mechanism of action may, in part, beanabolic and antiresorptive also is registered in Europe [58].There are abundant data on the efficacy and safety of these anabolic agents [44]. More data are needed on their use in sequence or combined with antiresorptive agents.

9.2 New and Emerging Antiresorptives

9.2.1 Denosumab

A new therapeutic advancement in the treatment of postmenopausal osteoporosis (PMO) is denosumab (Prolia™), a fully human monoclonal antibody to an activator of osteoclastic differentiation and activity, soluble Rank-Ligand (Rank-L). Rank-Ligand is receptor activator (Rank being the receptor on osteoclasts, also called NF-kB). Rank-L, a glycoprotein produced in the osteoblast, is a member of the superfamily of ligands and is also known as TNF – activation-induced cytokine and osteoclast activator [11, 19, 68]. Also produced in the osteoblast is the decoy receptor for Rank-Ligand, osteoprotegerin (OPG). Rank-Ligand and OPG are molecular competitors to each other and are either upregulated or downregulated by opposing biological control systems. For example, in the estrogen deficient state, there is an upregulation of Rank-L (i.e., more Rank-L is produced). When Rank-L concentrations in the bone marrow microenvironment exceed the concentration of OPG, then more Rank-L can bind to its receptor on the osteoclast, Rank. When this Rank-L-Rank binding occurs, there is a marked increase of osteoclast differentiation and activity and, thus, increase in bone resorption. If there is a greater concentration of OPG produced by the osteoblast, then less Rank-L is assessable to the osteoclast receptor, Rank, and there is more inhibition of osteoclast differentiation and activity and less bone resorption. Hence the balance between osteoblast produced Rank-L and OPG are the determining factors for the internal bone microenvironment regulation of bone resorption (Fig. 9.1) [11]. Denosumab (anti-rank ligand antibody) thus acts like OPG, preventing Rank-L from binding to Rank and reducing bone resorption.

In the initial basic science development of these remarkable bone biological regulatory pathways, the development company, Amgen™ (Thousand Oaks, California, USA) first introduced parenteral administration of OPG as a means of reducing bone resorption, by then allowing less Rank-L to become available to the osteoclast receptor, Rank [2, 3]. However, the development of neutralizing antibodies to OPG prevented its development as a therapeutic agent, something that has not been seen with the administration of anti-Rank Ligand antibody, denosumab. As a culmination of this pioneering basic science work and the solid antifracture data observed in the pivotal registration trial, denosumab received international registration for the treatment of PMO in June 2010 at a dose of 60 mg subcutaneous (SQ) every 6 months [17].

9.2.2 The Phase 2 Denosumab Dose-Ranging Clinical Trials: The Longest Term Denosumab Data Available: 2-, 4-, 6-, and 8-Year Data

The initial dose-ranging studies in postmenopausal women randomized patients to seven different doses of denosumab given at different

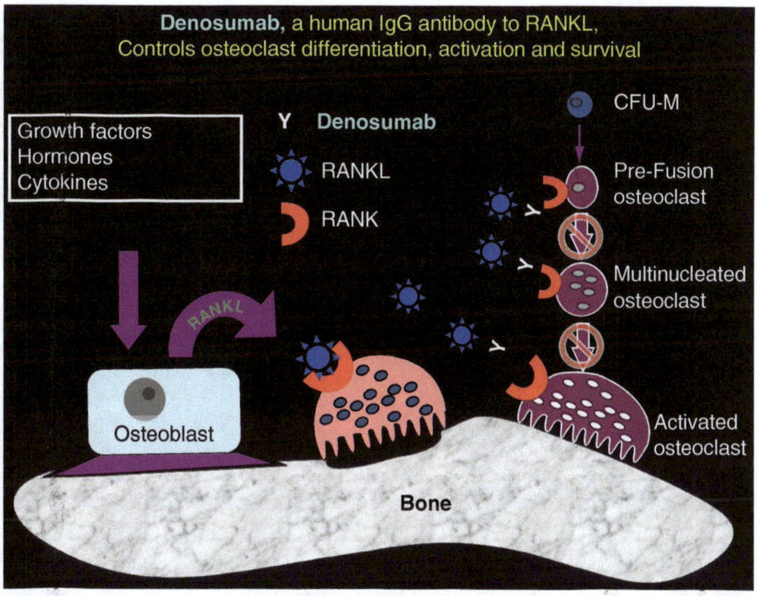

Fig. 9.1 The basic bone biology showing the local regulation of bone remodeling by the RANK ligand, osteoprotogerin, RANK system (Modified from Boyle et al. [11])

intervals versus alendronate (70 mg/week) versus placebo [41]. This initial 1-year data as well as the 2-year data showed that these doses increased bone mineral density (BMD) at all skeletal sites and reduced biochemical markers of bone turnover more than did alendronate or placebo [36]. This initial 2-year study then was extended to 4, 6, and now 8 years [42, 48, 49]. The 4- and 8-year data show a few unique highlights: the 4-year group had a subgroup that discontinued denosumab for 2 years after the initial 2 years of treatment and a group that, after 1 year of discontinuation, were rechallenged with denosumab. In the continuous discontinuation group, the bone resorption marker (CTX) increased and even went above the pretreatment baseline by the sixth month after discontinuation, reached a peak at month 36, but returned to baseline during the fourth year without any further treatment (Fig. 9.2) [48]. Likewise, the BMD responses were the mirror image of the bone turnover markers. The reason(s) for the return of CTX and BMD back to baseline without any additional denosumab being provided are unknown but might be related to the bone mechanostat mechanism [10, 57]. In addition, in the retreatment group, the response to denosumab was retained, such that upon rechallenge with denosumab, the BMD increased and the CTX declined with these responsive changes, having the same slope as seen in the first year of treatment (Fig. 9.3) [48]. Thus, as expected from the initial pharmacokinetic and pharmacodynamics data, the human biological data show that the effect of denosumab is reversible yet retains responsiveness after treatment, discontinuation, and retreatment.

The 6-year and 8-year phase 2 data provide some additional interesting insights into denosumab pharmacodynamics [42, 49]. During these periods, the lumbar spine and total hip BMD continue to increase and not plateau as is seen with other antiresorptive agents. The mechanism(s) for this progressive increase in BMD is not yet defined, but may be related to the larger degree of suppression of bone turnover than that seen with the bisphosphonate, alendronate. In addition, the serum bone resorption marker carboxy-terminal collagen cross-links (CTX) does not continue to decline with repeated doses of denosumab, and in fact has a trend to increase over time though remain within the premenopausal normal reference range (Fig. 9.4) [49]. These data are reassuring in that continuous administration of denosumab is not associated with sustained reduction of bone turnover markers (BTM) to levels below the normal premenopausal reference range.

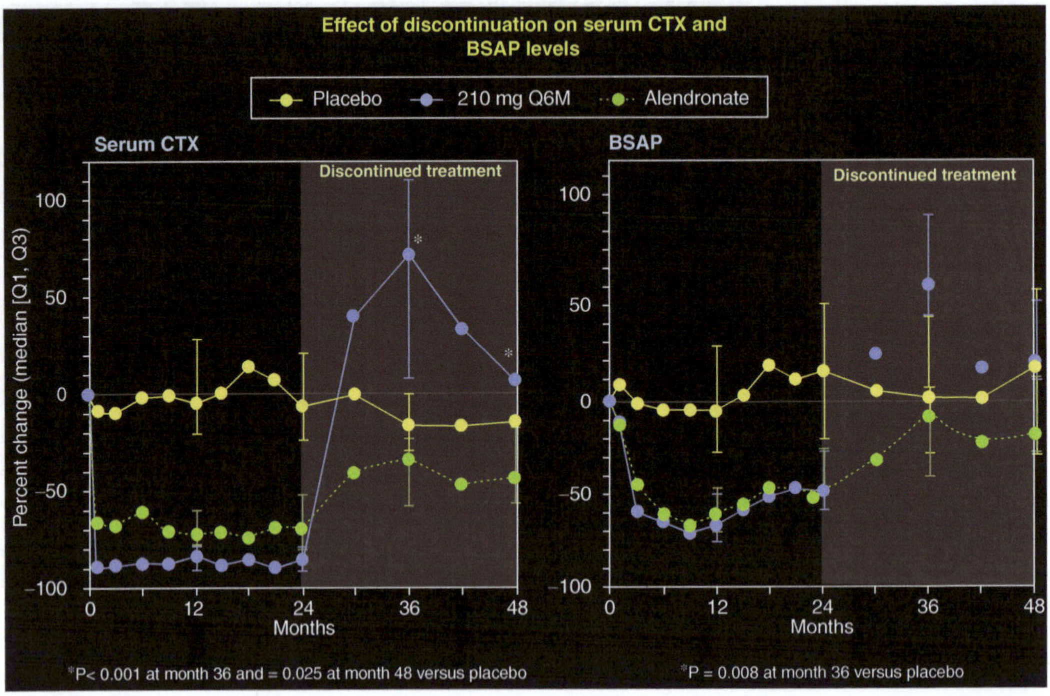

Fig. 9.2 The phase 2 denosumab clinical trial showing the rapid offset of bone remodeling upon discontinuation of denosumab and the return of the bone turnover to baseline without any additional denosumab as measured by two biochemical markers of bone turnover (Adapted from Miller et al. [48], Copyright 2008, with permission from Elsevier)

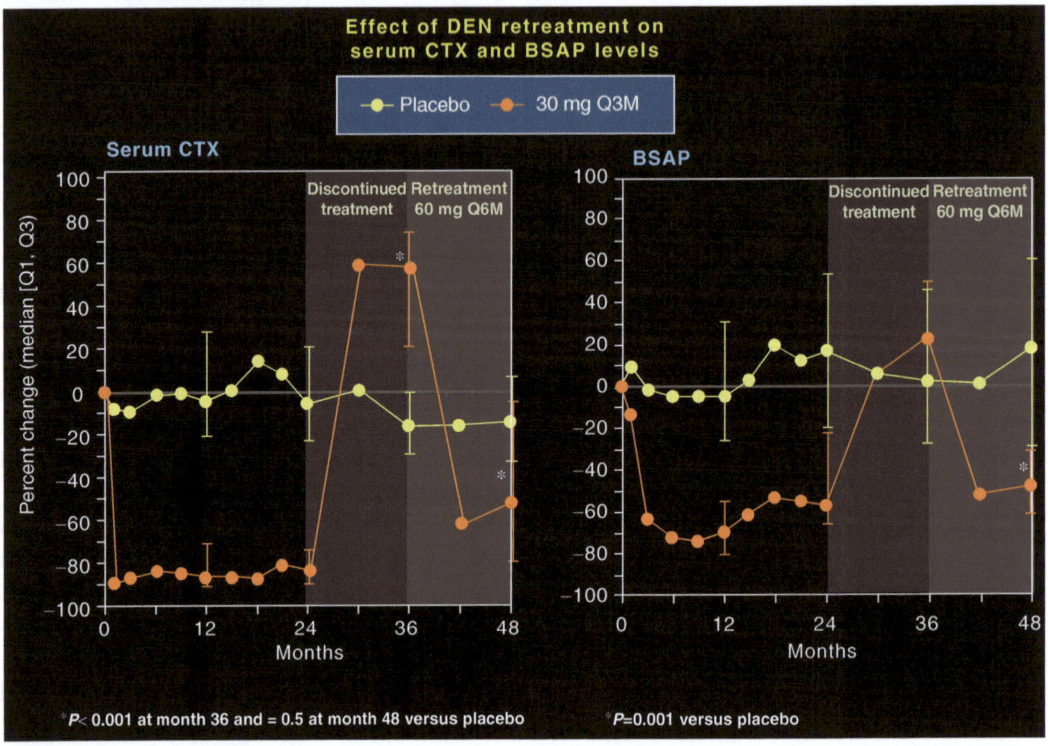

Fig. 9.3 The effect of discontinuation and then retreatment with denosumab on bone turnover markers. The rise of bone turnover above baseline was accompanied by a rapid return of bone turnover to baseline with retreatment (Adapted from Miller et al. [48], Copyright 2008, with permission from Elsevier)

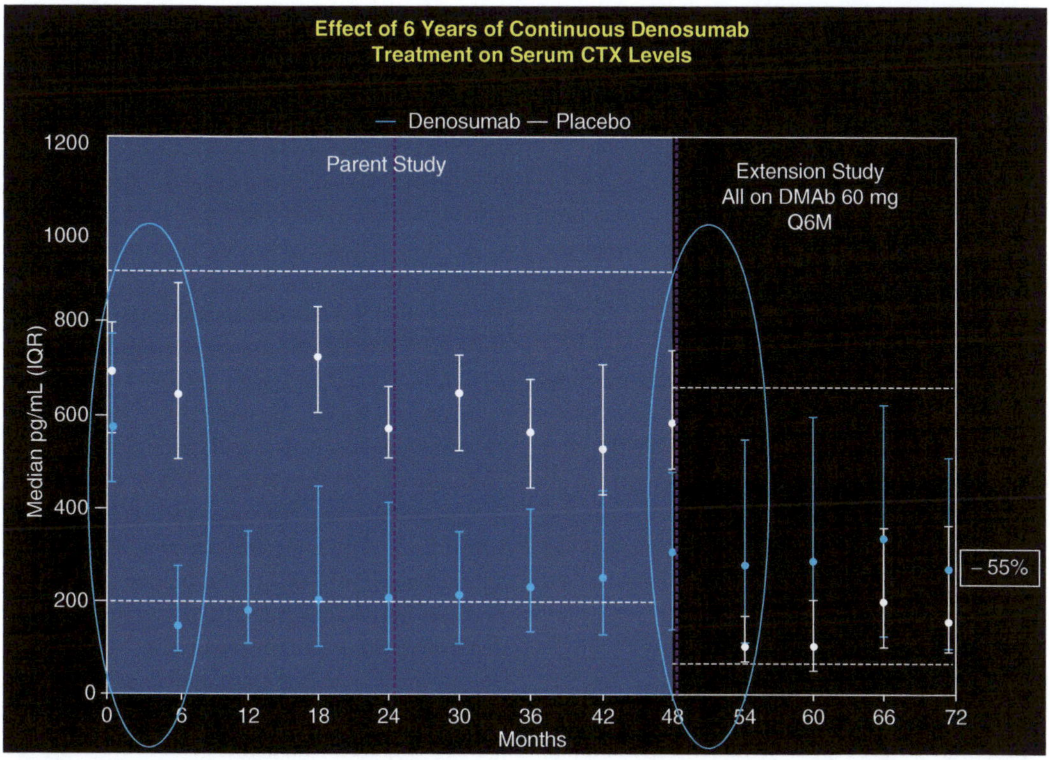

Fig. 9.4 The 6-year phase 2 denosumab data showing the bone turnover marker (serum CTX) staying within the premenopausal reference range and a slight attenuation of the reduction in CTX despite 6 years of denosumab continuation (Adapted from Miller et al. [49])

9.2.3 The Phase 3 Clinical Trials: "DEFEND," "DECIDE," "STAND," and the Registration Trial "FREEDOM"

9.2.3.1 DEFEND

The "DEFEND" trial was a prevention trial. 332 early postmenopausal younger Caucasian women, mean age: 56 years of age [7]. These patients were treatment naive, at low risk for fracture (mean lumbar spine T-score: −1.6), postmenopausal and were randomized to either denosumab (60 mg SQ Q6Mos) or SQ placebo in a 1:1 ratio. The first 2 years of the study showed that denosumab significantly increased BMD at all skeletal sites both from baseline and compared to placebo and significantly reduced the level of bone turnover markers. After the first 2 years of the "DEFEND" trial, 252 of the initial study participants continued into an extension study for an additional 2 years [8]. During these "treatment-off" 2 years, all patients were administered placebo, so the initial study placebo group had a total of 4 years of placebo and the initial denosumab treated group came off therapy to receive 2 years of placebo. During the extension study, the BMD in the initial denosumab-treated group declined to baseline at all skeletal sites during months 24–36, but then leveled off and plateaued at the lumbar spine while it continued to decline at the total hip and 1/3 radius. Likewise, the BTM increased to and then above baseline within 6 months of discontinuation (as was seen in the phase 2 trials), but then returned to baseline during the fourth year without any additional therapy (also as was seen in the phase 2 trials). Thus, examining the registered dose (60 mg SQ Q6Mos) for this entire 4-year study showed that the effects of denosumab are reversible upon discontinuation and suggest that treatment may need to be continued to maintain an effect on BMD and BTM. What is unknown in this phase 3 study, like the phase 2 trial, is what the effect on bone strength (fractures) is upon discontinuation of denosumab.

9.2.3.2 DECIDE

The "DECIDE" trial was a prospective randomized comparison of alendronate (70 mg/week) to denosumab (60 mg SQ Q6 MOS) in 1,189 early postmenopausal women with low bone mass [12]. At the total hip, denosumab resulted in a significantly greater increase in BMD as compared to alendronate (3.5% versus 2.6%, $P<0.0001$). The larger increases in BMD with denosumab administration also were seen at all skeletal sites measured. In addition, denosumab induced a significantly greater reduction in BTM as compared to alendronate. There is no prespecified fracture data in DECIDE.

9.2.3.3 STAND

The "STAND" study (study of transitioning from alendronate to denosumab) was an international, multicenter, randomized, double-dummy, parallel-group phase 3 trial [32]. Five hundred and four postmenopausal women (average age: 67 years) previously taking alendronate (median: 36 months, range: 6–192 months) were randomized to receive either brand name alendronate (Fosamax™) (70 mg/week) or placebo injections or denosumab (60 mg Q 6 months) or placebo alendronate for 12 months. A repeated-measures model was used as the primary analysis method for the percent change in BMD at months 6 and 12. The model included treatment, time of BMD assessment, treatment-by-time-of-BMD-assessment interaction, baseline BMD value, time-on-prior-alendronate-therapy stratum, dual-emission X-ray absorptiometry (DXA) instrument type, and baseline-BMD-value-and-instrument type interaction. The primary hypothesis was that denosumab was not inferior to alendronate with respect to the mean percentage change in total hip BMD at month 12. BMD at the total hip increased by 1.90% (95% CI 1.61–2.18%) at month 12 in subjects transitioned to denosumab compared with a 1.05% (95% CI 0.76–1.34%) increase from baseline in subjects continuing on alendronate therapy (Fig. 9.2). The difference between treatment groups was 0.85% (95% CI 0.44–1.25%) greater with denosumab; the lower limit of the confidence interval excluded the prespecified noninferiority margin (0.35%), thus showing the noninferiority of denosumab compared with alendronate. Superiority testing demonstrated the BMD increase with denosumab at the total hip was statistically superior to the change with alendronate ($P<0.0001$).

At the lumbar spine, denosumab increased BMD by 3.03% (95% CI 2.63–3.44%) at month 12, and alendronate increased BMD by 1.85% (95% CI 1.44–2.26%), for a difference of 1.18% (95% CI 0.63–1.73%), with the lower limit of the confidence interval excluding the noninferiority margin of 0.22. These data demonstrate the noninferiority of denosumab versus alendronate at this skeletal site. The increase in BMD with denosumab versus alendronate was statistically significant ($P<0.0001$). Significantly greater increases in BMD with denosumab compared with alendronate also were observed at month 12 at the femoral neck and one-third radius ($P<0.0121$). Furthermore, significant BMD increases for denosumab compared with alendronate were observed as early as month 6 at the lumbar spine and all measured femoral sites ($P<0.05$). Thus, the data show that in patients previously on alendronate, changing to denosumab is accompanied by at least stabilization, if not further increases in BMD.

9.2.3.4 FREEDOM

The large phase 3 registration trial randomized 7,808 postmenopausal women (mean age: 72.3 years, average lumbar spine T score: −2.8 (WHO-defined osteoporosis)), and 23% of whom had a prevalent vertebral fracture [17]. One-half received denosumab (60 mg SQ Q6 Mos) and the other half SQ placebo. Over 3 years of the study, denosumab reduced the incidence of morphometric vertebral fractures, the primary end-point (Fig. 9.5) [17] (RR reduction: 68%, $P<0.0001$ versus placebo), nonvertebral fractures (RR reduction: 20%, $P<0.01$ versus placebo), and hip fractures (RR reduction: 40%, $P<0.04$).

The FREEDOM trial is designed to extend to 10 years. The initial 5-year data of the extension has recently been presented as well [55]. The design of the extension trial is as follows: after the initial 3 years, 2,343 patients from the initial 3,902 patients randomized continued into the continuous treatment arm of denosumab (continuing 60 mg SQ Q6

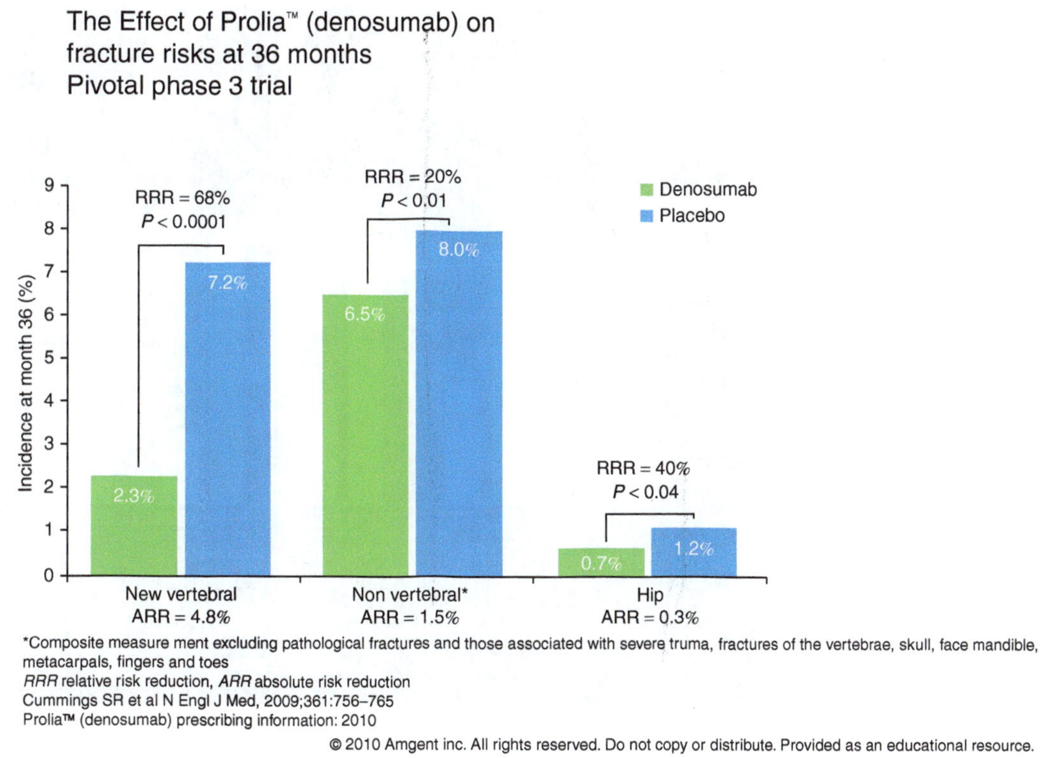

Fig. 9.5 The effect of denosumab (60 mg SQ Q6 MOS) on incident fractures (spine, hip, and nonvertebral) as compared to placebo from the randomized phase 3 registration clinical trial (Adapted from Cummings et al. [17])

MOS). From the initial randomized placebo arm of 3,906 patients, 2,207 patients switched over to treatment with denosumab (60 mg SQ Q6 MOS). In those that continued 5 years of denosumab, the fracture rates continued to remain reduced from the end of the registration trial, and the BMD continued to increase at both the spine and hip. In the initial placebo group that went onto denosumab, the BMD increased and the fracture rates declined similar to those in the initial 3 years of FREEDOM.

9.2.4 Safety Data on Denosumab

In the collective data from the phase 2 and phase 3 clinical trials, denosumab has been safe [45]. The clinical concern, due to the ubiquitous presence of RankL throughout many tissues, has been the potential risk for infections. In the pivotal registration trial, only the serious adverse events (SAE) that were significantly greater than placebo were skin infections (termed either "cellulitis" or "erysipelas"), 0.3% versus <0.01%, $P<0.002$. In the AE reports, there were 54 events in the denosumab versus 53 in placebo. These areas of inflammation could occur at any time after the injection and a distant site of the injection and all responded to conservative management. There were no unusual opportunistic infections reported. There have not been studies examining the potential for infections in patients who are immunosuppressed or on other biologics. However, in the oncology trials in which denosumab has recently received registration to reduce the risk of fractures in patients with metastatic carcinoma to bone, there was no increased risk of infection seen in this group of patients who have more compromised immune systems and receive a much larger dose of denosumab for this indication (120 mg/month) [67]. In addition, in the extension data from FREEDOM, the continual exposure to denosumab through 5 years was lower than the incident in the first 3 years of the registration trial (<0.1% versus 0.1%). Vigilance is a key word as this very effective human monoclonal antibody becomes used in

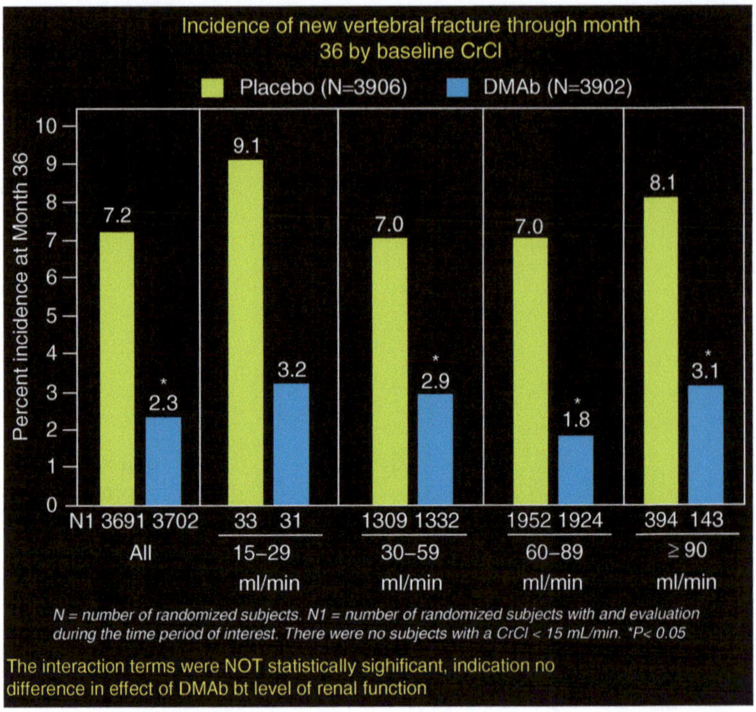

Fig. 9.6 The post hoc analysis of the effect of denosumab on incident vertebral fractures in the pivotal registration clinical trial by baseline quartiles of estimated glomerular filtration rate (eGFR) (Adapted from Jamal et al. [29])

large population numbers so that any trends in adverse events can be reported to the FDA.

The FDA label for the postmenopausal osteoporosis indication does not have any lower cutoff for renal function. This is because denosumab is not cleared by the kidney, but by the reticuloendothelial system, and may not have any adverse renal effects as may be seen, though rarely, with intravenous bisphosphonates [46]. In a post hoc analysis of FREEDOM where the registration population had estimated glomerular filtration rates (eGFR) divided into quartiles (>90 to 15–29 ml/min), denosumab had evidence of reduction in incident vertebral fractures across these quartiles without any adverse renal effects (e.g., change in eGFR over 3 years) (Fig. 9.6) [29]. There is no data on changes in BMD or fractures in patients with GFR < 15 ml/min. In this latter population, the diagnosis of osteoporosis becomes far more difficult to establish, and there is concern that in patients with preexisting adynamic renal bone disease, reducing bone turnover further may be associated with an increase in cardiovascular calcification [28]. This theoretical interaction is predicated on the knowledge that absorbed calcium and/or phosphorus cannot be adequately eliminated by renal clearance, and if bone turnover is low, the capacity of bone to take up these ions is restricted, leaving vascular tissue exposed to calcium-phosphorus and risk for vascular calcification. One study has examined the effect of denosumab on vascular calcification in the FREEDOM trial and found that across the quartiles of eGFR, there was not greater increase in vascular calcification with denosumab versus placebo, at least when assessed by lateral lumbar X-ray assessment of aortic calcification [18].

The FDA label cautions the physician concerning the possibility of hypocalcemia after denosumab administration. While all antiresorptive agents may induce a small and transient hypocalcemia after administration, clinically significant hypocalcemia (associated with tetany or paresthesias) is not observed in patients with adequate calcium and vitamin D intake and with intact parathyroid hormone (PTH) responses to normalize the transient hypocalcemia. In that regard, hypocalcemia in the FREEDOM trial was no different between the treated versus placebo groups either in the registration (first 3 years) or the extension trial. It is important in patient management to ensure that an adequate amount of calcium and vitamin D are provided.

The effect of denosumab on bone turnover is pronounced. While, as stated, BTM do not remain suppressed below the normal premenopausal reference range in the long-term denosumab trials and rise rapidly after discontinuation of denosumab, the quantitative bone histomorphometry data show absent tetracycline labels, an indicator of new bone mineralization in a small number of a subset of patients in whom bone biopsies were performed. Absent single tetracycline labels were seen in zero of the 62 placebo biopsies, while 19 of 33 (36%) of the biopsies in patients on denosumab had no single labels [60]. The clinical significance of these findings is unknown. It is reassuring that in these biopsy patients, the serum CTX overlapped and were no different between the biopsies that had no labels versus biopsies that had single or double labels. The tetracycline labels (and, therefore, mineralization) would be expected to return after denosumab discontinuation because the BTM increase. However, this has yet to be studied. Bone biopsies have been done in patients treated with denosumab and then taken off from the DECIDE study and have shown normal labels. However, it is unknown if any of these patients had absent labels to start with. The maintenance of the low fracture incidence in the extension of FREEDOM is reassuring that 5-year use is not associated with any rise in fracture events.

From the safety viewpoint, there have been no cases of osteonecrosis of the jaw (ONJ) or atypical subtrochanteric femur fractures reported in the registration osteoporosis clinical trials. In the extension trial of FREEDOM, there have been two adjudicated cases of ONJ – 2 in the continuous treatment group and two in the placebo then denosumab group. There has been a low but similar incidence of ONJ in the oncology trials using monthly denosumab versus monthly intravenous bisphosphonate, zoledronic acid (1.3% versus 1.8% over 3 years). Postmarketing data will let us know in time if these rare events may occur in the osteoporosis population and with the lower doses of denosumab used in this population.

9.3 Cathepsin K Inhibitors

Cathepsin K, an enzyme that is secreted from the osteoclast into the subcellular osteoclast space (between the osteoclast and the bone matrix), degrades the organic matrix of bone and, thus, helps to define the depth of bone-remodeling space [35] (Fig. 9.7). The cathepsin K inhibitor, odanacatib, renders the osteoclast effectively dysfunctional in this regard, but does not appear to impair other properties of the osteoclast, such as intercellular communication with the osteoblast, apoptosis, or other osteoclast cellular activities [35]. Animal studies have shown that the osteoclastic resorption pits are more shallow under the influence of odanacatib and that osteoclasts remain present and numerous [56]. In the dose-ranging phase 2 clinical trials conducted in postmenopausal women, the daily oral formulation of 50 mg/week had the greatest effect on increasing BMD [5] (Fig. 9.8) and reducing bone resorption markers than the other doses and had a rapid offset as shown by the rebound in resorption markers to and above baseline upon discontinuation [5] (Fig. 9.9). In addition, bone formation does not appear to be reduced to the same extent as it is with bisphosphonates or denosumab in non-head-to-head data. Clinical experience with this drug in phase 2 trials appears to bear out this observation by reductions in bone formation that are small relative to reductions in bone resorption [5, 9]. This observation suggests that with odanacatib, the functional properties of the osteoblast may be maintained to a greater extent than is typically seen with other classes of antiresorptives [37]. Throughout the phase 2 trials, there were no safety signals observed. The phase 3 fracture study of odanacatib currently is being conducted.

9.4 Newer Anabolic Agents

9.4.1 Parathyroid Hormone – Exogenous or Endogenous: Beyond Subcutaneous Route of Administration

Teriparatide (recombinant human 1–34 PTH, TPTD) and PTH (1–84) are administered by daily subcutaneous injection. Two alternative delivery systems to circumvent this inconvenient feature are being studied at this time. A transdermal delivery system administers TPTD through the skin [16]. Cosman et al. have shown that the pharmacokinetic profile of transdermal TPTD displays very favorable kinetics with rapid uptake and rapid disappearance from the circulation, features

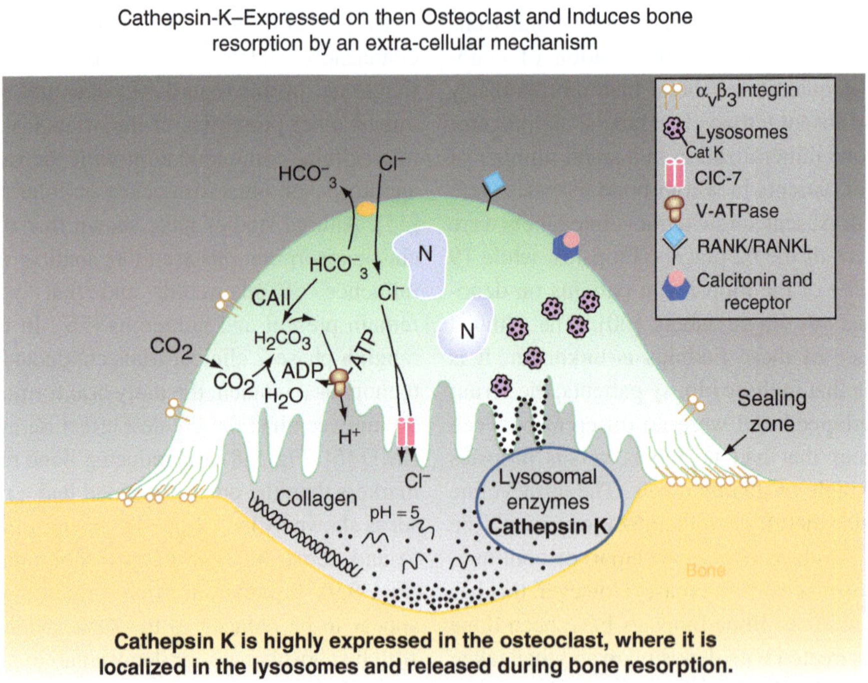

Fig. 9.7 The mechanism of action of the osteoclast-derived enzyme, cathepsin K, to induce bone resorption (Adapted from Leung et al. [35])

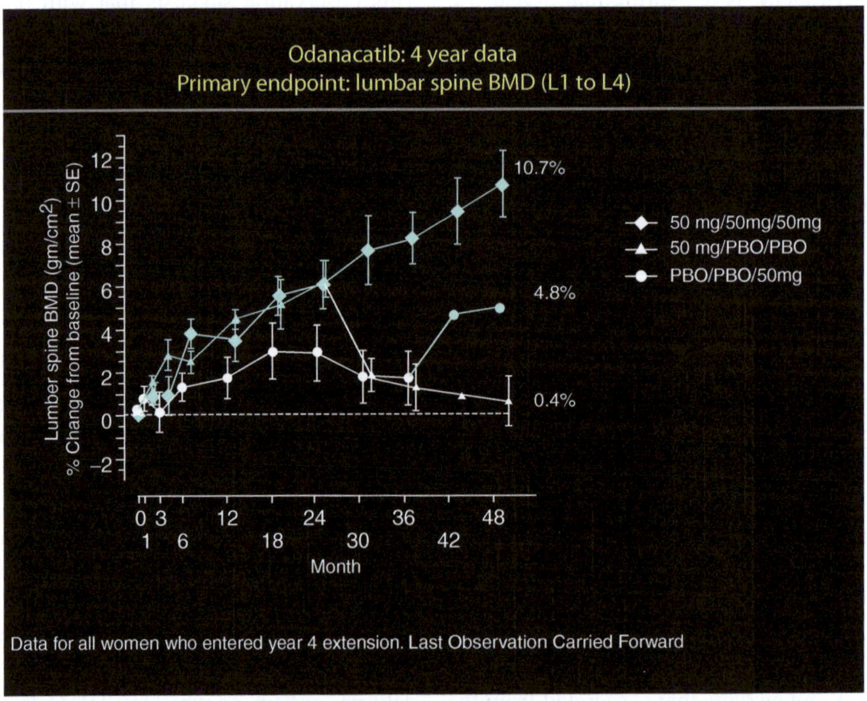

Fig. 9.8 The data from the phase 2 cathepsin K inhibitor (odanacatib) clinical trial showing the continuous increase in lumbar spine bone mineral density with the 50 mg/week dosage (Adapted from Binkley et al. [5])

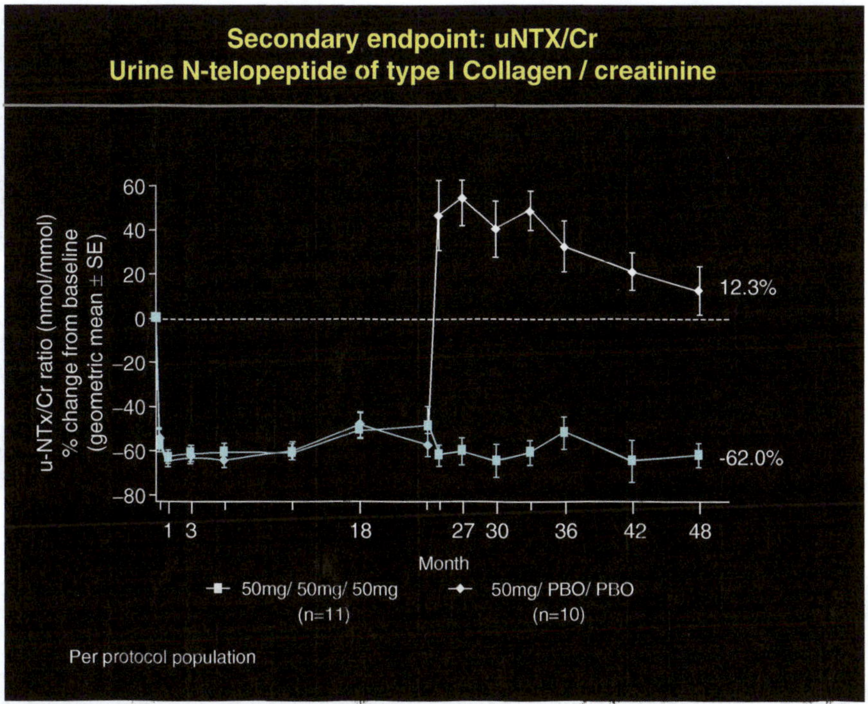

Fig. 9.9 The data from the phase 2 cathepsin K inhibitor (odanacatib) clinical trial showing the rapid offset of effect upon discontinuation as measured by an increase in the bone resorption marker urinary NTX. (Adapted from Binkley et al. [5])

that are believed to be important for the anabolic effects of the drug [16]. Another approach to more facile administration of PTH is the use of oral agents that inhibit the calcium-sensing receptor on the parathyroid cell. These so-called calcilytics lead to stimulation of the parathyroid cell to synthesize and secrete endogenous PTH. Preliminary reports with the calcilytic, ronacaleret, were promising, but more recent observations suggest that the pharmacokinetic profile may not be ideal [21, 22]. Finally, parathyroid hormone-related protein (PTHrP) is being studied as a potential PTH-like therapeutic agent [27].

9.4.2 Sclerostin Inhibition

Sclerostin is an osteocyte-produced glycoprotein that inhibits osteoblast activity by inserting itself in the Wnt pathway [10] (Fig. 9.10). Recent data suggest that one of the mechanisms by which PTH may be anabolic is by inhibiting sclerostin, a powerful inhibitor of the anabolic Wnt-signaling pathway [1, 26, 50, 65]. This concept has led to the development of an antibody that inhibits sclerostin. Data by Li et al. [38] have shown that the antisclerostin antibody is a powerful stimulator of periosteal and endocortical bone, while it has little ability to stimulate osteoclast activity [38] (Fig. 9.11). The phase 2 clinical trials are completed, and results soon will be presented. The phase 3 registration trials are being designed for a 2012 startup date.

9.4.3 Anti-DKK1

DKK1 is an inhibitor of the Wnt pathway and osteoblast activity. It is predominantly secreted by myeloma cells and their precursors. A monoclonal antibody has been developed against DKK1 to attempt to inhibit the bone loss, osteolytic lesions, and fractures seen in patients with multiple myeloma. To date, results look promising and in models to improve bone mass as a potential therapy for diseases of low bone mass [24, 71].

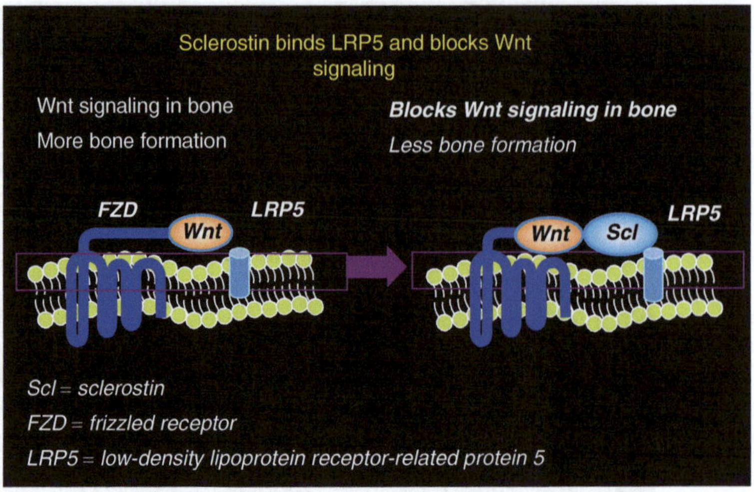

Fig. 9.10 The effect whereby osteocyte-derived sclerostin inhibits osteoblast activity, inserting itself between cofactors LRP5 and Wnt on the osteoblast membrane (Adapted from Bonewald [10])

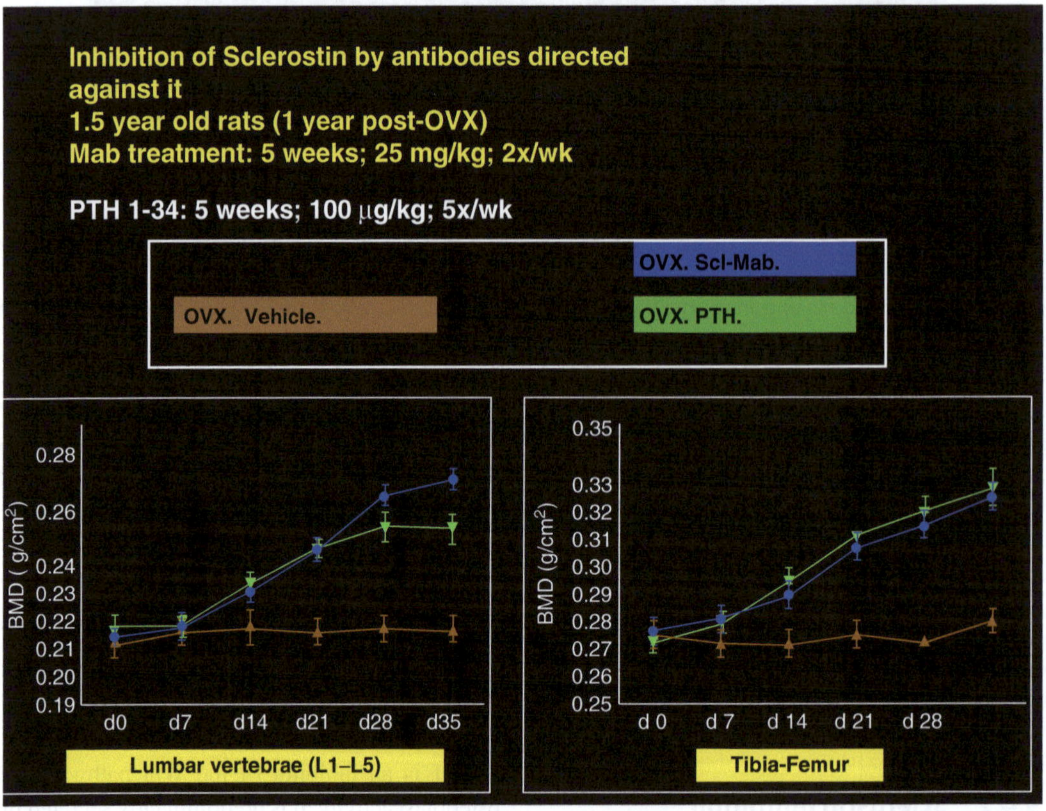

Fig. 9.11 The effect of a monoclonal antibody to sclerostin on spine and hip BMD in a rat model (Adapted from Li et al. [38])

9.4.4 Serotonin Antagonism

Two serotonin systems are thought to regulate skeletal mass [72, 73]. In the central nervous system, serotonin is synthesized by the enzyme tryptophan synthase 2 (Tph2). It is associated with the stimulation of bone formation and may mediate its effects indirectly via the sympathetic nervous system that decreases bone formation. Data suggest that in the hypothalamus, leptin increases sympathetic tone, which would lead to a decrease in bone formation. Serotonin seems to inhibit the binding of leptin to the hypothalamus, which, in turn, decreases sympathetic tone and increases bone formation [31]. CNS serotonin does not cross the blood–brain barrier. The mechanism for the increase in fracture risk observed in cohort studies in patients receiving the central nervous system selective serotonin receptor uptake inhibitors remains undefined. It is unknown if the effect is central or peripheral, though the fracture risk seems to be seen despite adjusting for fall frequency and BMD. In the gastrointestinal tract where most of the body's serotonin is made mostly in the gastrointestinal tract luminal cells, the responsible enzyme is tryptophan synthase 1 (Tph1). It is associated with inhibition of bone formation [30]. Animal studies employing a specific Tph1 inhibitor have shown a remarkable effect to stimulate bone formation as powerfully as PTH in ovariectomized rats [72, 73]. The interactions between the gut-brain-bone remain an exciting area for investigation and the development of LRP5, Tph1, and serotonin-modifying pathways to influence bone remodeling and risk for fracture [23].

9.5 Future Molecules

In preclinical development are molecules that influence bone remodeling, which include a relatively osteoclast-selective inhibitor, H+ATPase inhibitor which inhibits ovariectomy-induced bone loss in rats by inhibiting the active transport of protons necessary in the bone resorption process [69]. Similar inhibition of bone resorption without an apparent inhibition of bone formation also has been seen in mice with mutation-induced deficiencies of c-src or chloride-7 channel (CLCN7) necessary for osteoclatst to form ruffled borders. The low-density lipoprotein receptor-related protein (LRP5) is a Wnt coreceptor necessary for increasing osteoblast function. Increasing LRP5 signaling in mature bone cells may be a way of treating human disorders associated with low bone mass [1]. Finally, inhibition of GSK-3 (glycogen synthetase kinase 3), an enzyme involved the osteoblast Β-catenin pathway, could lead to an increase in bone strength through a number of mechanisms.

Conclusion

Current therapies to treat osteoporosis are effective, have a very high benefit to risk ratio, and, when used in the right population for the right duration, reduce the individual as well as population burden that accompanies untreated osteoporosis.

Newer molecules are being developed to improve on what is currently available and to take advantage of bone cell pathways of activation and inhibition. In the course of exploring these new approaches, it is important to bear in mind the ever-present goals of providing specificity and safety along with efficacy. Osteoporotic fractures in both genders and among all ethnicities are associated with a high morbidity and mortality regardless of the location of the fracture. Both basic and clinical scientists should strive to improve outcomes and safety.

References

1. Baron R, Rawadi GA. Wnt signaling and the regulation of bone mass. Curr Osteoporos Rep. 2007;5(2):73–80.
2. Bekker PJ, Holloway DL, Rasmussen AS, Murphy R, Martin SW, Leese PT, Holmes GB, Dunstan CR, DePaoli AM. Single-dose placebo-controlled study of AMG 162, a fully human monoclonal antibody to RANKL, in postmenopausal women. J Bone Miner Res. 2004;19:1059–66.
3. Bekker PJ, Holloway D, Nakanishi A, Arrighi M, Leese PT, Dunstan CR. The effect of a single dose of osteoprotogerin in postmenopausal women. J Bone Miner Res. 2001;16(2):348–60.

4. Bilezikian JP, Kurland ES. Therapy of male osteoporosis with parathyroid hormone. Calcif Tissue Int. 2001;69(4):248–51.
5. Binkley N, Bone H, Eisman J, Hosking D et al (2010) Effect of odanacatib on bone density and bone turnover markers in postmenopausal women with low bone mineral density: year 4 results. J Bone Miner Res; American Society of Bone and Mineral Research
6. Black DM, Cummings SR, Karpf DB, Cauley JA, Thompson DE, Nevitt MC, Bauer DC, Genant HK, Haskell WL, Marcus R, Ott SM, Torner JC, Quandt SA, Reiss TF, Ensrud KE. Randomised trial of effect of alendronate on risk of fracture in women with existing vertebral fractures. Fracture Intervention Trial Research Group. Lancet. 1996;348(9041):1535–41.
7. Bone HG, Bolognese MA, Yuen CK, Kendler DL, Wang H, Liu Y, San Martin J. Effects of denosumab on bone mineral density and bone turnover in postmenopausal women. J Clin Endocrinol Metab. 2008;93:2149–57.
8. Bone HG, Bolognese MA, Yuen CK, Kendler DL, Miller PD, Yang YC, Grazette L, San Martin J, Gallagher CJ. Effects of denosumab treatment and discontinuation on bone mineral density and bone turnover markers in postmenopausal women with low bone mass. J Clin Endocrinol Metab. 2011;96(4):972–80.
9. Bone HG, McClung MR, Roux C, et al. Odanacatib, a cathepsin-K inhibitor for osteoporosis: a two-year study in postmenopausal women with low bone density. J Bone Miner Res. 2010;25(5):937–47.
10. Bonewald L. The amazing osteocyte. J Bone Miner Res. 2011;60:305–17.
11. Boyle WJ, Simonet WS, Lacey DL. Osteoclast differentiation and activation. Nature. 2003;423:337–42.
12. Brown JP, Prince RI, Deal C, et al. Comparison of the effect of denosumab and alendronate on BMD and biochemical markers of bone turnover in postmenopausal women with low bone mass: a randomized, blinded, phase 3 trial. J Bone Miner Res. 2009;24:153–61.
13. Canalis E, Mazziotti G, Giustina A, Bilezikian JP. Glucocorticoid-induced osteoporosis: pathophysiology and therapy. Osteoporos Int. 2007;18(10):1319–28.
14. Chesnut III CH, Silverman S, Andriano K, et al. A randomized trial of nasal spray salmon calcitonin in postmenopausal women with established osteoporosis: the Prevent Recurrence of Osteoporotic Fractures study. Am J Med. 2000;102:267–76.
15. Coleman RE, McCloskey EV. Bisphosphonates in oncology. Bone. 2011;49(1):71–5.
16. Cosman F, Lane NE, Bolognese MA, et al. Effect of transdermal teriparatide administration on bone mineral density in postmenopausal women. J Clin Endocrinol Metab. 2010;95(1):151–8.
17. Cummings SR, San Martin J, McClung MR, Siris ES, Eastell R, Reid IR, Delmas PD, Zoog HB, Austin M, Wang A, Kutilek S, Adami S, Zanchetta J, Libanati C, Siddhanti S, Christiansen C, The FREEDOM Trial. Denosumab for prevention of fractures in postmenopausal women with osteoporosis. N Engl J Med. 2009;361(8):756–65.
18. Egbuna OI, Cheung AM, Siddhanti S, Wang A, Daizadeh N, Anthony M, Grazette L, Miller PD (2010) Treatment of osteoporosis by RANKL inhibition with denosumab in women at high cardiovascular risk and with renal impairment does not accelerate vascular calcification. Abstract book of the 43rd annual meeting of the American Society of Nephrology, Denver
19. Eghbali-Fatourechi G, Khosla S, Sanyal A, Boyle WJ, Lacey DL, Riggs BL. Role of RANK ligand in mediating increased bone resorption in early postmenopausal women. J Clin Invest. 2003;111:1221–30.
20. Ettinger B, Black DM, Mitlak BH, Knickerbocker RK, Nickelsen T, Genant HK, Christiansen C, Delmas PD, Zanchetta JR, Stakkestad J, Gluer CC, Krueger K, Cohen FJ, Eckert S, Ensrud KE, Avioli LV, Lips P, Cummings SR, Multiple Outcomes of Raloxifene Evaluation (MORE) Investigators. Reduction of vertebralfracture risk in postmenopausal women with osteoporosis treated with raloxifene: results from a 3-year randomized clinical trial. JAMA. 1999;282: 637–45.
21. Fitzpatrick LA, Brennen E, Kumar S, et al. Ronacaleret, a novel calcium-sensing receptor antagonist, demonstrates potential as an oral bone-forming therapy in healthy postmenopausal women. J Bone Miner Res. 2008;23 Suppl 1:S50.
22. Fitzpatrick LA, Dabrowski CE, Cicconetti G, Gordon DN, Fuerst T, Engelke KA, Genant HK. Ronacaleret, a calcium-sensing receptor antagonist, increases trabecular but not cortical bone in postmenopausal women. J Bone Miner Res. 2011 Nov 2. doi:10.1002/jbmr.554
23. Frost M, Andersen TE, Yadav V, Brixen K, Karsenty G, Kassem M. Patients with high-bone-mass phenotype owing to Lrp5-T253I mutation have low plasma levels of serotonin. J Bone Miner Res. 2010;25(3): 673–5.
24. Glantschnig H, Hampton RA, Lu P, Zhao JZ, Vitelli S, Huang L, Haytko P, Cusick T, Ireland C, Jarantow SW, Ernst R, Wei N, Nantermet P, Scott KR, Fisher JE, Talamo F, Orsatti L, Reszka AA, Sandhu P, Kimmel D, Flores O, Strohl W, An Z, Wang F. Generation and selection of novel fully human minoclonal antibodies that neutralize Dickkopf-1 (DKK1) inhibitory function in vitro and increase bone mass in vivo. J Biol Chem. 2010;285(51):40145–7.
25. Greenspan SL, Bone HG, Macciott TB, et al. Preventing the first vertebral fracture in postmenopausal women with low bone mass using PTH (1–84): results from the TOP study. J Bone Miner Res. 2005; 20 Suppl 1:S56.
26. Hoeppner LH, Secreto FJ, Westendorf JJ. Wnt signaling as a therapeutic target for bone diseases. Expert OpinTherTargets. 2009;13(4):485–96.
27. Horwitz MJ, Tedesco MB, Garcia-Ocana A, et al. Parathyroid hormone-related protein for the treatment of postmenopausal osteoporosis: defining the maximal tolerable dose. J Clin Endocrinol Metab. 2010; 95(3):1279–87.

28. Hruska KA, Mathew S, Lund R, et al. The pathogenesis of vascular calcification in the chronic kidney disease mineral bone disorder: the links between bone and the vasculature. Semin Nephrol. 2009;29(2): 156–65.
29. Jamal SA, Ljunggren O, Stehman-Breen C, Cummings SR, McClung MR, Goemaere S, Ebeling PR, Franek E, Yang Y, Egbuna OI, Boonen S, Miller PD. The effects of denosumab on fracture and bone mineral density by level of kidney function. J Bone Miner Res. 2011;26(8):1829–35.
30. Karsenty G, Gershon MD. The importance of the gastrointestinal tract in the control of bone mass accrual. Gastroenterology. 2011;141(2):439–42. Epub 2011 Jun 17.
31. Karsenty G, Oury F. The central regulation of bone mass. The first link between bone remodeling and energy metabolism. J Clin Endocrinol Metab. 2010; 95(11):4795–801.
32. Kendler DL, Roux C, Benhamou CL, Brown JP, Lillestol M, Siddhanti S, Ho-Shen M, Martin JA, Bone HG. Effects of denosumab on bone mineral density and bone turnover in postmenopausal women transitioning from alendronate. J Bone Miner Res. 2010;25:72–81.
33. Khosla S, Burr D, Cauley J, et al. Bisphosphonate-associated osteonecrosis of the jaw: report of a Task Force of the American Society for Bone and Mineral Research ASBMR Task Force on Bisphosphonate-Associated ONJ. J Bone Miner Res. 2007;22(10): 1479–91.
34. Kousteni S, Bilezikian JP. The cell biology of parathyroid hormone in osteoblasts. Curr Osteoporos Rep. 2008;6(2):72–6.
35. Leung P, Pickarski M, Zhuo Y, Masarachia PJ. Duong LT (2011) The effects of the cathepsin K inhibitor odanacatib on osteoclastic bone resorption and vesicular trafficking. Bone. 2011;49(4):623–35. Epub 2011 Jun 22.
36. Lewiecki EM, Miller PD, McClung MR, et al. Two-year treatment with denosumab (AMG 162) in a randomized phase 2 study of postmenopausal women with low bone mineral density. J Bone Miner Res. 2007;22:1832–41.
37. Lewiecki EM. Odanacatib, a cathepsin K inhibitor for the treatment of osteoporosis and other skeletal disorders associated with excessive bone remodeling. Drugs. 2009;12(12):799–809.
38. Li X, Ominsky MS, Warmington KS, et al. Sclerostin antibody treatment increases bone formation, bone mass, and bone strength in a rat model of postmenopausal osteoporosis. J Bone Miner Res. 2009; 24(4):578–88.
39. Lindsay R. The menopause and osteoporosis. Obstet Gynecol. 1996;87 Suppl 2:S16–9.
40. Lindsay R. Hormones and bone health in postmenopausal women. Endocrine. 2004;24(3):223–30.
41. McClung MR, Lewiecki EM, Cohen SB, Bolognese MA, Woodson GC, Moffett AH, Peacock M, Miller PD, Lederman SN, Chesnut CH, Lain D, Kivitz AJ, Holloway DL, Zhang C, Peterson MC, Bekker PJ. Denosumab in postmenopausal women with low bone mineral density. N Engl J Med. 2006;354:821–31.
42. McClung MR, Lewiecki EM, Bolognese M, Peacock M, Weimstein RL, Ding B, Geller ML, Grauer A, Wagman RB, Miller PD (2011) Effect of densoumab on bone mineral density and biochemical markers of bone turnover" results of an 8 year phase 2 clinical trial. J Clin Endocrinol Metab (in press)
43. Miller PD. Anti-resorptives in the management of osteoporosis. Best Pract Res Clin Endocrinol Metab. 2008;22(5):849–68.
44. Miller PD. Safety of parathyroid hormone for the treatment of osteoporosis. Curr Osteoporos Rep. 2008;6:12–6.
45. Miller PD. Denosumab: anti-RANKL antibody. Curr Osteoporos Rep. 2009;7(1):18–22.
46. Miller PD. Fragility fractures in chronic kidney disease: an opinion-based approach. Cleve Clin J Med. 2009;76:715–23.
47. Miller PD, Derman R. What is the best balance of benefits and risks among anti-resorptive therapies for postmenopausal osteoporosis? Osteoporos Int. 2010;21(11):1793–802. Epub 2010 Mar 23.
48. Miller PD, Bolognese MA, Lewiecki EM, et al. Effect of denosumab on bone density and turnover in postmenopausal women with low bone mass after long-term continued, discontinued, and restarting of therapy: a randomized blinded phase 2 clinical trial. Bone. 2008;43(2):222–9.
49. Miller PD, Wagman RB, Peacock M, Lewiecki EM, Bolognese MA, Weinstein RL, Martin JS, McClung MR. Effect of denosumab on bone mineral density and biochemical markers of bone turnover: six-year results of a phase 2 clinical trial. J Clin Endocrinol Metab. 2011;96(2):1–6.
50. Mirza FS, Padhi ID, Raisz LG, Lorenzo JA. Serum sclerostin levels negatively correlate with parathyroid hormone levels and free estrogen index in postmenopausal women. J Clin Endocrinol Metab. 2010;95(4):1991–7.
51. Neer RM, Arnaud CD, Zanchetta JR, et al. Effect of parathyroid hormone (1–34) on fractures and bone mineraldensity in postmenopausal women with osteoporosis. N Engl J Med. 2001;344:1434–41.
52. O'Brien CA, Plotkin LI, Galli C, et al. Control of bone mass and remodeling by PTH receptor signaling in osteocytes. PLoS One. 2008;3(8):e2942.
53. Orwoll ES, Miller PD, Adachi JD, Brown J, Adler RA, Kendler D, Bucci-Rechtweg C, Readie A, Mesenbrink P, Weinstein RS. Efficacy and safety of a once-yearly i.v. Infusion of zoledronic acid 5 mg versus a once-weekly 70-mg oral alendronate in the treatment of male osteoporosis: a randomized, multicenter, double-blind, active-controlled study. J Bone Miner Res. 2010;25(10):2239–50.
54. Orwoll ES, Scheele WH, Paul S, et al. The effect of teriparatide [human parathyroid hormone (1–34)] therapy on bone density in men with osteoporosis. J Bone Miner Res. 2003;18:9–17.

55. Papapoulos S, Chapurlat R, Libanati C, Brandi M, Brown J, Czerwiński E, Krieg MA, Man Z, Mellström D, Radominski S, Reginster JY, Resch H, Román J, Roux C, Vittinghoff E, Austin M, Daizadeh N, Bradley M, Grauer A, Cummings S, Bone H. Five years of denosumab exposure in women with postmenopausal osteoporosis: Results from the first two years of the FREEDOM extension. J Bone Miner Res. 2011 Nov 23. doi:10.1002/jbmr.1479.
56. Pennypacker B, Shea M, Liu Q, et al. Bone density, strength, and formation in adult cathepsin K (–/–) mice. Bone. 2009;44(2):199–207.
57. Price JS, Sugiyama T, Galea GL, Meakin LB, Sunters A, Lanyon LB. Role of endocrine and paracrine factors in the adaptation of bone to mechanical loading. Curr Osteoporos Reports. 2011;9:72–6.
58. Reginster JY, Seeman E, De Vernejoul MC, Adami S, Compston J, Phenekos C, et al. Strontium ranelate reduces the risk of nonvertebral fractures in postmenopausal women with osteoporosis: Treatment of Peripheral Osteoporosis (TROPOS) study. J Clin Endocrinol Metab. 2005;90(5):2816–22.
59. Reid IR, Hosking DJ. Bisphosphonates in Paget's disease. Bone. 2011;49(1):89–94.
60. Reid IR, Miller PD, Brown JP, Kendler DL, Fahrleitner-Pammer A, Valter AI, Maasalu K, Bolognese MA, Woodson G, Bone H, Ding B, Wagman RB, Martin S, Ominsky MS, Dempster DW, on behalf of the Denosumab Phase 3 Bone Histology Study Group. Effects of denosumab on bone histomorphometry: the freedom and stand studies. J Bone Min Res. 2010;25:2256–65.
61. Russell G, Burr D. 40th Anniversary of bisphosphonates. Bone. 2011;49(1):2–19.
62. Russell RG, Watts NB, Ebetino FH, Rogers MJ. Mechanisms of action of bisphosphonates: similarities and differences and their potential influence on clinical efficacy. Osteoporos Int. 2008;19:733–59.
63. Saag KG, Shane E, Boonen S, et al. Teriparatide oralendronate in glucocorticoid-induced osteoporosis. N Engl J Med. 2007;357:2028–39.
64. Shane E, Burr D, Ebeling P, et al. Atypical subtrochanteric and diaphyseal femoral fractures: report of a task force of The American Society for Bone and Mineral Research. J Bone Miner Res. 2010;25:1–28.
65. Silvestrini G, Ballanti P, Leopizzi M, et al. Effects of intermittent parathyroid hormone (PTH) administration on SOST mRNA and protein in rat bone. J Mol Histol. 2007;38(4):261–9.
66. Siris E, Pasquale MK, Wang Y, Watts NB. Estimating bisphosphonate use and fracture reduction in US women aged 45 and older: 2001–2008. Bone. 2011;26: 3–11.
67. Stopeck AT, Lipton A, Body J-J, et al. Densoumab compared with zoledronic acid for the treatment of bone metastisis in patients with advanced breast cancer: a randomized, double-blind study. J Clin Oncol. 2010;28(35):5132–9.
68. Suda T, Takahashi N, Udagawa N, Jimi E, Gillespie MT, Martin TJ. Modulation of osteoclast differentiation and function by the new members of the tumor necrosis factor receptor and ligand families. Endocr Rev. 1999;20:345–57.
69. Visentin L, Dodds RA, Valente M, et al. A selective inhibitor of the osteoclastic V-H(+)- ATPase prevents bone loss in both thyroparathyroidectomized and ovaricetomized rats. J Clin Invest. 2000;106:309–18.
70. Watts NB. Long term use of bisphosphonates in osteoporosis. J Clin Endocrinol Metab. 2010;95:1555–65.
71. Yaccoby S, Ling W, Zhan F, Walker R, Barlogie B, Shaughnessy Jr JD. Antibody-based inhibition of DKK1 suppresses tumor-induced bone resorption and multiple myeloma growth in vivo. Blood. 2007;109: 2106–11.
72. Yadav VK, Ducy P. Lrp5 and bone formation: a serotonin-dependent pathway. Ann N Y Acad Sci. 2010; 1192(1):103–9.
73. Yadav VK, Balaji S, Suresh PS, et al. Pharmacological inhibition of gut-derived serotonin synthesis is a potential bone anabolic treatment for osteoporosis. Nat Med. 2010;16(3):308–12.

Renal Diseases and Bone: Emerging Therapeutics

10

Nancy S. Krieger and David A. Bushinsky

Keywords
Metabolic acidosis • Chronic kidney disease • Bone resorption $1,25(OH)_2D_3$ • Phosphate • Calcimimetics

10.1 Introduction

Disorders of bone metabolism occur relatively early in the presence of chronic kidney disease (CKD). They become more prevalent as kidney function declines and are common in dialysis patients. A new designation, chronic kidney disease–mineral and bone disorders (CKD-MBD), has been advocated by the Kidney Disease: Improving Global Outcomes (KDIGO) group to broadly describe the interrelationship of the disorders that involve mineral metabolism, skeletal disorders, and soft tissue calcification associated with CKD [79]. In addition to characterizing the effect of renal diseases on skeletal homeostasis, we will also discuss both current and emerging strategies aimed at correcting the biochemical parameters that lead to the resultant mineral and bone disorders. The clinician must recognize that the approach to a patient with CKD-MBD involves multiple considerations and interventions; there is no one pharmacologic therapy that will independently correct the disordered mineral metabolism of CKD. This chapter will concentrate on the skeletal disorders associated with metabolic acidosis [45, 46].

10.2 Metabolic Acidosis

Human metabolism leads to production of ~1 mmol/kg of acid (protons, H^+) per day that is termed endogenous acid production [25, 93]. Additional endogenous acid production occurs during disorders such as diarrhea, diabetic ketoacidosis, and lactic acidosis. This additional acid results in a reduction of systemic pH, secondary to a reduction in blood bicarbonate concentration [HCO_3^-] that is termed metabolic acidosis [45, 46]. The physiologic response to metabolic acidosis is to rapidly increase extracellular fluid pH toward the physiologic neutral of 7.40 in order to maintain optimal cellular function [93]. The homeostatic response to metabolic acidosis involves first buffering the acid, then increasing the respiratory rate to lower the partial

N.S. Krieger, Ph.D. • D.A. Bushinsky, M.D. (✉)
Department of Medicine,
University of Rochester School of Medicine,
601 Elmwood Ave., Box 675,
Rochester, NY 14642, USA
e-mail: david_bushinsky@urmc.rochester.edu

F. Bronner et al. (eds.), *Bone-Metabolic Functions and Modulators,* Topics in Bone Biology,
DOI 10.1007/978-1-4471-2745-1_10, © Springer-Verlag London 2012

pressure of carbon dioxide (PCO_2), and finally renal excretion of the additional acid. The initial step, buffering of the additional acid, is critical to the immediate restoration toward neutral pH allowing the preservation of life. The final step, renal excretion of the acid, begins hours after the acid challenge and is complete only days later. Renal acid excretion relies upon normal kidney function; as we age, our ability to excrete acid declines and all older individuals become slightly, but significantly, more acidemic [65].

During acute metabolic acidosis in vivo, ~60% of the excess hydrogen ions are buffered by soft tissue and by bone. The evidence that bone acutely buffers hydrogen ions in vivo, and releases calcium (Ca) during that process, comes primarily from the observation of an increase in serum Ca and sodium observed during acute metabolic acidosis [6, 9]. As the vast majority of body Ca is contained within the bone mineral, the increase in serum Ca almost certainly is derived from mineral in the skeleton. Animal studies suggest that acute metabolic acidosis affects the cardiovascular system most critically [81].

Chronic metabolic acidosis, found in patients with CKD and renal tubular acidosis, has its most prominent effects on the musculoskeletal system. Metabolic acidosis can produce or exacerbate existing bone disease by increasing urinary Ca excretion secondary to a direct reduction in renal tubular Ca reabsorption [46, 93]. There is little, if any, increase in intestinal Ca absorption. The increase in urinary excretion without a concomitant increase in intestinal absorption results in a net loss of body Ca [93]. As bone contains ~99% of total body Ca, the source of much of this additional urinary Ca appears to be acid-mediated dissolution and resorption of bone mineral [5, 93]. Chronic metabolic acidosis appears to decrease bone mineral content [5] and has been shown to significantly decrease bone density, formation, and growth [57]. Patients with proximal renal tubular acidosis, a defect in renal acid excretion, are shorter in height and have decreased radial bone densities and thinner iliac cortices than unaffected relatives [92]. Patients with distal renal tubular acidosis have a lower bone mineral density in most skeletal areas when compared with normal controls and also have a decreased bone formation rate [57].

During the sustained metabolic acidosis of severe CKD, blood pH remains stable, although substantially reduced, in spite of progressive acid retention, suggesting the availability of large stores of proton buffers [93]. During renal failure, significant clinical evidence indicates that acidosis adversely affects bone density. Bone carbonate is decreased in acidic, uremic patients [106], which may represent dissolution of bone carbonate or replacement by phosphate, resulting in the incorporation of acid into the mineral. In view of the deleterious effect of metabolic acidosis on bone, the National Kidney Foundation has issued evidence-based guidelines that recommend treatment of metabolic acidosis to help prevent what is now termed chronic kidney disease–mineral bone disorders (CKD-MBD) [102].

In addition to its effects on existing bone, metabolic acidosis also decreases de novo bone formation. This independent effect of metabolic acidosis to suppress bone formation has been demonstrated in pediatric patients with renal tubular acidosis [97]. It was found that six of ten children with renal tubular acidosis were short (height < 2.5 SD), two of the ten were less than 2 weeks old, so shortness could not be determined, and the remaining two had not previously been acidemic. After treatment with alkali, each child attained and maintained normal stature, the mean height increased from 1.4 to the 37th percentile, and the growth rate increased two- to three-fold.

The common high-protein diet of North Americans, coupled with the known effects of bone to buffer an acid load [26, 93] and the age-related decline in renal function which prevents quantitative excretion of this acid [64, 65], has led to the suggestion that excess dietary acid may play a role in the etiology of osteoporosis [3–5, 26, 63, 93]. Adequate dietary protein intake is necessary for optimal bone health [115]. Treatment of postmenopausal women with the base $KHCO_3$, which neutralizes endogenous H^+ production, leads to improved Ca retention, reduced bone resorption, and increased bone formation [63, 91, 116, 120]. Severe, life-threatening metabolic acidosis must be treated [19];

however, the mild metabolic acidosis present in the initial stages of CKD [93, 118, 119] and in aging [64, 65], worsened in the latter case by an animal protein-rich diet [63, 87, 93], is rarely treated [19, 26, 93]. While this hypothesis is controversial [61, 62], there is no controversy that patients with CKD have sustained metabolic acidosis due to a decreased ability to excrete H^+ and the resultant bone disease is associated with fractures [1, 21, 23, 24, 46, 77, 93, 99].

10.2.1 Acute Acidosis, In Vitro Studies

10.2.1.1 Calcium Release

Using a model system of cultured neonatal mouse calvariae, we have found that these bones exhibit acid-dependent net Ca efflux during both acute (3-h) [33] and more chronic (>24–99-h) incubations [18, 32, 37, 68, 70, 71, 84–86]. The mechanism of acid-mediated Ca efflux from bone during acute incubations is direct physicochemical bone dissolution and is not cell-mediated [32]. This finding was confirmed by demonstrating Ca efflux from synthetic carbonated apatite (CAP) disks, a cell-free model of bone mineral, cultured in physiologically acid medium [40].

The type of bone mineral in equilibrium with the medium and thus altered by physicochemical forces might be carbonate or phosphate in association with Ca. It was found that bone carbonate is solubilized during an acute reduction in pH leading to a release of Ca [34, 35]. Further support for the role of carbonate in acid-mediated bone mineral dissolution comes from the observation that at a constant pH, whether physiologically neutral or acid, Ca flux from bone is dependent on the medium [HCO_3^-]; the lower the [HCO_3^-], the greater the Ca efflux [39].

10.2.1.2 Hydrogen Ion Buffering

The in vitro evidence for acid buffering by bone is derived from studies of acidosis-induced proton flux into bone [17, 33, 35, 43], high-resolution ion microprobe evidence for a depletion of bone sodium and potassium during acute acidosis [30, 31, 36, 43, 44], and from a depletion of bone carbonate and phosphate during acidosis [43]. When calvariae are cultured in medium acidified by a decrease in [HCO_3^-], a net influx of protons into bone is seen that decreases medium acidity. This indicates that the additional acid is being buffered by bone, ultimately leading to an increase in medium pH [33, 35, 43]. During acute acidosis, there appear to be two principal mechanisms by which the acid is buffered: proton for sodium and/or potassium exchange [30, 36, 43, 44] and consumption of the buffers carbonate and phosphate [28, 33, 35, 39, 43].

10.2.1.3 Proton for Sodium and/or Potassium Exchange

In addition to Ca, bone is a reservoir for sodium and potassium, and its surface has fixed negative sites which normally complex with sodium, potassium, and hydrogen [137]. The calvarial surface actually has more sodium and potassium relative to Ca [28, 30, 31, 36, 43, 44, 50, 100]. A high-resolution ion microprobe was used to determine how protons alter the ion composition of bone mineral. The excess mineral potassium is maintained through cell-mediated processes [29]. A model of metabolic acidosis caused release of bone Ca and led to a decrease in the surface ratio of sodium to Ca and potassium to Ca, indicating a greater relative release of mineral sodium and potassium than Ca in response to the acid challenge [30, 36].

10.2.1.4 Fall in Bone Carbonate and Phosphate

Bone contains ≈80% of the total body carbon dioxide, and acute metabolic acidosis decreases total bone carbon dioxide [8]. Bone also contains a substantial amount of the total body phosphate, estimated to be ~90% [27] largely in the form of hydroxyapatite ($Ca_{10}(PO_4)_6(OH)_2$) and other forms of apatite [103]. During metabolic acidosis, protonation of the phosphate in apatite will consume protons and help restore the pH toward normal [25, 93]. Using chemical analysis, a model of metabolic acidosis was found to induce the release of bone Ca and carbonate [35], leading to a progressive loss of bone carbonate [34].

The high-resolution scanning ion microprobe was used to study the bone content of carbonate and phosphate in response to acute metabolic acidosis [43]. A marked preferential loss of surface HCO_3^- and of cross-sectional phosphate was seen. When the in vitro and in vivo studies are considered together, there is clear evidence that bone is a proton buffer capable of maintaining the extracellular fluid pH near the physiologic normal. The loss of bone sodium, potassium, carbonate, and phosphate suggests that in addition to sodium and potassium for proton exchange, bone carbonate and phosphate are lost from the mineral in response to acidosis, each of which helps to restore the pH toward normal.

10.2.2 Chronic Acidosis, In Vitro Studies

10.2.2.1 Increased Bone Resorption

Chronic metabolic acidosis causes the release of bone Ca from neonatal mouse calvariae in vitro, predominantly by enhanced cell-mediated bone resorption combined with decreased bone formation [18, 31, 37, 68, 84, 85]. There also continues to be a component of direct physicochemical acid-induced mineral dissolution [32, 33, 35, 39, 40, 43, 44]. Osteoblastic collagen synthesis and alkaline phosphatase activity both are decreased after 48-h incubation in a model of metabolic acidosis compared to neutral medium [85], while receptor activator of NFκb ligand (RANKL) synthesis was increased [68]. Release of osteoclastic β-glucuronidase, a lysosomal enzyme whose secretion correlates with osteoclast-mediated bone resorption, is increased during in vitro metabolic acidosis. Conversely, an increase in [HCO_3^-], modeling metabolic alkalosis, decreases Ca efflux from bone through an increase in osteoblastic bone formation and a decrease in osteoclastic bone resorption [22].

Further support for a direct effect of metabolic acidosis to inhibit osteoblastic bone formation was obtained using primary cells isolated from the calvariae. These isolated cells, almost exclusively osteoblasts, synthesize collagen and form nodules of apatitic bone [123]. Compared to cells incubated in neutral medium, cells incubated in a model of metabolic acidosis produced fewer nodules and had decreased Ca influx into the nodules [123].

In addition to the acidosis that occurs during clinical chronic kidney disease, an increase in PTH secretion also occurs often [94]. In in vitro studies, acidosis and PTH independently stimulated Ca efflux from bone, inhibited osteoblastic collagen synthesis, and stimulated osteoclastic β-glucuronidase secretion. The combination of both acidosis and PTH had a greater effect on each of these parameters than either alone, suggesting an additive deleterious effect of PTH and acidosis on bone [37].

10.2.2.2 Mechanism of Proton Signaling

Bone responds to metabolic acidosis through a coordinated homeostatic response aimed at normalizing systemic pH, often at the cost of decreased mineral content; however, the mechanism by which extracellular pH is sensed was previously not clear. A novel class of G-protein-coupled receptors that respond to protons has been recently characterized [96, 134]. This family includes the ovarian G-protein-coupled receptor 1 (OGR1), GPR4, T-cell-death-associated gene 8 (TDAG8), and G2A, which share 40–50% homology. Activation of OGR1 and G2A by decreased pH leads to inositol phosphate accumulation and Ca signaling, while GPR4 and TDAG8 are coupled to cAMP formation. However, the activation of G2A shows little pH dependence, and H^+ sensing may be a minor role for this receptor.

We have found that one of the first responses of the osteoblast to metabolic acidosis is an increase in intracellular Ca [71]. Because the proton receptor OGR1 has been shown to be coupled to Gq and activates intracellular Ca signaling, we tested the hypothesis that OGR1 acts as an H^+ sensing receptor in bone cells. It was found that OGR1 was present in cultured neonatal mouse calvariae and an inhibitor of OGR1 ($CuCl_2$) could inhibit acidosis-induced Ca efflux from bone [71]. In addition, primary mouse calvarial bone cells respond to a decrease in extracellular pH with an increase in intracellular Ca, while Chinese hamster ovary fibroblasts (CHO cells) increased intracellular Ca in response to a model of metabolic acidosis only after being transfected with mouse OGR1 cDNA [71]. Thus, OGR1 appears to have a primary role as a proton sensor in bone cells.

10.2.2.3 Role of PGE_2

Prostaglandin E_2 (PGE_2) levels increase in response to chronic metabolic acidosis, leading to enhanced renal acid excretion, and acidosis increases the level of prostaglandins in a variety of experimental model systems [84]. Prostaglandins, especially PGE_2, are potent multifunctional regulators with effects on both bone resorption and formation [113]. Prostaglandins have been shown to promote new bone formation in vivo and in isolated osteoblasts. However, in bone organ culture, PGE_2 has been shown to directly stimulate bone resorption [84] and to stimulate RANKL expression in calvarial osteoblasts [68]. The relative effects of prostaglandins on bone may be dependent on timing or magnitude of dose [114], as has been found for PTH, or dependent on stage of osteoblast differentiation.

Incubation of neonatal mouse calvariae in medium-simulating metabolic acidosis increases medium PGE_2 in parallel with an increase in net Ca efflux [84]. Inhibition of PGE_2 production by indomethacin strongly limited this acidosis-induced bone Ca release as well as acid stimulation of RANKL [68]. Incubation of primary mouse calvarial bone cells, which consist mostly of osteoblasts [83], in a model of metabolic acidosis, led to a marked increase in medium PGE_2 levels that was again completely suppressed by indomethacin [84]. Cortisol inhibits acid-induced bone resorption through a decrease in osteoblastic PGE_2 production [82]. These results suggest that acid-induced, cell-mediated Ca efflux from bone is regulated, at least in part, by an increase in endogenous PGE_2 production in the osteoblast leading to an increase in RANKL.

Prostaglandin synthesis is regulated by the release of arachidonic acid from membrane phospholipids. The rate-limiting step converting arachidonic acid to specific prostanoids is catalyzed by prostaglandin G/H synthase or cyclooxygenase (COX) [122]. There are two forms of COX: COX1, which is constitutively expressed, and COX2, which is the inducible form of the enzyme [122]. Both forms of COX are expressed in osteoblasts, but COX2 appears to be the enzyme most responsible for the prostaglandin response in osteoblasts [108]. COX2 expression is regulated by several bone-resorbing factors, including interleukin-1, PTH, interleukin-6, TGF-α, and basic fibroblast growth factor, as well as fluid flow [112]. NS-398, a specific COX2 isozyme inhibitor, significantly inhibits H^+-induced Ca release from calvariae, which supports the hypothesis that this enzyme is stimulated by acidosis [86]. Further support for the importance of COX2 as an intermediate in the response of the osteoblast to acid derives from a study of the effects of COX2 gene deletion using calvariae from the offspring of matings of COX2 +/− mice and correlating genotype and phenotype. We found COX2 is necessary for acid-induced bone Ca release, and it appears that the gene dosage of COX2 sets the level of basal and of H^+-induced bone resorption. Direct measurement of RNA expression in primary osteoblasts also indicates that metabolic acidosis causes greater stimulation of COX2 RNA levels than neutral medium, with no change in COX1 [86].

10.2.2.4 Regulation of Gene Expression

External pH modulates gene expression in several cell types. To determine if metabolic acidosis would alter specific gene expression in osteoblasts, we examined several immediate early response genes in primary neonatal mouse calvarial cells, including egr-1, junB, c-jun, junD, and c-fos. In response to incubation in acidic medium, only the magnitude of egr-1 stimulation was dependent on medium pH [69]. Osteoblasts express type 1 collagen as the major component of the bone extracellular matrix, which subsequently becomes mineralized. Similarly to egr-1, type I collagen RNA synthesis was decreased by acidosis and increased by alkalosis [69].

Primary mouse calvarial cells differentiate in culture to form bone nodules. These osteoblastic cells express a number of bone specific matrix proteins, including bone sialoprotein, osteocalcin, osteonectin (ON), osteopontin (OP), and matrix gla protein (MGP) [126]. Because acidic medium decreases bone nodule number, size, and

Ca content [124], we hypothesized that acidosis would alter the pattern of matrix gene expression in these long-term cell cultures. After 3–4 weeks in neutral medium, OP RNA levels increased while incubation in acid medium completely inhibited this increase [66]. The RNA levels of two other proteins, ON and transforming growth factor β_1, did not vary with pH. RNA for MGP also was induced by incubation in neutral medium differentiation medium while acidic medium almost totally prevented the increase in MGP RNA levels. The inhibition of MGP and OP RNA levels by acidosis was found to be reversible [66].

We hypothesized that the acidosis-induced bone resorption was a result of alterations in osteoblastic expression of osteoclastogenic factors. Such factors include macrophage colony-stimulating factor (M-CSF), a growth factor for osteoclast precursor cells, RANKL, RANK, and osteoprotegerin (OPG), a decoy receptor for RANKL. Activation of RANK by RANKL initiates a differentiation cascade that culminates in mature, bone-resorbing osteoclasts as well as stimulation of mature osteoclast activity. Analysis of RNA extracted from calvariae incubated for 24 or 48 h in neutral or acidic medium indicated that expression of RANKL RNA was upregulated by acidosis, while expression of M-CSF, OPG, and β-actin were not altered [68]. Analysis of culture supernatants by ELISA demonstrated that calvariae in acidic medium produced greater amounts of soluble RANKL protein than calvariae cultured at neutral pH; production of OPG was not affected [70].

To examine the role of PGE_2 synthesis in RANKL expression, calvariae were incubated in the absence or presence of indomethacin to inhibit COX activity; Ca flux was determined as well as RANKL RNA content by northern analysis. Indomethacin significantly inhibited acid-induced Ca flux and completely suppressed the induction of RANKL RNA by Met [68]. Thus, acidosis-induced synthesis of PGE_2 causes an autocrine or paracrine stimulation of osteoblastic prostaglandin receptors. Activation of these receptors consequently induces an increase in RANKL RNA expression, which in turn increases osteoclastogenesis and activation of mature osteoclasts.

10.2.3 Comparison of Metabolic and Respiratory Acidosis

Most studies have used NH_4Cl (in vivo) or HCl (in vitro) to decrease [HCO_3^-] as a model of metabolic acidosis. This non-anion gap acidosis mimics the clinical disorder of renal tubular acidosis, moderate to severe diarrhea, and early renal failure. The Henderson-Hasselbalch equation predicts that pH is a function of [HCO_3^-] and the partial pressure of carbon dioxide (PCO_2) so that pH also can be lowered by an increase in PCO_2 to model respiratory acidosis.

There are significant differences between the effects of metabolic and respiratory acidosis on net bone release and proton buffering. In contrast to metabolic acidosis, chronic respiratory acidosis has little or no effect on urine Ca excretion in vivo [49, 88, 117], and an isohydric reduction in pH in vitro, achieved by increasing the PCO_2, does not stimulate net Ca efflux from cultured calvariae [17, 18, 20, 34, 38, 67]. We have shown that the decreased net Ca efflux in an in vitro model of respiratory, compared with metabolic, acidosis is due to decreased unidirectional Ca efflux from the mineral coupled to deposition of medium Ca on the bone surface during hypercapnia [41]. Bone carbonate also decreases in response to a model of metabolic, but not respiratory, acidosis [34]. Over short time periods, the decreased [HCO_3^-] of metabolic acidosis favors dissolution of bone mineral, while during respiratory acidosis the increased PCO_2 and higher [HCO_3^-] favors deposition of carbonated apatite [35]. Indeed, there is no net proton influx into bone during respiratory acidosis [17].

During more chronic incubations of bones in vitro, there is cell-mediated net Ca efflux from bone during metabolic, but not respiratory, acidosis. In our model of respiratory acidosis, there also was no stimulation of osteoblastic PGE_2 production and no decrease in osteoblastic collagen synthesis, both responses that are observed with metabolic acidosis [20, 38]. Thus, there is a fundamental difference between an isohydric lowering of pH by decreasing the [HCO_3^-] compared with increasing the PCO_2. Perhaps the newly characterized proton-sensing receptor signaling is modulated by [HCO_3^-] to account for these differences.

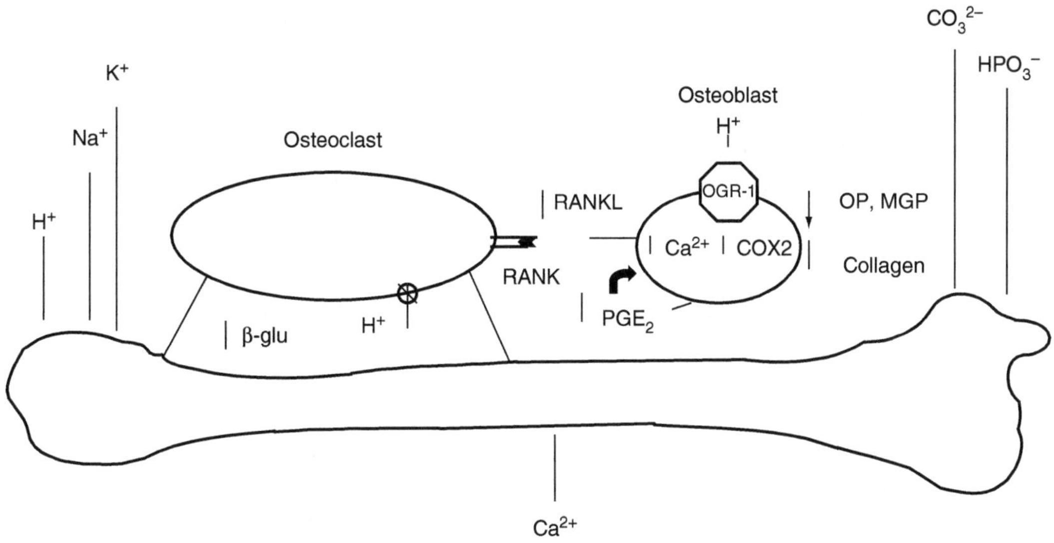

Fig. 10.1 Model of the effects of metabolic acidosis on bone. *Abbreviations*: H^+ hydrogen ion, Na^+ sodium, K^+ potassium, β-glucuronidase, *RANK* receptor activator of NFκB, *RANKL* receptor activator of NFκB ligand, PGE_2 prostaglandin E_2, Ca^{2+} calcium, *COX2* cyclooxygenase 2, *OPN* osteopontin, *MGP* matrix Gla protein, CO_3^{2-} carbonate, HPO_3^- phosphate (From Bushinsky [46])

10.2.4 Overview of the Response of Bone to Acid

Thus, metabolic acidosis induces changes in the bone mineral, which are consistent with its role as an H^+ buffer [46] (Fig. 10.1). Over the first few hours, buffering of the acidic medium pH occurs through physicochemical bone mineral dissolution [33, 35, 44], releasing Ca as well as the buffers, carbonate, and phosphate [39, 43], and there is exchange of bone sodium and potassium for hydrogen [30, 36, 43, 44]. Hours later, cellular mechanisms increase bone resorption and decrease bone formation, both of which normalize systemic pH [32, 85]. Increased bone resorption further releases bone carbonate and phosphate [28, 42], and decreased bone formation lessens the amount of acid produced during bone mineralization. In cells, the acidic pH is sensed by the H^+ receptor OGR1 [71], and acidosis alters expression of a number of genes in osteoblasts [66, 68, 69]. Acidosis increases osteoblastic PGE_2 synthesis [38, 84, 86] leading to an increase in RANKL expression and osteoclastic bone resorption [68, 70], which can account for the bone loss associated with this disease state.

10.2.5 Bicarbonate as Emerging Therapeutic for Acidosis-Induced Bone Disease

During CKD, there is ample clinical evidence that acidosis adversely affects bone [72, 90, 95, 101], which may be corrected by HCO_3^- treatment [10, 53, 80, 89, 98]. Bone carbonate is decreased in acidic, uremic patients [78, 106, 107], which may represent dissolution of bone carbonate or replacement by phosphate, resulting in the incorporation of H^+ into the mineral [8, 34, 35]. As mentioned above, treating patients with distal RTA with the base $KHCO_3$ for 1 year led to a significant improvement in bone mineral density in the trochanter, and total femur and bone formation rate normalized [58]. Although the role of mild acidosis on osteoporosis is controversial, it has been found that treatment of postmenopausal women with the base $KHCO_3$, which neutralizes endogenous acid production, leads to improved Ca retention, reduced bone resorption, and increased bone formation [63, 91, 116, 120]. These findings suggest that bicarbonate administration could minimize the bone mineral loss associated with metabolic acidosis and CKD.

10.3 Renal Bone Disease

As kidney function declines, the clearance of phosphorus (P) becomes impaired. The phosphaturic hormone FGF-23, produced in bone [7, 110], is increased and acts cooperatively with the coreceptor klotho to decrease production of the active metabolite of vitamin D, 1,25 dihydroxyvitamin D_3 (1,25$(OH)_2D_3$), and to inhibit proximal tubular reabsorption of P to help normalize serum P levels [7, 59, 110]. The increase in P and loss of renal mass further decrease 1,25$(OH)_2D_3$ production, leading to less Ca absorption and a decrease in serum Ca. Independently, the low serum Ca, high serum P, and low 1,25$(OH)_2D_3$ act on the parathyroid gland to increase PTH secretion and stimulate parathyroid gland hyperplasia. As renal function decreases further, the kidney is unable to quantitatively excrete the absorbed P in spite of elevated levels of the phosphaturic hormones PTH and FGF-23. Loss of functioning renal mass and elevated FGF-23 levels prevent PTH stimulation of 1,25$(OH)_2D_3$, which would provide a feedback mechanism to limit hyperparathyroidism. With progressive CKD, the decline in GFR leads to further increases in PTH and FGF-23 and reductions in 1,25$(OH)_2D_3$, while serum P progressively increases and serum Ca continues to decrease. The increase in FGF-23 is evident with a minimal decline in renal function. The decrease in 1,25$(OH)_2D_3$ and increase in PTH becomes evident with a GFR of ~50 ml/min, while the fall in serum Ca and rise in serum P may not be evident until the GFR is less than 30 ml/min [73, 94]. In a number of retrospective studies, a significant increase in mortality was associated with increased FGF-23 levels, increased P, and decreased serum Ca [11, 12, 73]. It is unclear if correction of these abnormalities will decrease mortality in affected individuals.

This secondary hyperparathyroidism resulting from CKD is associated with high turnover bone disease [60]. The excess PTH stimulates bone resorption to increase serum Ca, but serum P levels also increase further. The high turnover disease is characterized by rapid turnover bone formation and impaired osteoid mineralization and bone loss, mainly in cortical bone. Patients on dialysis have a significantly increased risk of hip fracture the longer they remain on dialysis, which contributes to their overall mortality risk [104]. Thus, a major clinical consequence of the initial renal disease is abnormal bone morphology, including abnormal bone turnover, decreased mineralization and bone volume, as well as decreased bone growth and bone strength. Clinical outcomes are further impaired by vascular and soft tissue calcification. These abnormalities of mineral metabolism related to secondary hyperparathyroidism are associated with increased morbidity and mortality [12]. Monitoring and maintaining control of serum levels of PTH, P, and Ca over time remains central to the management of secondary hyperparathyroidism.

The abnormalities of mineral metabolism associated with decreased renal function often are established in many patients by the time they start dialysis. According to current recommendations, PTH levels in dialysis patients should be maintained between about 130 and 600 pg/ml; however, increased mortality risk is associated with PTH levels greater than 400 pg/ml [79, 135]. Conversely, oversuppression of PTH leads to a marked decrease in osteoclastic and osteoblastic activity, which is the hallmark of adynamic bone disease. As yet, no hard evidence exists to define the exact level at which PTH should be maintained nor if correction to the recommended levels will improve mortality. Serum Ca and P should be maintained in the normal range to promote normal bone turnover and mineralization.

10.3.1 Phosphate Binders

In CKD, phosphate retention, often leading to hyperphosphatemia, is central to development of secondary hyperparathyroidism and is a principal factor leading to vascular cell transformation into collagen secreting osteoblasts resulting in vascular calcification. Dietary phosphate restriction often results in less than adequate protein intake, especially in end-stage renal disease. Dialysis three times a week is not adequate to remove sufficient phosphate to maintain neutral phosphate balance. An elevation in serum P stimulates PTH and FGF-23 secretion. Normally, the PTH- and FGF-23-induced phosphaturia would lower serum P into the normal range; however, in the absence of a sufficient filtered load of P, the kidney is unable to excrete adequate P, and serum P remains elevated. Elevated levels of PTH stimulate bone resorption, adding phosphate to the systemic circulation exacerbating the hyperphosphatemia.

A primary therapeutic intervention to limit phosphate retention and hyperphosphatemia in CKD is the use of intestinal phosphate binders. Phosphate binders currently available to decrease serum P levels can be divided into those that contain Ca and those that do not.

Calcium containing phosphate binders, such as Ca acetate and Ca carbonate, are inexpensive and can also correct hypocalcemia, which will aid in the suppression of PTH secretion. However, these binders often result in patients retaining more Ca than they excrete, which is termed positive Ca balance. Modeling has demonstrated that higher doses of these binders often lead to Ca retention [47]. The use of active vitamin D analogs will increase Ca absorption and lead to further Ca retention. As Ca is retained, it first will deposit into unmineralized matrix and then into the soft tissues. The vast majority of dialysis patients, especially those with diabetes, have readily evident vascular calcification.

Although a more expensive alternative, Ca-free phosphate binders are now available which reduce serum P without inducing Ca retention [47, 54]. In two studies, sevelamer hydrochloride has been shown to attenuate progression of vascular calcification in hemodialysis patients while lowering both serum P and Ca [13, 51]; however, other studies fail to demonstrate a change in calcification with sevelamer [2, 111, 128]. However, no study has ever demonstrated that Ca-based phosphate binders reduce vascular calcification, only that they may not be inferior to Ca-free phosphate binders. Lanthanum carbonate, another Ca-free binder, also effectively decreases hyperphosphatemia although its role in prevention of vascular calcification in not known [54].

Future therapeutic options to prevent phosphate retention include trivalent iron preparations and nicotinamide. The latter agent already is used as a lipid-lowering agent; however, its ability to inhibit intestinal sodium-dependent phosphate cotransport suggests a potential role in preventing phosphate retention [129].

10.3.2 Repletion of $1{,}25(OH)_2D_3$

Vitamin D either is acquired through the diet or produced in skin exposed to ultraviolet radiation. Vitamin D then is transported to the liver where it is converted to 25-hydroxyvitamin D, the main storage form of the hormone, which circulates primarily bound to a vitamin D-binding protein. This complex then is filtered by the kidney, taken up in the proximal convoluted tubule where it is hydroxylated in the 1-α position to become the fully activated hormone. With kidney disease, the endogenous production of $1{,}25(OH)_2D_3$ is greatly reduced [74, 109]. $1{,}25(OH)_2D_3$ stimulates absorption of Ca and P and provides feedback inhibition of PTH synthesis. Adequate $1{,}25(OH)_2D_3$ is necessary to normalize serum Ca and P and promote bone accretion. In excess, $1{,}25(OH)_2D_3$ stimulates bone resorption. There is a general consensus that all patients should be 25-(OH) vitamin D replete, though the level at which people are considered replete is not yet clear. A recent Institute of Medicine study suggested that levels of 20 ng/ml were sufficient in patients without kidney disease [75]. The optimal level of 25-(OH) vitamin D in patients with CKD is not yet known.

All active vitamin D sterols, including calcitriol, paracalcitol, and doxercalciferol, effectively lower PTH and appear, in humans, to have similar physiologic effects on Ca and P homeostasis. Thus, utilization of large amounts of these activated vitamin D sterols has the potential to increase Ca and P absorption and promote retention. Several retrospective analyses demonstrate that repletion of activated vitamin D is associated with increased survival [76, 121, 127, 130–132], while others fail to do so [48, 105, 125, 133]. Prospective studies are clearly needed to define the role of active vitamin D repletion.

10.3.3 Calcimimetics

Calcimimetics allosterically increase the sensitivity of the Ca-sensing receptor to extracellular Ca, primarily in the parathyroid glands [16]. As PTH production and secretion is inhibited by Ca, the calcimimetic-induced increased sensitivity of the Ca receptor leads to a decrease in PTH secretion [15]. The calcimimetic-induced reduction of PTH will lessen bone resorption and increase Ca and P incorporation into the bone mineral; serum Ca and P levels will fall.

In secondary hyperparathyroidism, calcimimetics lower PTH levels. There is no specific level of PTH at which it is imperative to intervene; however, guidelines specify that significant changes of PTH within the 130–600-pg/ml range should trigger a response to prevent a future level outside of the range [79, 135]. If serum Ca is high, calcimimetics are clearly the drug of choice to manage PTH levels. If serum Ca is within the normal range, either calcimimetics or active vitamin D sterols are appropriate [79].

In an animal model of secondary hyperparathyroidism, the calcimimetic cinacalcet improved control of PTH levels and reduced parathyroid cell proliferation and gland hyperplasia [136]. A retrospective clinical study has shown that cinacalcet therapy significantly reduces the risk of surgical parathyroidectomy, fracture, and hospitalization for cardiovascular disease [55]. Treatment with cinacalcet was associated with favorable changes in the biochemical markers of bone formation (bone-specific alkaline phosphatase) and resorption (serum N-telopeptide), as well as improved bone turnover parameters. In a prospective observational study, hemodialysis patients treated with cinacalcet in addition to the traditional treatment of phosphate binders and vitamin D were compared to controls on traditional treatment and found to have a significant reduction in fractures, which is consistent with an improvement in high bone turnover and increased bone mineral density and strength in response to the calcimimetic [14]. In this observational study, the combination of cinacalcet and vitamin D sterols was associated with a significant survival benefit.

A prospective, multicenter, randomized, double-blind, placebo-controlled study designed to assess the effects of cinacalcet on mortality and cardiovascular morbidity in subjects on dialysis with CKD (EVOLVE study) [52] is currently underway. A recent study demonstrated that consistent control of PTH, serum Ca, and P in patients beginning hemodialysis was a strong predictor of overall survival over at least 2 years [56]. A reasonable approach to the control of PTH, Ca, and P is to use calcimimetics to lower PTH, activated vitamin to replace the missing hormone, and Ca-free phosphate binders to prevent phosphate accumulation.

References

1. Alem AM, Sherrard DJ, Gillen DL, Weiss NS, Beresford SA, Heckbert SR, Wong C, Stehman-Breen C. Increased risk of hip fracture among patients with end-stage renal disease. Kidney Int. 2000;58:396–9.
2. Barreto DV, Fd B, de Carvalho AB, Cuppari L, Draibe SA, Dalboni MA, Moyses RM, Neves KR, Jorgetti V, Miname M, Santos RD, Canziani ME. Phosphate binder impact on bone remodeling and coronary calcification – results from the BRiC study. Nephron Clin Pract. 2008;110:c273–283283.
3. Barzel US. The role of bone in acid base metabolism. In: Barzel US, editor. Osteoporosis. New York: Grune and Stratton; 1970. p. 199.
4. Barzel US. Osteoporosis II: an overview. In: Barzel US, editor. Osteoporosis II. New York: Grune and Stratton; 1976. p. 1.
5. Barzel US. The skeleton as an ion exchange system: Implications for the role of acid–base imbalance in the genesis of osteoporosis. J Bone Miner Res. 1995;10:1431–6.
6. Beck N, Webster SK. Effects of acute metabolic acidosis on parathyroid hormone action and calcium mobilization. Am J Physiol. 1976;230:127–31.
7. Bergwitz C, Juppner H. Regulation of phosphate homeostasis by PTH, vitamin D, and FGF23. Annu Rev Med. 2010;61:91–104.
8. Bettice JA. Skeletal carbon dioxide stores during metabolic acidosis. Am J Physiol (Renal Fluid Electrolyte Physiol 16). 1984;247:F326–30.
9. Bettice JA, Gamble Jr JL. Skeletal buffering of acute metabolic acidosis. Am J Physiol. 1975;229:1618–24.
10. Bishop MC, Ledingham JG. Alkali treatment of renal osteodystrophy. Br Med J. 1972;4:529.
11. Block GA, Hulbert-Shearon TE, Levin NW, Port FK. Association of serum phosphorus and calcium x phosphate product with mortality risk in chronic hemodialysis patients: a national study. Am J Kidney Dis. 1998;31:607–17.

12. Block GA, Klassen PS, Lazarus JM, Ofsthun N, Lowrie EG, Chertow GM. Mineral metabolism, mortality, and morbidity in maintenance hemodialysis. J Am Soc Nephrol. 2004;15:2208–18.
13. Block GA, Spiegel DM, Erlich J, Mehta R, Lindbergh J, Dreisbach A, Raggi P. Effects of sevelamer and calcium on coronary artery calcification in patients new to hemodialysis. Kidney Int. 2005;68:1815–24.
14. Block GA, Zaun D, Smits G, Persky M, Brillhart S, Nieman K, Liu J, St Peter WL. Cinacalcet hydrochloride treatment significantly improves all-cause and cardiovascular survival in a large cohort of hemodialysis patients. Kidney Int. 2010;78:578–89.
15. Brown EM. Clinical lessons from the calcium-sensing receptor. Nat Clin Pract Endocrinol Metab. 2007; 3:122–33.
16. Brown EM. Clinical utility of calcimimetics targeting the extracellular calcium-sensing receptor (CaSR). Biochem Pharmacol. 2010;80:297–307.
17. Bushinsky DA. Net proton influx into bone during metabolic, but not respiratory, acidosis. Am J Physiol (Renal Fluid Electrolyte Physiol 23). 1988;254: F306–10.
18. Bushinsky DA. Net calcium efflux from live bone during chronic metabolic, but not respiratory, acidosis. Am J Physiol (Renal Fluid Electrolyte Physiol 25). 1989;256:F836–42.
19. Bushinsky DA. Metabolic acidosis. In: Jacobson HR, Striker GE, Klahr S, editors. The principles and practice of nephrology. St. Louis: Mosby; 1995. p. 924–32.
20. Bushinsky DA. Stimulated osteoclastic and suppressed osteoblastic activity in metabolic but not respiratory acidosis. Am J Physiol Cell Physiol. 1995;268:C80–8.
21. Bushinsky DA. The contribution of acidosis to renal osteodystrophy. Kidney Int. 1995;47:1816–32.
22. Bushinsky DA. Metabolic alkalosis decreases bone calcium efflux by suppressing osteoclasts and stimulating osteoblasts. Am J Physiol (Renal Fluid Electrolyte Physiol 40). 1996;271:F216–22.
23. Bushinsky DA. Bone disease in moderate renal failure: cause, nature and prevention. Annu Rev Med. 1997; 48:167–76.
24. Bushinsky DA. Renal osteodystrophy. Philadelphia: Lippincott-Raven; 1998. p. 1–514.
25. Bushinsky DA. Acid–base imbalance and the skeleton. Eur J Nutr. 2001;40:238–44.
26. Bushinsky DA. Acid–base balance and bone health. In: Holick MF, Dawson-Hughes B, editors. Nutrition and bone health. Totowa: Humana Press, Inc.; 2004. p. 279–304.
27. Bushinsky DA. Disorders of calcium and phosphorus homeostasis. In: Greenberg A, editor. Primer on kidney diseases. 4th ed. San Diego: Academic; 2005. p. 120–30.
28. Bushinsky DA, Chabala JM, Gavrilov KL, Levi-Setti R. Effects of *in vivo* metabolic acidosis on midcortical bone ion composition. Am J Physiol Renal Physiol. 1999;277:F813–9.
29. Bushinsky DA, Chabala JM, Levi-Setti R. Ion microprobe analysis of mouse calvariae in vitro: evidence for a "bone membrane". Am J Physiol Endocrinol Metab. 1989;256:E152–8.
30. Bushinsky DA, Gavrilov K, Chabala JM, Featherstone JDB, Levi-Setti R. Effect of metabolic acidosis on the potassium content of bone. J Bone Miner Res. 1997;12:1664–71.
31. Bushinsky DA, Gavrilov K, Stathopoulos VM, Krieger NS, Chabala JM, Levi-Setti R. Effects of osteoclastic resorption on bone surface ion composition. Am J Physiol Cell Physiol. 1996;271: C1025–31.
32. Bushinsky DA, Goldring JM, Coe FL. Cellular contribution to pH-mediated calcium flux in neonatal mouse calvariae. Am J Physiol (Renal Fluid Electrolyte Physiol 17). 1985;248:F785–9.
33. Bushinsky DA, Krieger NS, Geisser DI, Grossman EB, Coe FL. Effects of pH on bone calcium and proton fluxes in vitro. Am J Physiol (Renal Fluid Electrolyte Physiol 14). 1983;245:F204–9.
34. Bushinsky DA, Lam BC, Nespeca R, Sessler NE, Grynpas MD. Decreased bone carbonate content in response to metabolic, but not respiratory, acidosis. Am J Physiol (Renal Fluid Electrolyte Physiol 34). 1993;265:F530–6.
35. Bushinsky DA, Lechleider RJ. Mechanism of proton-induced bone calcium release: calcium carbonate-dissolution. Am J Physiol (Renal Fluid Electrolyte Physiol 22). 1987;253:F998–1005.
36. Bushinsky DA, Levi-Setti R, Coe FL. Ion microprobe determination of bone surface elements: effects of reduced medium pH. Am J Physiol (Renal Fluid Electrolyte Physiol 19). 1986;250:F1090–7.
37. Bushinsky DA, Nilsson EL. Additive effects of acidosis and parathyroid hormone on mouse osteoblastic and osteoclastic function. Am J Physiol Cell Physiol. 1995;269:C1364–70.
38. Bushinsky DA, Parker WR, Alexander KM, Krieger NS. Metabolic, but not respiratory, acidosis increases bone PGE_2 levels and calcium release. Am J Physiol (Renal Fluid Electrolyte Physiol). 2001;281: F1058–66.
39. Bushinsky DA, Sessler NE. Critical role of bicarbonate in calcium release from bone. Am J Physiol (Renal Fluid Electrolyte Physiol 32). 1992;263: F510–5.
40. Bushinsky DA, Sessler NE, Glena RE, Featherstone JDB. Proton-induced physicochemical calcium release from ceramic apatite disks. J Bone Miner Res. 1994;9:213–20.
41. Bushinsky DA, Sessler NE, Krieger NS. Greater unidirectional calcium efflux from bone during metabolic, compared with respiratory, acidosis. Am J Physiol (Renal Fluid Electrolyte Physiol 31). 1992; 262:F425–31.
42. Bushinsky DA, Smith SB, Gavrilov KL, Gavrilov LF, Levi-Setti R. Chronic acidosis-induced alteration in bone bicarbonate and phosphate. Am J Physiol Renal Physiol. 2003;285:F532–9.

43. Bushinsky DA, Smith SB, Gavrilov KL, Gavrilov LF, Li J, Levi-Setti R. Acute acidosis-induced alteration in bone bicarbonate and phosphate. Am J Physiol Renal Physiol. 2002;283:F1091–7.
44. Bushinsky DA, Wolbach W, Sessler NE, Mogilevsky R, Levi-Setti R. Physicochemical effects of acidosis on bone calcium flux and surface ion composition. J Bone Miner Res. 1993;8:93–102.
45. Bushinsky DA. Acidosis and bone. In: Burckhardt P, Dawson-Hughes B, Weaver CM, editors. Nutritional influences on bone health. 1st ed. London: Springer; 2010. p. 161–7.
46. Bushinsky DA. Acidosis and renal bone disease. In: Olgaard K, Salusky IB, Silver J, editors. The spectrum of mineral and bone disorders in chronic kidney disease. 2nd ed. New York: Oxford University Press; 2010. p. 253–65.
47. Bushinsky DA. Contribution of intestine, bone, kidney, and dialysis to extracellular fluid calcium content. Clin J Am Soc Nephrol. 2010;5:S12–22.
48. Cantor TL. Lack of evidence for administering vitamin D analogs to kidney failure patients to improve survivability. Clin Nephrol. 2009;72:97–104.
49. Canzanello VJ, Bodvarsson M, Kraut JA, Johns CA, Slatopolsky E, Madias NE. Effect of chronic respiratory acidosis on urinary calcium excretion in the dog. Kidney Int. 1990;38:409–16.
50. Chabala JM, Levi-Setti R, Bushinsky DA. Alteration in surface ion composition of cultured bone during metabolic, but not respiratory, acidosis. Am J Physiol (Renal Fluid Electrolyte Physiol 30). 1991;261:F76–84.
51. Chertow GM, Burke SK, Raggi P. Sevelamer attenuates the progression of coronary and aortic calcification in hemodialysis patients. Kidney Int. 2002;62:245–52.
52. Chertow GM, Pupim LB, Block GA, Correa-Rotter R, Drueke TB, Floege J, Goodman WG, London GM, Mahaffey KW, Moe SM, Wheeler DC, Albizem M, Olson K, Klassen P, Parfrey P. Evaluation of cinacalcet therapy to lower cardiovascular events (EVOLVE): rationale and design overview. Clin J Am Soc Nephrol. 2007;2:898–905.
53. Cochran M, Wilkinson R. Effect of correction of metabolic acidosis on bone mineralization rates in patients with renal osteomalacia. Nephron. 1975;15:98–110.
54. Connor A. Novel therapeutic agents and strategies for the management of chronic kidney disease mineral and bone disorder. Postgrad Med J. 2009;85:274–9.
55. Cunningham J, Danese M, Olson K, Klassen P, Chertow GM. Effects of the calcimimetic cinacalcet HCl on cardiovascular disease, fracture, and health-related quality of life in secondary hyperparathyroidism. Kidney Int. 2005;68:1793–800.
56. Danese MD, Belozeroff V, Smirnakis K, Rothman KJ. Consistent control of mineral and bone disorder in incident hemodialysis patients. Clin J Am Soc Nephrol. 2008;3:1423–9.
57. Domrongkitchaiporn S, Pongsakul C, Stitchantrakul W, Sirikulchayanonta V, Ongphiphadhanakul B, Radinahamed P, Karnsombut P, Kunkitti N, Ruang-raksa C, Rajatanavin R. Bone mineral density and histology in distal renal tubular acidosis. Kidney Int. 2001;59:1086–93.
58. Domrongkitchaiporn S, Pongskul C, Sirikulchayanonta V, Stitchantrakul W, Leeprasert V, Ongphiphadhanakul B, Radinahamed P, Rajatanavin R. Bone histology and bone mineral density after correction of acidosis in distal renal tubular acidosis. Kidney Int. 2002;62:2160–6.
59. Drueke TB. Klotho, FGF23, and FGF receptors in chronic kidney disease: a yin-yang situation? Kidney Int. 2010;78:1057–60.
60. Elder G. Pathophysiology and recent advances in the management of renal osteodystrophy. J Bone Miner Res. 2002;17:2094–105.
61. Fenton TR, Eliasziw M, Lyon AW, Tough SC, Hanley DA. Meta-analysis of the quantity of calcium excretion associated with the net acid excretion of the modern diet under the acid-ash diet hypothesis. Am J Clin Nutr. 2008;88:1159–66.
62. Fenton TR, Lyon AW, Eliasziw M, Tough SC, Hanley DA. Meta-analysis of the effect of the acid-ash hypothesis of osteoporosis on calcium balance. J Bone Miner Res. 2009;24(11):1835–40.
63. Frassetto L, JrRC M, Sebastian A. Long-term persistence of the urine calcium-lowering effect of potassium bicarbonate in postmenopausal women. J Clin Endocrinol Metab. 2005;90:831–4.
64. Frassetto L, Sebastian A. Age and systemic acid–base equilibrium: analysis of published data. J Gerontol A Biol Sci Med Sci. 1996;51:B91–9.
65. Frassetto LA, Morris Jr RC, Sebastian A. Effect of age on blood acid–base composition in adult humans: role of age-related renal functional decline. Am J Physiol (Renal Fluid Electrolyte Physiol 40). 1996;271:F1114–22.
66. Frick KK, Bushinsky DA. Chronic metabolic acidosis reversibly inhibits extracellular matrix gene expression in mouse osteoblasts. Am J Physiol Renal Physiol. 1998;275:F840–7.
67. Frick KK, Bushinsky DA. In vitro metabolic and respiratory acidosis selectively inhibit osteoblastic matrix gene expression. Am J Physiol Renal Physiol. 1999;277:F750–5.
68. Frick KK, Bushinsky DA. Metabolic acidosis stimulates RANK ligand RNA expression in bone through a cyclooxygenase dependent mechanism. J Bone Miner Res. 2003;18:1317–25.
69. Frick KK, Jiang L, Bushinsky DA. Acute metabolic acidosis inhibits the induction of osteoblastic *egr*-1 and type 1 collagen. Am J Physiol Cell Physiol. 1997;272:C1450–6.
70. Frick KK, LaPlante K, Bushinsky DA. RANK ligand and TNF-α mediate acid-induced bone calcium efflux in vitro. Am J Physiol Renal Physiol. 2005;289:F1005–11.
71. Frick KK, Krieger NS, Nehrke K, Bushinsky DA. Metabolic acidosis increases intracellular calcium in bone cells through activation of the proton receptor OGR1. J Bone Miner Res. 2009;24:305–13.

72. Goodman AD, Lemann Jr J, Lennon EJ, Relman AS. Production, excretion, and net balance of fixed acid in patients with renal acidosis. J Clin Invest. 1965;44: 495–506.
73. Gutiérrez OM, Mannstadt M, Isakova T, Rauh-Hain JA, Tamez H, Shah A, Smith K, Lee H, Thadhani R, Jüppner H, Wolf M. Fibroblast growth factor 23 and mortality among patients undergoing hemodialysis. N Engl J Med. 2008;359:584–92.
74. Holick MF. Resurrection of vitamin D deficiency and rickets. J Clin Invest. 2006;116:2062–72.
75. Institute of Medicine (IOM). Dietary reference intakes for calcium and vitamin D. Washington, D.C.: National Academies Press; 2010.
76. Kalantar-Zadeh K, Kuwae N, Regidor DL, Kovesdy CP, Kilpatrick RD, Shinaberger CS, McAllister CJ, Budoff MJ, Salusky IB, Kopple JD. Survival predictability of time-varying indicators of bone disease in maintenance hemodialysis patients. Kidney Int. 2006;70:771–80.
77. Kaneko TM, Foley RN, Gilbertson DT, Collins AJ. Clinical epidemiology of long-bone fracture in patients receiving hemodialysis. Clin Orthop Relat Res. 2007;457:188–93.
78. Kaye M, Frueth AJ, Silverman M. A study of vertebral bone powder from patients with chronic renal failure. J Clin Invest. 1970;49:442–53.
79. Kidney Disease: Improving Global Outcomes CKD-MBD work group. KDIGO clinical practice guideline for the diagnosis, evaluation, prevention and treatment of Chronic Kidney-Disease-Mineral Bone Disorder (CKD-MBD). Kidney Int. 2009;79:S1–130.
80. Kraut JA, Kurtz I. Metabolic acidosis of CKD: diagnosis, clinical characteristics, and treatment. Am J Kidney Dis. 2005;45:978–93.
81. Kraut JA, Madias NE. Metabolic acidosis: pathophysiology, diagnosis and management. Nat Rev Nephrol. 2010;6:274–85.
82. Krieger NS, Frick KK, Bushinsky DA. Cortisol inhibits acid-induced bone resorption in vitro. J Am Soc Nephrol. 2002;13:2534–9.
83. Krieger NS, Hefley TJ. Differential effects of parathyroid hormone on protein phosphorylation in two osteoblast-like cell populations isolated from neonatal mouse calvaria. Calcif Tissue Int. 1989;44:192–9.
84. Krieger NS, Parker WR, Alexander KM, Bushinsky DA. Prostaglandins regulate acid-induced cell-mediated bone resorption. Am J Physiol Renal Physiol. 2000; 279:F1077–82.
85. Krieger NS, Sessler NE, Bushinsky DA. Acidosis inhibits osteoblastic and stimulates osteoclastic activity in vitro. Am J Physiol (Renal Fluid Electrolyte Physiol 31). 1992;262:F442–8.
86. Krieger NS, Frick KK, LaPlante SK, Michalenka A, Bushinsky DA. Regulation of COX-2 mediates acid-induced bone calcium efflux in vitro. J Bone Miner Res. 2007;22:907–17.
87. Kurtz I, Maher T, Hulter HN, Schambelan M, Sebastian A. Effect of diet on plasma acid–base composition in normal humans. Kidney Int. 1983;24: 670–80.
88. Lau K, Rodriquez Nichols F, Tannen RL. Renal excretion of divalent ions in response to chronic acidosis: evidence that systemic pH is not the controlling variable. J Lab Clin Med. 1987;109:27–33.
89. Lefebvre A, de Vernejoul MC, Gueris J, Goldfarb B, Graulet AM, Morieux C. Optimal correction of acidosis changes progression of dialysis osteodystrophy. Kidney Int. 1989;36:1112–8.
90. Lemann Jr J. The urinary excretion of calcium, magnesium and phosphorus. In: Favus MJ, editor. Primer on the metabolic bone diseases and disorders of mineral metabolism. Kelseyville: American Society for Bone and Mineral Research; 1990. p. 36–9.
91. Lemann Jr J, Gray RW, Pleuss JA. Potassium bicarbonate, but not sodium bicarbonate, reduces urinary calcium excretion and improves calcium balance in healthy men. Kidney Int. 1989;35:688–95.
92. Lemann Jr J, Adams ND, Wilz DR, Brenes LG. Acid and mineral balances and bone in familial proximal renal tubular acidosis. Kidney Int. 2000;58: 1267–77.
93. Lemann Jr J, Bushinsky DA, Hamm LL. Bone buffering of acid and base in humans. Am J Physiol Renal Physiol. 2003;285:F811–32.
94. Levin A, Bakris GL, Molitch M, Smulders M, Tian J, Williams LA, Andress DL. Prevalence of abnormal serum vitamin D, PTH, calcium, and phosphorus in patients with chronic kidney disease: results of the study to evaluate early kidney disease. Kidney Int. 2006;71:31–8.
95. Litzow JR, Lemann Jr J, Lennon EJ. The effect of treatment of acidosis on calcium balance in patients with chronic azotemic renal disease. J Clin Invest. 1967;46:280–6.
96. Ludwig MG, Vanek M, Gueirine D, Gasser JA, Jones CE, Junker U, Hofstetter H, Wolf RM, Seuwen K. Proton-sensing G-protein-coupled receptors. Nature. 2003;425:93–8.
97. McSherry E. Acidosis and growth in nonuremic renal disease. Kidney Int. 1978;14:349–54.
98. Mitch WE. Metabolic and clinical consequences of metabolic acidosis. J Nephrol. 2006;19 suppl 9:S70–7575.
99. Mittalhenkle A, Gillen DL, Steigbigel RT. Increased risk of mortality associated with hip fracture in the dialysis population. Am J Kidney Dis. 2004;44: 672–9.
100. Miyazaki Y, Setoguchi M, Yoshida S, Higuchi Y, Akizuki S, Yamamoto S. The mouse osteopontin gene. Expression in monocytic lineages and complete nucleotide sequence. J Biol Chem. 1990;265: 14432–8.
101. Mora Palma FJ, Ellis HA, Cook DB, Dewar JH, Ward MK, Wilkinson R, Kerr DNS. Osteomalacia in patients with chronic renal failure before dialysis or transplantation. Q J Med. 1983;52:332–48.
102. National Kidney Foundation. K/DOQI clinical practice guidelines for bone metabolism and disease in chronic kidney disease. Am J Kidney Dis. 2003; 42:S1–201.

103. Neuman WF, Neuman MW. The chemical dynamics of bone mineral. Chicago: University Chicago Press; 1958.
104. Ott SM. Review article: bone density in patients with chronic kidney disease stages 4–5. Nephrology (Carlton). 2009;14:395–403.
105. Palmer SC, McGregor DO, Macaskill P, Craig JC, Elder GJ, Strippoli GF. Meta-analysis: vitamin D compounds in chronic kidney disease. Ann Intern Med. 2007;147:840–53.
106. Pellegrino ED, Blitz RM. The composition of human bone in uremia. Medicine. 1965;44:397–418.
107. Pellegrino ED, Blitz RM, Letteri JM. Interrelationships of carbonate, phosphate, monohydrogen phosphate, calcium, magnesium, and sodium in uraemic bone: comparison of dialyzed and non-dialyzed patients. Clin Sci Mol Med. 1977;53:307–16.
108. Pilbeam CC, Kawaguchi H, Hakeda Y, Voznesensky O, Alander CB, Raisz LG. Differential regulation of the inducible and constitutive prostaglandin endoperoxide synthase in osteoblastic MC3T3-E1 cells. J Biol Chem. 1993;268:25643–9.
109. Qazi RA, Martin KJ. Vitamin D in kidney disease: pathophysiology and the utility of treatment. Endocrinol Metab Clin North Am. 2010;39:355–63.
110. Quarles DL. Endocrine functions of bone in mineral metabolism regulation. J Clin Invest. 2009;118: 3820–8.
111. Qunibi W, Moustafa M, Muenz LR, He DY, Kessler PD, Diaz-Buxo JA, Budoff M. A 1-year randomized trial of calcium acetate versus sevelamer on progression of coronary artery calcification in hemodialysis patients with comparable lipid control: the calcium acetate Renagel evaluation-2 (CARE-2) study. Am J Kidney Dis. 2008;51:952–65.
112. Raisz LG. Physiologic and pathologic roles of prostaglandins and other eicosanoids in bone metabolism. J Nutr. 1995;125:2024S–7.
113. Raisz LG. Prostaglandins and bone: physiology and pathophysiology. Osteoarthritis Cartilage. 1999;7: 419–21.
114. Raisz LG, Fall PM, Petersen DN, Lichtler A, Kream BE. Prostaglandin E_2 inhibits alpha 1(1) procollagen gene transcription and promoter activity in the immortalized rat osteoblastic clonal cell line Py1a. Mol Endocrinol. 1993;7:17–22.
115. Rizzoli R, Bonjour JP. Dietary protein and bone health. J Bone Miner Res. 2004;19:527–31.
116. Sakhaee K, Nicar M, Hill K, Pak CY. Contrasting effects of potassium citrate and sodium citrate therapies on urinary chemistries and crystallization of stone-forming salts. Kidney Int. 1983;24:348–52.
117. Schaefer KE, Pasquale S, Messier AA, Shea M. Phasic changes in bone CO_2 fractions, calcium, and phosphorus during chronic hypercapnia. J Appl Physiol. 1980;48:802–11.
118. Schwartz WB, Hall III PW, Hays RM, Relman AS. On the mechanism of acidosis in chronic renal disease. J Clin Invest. 1959;38:39–52.
119. Schwartz WB, Relman AS. Acidosis in renal disease. N Eng J Med. 1957;256:1184–6.
120. Sebastian A, Harris ST, Ottaway JH, Todd KM, Morris Jr RC. Improved mineral balance and skeletal metabolism in postmenopausal women treated with potassium bicarbonate. N Engl J Med. 1994;330: 1776–81.
121. Shoben AB, Rudser KD, de Boer IH, Young B, Kestenbaum B. Association of oral calcitriol with improved survival in nondialyzed CKD. J Am Soc Nephrol. 2008;19:1613–9.
122. Smith WL. Prostanoid biosynthesis and mechanisms of action. Am J Physiol. 1992;263:F181–91.
123. Sprague SM, Krieger NS, Bushinsky DA. Aluminum inhibits bone nodule formation and calcification in vitro. Am J Physiol (Renal Fluid Electrolyte Physiol 33). 1993;264:F882–90.
124. Sprague SM, Krieger NS, Bushinsky DA. Greater inhibition of in vitro bone mineralization with metabolic than respiratory acidosis. Kidney Int. 1994;46: 1199–206.
125. St Peter WL, Li S, Liu J, Gilbertson DT, Arneson TJ, Collins AJ. Effects of monthly dose and regular dosing of intravenous active vitamin D use on mortality among patients undergoing hemodialysis. Pharmacotherapy. 2009;29:154–64.
126. Stein GS, Lian JB, Stein JL, van Wijnen AJ, Montecino M. Transcriptional control of osteoblast growth and differentiation (Review). Physiol Rev. 1996;76:593–629.
127. Sugiura S, Inaguma D, Kitagawa A, Murata M, Kamimura Y, Sendo S, Hamaguchi K, Nagaya H, Tatematsu M, Kurata K, Yuzawa Y, Matsuo S. Administration of alfacalcidol for patients with predialysis chronic kidney disease may reduce cardiovascular disease events. Clin Exp Nephrol. 2010;14:43–50.
128. Suki WN, Zabaneh R, Cangiano JL, Reed J, Fischer D, Garrett L, Ling BN, Chasan-Taber S, Dillon MA, Blair AT, Burke SK. Effects of sevelamer and calcium-based phosphate binders on mortality in hemodialysis patients. Kidney Int. 2007;72:1130–7.
129. Takahashi Y, Tanaka A, Nakamura T, Fukuwatari T, Shibata K, Shimada N, Ebihara I, Koide H. Nicotinamide suppresses hyperphosphatemia in hemodialysis patients. Kidney Int. 2004;65: 1099–104.
130. Teng M, Wolf M, Lowrie E, Ofsthun N, Lazarus JM, Thadhani R. Survival of patients undergoing hemodialysis with paricalcitol or calcitriol therapy. N Engl J Med. 2003;349:446–56.
131. Teng M, Wolf M, Ofsthun MN, Lazarus JM, Hernan MA, Camargo Jr CA, Thadhani R. Activated injectable vitamin D and hemodialysis survival: a historical cohort study. J Am Soc Nephrol. 2005;16:1115–25.
132. Tentori F, Hunt WC, Stidley CA, Rohrscheib MR, Bedrick EJ, Meyer KB, Johnson HK, Zager PG. Mortality risk among hemodialysis patients receiving different vitamin D analogs. Kidney Int. 2006;70:1858–65.

133. Tentori F, Albert JM, Young EW, Blayney MJ, Robinson BM, Pisoni RL, Akiba T, Greenwood RN, Kimata N, Levin NW, Piera LM, Saran R, Wolfe RA, Port FK. The survival advantage for haemodialysis patients taking vitamin D is questioned: findings from the dialysis outcomes and practice patterns study. Nephrol Dial Transplant. 2009;24:963–72.
134. Tomura H, Mogi C, Sato K, Okajima F. Proton-sensing and lysolipid-sensitive G-protein-coupled receptors: a novel type of multi-functional receptors. Cell Signal. 2005;17:1466–76.
135. Uhlig K, Berns JS, Kestenbaum B, Kumar R, Leonard MB, Martin KJ, Sprague SM, Goldfarb S. KDOQI US commentary on the 2009 KDIGO clinical practice guideline for the diagnosis, evaluation, and treatment of CKD-mineral and bone disorder (CKD-MBD). Am J Kidney Dis. 2010;55: 773–99.
136. Wada M, Nagano N, Furuya Y, Chin J, Nemeth EF, Fox J. Calcimimetic NPS R-568 prevents parathyroid hyperplasia in rats with severe secondary hyperparathyroidism. Kidney Int. 2000;57:50–8.
137. Widdowson EM, Dickerson JWT. Chemical composition of the body. In: Comar CL, Bronner F, editors. Mineral metabolism. New York: Academic Press, Inc.; 1964. p. 1–247.

Wasting Diseases and Metabolic Impact on Bone: Emerging Therapeutics and Treatment Options

11

Linda A. DiMeglio

Keywords
Wasting disorders • Muscle function • Bone strength • Muscular dystrophy
Inflammatory bowel disease • HIV • Cystic fibrosis • Cerebral palsy

11.1 Introduction

Many chronic diseases have adverse bone effects, often arising both from the disease process and from the pharmacologic therapies employed as treatments. Persons with wasting disorders have a particularly high risk of bone disease, due to their direct impact on lean muscle mass, which is both a key determinant of childhood bone accrual and is important for the maintenance of bone mineral density (BMD) and bone mineral content (BMC) in adults.

The negative impact of wasting diseases on the skeleton is particularly pronounced in pediatric populations. As children grow, they typically gain muscle mass, increase body weight, and increase muscle strength. This growth leads to the development of skeletons with sufficient strength to resist mechanical failure under conditions of normal physiologic loading. Disruptions of muscle function with mechanical unloading diminish bone growth and mineral accrual and maintenance [34]. Skeletal immobilization is especially deleterious; bone loss is seen even in able-bodied persons subjected to periods of prolonged bed rest [31].

Nearly 80% of bone strength is determined by the amount of bone [96]. Bone mass is highly related to muscle mass because skeletal strength increases primarily as an adaptation to the strains of routinely applied mechanical loads [41]. Total body BMC is more strongly associated with lean mass than with either total mass or fat mass [65]. Osteocytes and osteoblasts are mechanoresponsive cells of the mesenchymal lineage, adapting in vivo to changes in strain as well as to strain-generated changes in the surrounding fluid. Continued mechanical strains are important for bone accrual to occur during childhood. The matching of bone capacity to the perceived mechanical needs of the individual continues into adulthood. Muscle also produces a variety of factors (known as "myokines") that are released in response to physical activity and have beneficial paracrine and/or endocrine effects, including induction of lipolysis and angiogenesis [80].

Not all of the adverse effects on bone of the wasting diseases are mediated through the mechanostat system. Some wasting disorders (including cystic fibrosis and the inflammatory bowel diseases)

L.A. DiMeglio, M.D., M.P.H.
Department of Pediatrics,
Indiana University School of Medicine,
705 Riley Hospital Drive, Indianapolis, IN 46202, USA
e-mail: dimeglio@iupui.edu

F. Bronner et al. (eds.), *Bone-Metabolic Functions and Modulators*, Topics in Bone Biology,
DOI 10.1007/978-1-4471-2745-1_11, © Springer-Verlag London 2012

also are associated with chronic infection and/or inflammation. Cytokines typically affect bone metabolism by decreasing bone formation and increasing bone resorption [72]. Several wasting disorders (including the muscular dystrophies, cystic fibrosis, and inflammatory bowel disease) are treated with glucocorticoids, which adversely affect bones by a variety of complex, incompletely understood mechanisms. Their primary effect is to reduce bone formation by decreasing osteoblast number and activity and suppressing insulin-like growth factor (IGF)-1. Glucocorticoids also decrease sex hormone production, inhibit intestinal calcium absorption (by interfering with the action of 1,25-OH vitamin D), and increase renal tubular calcium excretion [2]. They also can induce secondary hyperparathyroidism and enhance interleukin (IL)-1-induced osteoclastic bone resorption. Glucocorticoid use results in a low bone turnover state with poor bone formation. Steroids tend to have the greatest adverse impact during the first few months of treatment and at sites with high amounts of trabecular bone (spine and ribs), rather than those sites with more cortical bone (long bones).

Decreases in bone mineralization often translate into osteoporosis and consequent skeletal fragility. The World Health Organization has defined osteoporosis as a "systemic skeletal disease characterized by low bone mass and microarchitectural deterioration of bone tissue, with a consequent increase in bone fragility and susceptibility to fracture" [107]. In adults, osteoporosis is defined by T-score comparisons to young adult normative data. The diagnosis of osteoporosis in children requires both a low Z-score (age and sex matched standard deviation score) and a significant fracture history [83]. Osteoporosis also can be accompanied by defective mineralization of newly formed osteoid, a condition known as osteomalacia. Both osteoporosis and osteomalacia lower BMD.

Regardless of the mechanisms, the adverse effects on bone in persons with wasting disorders increase the predisposition to fractures. Not only is the number of fractures increased but the mechanisms and distribution of fractures are dissimilar to those that occur in healthy individuals. In healthy children, the most common site for fracture is the forearm, which accounts for 80% or more of all fractures [27]. The fracture pattern in nonambulatory children with disabilities is very different, with >70% of fractures occurring in the legs and ~50% in the femurs [52]. In healthy individuals, the most common mechanisms for fractures involve falls and significant force or trauma. In persons with wasting disorders, fractures can occur with minimal force, such as that experienced during routine handling or physical therapy maneuvers. Children with chronic illnesses also are more likely to suffer from vertebral compression fractures than their healthy peers.

This chapter will briefly outline several of the most common wasting disorders (muscular dystrophy, human immunodeficiency virus (HIV), cystic fibrosis, inflammatory bowel disease, and cerebral palsy) and the impact each of these disorders has on bone health. Conventional and novel treatments for low bone mass related to these types of conditions then will be explored.

11.2 Muscular Dystrophy

The muscular dystrophies are multisystem disorders characterized by progressive and predictable loss of muscle mass and function [37]. Two major types occur: Duchenne (OMIM 310200) and Becker (OMIM 300376). Both forms are due to mutations in the gene encoding dystrophin and are inherited in an X-linked recessive manner. Duchenne muscular dystrophy (DMD) has a birth incidence of 1:3,500 boys [36]. Boys with DMD manifest proximal muscular weakness at 3–6 years of age. They lose the ability to ambulate by 6–12 years of age and generally die during the third decade of life from respiratory or cardiac failure.

Becker muscular dystrophy is less severe and less common (1:18,000 male births). Boys with Becker muscular dystrophy first demonstrate weakness at age 12 or later, lose the ability to walk during adolescence or later, and die in the fourth or fifth decade of life. There are fewer data on bone health in Becker muscular dystrophy than DMD; therefore, the remainder of this chapter will refer simply to DMD, with the understanding that the principles outlined can be applied to the later stages of Becker muscular dystrophy.

Persons with muscular dystrophy have low BMD for age, and this tends to worsen as they get older [97]. Although bone loss and/or failure to accrue bone are primarily due to the decrease in weight-bearing activities, repeated assessments demonstrate progressive decreases in BMD over time, even before striking impairments in ambulation occur [68]. This low BMD increases the incidence of spontaneous and low trauma fractures. The incidence of fractures in DMD has been reported to be as high as 44% in affected boys [68]. The most common fracture sites are the vertebrae and the legs. With time, these fractures can worsen the loss of mobility due to prolonged inactivity. Significant, progressive scoliosis also is common.

Corticosteroids are frequently being used as therapy in boys with DMD. Standard initial doses are 0.75 mg/kg/day of prednisone or 0.9 mg/kg/day of deflazacort [73]. Although corticosteroids are generally considered detrimental to bone health in most chronic diseases and steroids appear to suppress bone turnover in boys with DMD [97], steroid therapy does not seem to be adverse to bone health in DMD primarily because the steroids ameliorate some of the muscle wasting. Steroid treatment can prolong the period of independent ambulation by approximately 3 years, improving both muscle strength and function [64]. Even though steroid treatment is associated with a loss of "total body less head" BMC assessed by dual-energy x-ray absorptiometry (DXA), the retention of muscle function results in favorable increases both in subcranial bone area and in lumbar spine bone mineral apparent density (BMAD) [29]. Boys treated with steroids also have a lower incidence of scoliosis requiring surgical therapy than boys not on steroid therapy [11].

Guidelines for assessment and management of bone health in boys with DMD have been published and include measurements of bone mineral and vitamin D status, DXA assessments starting at age 3 years, and spine X-rays for scoliosis or back pain [18].

11.3 HIV

Human immunodeficiency virus (HIV) now affects 0.6% of the world's population. With the advent of increasingly effective antiretroviral therapy, HIV in Western nations increasingly is becoming a chronic disease, with dramatic declines in acute mortality rates. Recent estimates place the median survival time for young adults diagnosed with HIV as greater than 35 years, a figure that will likely continue to increase [71]. With this improvement in lifespan has come increasing awareness of the long-term complications of the disease and its therapies, including the adverse effects on bone health.

Low BMD is observed frequently in persons who are HIV-infected. Perinatally infected children (particularly boys) have lower BMD at the end of puberty than do their HIV-uninfected peers [61]. A recent meta-analysis demonstrated a 15% prevalence of osteoporosis and a 52% prevalence of osteopenia in HIV-infected adults [78]. These decreases in BMD appear to translate into increases in fracture rates. Even those HIV-infected individuals with normal BMD appear to be at increased risk of fracture. Population-based data suggest that young women infected with HIV have a higher likelihood of fragility fractures than do their HIV-negative peers (odds ratio 1.7) despite having normal BMD [82]. These data, coupled with the aging of the HIV-infected population, raise concerns of a possible fracture epidemic in persons living with HIV.

Risk factors for low BMD in persons with HIV are numerous and include the chronic HIV infection itself; acquired immunodeficiency syndrome (AIDS)-associated diseases such as AIDS wasting, hypogonadism, and renal disease; effects of various highly active antiretroviral therapies (HAART); as well as traditional osteoporosis risk factors, such as vitamin D deficiency, smoking, and alcohol use. Evidence that the HIV infection itself contributes to the bone loss includes data from an HIV-1 transgenic rat model that demonstrates increased osteoclastic bone resorption leading to lower BMD along with decreases in cortical and trabecular bone volume [102]. These data are supported by human data demonstrating high levels of bone turnover markers (N-telopeptide cross-links (NTX) and C-telopeptide cross-links (CTX)) in postmenopausal, HIV-infected women [111]. Very limited pediatric data suggest that low bone formation (assessed by osteocalcin) may be an initial sign of poor bone status in children with HIV [112].

11.4 Cystic Fibrosis

Cystic fibrosis (CF) (OMIM 219700) is a recessively inherited, chronic lung disease arising from mutations in the CF transmembrane conductance regulator (CFTR) protein. As survival improves for persons with CF, bone disease is an increasingly significant comorbidity, with manifestations that include low BMD, bone pain, kyphosis, and fractures. A variety of factors have been implicated for bone loss in this population, including overall malnutrition; vitamin D, vitamin K, and calcium deficiencies; chronic infection and inflammation; glucocorticoid treatment; hypogonadism; low physical activity and lean body mass (LBM); CF-related diabetes; and direct bone effects of CFTR mutations. Despite routine recommendations for supplementation, vitamin D deficiency, in particular, is prevalent in persons with CF. In an observational study of 81 relatively well-nourished pediatric CF patients with mild to moderate lung disease, 95% had 25-OH vitamin D levels below 75 nmol/l (30 ng/ml), and half had values less than 40 nmol/l (16 ng/ml) [44]. The majority of adults with CF also have 25-OH vitamin D levels less than 75 nmol/l [8].

Early diagnosis of CF-related bone disease is critical for effective prophylaxis and management. Diagnosis begins with DXA screening. Guidelines for care of persons with CF recommend DXA for all adults and for children over 8 years of age if they have risk factors for low BMD, including fracture, high glucocorticoid use, low body weight, delayed puberty, or low forced expiratory volume (FEV)-1 [8].

11.5 Inflammatory Bowel Disease

Crohn disease is an autoimmune, intestinal disorder that results in inflammation that is transmural (affecting the entire gut wall). Affected regions can be seen anywhere along the gastrointestinal tract but most commonly are located in the distal ileum and colon. Symptoms of Crohn disease include diarrhea, fever, abdominal pain, and anorexia. Persons with Crohn disease experience a chronic disease course, with intermittent exacerbations and remissions. Therapy consists of steroids followed by nonsteroidal immune modulating agents.

Metabolic bone disease is found in up to 80% of persons with Crohn disease. The cause of decreased bone mass in persons with Crohn disease is multifactorial and includes inflammation from the underlying disease, nutritional deficits (cachexia, poor absorption and utilization of nutrients, particularly calcium and vitamin D), growth and pubertal delays, deficits in lean body mass, and glucocorticoid therapy [43]. Inflammatory cytokines such as the interleukins IL-1α, IL-1β, IL-6, IL-11, IL-17, epidermal growth factor, prostaglandin E_2, tumor necrosis factor (TNF)-α, and TNF-β all have been shown to activate osteoclasts and increase bone resorption [14].

Persons with Crohn disease often have decreased BMC and BMD [33]. Bone formation is markedly suppressed, even at the time of diagnosis, leading to altered bone accrual. This failure of bone accrual appears to lead to an increased risk of fragility fractures, particularly vertebral and hip fractures [19, 93], although this does not manifest as a very high overall fracture rate in this population. Estimates place the risk of fracture at approximately one fracture per 100 patient years [13]. High-dose steroid therapy also adversely affects bones, although low-dose steroids may not impact bone as significantly in part because these agents also suppress inflammation. The glucocorticoid therapy used for Crohn disease can also lead to avascular necrosis of bones, particularly the hip, but also the shoulder, knee, and talus.

Limited data exist on the strategies designed to prevent bone loss in persons with Crohn disease. Overall, interventions to ameliorate bone loss in persons with Crohn disease focus on reducing the risk factors. Studies suggest that low body weight and body mass index (BMI) consistently are associated with low bone mass in persons with Crohn disease; therefore, optimizing nutrition is beneficial for bone health. Reducing or limiting the use of bone-compromising agents (such as systemic corticosteroids) by using topical steroid treatments (budesonide) or nonsteroid agents (such as infliximab) also can be helpful. Therapies for those with established bone loss are discussed below.

11.6 Cerebral Palsy/Immobilization Osteoporosis

Cerebral palsy (CP) is a static neurologic condition resulting from a congenital anomaly or in utero or postpartum insult to the developing brain. It is relatively common, affecting approximately 0.24% of children aged 3–10 years [66]. The motor disorders of CP generally limit or preclude the ability to ambulate. These moderate to severe functional limitations are classified using the gross motor function classification system (GMFCS). Children at GMFCS levels III, IV, and V are particularly susceptible to bone issues due to muscle disuse and decreased skeletal loading. Persons with CP also can have spasticity with joint contractures and subluxations.

The low BMD observed in CP patients is generally multifactorial and related to poor overall growth, reduced mobility, poor nutritional status, low 25-OH vitamin D levels, and use of anticonvulsant medications, which may directly impact bone or may accelerate vitamin D metabolism [55]. The frequency of poor BMD in children with moderate to severe CP increases with increasing age and increasing GMFCS scores. At 10 years of age, 95% of children with GMFCS of IV–V have DXA Z-scores of ≤–2.0 [51]. However, a direct correlation between DXA measures and risk of fracture in children with CP has not been demonstrated [75].

Poor bone mineralization can predispose to spontaneous fractures as well as fractures after minimal trauma. Prospective, longitudinal reports demonstrate annual fracture rates in children with CP of 5%, a rate more than twice that of healthy children [50]. Estimates are that annual costs from these fractures may reach $150 million dollars [63]. Many fractures in persons with CP occur at the femoral diaphyses; the tibiae are the second most common site. Fracture diagnoses are sometimes delayed, due to communication difficulties, neurosensory deficits, and possible decreases in pain perception [105]. Fractures can further limit mobility, leading to further disuse muscle wasting.

Other factors that contribute to poor bone development in children with CP include issues with nutritional intake, vitamin D deficiency, and anticonvulsant use [105].

11.7 Evaluation of Bone Status in Persons with Wasting Disorders

Prophylactic treatment of bone disease in persons with wasting disorders aims to prevent fracture, bony deformity, and bone pain. Early diagnosis is important for effective management. Evaluation for any child or adult with a wasting disorder suspected of having low BMD for age begins with a careful assessment of traditional risk factors for low bone mass. These include personal history of fractures, family history of osteoporosis or fractures, aging, menopause, smoking, poor calcium intake, poor vitamin D status (low intake and low sun exposure), overall malnutrition, and limited weight-bearing exercise.

The next step in any evaluation of suspected osteoporosis in a person with a wasting disorder is a targeted laboratory assessment, tailored according to the disease state and the differential diagnosis. In general, laboratory studies of mineral homeostasis (calcium, phosphorus, parathyroid hormone (PTH), urine calcium/creatinine ratio), renal function (creatinine), vitamin D status (25-OH vitamin D), and bone turnover (alkaline phosphatase, serum or urine NTX) are useful assessments.

The next step in the evaluation may require an assessment of bone mass and/or bone quality. The "gold standard" for bone assessment is bone biopsy. However, this procedure is invasive and often subjectively interpreted. Fortunately, there are several noninvasive methods available for BMD evaluation. Noninvasive quantitation of bone mass is important for several reasons. Accurate assessment of BMD allows quantification of the amount of bone deficiency; it also is important for following the treated or untreated individual longitudinally.

Evaluations of conventional radiographs are useful for bone assessment and can demonstrate osteopenia. Persons with wasting disorders may have thin cortices. However, X-rays are an insensitive means of examining bone mass, as BMD can decrease by 30–50% before bone loss can be appreciated [38].

Dual-energy X-ray absorptiometry (DXA) is, therefore, the most commonly used clinical tool for bone density measurements and can document the extent of low bone mass in persons with wasting disorders. The accuracy and reproducibility of DXA in persons with wasting disorders may be limited, however, by the inability of the patient to cooperate with the procedure (which involves lying still while the scanning arm acquires images), by uncontrolled movement, and/or by the presence of joint contractures, hip dysplasia, severe scoliosis, or metal implants. As a way to clinically measure BMD in a technically feasible manner, several centers are developing expertise using distal femur BMD measurements in persons with impaired mobility [52]. DXA interpretation must also take into account the size of the subject because DXA-acquired BMD measurements are strongly influenced by bone size, with smaller children having falsely low areal BMD (g/cm^2) despite a normal volumetric BMD (g/cm^3).

It is important to recognize that the magnitude of an intervention or treatment's effect on bone depends on the area of the skeleton that is being assessed. Trabecular bone, present in the lumbar spine and in the ends of long bones, is more metabolically active than cortical bone and therefore responds more rapidly to perturbations in bone status. It is also important to recognize that in patients with immobilization, spine BMD may not correlate well with BMD in the extremities [54].

11.8 Therapy of Bone Disease in Persons with Wasting Disorders

Therapy for each of the wasting conditions starts with amelioration of the primary disease, when possible. Improving body weight and muscle strength can readily improve BMD. Over the years, a number of different bone-specific therapies have been employed for bone disease in each of these disorders, with variable degrees of effectiveness. Approaches to management are outlined below.

11.8.1 Physical Activity

Physical activity, through mechanical loading, increases pediatric bone mineral acquisition primarily by augmenting bony modeling. Adolescent physical activity patterns may explain up to 22% of adult BMD variability. Exercise also is important for maintaining bone mass in adulthood. The best forms of exercise for bone formation and bone maintenance are not known. Whether the increases in BMD observed with interventions translate into increases in bone strength or are maintained after the training regimen attenuates also is unclear. It is also important to balance the need for exercise with the risk of fractures from overvigorous physical therapy.

Short-term, controlled activity intervention trials in children demonstrate gains in rates of bone mineral accrual if the activity is intense in nature [10]. These data are borne out in longitudinal studies that show that elite athletes who engage in intensive, weight-bearing activities during childhood have significantly greater volumetric BMD than do their peers [70]. Further evidence suggests that even very low-magnitude (<10 μstrain) mechanical signals, when induced at a high frequency (20–50 Hz), also stimulate bone activity. Such strains are continually present during more subtle physical activities such as active standing [104].

Few studies have examined the impact of exercise programs on bone in persons with wasting diseases. In DMD, although exercise has the potential to reduce muscle wasting, it also can injure the diseased skeletal muscle, and therefore, caution is necessary [20]. Exercise training has been employed as an anabolic therapy in persons with AIDS. Small studies have shown improvements in muscle strength and lean body mass after implementation of exercise programs including resistance training, cycling, and/or strength training. Although these improvements also likely benefit bone mass, studies have not yet explored this as an outcome [28].

There have been no randomized trials of effects of exercise on bone health in persons with CF, but several observational studies suggest associations between exercise and bone health [57]. Energy expenditure [16, 35], physical activity [25, 49], and exercise capacity [40] all have been positively related to BMD in persons with CF. Prospective, intervention studies are needed to establish the relationship between exercise and bone health in persons with CF and to determine the best forms and frequency of exercise for skeletal benefit [57].

A randomized study of a low-impact, increasing intensity exercise program in adults with Crohn disease showed significant improvements in BMD in those compliant with therapy, with a significant correlation between the number of exercise sessions completed and the magnitude of the BMD increase [87]. Exercise in persons with Crohn disease also is associated with improvements in quality of life measures [76].

There are limited studies of exercise in children with CP, even though poor mechanical loading is a primary reason for their increased fracture risk. A small 8-month study of upper body, lower body, and trunk exercises in children with CP showed increases in proximal femur and femoral neck estimated volumetric BMD [22]. In children with cerebral palsy, and in those with other central nervous system disorders, static standing equipment often is used in an attempt to improve bone and muscle health. Increasing standing time in these devices has been shown to improve lumbar spine BMD but not proximal tibial BMD, with the tibiae being a more relevant site for fracture in these children [21]. Dynamic standing frames also have been employed. It is important to note that the amount of weight borne by the skeleton when children with CP stand in frames is highly variable [56]. Studies on devices that allow children with CP to move from sitting to standing have shown benefits for functional muscle strength and bone health [69]. It is not known if bone development and prevention of bone resorption are better facilitated by direct loading of bone or by muscle activity [91].

11.8.2 Calcium

Adequate calcium intake, particularly during puberty, is an important determinant of final peak bone mass. Later in life, calcium is important for maintaining the accrued bone. Data suggest that children with higher calcium intake complete bone mineralization sooner than those with lower calcium intakes [1] and that higher calcium intake may accelerate the onset of pubertal maturation, helping to generate a higher peak bone mass [23]. However, calcium is a "threshold" nutrient; taking calcium beyond "sufficient" intake levels does not further augment bone mass [42]. Calcium consumption, particularly in the youth population, is declining as carbonated soft drinks and bottled water displace milk consumption. Calcium intake from dietary sources and supplements should supply at least the minimum recommended for age, ranging from 700 mg/day in children aged 1–3 years to 1,300 mg/day in adolescents [90]. The availability of ingested calcium also is impacted by the rates of intestinal calcium absorption and of urinary calcium excretion. Limited data suggest that physical activity and calcium intake are synergistic in promoting bone health.

Persons on glucocorticoids may have hypercalciuria accompanied by hyperoxaluria and may have a high risk of calcium oxalate stones. When urine calcium levels are elevated, a low oxalate diet or a thiazide diuretic to decrease urinary calcium excretion may be indicated [14]. Current recommendations call for persons with DMD to take in at least 750 mg of calcium daily, especially if on steroids [30].

Although calcium intake is important for bone mineral accrual, there have been no randomized controlled studies of calcium supplements in CF to date. The current recommendation is for intakes of 1,300–1,500 mg/day [8]. The rate of calcium deposition in bone in children with CF also appears to be low, contributing to low bone accrual. In a calcium kinetics analysis, calcium deposition in bone was found to be lower among a group of girls with CF compared to healthy children consuming comparable calcium intakes [92].

Limited data suggest fractional calcium absorption is normal in at least some individuals with stable Crohn disease [67]; however, persons with inflammatory bowel disease may still benefit from supplementation as, on average, they appear to ingest considerably less than the recommended amounts of dietary calcium [15].

Studies of calcium supplementation's effects on BMD in children with CP have not examined calcium itself but have used calcium in conjunction with other medications, such as vitamin D, growth hormone, and bisphosphonates [59].

11.8.3 Vitamin D

Vitamin D can be synthesized in the skin with ultraviolet B light exposure or absorbed from dietary sources. Recent guidelines recommended an allowance of vitamin D from diet and supplements for individuals aged 1–70 years of 600 international units (IU) per day. For infants, the recommended allowance is 400 IU/day and 800 IU/day for those over 70 [90]. The storage form of vitamin D, 25-OH vitamin D, is then synthesized in the liver from vitamin D. 25-OH vitamin D then is converted in the kidneys to the highly active form, 1,25-OH vitamin D. Low serum 25-OH vitamin D levels are common in persons with wasting diseases [74], who may ingest less than the recommended daily intake and also have decreases in sun exposure. Vitamin D supplementation can be achieved with either ergocalciferol (vitamin D_2) or cholecalciferol (vitamin D_3).

Vitamin D is essential for intestinal calcium absorption and skeletal mineralization. It also plays a role in improving muscle strength. By making more calcium available to the skeleton and increasing the mechanical stress on bones, vitamin D improves bone quality. Vitamin D has additional nonskeletal effects, including benefits to cardiovascular health, glucose homeostasis, and innate immunity.

Numerous studies have demonstrated correlations between low serum 25-OH vitamin D levels and fractures [89]. All individuals with wasting diseases should have serum 25-OH vitamin D concentrations measured [18]. Serum 25-OH vitamin D levels are the best indicator of overall vitamin D status because they reflect dietary intake, synthesis after sun exposure, and adipose stores of vitamin D. Supplementation should be given as needed to reach target levels of 75–150 nmol/l (30–60 ng/ml) [8]. Measurement of 1,25-OH vitamin D is not valuable when evaluating vitamin D status.

It is important to realize that in wasting disorders associated with malabsorption (Crohn disease, CF) large vitamin D doses may be needed to optimize serum 25-OH vitamin D concentrations [17], although therapy needs to be individualized and monitored. For persons with CF, intake of 400 IU of ergocalciferol by infants and 800 IU by individuals older than 1 year is currently recommended. However, the best vitamin D preparation and dose required to achieve these levels needs further research.

Low 25-OH vitamin D levels have been reported in boys with DMD [97], this may be due either to dietary deficiencies or poor sunlight exposure. Current recommendations call for 1,000 IU of vitamin D daily [30], particularly for boys on steroid therapy.

Vitamin D deficiency also has been associated with bone loss in persons with HIV [110]. A number of studies have reported a higher prevalence of vitamin D deficiency in HIV-positive individuals than in HIV-negative persons [98]. Black race, CD4 cell counts <200, current use of

HAART, and winter sampling all are significant risk factors. Nonnucleoside reverse transcriptase inhibitor use, particularly efavirenz, is specifically implicated, suggesting that particular antiretroviral therapies might influence bone turnover. No data on vitamin D status and fracture rates nor any studies of vitamin D therapy for bone disease in HIV have been yet reported.

Vitamin D has been given to children with CP in a number of studies but mostly to replace deficiencies in both control and intervention groups. One study has examined use of 1,25-OH vitamin D_3 (0.25 mcg/day) with calcium (500 mg/day) in a group of persons with nonambulatory CP; the intervention increased lumbar spine BMD [62].

11.8.4 Vitamin K

Vitamin K plays a key role in bone formation, promoting vitamin-D-induced osteoblast mineralization in vitro [106]. Vitamin K serves as an essential cofactor for posttranslational γ-carboxylation of the three osteocalcin glutamyl residues. Uncarboxylated and undercarboxylated osteocalcin has a greatly reduced affinity for hydroxyapatite calcium ions compared to carboxylated forms. Vitamin K is found naturally in dietary sources, including green vegetables and plant oils (vitamin K1) and dairy products (vitamin K2). Vitamin K2 also is synthesized by intestinal bacteria. Vitamin K (80 mcg/serving) is also a component of Viactiv® calcium soft chews, marketed for bone health.

Undercarboxylated osteocalcin measurement is a sensitive measure of vitamin K status. Vitamin K insufficiency is common in children and adults with wasting disorders associated with malabsorption. In a multicenter study of children and adolescents with CF, serum vitamin K levels were found to be low in 65% of patients, with 30% having undetectable levels [44]. Similar results were found in a study of 93 children with CF where 70% had suboptimal vitamin K levels [26]. High uncarboxylated osteocalcin levels reflecting vitamin K deficiency have been reported in individuals with CF [9, 39]. High levels of uncarboxylated osteocalcin also predicted lower lumbar spine BMD in a study of fourteen 8–12-year-old children with CF [39].

Vitamin K therapy may be useful in the wasting diseases. The current recommendation for individuals with CF is for a vitamin K supplement of 0.3–0.5 mg/day. Although literature on the appropriate dose to prevent vitamin K deficiency is limited, a study of 14 children with CF and pancreatic insufficiency supplemented with 1 mg or 5 mg of vitamin K daily showed that both doses restored normal serum vitamin K levels [32]. The efficacy of vitamin K supplementation for improving bone formation rates in children and adolescents with CF has been studied [77]. Twenty individuals aged 6–17 years were treated with a weekly 10 mg oral dose of vitamin K. Bone turnover markers were examined before and after therapy and compared with those in controls. Although BMD *Z*-scores did not improve with therapy, treated patients experienced an increase in serum levels of bone formation markers and a decrease in serum parathyroid hormone (PTH) levels, indicating a potential beneficial role.

Other than the data in CF, there are very few studies on vitamin K therapy for bone health in other wasting disorders. A single case report of an 8-year-old boy with CP treated with 15 mg of vitamin K daily for 8 months suggested improvements in tibial bone geometry that could translate to improvements in bone strength [99]. There are no published data on vitamin K for bone health in DMD, HIV, or Crohn disease. However, a second case report of vitamin K supplementation (10 mg/day for 6 weeks) in an astronaut on a 6 month space mission who demonstrated increases in the bone formation markers osteocalcin and bone-specific alkaline phosphatase suggested that vitamin K might counteract microgravity induced bone loss and could potentially have a anabolic role in immobilization or low-formation bone disorders [101]. Further investigation is warranted.

11.8.5 Parathyroid Hormone

As discussed in other chapters in this volume, PTH is an anabolic agent used for the treatment of low bone mass in adults. Although constant exposure to high levels of PTH increases bone resorption and leads to osteoporosis, intermittent, low-dose PTH stimulates osteoblastic cells. Two forms are available, teraparatide PTH [1–34] and full-length PTH [1–84] available in Europe. There is a black box warning advising against the use of PTH in pediatric populations. PTH doses are given daily subcutaneously, with a dose of 20 μg/day for teraparatide. PTH also augments IGF-1 synthesis, activates Wnt signaling, and inhibits sclerostin expression. PTH could have an advantage over other pharmacologic therapies in wasting disorders where the primary etiology of low bone mass is related to poor bone formation rather than high bone resorption, e.g., conditions with bone loss related to glucocorticoid use.

There are no published studies to date on the therapeutic use of PTH in DMD, HIV, CF, Crohn disease, or CP.

11.8.6 Bisphosphonates

Bisphosphonates are synthetic, stable analogues of pyrophosphate, in which a carbon replaces the oxygen that links the phosphates to give a "P-C-P" backbone [4]. This "P-C-P" both renders bisphosphonates resistant to enzymatic degradation and allows space for two (R1 and R2) side chain attachments [88]. R2 side chain variations affect the potency and therapeutic characteristics of the compounds, with introduction of nitrogen atoms (pamidronate, alendronate) particularly within a ring structure (zoledronic acid, risedronate), further increasing potency. In bone, bisphosphonates adsorb to hydroxyapatite crystals [4]. Once there, they inhibit osteoclasts from resorbing bone through mechanisms including preventing binding and activation, altering protein prenylation, increasing apoptosis, and limiting ruffled border development. Bisphosphonates also inhibit IL-6-mediated osteoclastogenesis. Bisphosphonate actions also may be partially mediated by osteoblast effects, such as stimulating an osteoblast-produced osteoclast inhibitory factor [85, 103]. At therapeutic doses, bisphosphonates primarily inhibit bone resorption; at higher doses, they also can inhibit bone mineralization. Choice of bisphosphonate for a given clinical indication depends on potency differences, the cost and availability of a particular compound, and prior experiences/labeling for that drug in a given patient population.

Bisphosphonates have been employed in the treatment of a variety of disorders of low bone mass, including wasting diseases, although data in the wasting diseases remain limited [88]. Primarily use has been in the wasting disorders that result in high bone resorption. A meta-analysis of four randomized, controlled trials examining alendronate use in persons with HIV and osteopenia or osteoporosis concluded that alendronate was an effective and preferred therapy [24]. Annual intravenous zoledronic acid may also be another option, with the benefit of not adding drugs with possible gastrointestinal side effects to the "pill burden" of persons with HIV [60].

Studies in small numbers of persons with DMD using daily [47] and weekly alendronate [5] show promising effects. DMD guidelines suggest that intravenous bisphosphonates be used for vertebral fractures but that prophylaxis with oral bisphosphonates is not routinely recommended for patients with muscular dystrophy [18].

Studies using bisphosphonates to improve BMD in adults with CF have yielded encouraging results. Intravenous pamidronate (30 mg every 3 months) was the first bisphosphonate used in adults with CF because intravenous administration avoided both the potential for decreased intestinal bioavailability due to malabsorption as well as the risk of esophagitis from gastroesophageal reflux of oral preparations. In a trial of 30 persons with CF, 6 months of pamidronate therapy resulted in significant gains in lumbar spine and total hip BMD (mean differences between pamidronate-treated and untreated groups of 5.8% and 3.0% respectively, $p<0.05$) [48]. Unfortunately, 73% of pamidronate-treated individuals experienced significant bone pain, requiring shortening of the trial. Because patients on glucocorticoids did not experience bone pain, pretreatment with prednisone may be useful. Pamidronate also was shown to improve BMD in patients with CF after lung transplantation [7]. Oral alendronate and etidronate therapies have shown promising results without adverse effects in a few studies [6, 79, 84].

Bisphosphonates also are useful for stemming the bone loss associated with glucocorticoid use and have been utilized even in disorders that affect bone formation. Although a randomized study of cyclic oral etidronate treatment in a large cohort of adults with osteopenia and Crohn disease (both active and inactive) failed to show benefits [95], subsequent studies examining pamidronate (intravenous) and alendronate (oral) therapy in adults with Crohn disease demonstrated increases in BMD [12, 45, 100].

Both oral and IV bisphosphonates also have been used in persons with cerebral palsy [50, 53, 94]. Although studies have consistently shown increases in BMD, the effect on fracture rates is uncertain. Cautious use of these medications is advisable because of long skeletal retention and concern about potential long-term adverse events, including osteonecrosis of the jaw and atypical subtrochanteric fracture. Further questions remain regarding optimal dosing and duration of treatment.

11.8.7 Growth Hormone

Growth hormone (GH) has been considered as an adjunctive therapy for the cardiomyopathy associated with DMD but not investigated as a bone anabolic agent in this disease. Similarly, none of the papers published on the effects of GH in HIV wasting or Crohn disease have focused on bone density as a primary outcome.

GH therapy has shown promising results on bone accrual in children with CF. In a multicenter, randomized, controlled crossover trial of 61 prepubertal children with CF, GH-treated patients demonstrated significant increases in height, weight, lean body mass, and BMC compared to the non-treated group [46]. Although BMC, not BMD, was measured, improvements remained significant even with correction for height increases, suggesting that GH improves bone mineral accrual. There has been a single published pilot study of the effects of GH in ten males with CP, which suggested improvements in spine BMD as well as augmented linear growth with 18 months of therapy [3]. However, several methodologic concerns were raised about this report, and further data are not yet available [81]; therefore, this is not yet an accepted therapy for these children.

11.8.8 Novel Emerging Therapies

Data are emerging on the use of vibrating platforms in some wasting conditions. These include the use of high-frequency, low-magnitude vibrating plates for skeletal stimulation. These plates offer a noninvasive home-based therapy. They expose bone to microstrains and may increase appendicular bone mass. In one published report, 20 children with CP stood for 10 min/day, 5 days/week for 6 months on vibrating platforms (90 Hz, 0.3 gravity) or placebo platforms [104]. Children using the active devices had a 6.3% increase in proximal tibial vTBMD, while those using sham devices showed an 11.9% decrease. A second preliminary study involving 6-month use of the plates (compared to a standing intervention) in 6–12-year-old children with CP demonstrated greater increase in appendicular cortical bone during the time of the vibration intervention [108].

Denosumab (Prolia®) is a fully human monoclonal antibody that binds to the cytokine known as receptor activator of nuclear factor κ B (RANK) ligand and prevents RANK ligand from interacting with the RANK receptor on osteoclasts and osteoclast precursors [86]. This action inhibits osteoclast formation, function, and survival. Denosumab is given as a subcutaneous injection of 60 mg every 6 months for therapy of adult women with postmenopausal osteoporosis. In this setting, it has been shown to reduce fracture rates at multiple sites. It also has been shown to reduce vertebral fractures in men undergoing androgen deprivation therapy as part of treatment for prostate cancer. Because RANK ligand also is expressed on immune cells, there is a possible increased risk of infection with denosumab use that should be monitored. Its use in wasting disorders has not yet been explored, but it has potential especially for those individuals characterized by high bone resorption.

Table 11.1 Treatment options for bone health in patients with wasting disorders

Treatment	Disorders studied	Status of therapy
Bisphosphonates	Fairly widely studied in many wasting disorders	Guidelines for considering use in DMD, CF. Therapy still individualized for all wasting diseases
Calcium	Supplementation recommended in DMD, CF Limited data suggesting supplementation benefits for CP, Crohn disease	DMD: ≥750 mg/day CF: 1,300–1,500 mg/day At least RDA for age for other wasting diseases
Glucocorticoids	DMD	Well established
Growth hormone	Studied in CF but results not sufficient for general recommendations for use. Used in HIV and Crohn but not with attention to bone outcomes Pilot studies in CP	Needs further study
Parathyroid hormone	Potential therapeutic agent. Black box warning precludes use in children	No published studies in wasting disorders
Physical activity/physical therapy	Limited studies in DMD, HIV, CF, Crohn, CP	Promising for all wasting disorders (with caution in DMD) but needs further study
Vitamin D	Reported as deficient/insufficient in populations across all wasting disorders	Individualized supplementation to target of 25-OH D of >30 ng/ml recommended. High doses may be needed in CF, Crohn
Vitamin K	Deficient in persons with CF. Very poorly studied in other wasting diseases	Recommended supplementation with 0.3–0.5 mg/day in CF (may not raise levels adequately). Other diseases need study
Vibrating platforms	Emerging data in CP	Needs further study
Denosumab, zinc, PTH-rP	Not yet studied	Need further study but potentially important therapy

Novel biologic therapies are also in development, including PTH-related peptide (PTH-rP) and zinc. PTH-rP, known to be essential for tooth eruption and mammary gland development, is now under study as a bone anabolic agent and has been shown to increase vertebral BMD in postmenopausal osteoporotic women [58]. Zinc is an essential nutrient that plays a key role in bone growth and development [109]. In conditions of dietary zinc deficiency, bone growth is retarded. Increasing zinc dietary intake increases bone mass. Zinc stimulates osteoblasts and inhibits osteoclast formation and survival. Various zinc compounds have been shown to have anabolic effects on bone. Zinc may prove useful for prevention and treatment of osteoporosis in wasting disorders.

Conclusion

Disorders of bone mineralization are common in many wasting diseases. Many of these disorders demonstrate progressive declines in bone mineralization over time. However, the wasting disorders are quite heterogeneous. Even within a given disorder, differences among individuals, particularly in disease severity and medical therapies, must be taken into consideration when determining the disease's potential impact on skeletal growth and development. This chapter has attempted to outline potential options, using the limited data available to date. These options are summarized in Table 11.1. Development of more evidence-based therapies will require adequately powered randomized controlled trials.

For now, optimal approaches to facilitating bone accrual and maintenance with a goal of reducing fractures requires first assessment of bone mineral status and, once that is done, a tailoring of available approaches and therapies to an individual's unique needs.

References

1. Abrams SA. Calcium supplementation during childhood: long-term effects on bone mineralization. Nutr Rev. 2005;63:251–5.
2. Ali NJ, Capewell S, Ward MJ. Bone turnover during high dose inhaled corticosteroid treatment. Thorax. 1991;46:160–4.
3. Ali O, Shim M, Fowler E, Greenberg M, Perkins D, Oppenheim W, Cohen P. Growth hormone therapy improves bone mineral density in children with cerebral palsy: a preliminary pilot study. J Clin Endocrinol Metab. 2007;92:932–7.
4. Allgrove J. Bisphosphonates. Arch Dis Child. 1997; 76:73–5.
5. Apkon S, Coll J. Use of weekly alendronate to treat osteoporosis in boys with muscular dystrophy. Am J Phys Med Rehabil. 2008;87:139–43.
6. Aris RM, Lester GE, Caminiti M, Blackwood AD, Hensler M, Lark RK, Hecker TM, Renner JB, Guillen U, Brown SA, Neuringer IP, Chalermskulrat W, Ontjes DA. Efficacy of alendronate in adults with cystic fibrosis with low bone density. Am J Respir Crit Care Med. 2004;169:77–82.
7. Aris RM, Lester GE, Renner JB, Winders A, Denene BA, Lark RK, Ontjes DA. Efficacy of pamidronate for osteoporosis in patients with cystic fibrosis following lung transplantation. Am J Respir Crit Care Med. 2000;162: 941–6.
8. Aris RM, Merkel PA, Bachrach LK, Borowitz DS, Boyle MP, Elkin SL, Guise TA, Hardin DS, Haworth CS, Holick MF, Joseph PM, O'Brien K, Tullis E, Watts NB, White TB. Guide to bone health and disease in cystic fibrosis. J Clin Endocrinol Metab. 2005;90:1888–96.
9. Aris RM, Ontjes DA, Brown SA, Chalermskulrat W, Neuringer I, Lester GE. Carboxylated osteocalcin levels in cystic fibrosis. Am J Respir Crit Care Med. 2003;168:1129.
10. Bachrach LK. Acquisition of optimal bone mass in childhood and adolescence. Trends Endocrinol Metab. 2001;12:22–8.
11. Balaban B, Matthews DJ, Clayton GH, Carry T. Corticosteroid treatment and functional improvement in Duchenne muscular dystrophy: long-term effect. Am J Phys Med Rehabil. 2005;84:843–50.
12. Bartram SA, Peaston RT, Rawlings DJ, Francis RM, Thompson NP. A randomized controlled trial of calcium with vitamin D, alone or in combination with intravenous pamidronate, for the treatment of low bone mineral density associated with Crohn's disease. Aliment Pharmacol Ther. 2003;18: 1121–7.
13. Bernstein CN, Blanchard JF, Leslie W, Wajda A, Yu BN. The incidence of fracture among patients with inflammatory bowel disease. A population-based cohort study. Ann Intern Med. 2000;133:795–9.
14. Bernstein CN, Leslie WD. Review article: osteoporosis and inflammatory bowel disease. Aliment Pharmacol Ther. 2004;19:941–52.
15. Bernstein CN, Seeger LL, Anton PA, Artinian L, Geffrey S, Goodman W, Belin TR, Shanahan F. A randomized, placebo-controlled trial of calcium supplementation for decreased bone density in corticosteroid-using patients with inflammatory bowel disease: a pilot study. Aliment Pharmacol Ther. 1996;10:777–86.
16. Bhudhikanok GS, Lim J, Marcus R, Harkins A, Moss RB, Bachrach LK. Correlates of osteopenia in patients with cystic fibrosis. Pediatrics. 1996;97:103–11.
17. Boyle MP, Noschese ML, Watts SL, Davis ME, Stenner SE, Lechtzin N. Failure of high-dose ergocalciferol to correct vitamin D deficiency in adults with cystic fibrosis. Am J Respir Crit Care Med. 2005;172: 212–7.
18. Bushby K, Finkel R, Birnkrant DJ, Case LE, Clemens PR, Cripe L, Kaul A, Kinnett K, McDonald C, Pandya S, Poysky J, Shapiro F, Tomezsko J, Constantin C. Diagnosis and management of Duchenne muscular dystrophy, part 2: implementation of multidisciplinary care. Lancet Neurol. 2010; 9:177–89.
19. Card T, West J, Hubbard R, Logan RF. Hip fractures in patients with inflammatory bowel disease and their relationship to corticosteroid use: a population based cohort study. Gut. 2004;53:251–5.
20. Carter GT, Wineinger MA, Walsh SA, Horasek SJ, Abresch RT, Fowler Jr WM. Effect of voluntary wheel-running exercise on muscles of the mdx mouse. Neuromuscul Disord. 1995;5:323–32.
21. Caulton JM, Ward KA, Alsop CW, Dunn G, Adams JE, Mughal MZ. A randomised controlled trial of standing programme on bone mineral density in non-ambulant children with cerebral palsy. Arch Dis Child. 2004;89:131–5.
22. Chad KE, Bailey DA, McKay HA, Zello GA, Snyder RE. The effect of a weight-bearing physical activity program on bone mineral content and estimated volumetric density in children with spastic cerebral palsy. J Pediatr. 1999;135:115–7.
23. Chevalley T, Rizzoli R, Hans D, Ferrari S, Bonjour JP. Interaction between calcium intake and menarcheal age on bone mass gain: an eight-year follow-up study from prepuberty to postmenarche. J Clin Endocrinol Metab. 2005;90:44–51.
24. Clay PG, Voss LE, Williams C, Daume EC. Valid treatment options for osteoporosis and osteopenia in HIV-infected persons. Ann Pharmacother. 2008;42:670–9.

25. Conway SP, Morton AM, Oldroyd B, Truscott JG, White H, Smith AH, Haigh I. Osteoporosis and osteopenia in adults and adolescents with cystic fibrosis: prevalence and associated factors. Thorax. 2000;55:798–804.
26. Conway SP, Wolfe SP, Brownlee KG, White H, Oldroyd B, Truscott JG, Harvey JM, Shearer MJ. Vitamin K status among children with cystic fibrosis and its relationship to bone mineral density and bone turnover. Pediatrics. 2005;115:1325–31.
27. Cooper C, Dennison EM, Leufkens HG, Bishop N, van Staa TP. Epidemiology of childhood fractures in Britain: a study using the general practice research database. J Bone Miner Res. 2004;19:1976–81.
28. Corcoran C, Grinspoon S. Treatments for wasting in patients with the acquired immunodeficiency syndrome. N Engl J Med. 1999;340:1740–50.
29. Crabtree NJ, Roper H, McMurchie H, Shaw NJ. Regional changes in bone area and bone mineral content in boys with Duchenne muscular dystrophy receiving corticosteroid therapy. J Pediatr. 2010;156: 450–5.
30. Davidson ZE, Truby H. A review of nutrition in Duchenne muscular dystrophy. J Hum Nutr Diet. 2009;22:383–93.
31. Donaldson CL, Hulley SB, Vogel JM, Hattner RS, Bayers JH, McMillan DE. Effect of prolonged bed rest on bone mineral. Metabolism. 1970;19:1071–84.
32. Drury D, Grey VL, Ferland G, Gundberg C, Lands LC. Efficacy of high dose phylloquinone in correcting vitamin K deficiency in cystic fibrosis. J Cyst Fibros. 2008;7:457–9.
33. Dubner SE, Shults J, Baldassano RN, Zemel BS, Thayu M, Burnham JM, Herskovitz RM, Howard KM, Leonard MB. Longitudinal assessment of bone density and structure in an incident cohort of children with Crohn's disease. Gastroenterology. 2009;136: 123–30.
34. Ehrlich PJ, Lanyon LE. Mechanical strain and bone cell function: a review. Osteoporos Int. 2002;13: 688–700.
35. Elkin SL, Fairney A, Burnett S, Kemp M, Kyd P, Burgess J, Compston JE, Hodson ME. Vertebral deformities and low bone mineral density in adults with cystic fibrosis: a cross-sectional study. Osteoporos Int. 2001;12:366–72.
36. Emery AE. Population frequencies of inherited neuromuscular diseases – a world survey. Neuromuscul Disord. 1991;1:19–29.
37. Emery AE. The muscular dystrophies. BMJ. 1998; 317:991–5.
38. Epstein DM, Dalinka MK, Kaplan FS, Arochick JM, Marinelli DL, Kundel HL. Observer variation in the detection of osteopenia. Skeletal Radiol. 1986;1986: 347–9.
39. Fewtrell MS, Benden C, Williams JE, Chomtho S, Ginty F, Nigdikar SV, Jaffe A. Undercarboxylated osteocalcin and bone mass in 8–12 year old children with cystic fibrosis. J Cyst Fibros. 2008;7:307–12.
40. Frangolias DD, Holloway CL, Vedal S, Wilcox PG. Role of exercise and lung function in predicting work status in cystic fibrosis. Am J Respir Crit Care Med. 2003;167:150–7.
41. Frost HM. Bone 'mass" and the "mechanostat": a proposal. Anat Rec. 1987;219:1–9.
42. Gibbons MJ, Gilchrist NL, Frampton C, Maguire P, Reilly PH, March RL, Wall CR. The effects of a high calcium dairy food on bone health in pre-pubertal children in New Zealand. Asia Pac J Clin Nutr. 2004;13:341–7.
43. Gordon CM. Boning up: exploring bone structure and strength in children with Crohn's disease. Gastroenterology. 2009;136:35–9.
44. Grey V, Atkinson S, Drury D, Casey L, Ferland G, Gundberg C, Lands LC. Prevalence of low bone mass and deficiencies of vitamins D and K in pediatric patients with cystic fibrosis from 3 Canadian centers. Pediatrics. 2008;122:1014–20.
45. Haderslev KV, Tjellesen L, Sorensen HA, Staun M. Alendronate increases lumbar spine bone mineral density in patients with Crohn's disease. Gastroenterology. 2000;119:639–46.
46. Hardin DS, ms-Huet B, Brown D, Chatfield B, Dyson M, Ferkol T, Howenstine M, Prestidge C, Royce F, Rice J, Seilheimer DK, Steelman J, Shepherds R. Growth hormone treatment improves growth and clinical status in prepubertal children with cystic fibrosis: results of a multicenter randomized controlled trial. J Clin Endocrinol Metab. 2006;91: 4925–9.
47. Hawker GA, Ridout R, Harris VA, Chase CC, Fielding LJ, Biggar WD. Alendronate in the treatment of low bone mass in steroid-treated boys with Duchennes muscular dystrophy. Arch Phys Med Rehabil. 2005;86:284–8.
48. Haworth CS, Selby PL, Adams JE, Mawer EB, Horrocks AW, Webb AK. Effect of intravenous pamidronate on bone mineral density in adults with cystic fibrosis. Thorax. 2001;56:314–6.
49. Haworth CS, Selby PL, Webb AK, Dodd ME, Musson H, McL NR, Economou G, Horrocks AW, Freemont AJ, Mawer EB, Adams JE. Low bone mineral density in adults with cystic fibrosis [see comments]. Thorax. 1999;54:961–7.
50. Henderson R. Low doses of pamidronate for the treatment of osteopenia in non-ambulatory children. Dev Med Child Neurol. 2006;48:708.
51. Henderson RC. Bone density and other possible predictors of fracture risk in children and adolescents with spastic quadriplegia. Dev Med Child Neurol. 1997;39:224–7.
52. Henderson RC, Berglund LM, May R, Zemel BS, Grossberg RI, Johnson J, Plotkin H, Stevenson RD, Szalay E, Wong B, Kecskemethy HH, Harcke HT. The relationship between fractures and DXA measures of BMD in the distal femur of children and adolescents with cerebral palsy or muscular dystrophy. J Bone Miner Res. 2010;25:520–6.

53. Henderson RC, Lark RK, Kecskemethy HH, Miller F, Harcke HT, Bachrach SJ. Bisphosphonates to treat osteopenia in children with quadriplegic cerebral palsy: a randomized, placebo-controlled clinical trial. J Pediatr. 2002;141:644–51.
54. Henderson RC, Lark RK, Newman JE, Kecskemthy H, Fung EB, Renner JB, Harcke HT. Pediatric reference data for dual X-ray absorptiometric measures of normal bone density in the distal femur. AJR Am J Roentgenol. 2002;178:439–43.
55. Henderson RC, Lin PP, Greene WB. Bone-mineral density in children and adolescents who have spastic cerebral palsy. J Bone Joint Surg Am. 1995;77:1671–81.
56. Herman D, May R, Vogel L, Johnson J, Henderson RC. Quantifying weight-bearing by children with cerebral palsy while in passive standers. Pediatr Phys Ther. 2007;19:283–7.
57. Hind K, Truscott JG, Conway SP. Exercise during childhood and adolescence: a prophylaxis against cystic fibrosis-related low bone mineral density? Exercise for bone health in children with cystic fibrosis. J Cyst Fibros. 2008;7:270–6.
58. Horwitz MJ, Tedesco MB, Garcia-Ocana A, Sereika SM, Prebehala L, Bisello A, Hollis BW, Gundberg CM, Stewart AF. Parathyroid hormone-related protein for the treatment of postmenopausal osteoporosis: defining the maximal tolerable dose. J Clin Endocrinol Metab. 2010;95:1279–87.
59. Hough JP, Boyd RN, Keating JL. Systematic review of interventions for low bone mineral density in children with cerebral palsy. Pediatrics. 2010;125:e670–8.
60. Huang J, Meixner L, Fernandez S, McCutchan JA. A double-blinded, randomized controlled trial of zoledronate therapy for HIV-associated osteopenia and osteoporosis. AIDS. 2009;23:51–7.
61. Jacobson DL, Lindsey JC, Gordon CM, Moye J, Hardin DS, Mulligan K, Aldrovandi GM. Total body and spinal bone mineral density across Tanner stage in perinatally HIV-infected and uninfected children and youth in PACTG 1045. AIDS. 2010;24:687–96.
62. Jekovec-Vrhovsek M, Kocijancic A, Prezelj J. Effect of vitamin D and calcium on bone mineral density in children with CP and epilepsy in full-time care. Dev Med Child Neurol. 2000;42:403–5.
63. King W, Levin R, Schmidt R, Oestreich A, Heubi JE. Prevalence of reduced bone mass in children and adults with spastic quadriplegia. Dev Med Child Neurol. 2003;45:12–6.
64. King WM, Ruttencutter R, Nagaraja HN, Matkovic V, Landoll J, Hoyle C, Mendell JR, Kissel JT. Orthopedic outcomes of long-term daily corticosteroid treatment in Duchenne muscular dystrophy. Neurology. 2007;68:1607–13.
65. Kohrt WM, Barry DW, Schwartz RS. Muscle forces or gravity: what predominates mechanical loading on bone? Med Sci Sports Exerc. 2009;41:2050–5.
66. Koman LA, Smith BP, Shilt JS. Cerebral palsy. Lancet. 2004;363:1619–31.
67. Kumari M, Khazai NB, Ziegler TR, Nanes MS, Abrams SA, Tangpricha V. Vitamin D-mediated calcium absorption in patients with clinically stable Crohn's disease: a pilot study. Mol Nutr Food Res. 2010;54:1085–91.
68. Larson CM, Henderson RC. Bone mineral density and fractures in boys with Duchenne muscular dystrophy. J Pediatr Orthop. 2000;20:71–4.
69. Liao HF, Liu YC, Liu WY, Lin YT. Effectiveness of loaded sit-to-stand resistance exercise for children with mild spastic diplegia: a randomized clinical trial. Arch Phys Med Rehabil. 2007;88:25–31.
70. Lloyd T, Beck TJ, Lin HM, Tulchinsky M, Eggli DF, Oreskovic TL, Cavanagh PR, Seeman E. Modifiable determinants of bone status in young women. Bone. 2002;30:416–21.
71. Lohse N, Hansen AB, Pedersen G, Kronborg G, Gerstoft J, Sorensen HT, Vaeth M, Obel N. Survival of persons with and without HIV infection in Denmark, 1995–2005. Ann Intern Med. 2007;146:87–95.
72. Manolagas SC. The role of IL-6 type cytokines and their receptors in bone. Ann N Y Acad Sci. 1998;840:194–204.
73. Moxley III RT, Ashwal S, Pandya S, Connolly A, Florence J, Mathews K, Baumbach L, McDonald C, Sussman M, Wade C. Practice parameter: corticosteroid treatment of Duchenne dystrophy: report of the Quality Standards Subcommittee of the American Academy of Neurology and the Practice Committee of the Child Neurology Society. Neurology. 2005;64:13–20.
74. Mueller NJ, Fux CA, Ledergerber B, Elzi L, Schmid P, Dang T, Magenta L, Calmy A, Vergopoulos A, Bischoff-Ferrari HA. High prevalence of severe vitamin D deficiency in combined antiretroviral therapy-naive and successfully treated Swiss HIV patients. AIDS. 2010;24:1127–34.
75. Munns CF, Cowell CT. Prevention and treatment of osteoporosis in chronically ill children. J Musculoskelet Neuronal Interact. 2005;5:262–72.
76. Ng V, Millard W, Lebrun C, Howard J. Low-intensity exercise improves quality of life in patients with Crohn's disease. Clin J Sport Med. 2007;17:384–8.
77. Nicolaidou P, Stavrinadis I, Loukou I, Papadopoulou A, Georgouli H, Douros K, Priftis KN, Gourgiotis D, Matsinos YG, Doudounakis S. The effect of vitamin K supplementation on biochemical markers of bone formation in children and adolescents with cystic fibrosis. Eur J Pediatr. 2006;165:540–5.
78. Paccou J, Viget N, Legrout-Gerot I, Yazdanpanah Y, Cortet B. Bone loss in patients with HIV infection. Joint Bone Spine. 2009;76:637–41.
79. Papaioannou A, Kennedy CC, Freitag A, Ioannidis G, O'Neill J, Webber C, Pui M, Berthiaume Y, Rabin HR, Paterson N, Jeanneret A, Matouk E, Villeneuve J, Nixon M, Adachi JD. Alendronate once weekly for the prevention and treatment of bone loss in Canadian

adult cystic fibrosis patients (CFOS trial). Chest. 2008;134:794–800.
80. Pedersen BK, Akerstrom TC, Nielsen AR, Fischer CP. Role of myokines in exercise and metabolism. J Appl Physiol. 2007;103:1093–8.
81. Porter JR, Shaw NJ. Growth hormone or bisphosphonate for cerebral palsy related osteoporosis. JCEM Online. 2007. http://jcem.endojournals.org/content/92/3/932/reply#jcem_el_2265.
82. Prior J, Burdge D, Maan E, Milner R, Hankins C, Klein M, Walmsley S. Fragility fractures and bone mineral density in HIV positive women: a case-control population-based study. Osteoporos Int. 2007;18: 1345–53.
83. Rauch F, Plotkin H, DiMeglio L, Engelbert RH, Henderson RC, Munns C, Wenkert D, Zeitler P. Fracture prediction and the definition of osteoporosis in children and adolescents: the ISCD 2007 pediatric official positions. J Clin Densitom. 2008;11:22–8.
84. Ringuier B, Leboucher B, Leblanc M, Troussier F, Duveau E, Audran M, Ginies JL. Effect of oral bisphosphonates in patients with cystic fibrosis and low bone mineral density. Arch Pediatr. 2004;11:1445–9.
85. Rizzoli R, Fleisch H, Bonjour J-P. Role of 1,25-dihydroxyvitamin D_3 on intestinal phosphate absorption in rats with a normal vitamin D supply. J Clin Invest. 1977;60:639.
86. Rizzoli R, Yasothan U, Kirkpatrick P. Denosumab. Nat Rev Drug Discov. 2010;9:591–2.
87. Robinson RJ, Krzywicki T, Almond L, al-Azzawi F, Abrams K, Iqbal SJ, Mayberry JF. Effect of a low-impact exercise program on bone mineral density in Crohn's disease: a randomized controlled trial. Gastroenterology. 1998;115:36–41.
88. Rodan GA. Mechanisms of action of bisphosphonates. Annu Rev Pharmacol Toxicol. 1998;38:375–88.
89. Rosen CJ. Vitamin D insufficiency. N Engl J Med. 2011;364:248–54.
90. Ross AC, Manson JE, Abrams SA, Aloia JF, Brannon PM, Clinton SK, Durazo-Arvizu RA, Gallagher JC, Gallo RL, Jones G, Kovacs CS, Mayne ST, Rosen CJ, Shapses SA. The 2011 report on dietary reference intakes for calcium and vitamin D from the Institute of Medicine: what clinicians need to know. J Clin Endocrinol Metab. 2011;96:53–8.
91. Rubin C, Judex S, Qin YX. Low-level mechanical signals and their potential as a non-pharmacological intervention for osteoporosis. Age Ageing. 2006;35 Suppl 2:ii32–6.
92. Schulze KJ, O'Brien KO, Germain-Lee EL, Booth SL, Leonard A, Rosenstein BJ. Calcium kinetics are altered in clinically stable girls with cystic fibrosis. J Clin Endocrinol Metab. 2004;89:3385–91.
93. Semeao EJ, Stallings VA, Peck SN, Piccoli DA. Vertebral compression fractures in pediatric patients with Crohn's disease. Gastroenterology. 1997;112: 1710–3.
94. Shaw NJ, White CP, Fraser WD, Rosenbloom L. Osteopenia in cerebral palsy. Arch Dis Child. 1994;71:235–8.
95. Siffledeen JS, Fedorak RN, Siminoski K, Jen H, Vaudan E, Abraham N, Steinhart H, Greenberg G. Randomized trial of etidronate plus calcium and vitamin D for treatment of low bone mineral density in Crohn's disease. Clin Gastroenterol Hepatol. 2005;3:122–32.
96. Smith CB, Smith DA. Relations between age, mineral density and mechanical properties of human femoral compacta. Acta Orthop Scand. 1976;47:496–502.
97. Soderpalm AC, Magnusson P, Ahlander AC, Karlsson J, Kroksmark AK, Tulinius M, Swolin-Eide D. Low bone mineral density and decreased bone turnover in Duchenne muscular dystrophy. Neuromuscul Disord. 2007;17:919–28.
98. Stone B, Dockrell D, Bowman C, McCloskey E. HIV and bone disease. Arch Biochem Biophys. 2010;503:66–77.
99. Sugiyama T, Takaki T, Saito T, Taguchi T. Vitamin K therapy for cortical bone fragility caused by reduced mechanical loading in a child with hemiplegia. J Musculoskelet Neuronal Interact. 2007;7:219–23.
100. Tsujikawa T, Andoh A, Inatomi O, Bamba S, Nakahara T, Sasaki M, Saito H, Fujiyama Y. Alendronate improves low bone mineral density induced by steroid therapy in Crohn's disease. Intern Med. 2009;48:933–7.
101. Vermeer C, Wolf J, Craciun AM, Knapen MH. Bone markers during a 6-month space flight: effects of vitamin K supplementation. J Gravit Physiol. 1998; 5:65–9.
102. Vikulina T, Fan X, Yamaguchi M, Roser-Page S, Zayzafoon M, Guidot DM, Ofotokun I, Weitzmann MN. Alterations in the immuno-skeletal interface drive bone destruction in HIV-1 transgenic rats. Proc Natl Acad Sci USA. 2010;107:13848–53.
103. Vitte C, Fleisch H, Guenther HL. Bisphosphonates induce osteoblasts to secrete an inhibitor of osteoclast-mediated resorption. Endocrinology. 1996;137: 2324–33.
104. Ward K, Alsop C, Caulton J, Rubin C, Adams J, Mughal Z. Low magnitude mechanical loading is osteogenic in children with disabling conditions. J Bone Miner Res. 2004;19:360–9.
105. Ward KA, Caulton JM, Adams JE, Mughal MZ. Perspective: cerebral palsy as a model of bone development in the absence of postnatal mechanical factors. J Musculoskelet Neuronal Interact. 2006;6:154–9.
106. Weber P. Vitamin K and bone health. Nutrition. 2001;17:880–7.
107. World Health Organization Study Group. Assessment of fracture risk and its application to screening for postmenopausal osteoporosis. World Health Organ Tech Rep Ser. 1994: 843:1–129.
108. Wren TA, Lee DC, Hara R, Rethlefsen SA, Kay RM, Dorey FJ, Gilsanz V. Effect of high-frequency, low-magnitude vibration on bone and muscle in children with cerebral palsy. J Pediatr Orthop. 2010;30:732–8.
109. Yamaguchi M. Role of nutritional zinc in the prevention of osteoporosis. Mol Cell Biochem. 2010; 338:241–54.

110. Yin MT, Lu D, Cremers S, Tien PC, Cohen MH, Shi Q, Shane E, Golub ET, Anastos K. Short-term bone loss in HIV-infected premenopausal women. J Acquir Immune Defic Syndr. 2010;53:202–8.
111. Yin MT, McMahon DJ, Ferris DC, Zhang CA, Shu A, Staron R, Colon I, Laurence J, Dobkin JF, Hammer SM, Shane E. Low bone mass and high bone turnover in postmenopausal human immunodeficiency virus-infected women. J Clin Endocrinol Metab. 2010;95:620–9.
112. Zamboni G, Antoniazzi F, Bertoldo F, Lauriola S, Antozzi L, Tato L. Altered bone metabolism in children infected with human immunodeficiency virus. Acta Paediatr. 2003;92:12–6.

Paget's Disease of Bone: Pathogenesis and Treatment

12

Frederick R. Singer and G. David Roodman

Keywords
Paget's disease of bone • Measles virus • Paramyxovirus • Nucleocapsid
Osteolytic lesions • Bone remodeling

12.1 Introduction

Paget's disease of bone (PDB) is a skeletal disorder that usually is diagnosed in patients over 50 years of age and affects one or several bones but not the entire skeleton. Radiological and pathological studies indicate that the underlying problem is an increase in osteoclastic activity, which initially produces dominant osteolytic lesions that move slowly throughout an affected bone. Over time, the osteolytic areas are replaced by osteosclerotic bone of increased size and chaotic structure. In the lower extremities, affected bones may become bowed due to impaired biomechanical properties of the bone. The overgrowth of bone is produced by a marked proliferation of osteoblasts.

A clue to the etiology of PDB was found in 1974 when it was discovered that nuclear inclusions were present in many of the osteoclasts in bone biopsies. These inclusions resembled nucleocapsids of the paramyxovirus family. Subsequently, some immunohistochemical and molecular studies indicated that measles virus (MV), respiratory syncytial virus (RSV), and canine distemper virus (CDV) were etiologic candidates, although other studies reported no evidence of these paramyxoviruses in specimens of PDB. More recently, an animal model of PDB has been developed in transgenic mice by inserting measles virus nucleocapsid protein (MVNP) into the genome. Other studies of the etiology of PDB were stimulated by the observation that a subset of patients inherited the disorder from a parent. The pattern of transmission was autosomal dominant, with incomplete penetrance. Mutations of the sequestosome 1 gene have been identified in about 30% of patients with familial PDB. The p62 protein encoded by this gene plays a role in nuclear factor-κB (NF-κB) signaling in osteoclasts, and variants of other genes that regulate osteoclasts may be factors involved in the

F.R. Singer, M.D. (✉)
Endocrine/Bone Disease Program,
John Wayne Cancer Institute, St. John's Health Center,
2200 Santa Monica Blvd, Santa Monica,
CA 90404, USA
e-mail: singerf@yahoo.com

G.D. Roodman, M.D., Ph.D.
Department of Medicine,
Director of Hematology/Oncology,
Indiana University,
980 W. Walnut, Suite C312,
Indianapolis, Indiana 46202, USA
e-mail: groodman@iupui.edu

F. Bronner et al. (eds.), *Bone-Metabolic Functions and Modulators*, Topics in Bone Biology,
DOI 10.1007/978-1-4471-2745-1_12, © Springer-Verlag London 2012

pathogenesis of PDB. However, transgenic mice that express the most common sequestosome 1 mutation develop osteopenia rather than PDB.

Many patients with PDB are asymptomatic and often will require no treatment. Bone pain, elective orthopedic surgery, hypercalcemia associated with immobilization, and hearing loss are indications for specific therapy. In younger individuals who remain asymptomatic, therapy might be considered to prevent future complications, particularly if the skull or weight-bearing bones are affected. Drugs that inhibit osteoclast activity have proven very effective in suppressing disease activity. Calcitonin was the first available drug used in the treatment of PDB, but subsequent development of potent bisphosphonates has led to these agents becoming the most common treatment. Oral or intravenous bisphosphonates effectively suppress disease activity as manifested by marked reduction or normalization of biochemical markers of bone turnover such as serum total alkaline phosphatase activity. The most impressive results have been produced by a single infusion of zoledronate, which can maintain normal serum total alkaline phosphatase activity for up to 6 years in 80% of treated patients.

12.2 What Is Paget's Disease of Bone?

PDB is a chronic skeletal disorder that produces an extremely heterogeneous clinical picture, which is predominantly seen in individuals over the age of 50 years and of European background. Sir James Paget published the first full description of the disorder he termed *osteitis deformans* in 1877 [86]. The disorder may affect one bone or several bones but not the entire skeleton. Population studies suggest that the disorder is asymptomatic in a high percentage of individuals found to have the condition [24]. In those with symptoms, bone pain and deformed, enlarged bones are common problems. A great variety of complications may occur, depending on which part of the skeleton is affected. Hearing loss and tinnitus may occur with skull involvement [61, 125]. Fractures generally develop in weight-bearing bones [103]. Arthritis is a very common complication in weight-bearing regions, particularly at the hip [28]. A combination of deformed lower extremity bones and arthritis may limit mobility. Sarcoma arising in bone affected by PDB is a rare complication [63]. Because of the increased vascularity of affected bone [23], an increased cardiac output is likely in patients with polyostotic disease [37]. This increase in cardiac output usually is not associated with congestive heart failure, although it could be a risk factor.

12.3 Pathogenesis of Paget's Disease of Bone

An examination of the natural history of PDP as determined by radiological evaluation and histological parameters strongly suggests that the osteoclast is the cell that triggers the disease process.

12.3.1 Radiology of Paget's Disease of Bone

Two years after the discovery of X-rays by Roentgen in 1895, Leopold-Levi [57] reported the postmortem X-ray appearance of sclerotic PDB in a femur from a female patient. The first description in a living patient was reported by Beclere [7] in 1901. Subsequently, numerous cross-sectional and long-term evolution studies of individual pagetic lesions have indicated that the disease progresses through predictable phases: an initial osteolytic phase, a mixed osteolytic-sclerotic phase, and a dominant sclerotic phase [62, 80].

The earliest osteolytic lesions are seldom observed because they usually are asymptomatic. Dominant osteolytic lesions most often are noted in the skull (Fig.12.1) and long bones of the extremities. While Schuller [100] first described the osteolytic lesion of the skull (*osteoporosis circumscripta*) in 1926, he did not appreciate that the patient had PDB. This connection was first recognized by Erdheim [26] in 1935. The lesions most commonly arise in the frontal and occipital bones and cross suture lines (Fig. 12.1). In 1938, Brailsford [13] was first to describe the osteolytic lesions in long

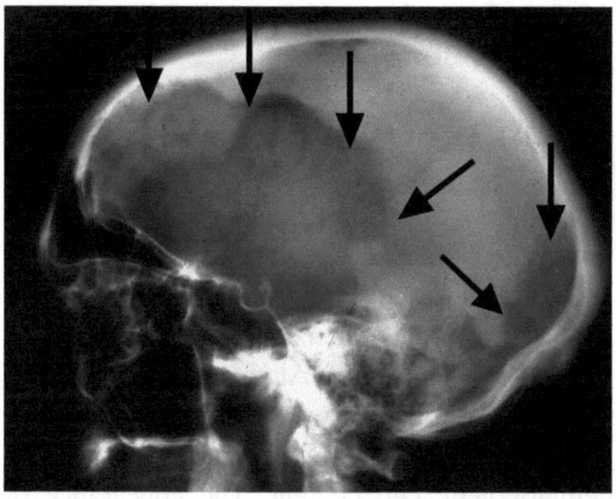

Fig. 12.1 Large osteolytic lesion in the frontal and temporal skull and small osteolytic lesion in the occipital region outlined by the *arrows* in a 64-year-old male

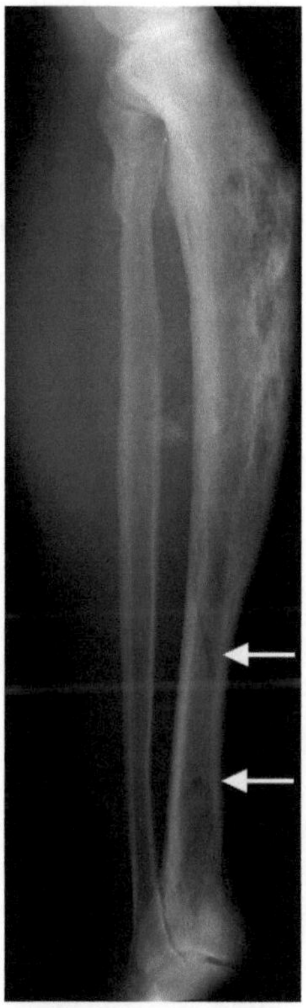

Fig. 12.2 Osteolytic front advancing distally in the mid- to distal tibia (*white arrows*) with sclerosis and secondary osteolytic fronts in the proximal and mid-tibia. Another osteolytic front is seen advancing proximally from the distal tibia (*white arrows*) in a 66-year-old male

bones. In the typical case of PDB, the osteolytic lesion advances from the metaphyseal to the diaphyseal region as a V-shaped cutting cone zone of resorption (Fig. 12.2). Less frequently, the osteolytic lesion may begin in the metaphyseal region and spread both distally and proximally. Rarely, two osteolytic lesions may progress from both the

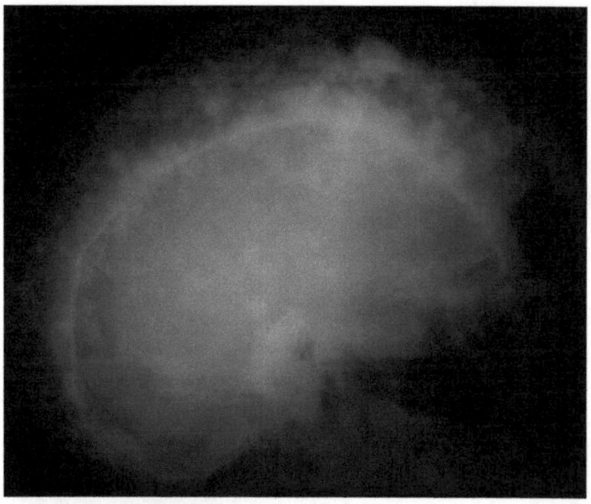

Fig. 12.3 Marked increase in size of the cranium with a "cotton wool patch" appearance of the sclerotic bone in a 68-year-old female

distal and proximal ends of a long bone (Fig. 12.2). In untreated patients, the process spreads at a maximal rate of 1 cm/year. The resorptive advance can be slowed or totally inhibited by effective antiresorptive therapy. In the untreated individual who survives to an advanced age, the process can eventually involve the whole bone.

As the osteolytic front advances through an affected bone, the previously osteolytic area exhibits coarsening of bone trabeculae, cortical thickening, and widening of the bone over time (Fig. 12.2). Secondary fronts of osteolytic activity may arise in the sclerotic bone (Fig. 12.2). This series of events is termed the mixed osteolytic/sclerotic phase.

In the final dominant sclerotic phase of PDB, the advancing edge of osteolytic activity is gone, although secondary fronts may be present. A bone may be markedly enlarged and deformed particularly in the lower extremities and the skull (Fig. 12.3). Nondisplaced, transverse fatigue fractures are quite common in the lateral cortex of the lower extremity long bones [80] (Fig. 12.4) and may lead to limb bowing. Transverse complete fractures of the long bones can accelerate and worsen the degree of deformity.

Patients who are immobilized for a prolonged period after a fracture or who are immobile for other reasons as well as patients who undergo surgery on a pagetic bone may experience a marked increase in osteolytic activity on X-ray evaluation.

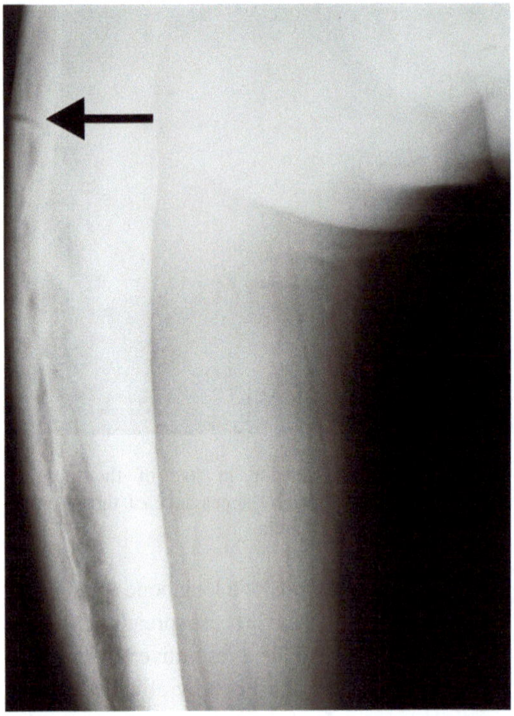

Fig. 12.4 Transverse fissure fracture (*arrow*) in the lateral cortex of the femur in a 60-year-old male

12.3.2 Pathology of Paget's Disease of Bone

12.3.2.1 Light Microscopy

Bone specimens from the advancing osteolytic lesion reveal numerous osteoclasts in Howship's lacunae. These cells often possess many more nuclei than are found in osteoclasts in normal bone [71] (Fig. 12.5). At the advancing front, there may be an increase in osteoblast numbers, but the adjacent bone marrow has normal fat and hematopoietic cell content. The appearance of the PDB bone can be distinguished from that of mild primary hyperparathyroidism by the presence of the large multinucleated osteoclasts.

Examination of bone more distal to the advancing front reveals a great increase in osteoblast numbers with hypertrophied osteoblasts present in Howship's lacunae where osteoclasts have vacated the lacunae [71] (Fig. 12.6). The marrow is hypervascular and mononuclear cells probably representing fibroblasts, preosteoclasts, and preosteoblasts have replaced variable amounts of the marrow (Fig. 12.6). The structure of the bone is

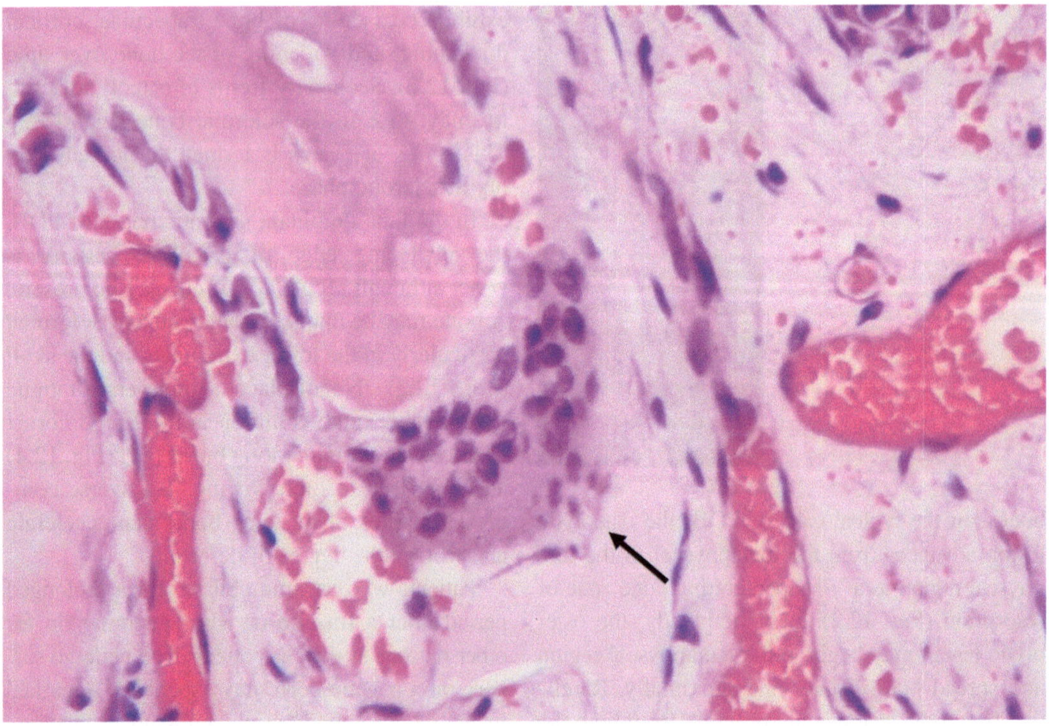

Fig. 12.5 Biopsy of Paget's disease exhibiting a large osteoclast (*arrow*) with at least 20 nuclei. H&E, ×20

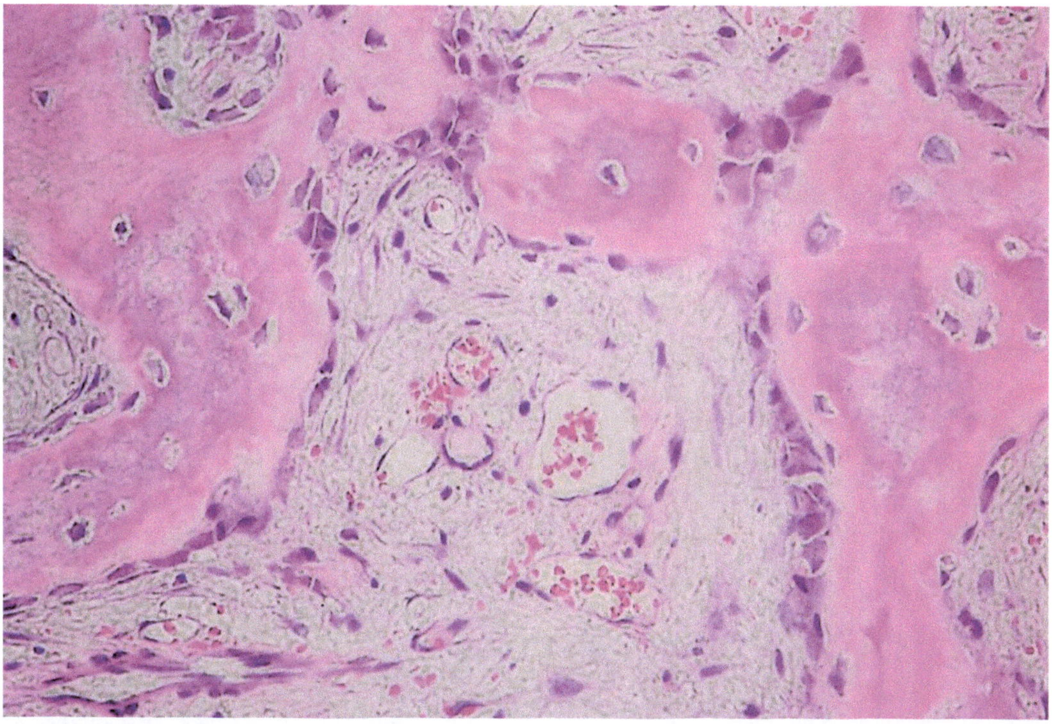

Fig. 12.6 Biopsy of Paget's disease exhibiting numerous osteoblasts lining the surface of thickened trabeculae that had likely undergone previous osteoclastic resorption. Normal bone marrow elements are replaced by fibrovascular tissue containing stromal cells, preosteoblasts, and preosteoclasts. H&E, ×20

now markedly abnormal. The trabeculae are markedly thickened, and, instead of the normal lamellar bone structure, a mosaic pattern of disorganized structure can be best seen under polarized light (Fig. 12.7). A significant component of woven bone is present and probably represents the most rapidly formed bone. Cortical widening is seen with involvement of the Haversian canals. Numerous large osteoclasts remain in resorbing bone, but at this stage, osteoblast activity exceeds osteoclast activity, accounting for the increase in the dimensions of the affected bone, albeit of highly abnormal structure. Bone formation rates calculated by the use of double labeling with tetracycline confirm a markedly increased rate of bone formation [73]. It has been suggested that enlarged lacunae surrounding some osteocytes indicate periosteocytic osteolysis, but it is more likely that these structures simply are a characteristic feature of osteocytes in woven bone.

In the last phase of PDB, the numbers of osteoclasts and osteoblasts are markedly reduced. It is unclear if the bone cell activity ever returns to a normal level in most patients. This last phase is associated with the most deformity of bone including bowing of long bones, skull enlargement, and kyphosis.

Just as potent antiresorptive agents can stop progression of osteolytic fronts noted on X-rays, these agents can markedly reduce the number of osteoclasts in bone. Secondarily, osteoblastic activity, as well as the hypervascularity of bone, also is reduced. Bone that is formed during antiresorptive therapy is lamellar. Despite this, it is unlikely that normal bone structure could be achieved in patients who present with significant sclerotic lesions.

12.3.2.2 Electron Microscopy

Osteoclasts

In the 1970s, investigators began to examine the ultrastructure of bone in patients with PDB to search for clues to its etiology. Rebel and colleagues in France first reported the presence of unusual nuclear inclusions in many of the osteoclasts in bone sections [90] (Fig. 12.8). This observation was subsequently confirmed in

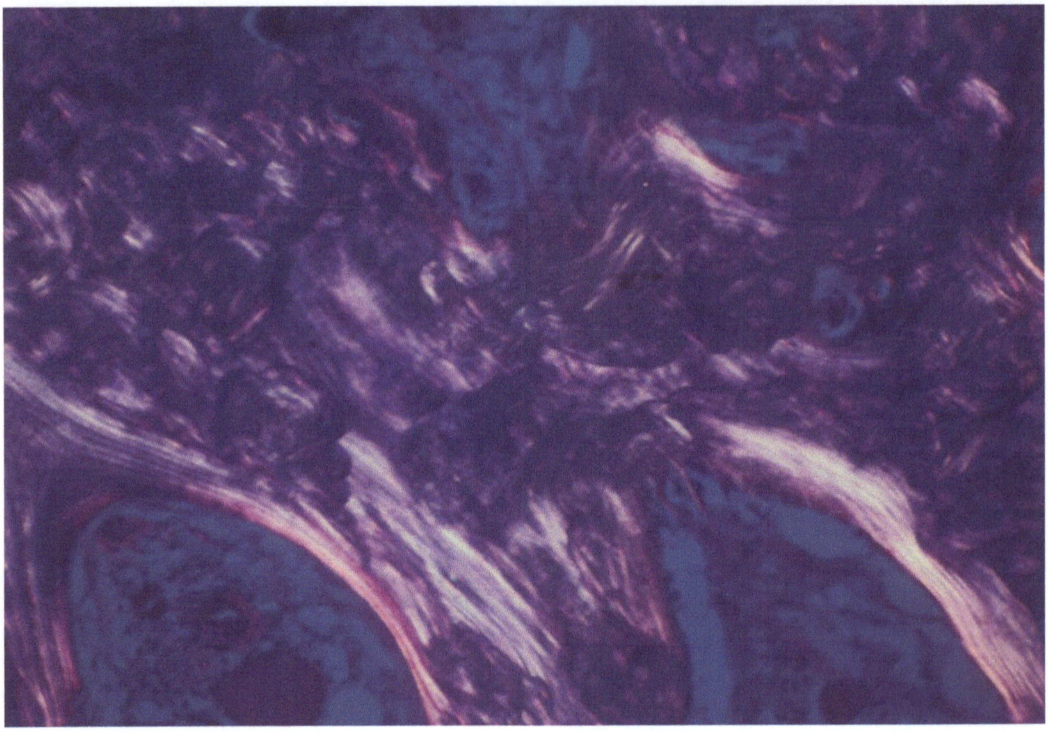

Fig. 12.7 Biopsy of iliac crest visualized under polarized light. Mosaic structure with mixture of lamellar and woven bone. ×40

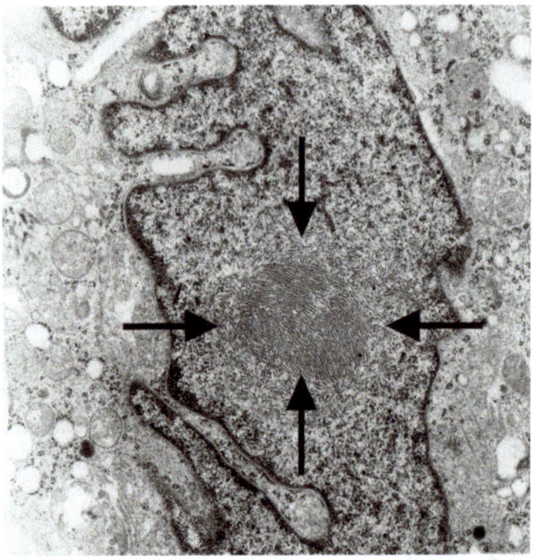

Fig. 12.8 Electron microscopy demonstrating the nucleus of an osteoclast in a patient with Paget's disease that has an inclusion in paracrystalline array. (Indicated by *black arrows*) Original magnification, ×9,000

patients from numerous countries including the United States, Germany, Italy, Canada, the United Kingdom, Japan, and Czechoslovakia [107]. The nuclear inclusions that have the form of microtubules are found in all patient specimens if enough osteoclasts are evaluated, but are not seen in osteoclasts from normal subjects. Inclusions are present in 20–40% of osteoclasts in a typical PDB specimen and in approximately 25% of the nuclei of osteoclasts that harbor an inclusion [76]. A variable distribution of the microtubules comprising the inclusions is seen, with a random distribution occupying 15% or more of the nucleus. Less frequently, the microtubules are packed into a paracrystalline array and occupy less than 5% of the nucleus. The inclusions are not membrane bound nor attached to nucleoli. Occasionally, the inclusions are associated with degenerating nuclei and can be seen in the gaps of the degenerating nuclear membranes and adjacent cell cytoplasm.

The external diameter measured in 94 individual microtubules was 12.4±0.4 nm, and under higher magnification, an electron-lucent central core with an internal diameter of 3.9±0.3 nm [41] was noted. Some of the microtubules were coated with a translucent ring. A cross section of the microtubules packed into paracrystalline array indicates a hexagonal arrangement of the microtubules.

Clearly, the inclusions are not normal components of osteoclasts, and similar structures have not been identified in the osteoclasts of patients with primary hyperparathyroidism, renal osteodystrophy, vitamin D-resistant rickets, osteomalacia, fibrous dysplasia, multiple myeloma, fibroosseous dysplasia, traumatic bone cyst, or cementoblastoma [76]. Not unexpectedly, the inclusions are readily found in the osteoclasts of giant cell tumors arising in the lesions of PDB [106]. Inclusions also have been found in a small minority of giant cell tumors of bone not arising in PDB [119], and in the osteoclasts of a few patients with pyknodysostosis [8], osteopetrosis [79], and familial expansile osteolysis [22]. Similar structures were identified in the giant cells of half (4/8) of patients with primary oxalosis [11].

Analysis of the ultrastructure of the osteoclast inclusions strongly suggests that they are nucleocapsids of the paramyxoviridae family. Howatson and Fornasier [41] carefully compared the structures of pagetic inclusions with nucleocapsids of MV and RSV in cells infected with the viruses and concluded that the inclusions of PDB were morphologically indistinguishable from the nucleocapsids of RSV, although RSV nucleocapsids are mainly found in elongated cytoplasmic processes of infected cells and not in the nucleus. The PDB microtubules are in the nuclei and to a lesser extent, the cytoplasm; a similar distribution is seen in the MV nucleocapsids. In one study, the microfilaments were noted either to be budding off from the peripheral cytoplasm or at the ruffled border of osteoclasts in two patients [1]. This observation would suggest the presence of an infectious virus in these patients. In no other study have such structures been observed.

Osteoblasts

The ultrastructure of the numerous osteoblasts found in active PDB lesions reveals well-developed rough endoplasmic reticulum with dilated cisternae, dense granular content, and a large circular Golgi complex. No nuclear inclusions have ever been described in the osteoblasts of PDB, and the cells are structurally indistinguishable from active osteoblasts in normal bone.

Osteocytes

Osteocytes have a more variable ultrastructure depending upon their localization in bone. Cells near a bone-forming surface frequently retain a well-developed endoplasmic reticulum indicating their origin from osteoblasts. Cells which are close to sites of osteoclast resorption have sparse cytoplasm with numerous vacuoles and minimal rough endoplasmic reticulum. These cells exhibit fine processes extending into canaliculi that interconnect with other osteocytes. These cells also have not been found to harbor nuclear inclusions.

12.3.3 Viral Studies

Because of resemblance of the nuclear inclusions to nucleocapsids of the paramyxovirus family, immunohistochemistry studies were undertaken using antibodies to several members of this viral family responsible for several common human infections. Basle and colleagues in France demonstrated the presence of MV antigen in the osteoclasts [4, 89], and this observation was confirmed in a large number of patients in the United States [78]. In a study of six patients in the United Kingdom, immunohistochemical analysis using one anti-MV antibody was negative [38].

Mills and colleagues initially found positive results with antibodies to RSV, which is a pneumovirus in the paramyxoviridae family [77]. Their initial results with one anti-MV antibody were negative, but several other anti-MV antibodies provided positive results and the unexpected observation that many of the patients that were studied had evidence of the presence of antigens from both MV and RSV, even in the same osteoclasts [78]. This could not be explained by cross-reacting antigens. No other laboratories have reported immunohistochemistry studies of RSV in PDB.

The initial molecular studies to identify a viral presence in PDB were reported by Basle and colleagues who utilized in situ hybridization to demonstrate MV ribonucleic acid (RNA) sequences not only in osteoclasts but also in osteoblasts, osteocytes, fibroblasts, lymphocytes, and monocytes [5]. From 80% to 90% of osteoclasts were positive, whereas 30–40% of the mononuclear cells were positive. The autoradiographic grains were noted in the cytoplasm and some of the nuclei of the osteoclasts. Reddy and colleagues confirmed the finding of MV RNA in pagetic bone marrow utilizing RT-PCR on cultured mononuclear cells from 5/6 PBD patients [92]. Full-length sequences of MVNP with a number of point mutations were identified clustered in the carboxy terminus of the protein. Subsequently, MV RNA was identified in a tiny proportion of cells in the circulation including monocytes and CFU-GM-derived colonies [91]. MV RNA also has been identified by one laboratory in 2/3 pagetic bone lesions and 2/3 pagetic osteosarcoma lesions [70]. Not all studies have found evidence of MV RNA in patients with PDB. Five laboratories have reported negative results [12, 33, 38, 65, 85].

Interest in CDV in PDB was stimulated by a study that suggested that dog owners were more likely to develop PDB [84]. Another study suggested that this was more likely if the dogs were not vaccinated [46]. Although a third study did not support this hypothesis [110], a series of studies by Sharpe, Mee, and colleagues reported evidence of CDV in bone using in situ hybridization, RT-PCR, and in situ RT-PCR in PDB patients [4, 33, 34, 42, 67, 68] and that CDV increased osteoclastogenesis from osteoclast progenitor cells in vitro [101]. Two other groups found no evidence of CDV in PDB [38, 65, 86].

12.3.4 Genetic Studies

PDB may affect multiple members of a family. From 15% to 40% of patients have a positive family history; men and women are equally likely to have the disorder, and there is an autosomal dominant transmission pattern with incomplete penetrance of the disorder. Because many individuals with PDB are asymptomatic, it is possible that the incidence of familial disease has been underestimated.

In 2002, Laurin and colleagues [56] reported the results of a genome wide-scan analysis of large French-Canadian families with PDB designed to identify genes associated with the disorder. They found a recurrent mutation in the sequestosome 1 gene whose 440 amino acid p62 protein was known to be involved in the NF-κB signaling pathway of osteoclasts. All but one of the family members with the mutation were heterozygotes. The finding of sequestosome1 mutations was confirmed by other studies of familial PDB, which found at least 22 different gene mutations in exon 7 and exon 8 in 29% of the families who were evaluated [95]. Patients with sequestosome 1 mutations have a somewhat younger age at presentation and more lesions than seen in sporadic patients [18, 115]. However, in the same family, one individual may have extensive disease and another, minimal disease. Mutations of the sequestosome 1 gene also have been reported in patients with apparent sporadic bone disease, ranging from 0% to 18.2% with an average of 6.1% in eight studies [95]. In the most recent report, 6% of apparently sporadic patients in New York City had sequestosome 1 mutations, and three new mutations were described in this study [75]. As mentioned previously, some of the patients labeled as sporadic could be members of a family in which PDB was not diagnosed due to the often asymptomatic nature of the disorder. In none of the studies were the parents or siblings of the patients clinically or genetically assessed.

Haplotype analysis in carriers of the most common sequestosome 1 mutation, P392L, has revealed that the French-Canadian patients had two haplotypes [95], H1(most common) and H2, while the great percentage of patients in European and United States populations had the H2 haplotype [16, 58, 75, 95], supporting the presence of an early founder effect for this mutation in these populations.

The majority of the sequestosome 1 mutations produce either missense or truncating mutations in the carboxy terminus of p62, the region of the ubiquitin-associated (UBA) domain. Evidence suggests that mutations within this region may reduce the ability of p62 to bind to ubiquitin, possibly increase RANK-NF-κB signaling, and then activate osteoclasts. Because mutations have been described outside of this region of the protein, other mechanisms may be involved in the activation of osteoclasts. There is increasing evidence that p62 is an important regulator of autophagy, the catabolic process involved in degradation of cytoplasmic proteins, protein aggregates and damaged cell organelles [60]. The exact mechanism by which an abnormality of autophagy might contribute to osteoclast hyperactivity remains to be determined.

In 2004, Watts and colleagues reported that mutations in the gene encoding valosin-containing protein (VCP) were responsible for the rare syndrome of inclusion body myopathy, PDB, and frontotemporal dementia (IBMPFD) [119]. This syndrome is an autosomal dominant disorder with incomplete penetrance of its components. Muscle disease is the most common finding and dementia is the least common. PDB is found in about 50% of members of affected families and is usually discovered at a younger age than in patients with classical PDB. Muscle biopsies in some patients contain rimmed vacuoles with filaments measuring 15–18 nm in diameter in the cytoplasm [50]. Muscle biopsies from three patients in separate studies were found to have mainly nuclear inclusions of filamentous nature [43, 48, 118]. In one study, the inclusions found in the osteoclasts of a family member with PDB were compared with those in muscle [48]. The inclusions in each tissue were similar in appearance, but detailed analyses of the ultrastructure in multiple specimens have not been performed. In a small number of brain specimens, nuclear inclusions have been found in neurons and dystrophic neurites that were ubiquitin positive, but rarely did the inclusions harbor the VCP protein [27]. A large study of patients with classical familial and sporadic PDB found no evidence of known disease-associated mutations of VCP in these patients [59].

VCP (also termed p97) is a member of the AAA-ATPase gene superfamily. VCP is believed to participate in the regulation of numerous cellular functions including ubiquitin-dependent protein degradation. The observation that the 13 unique mutations associated with IBMPFD cluster in a region proposed to associate with ubiquitin and ubiquitin-like domain containing proteins [120] suggests a common mechanism by which sequestosome 1 and VCP influence the pathogenesis of PDB. It also has been shown that there is a defect in autophagy associated with VCP mutations, which suggests a significant role for this process in IBMPFD [44]. As is the case with sequestosome 1 mutations, the mechanism by which impairment of autophagy would influence osteoclasts is uncertain.

Because sequestosome 1 mutations are only found in about 30% of families with classical PDB, investigators have continued to search for additional genetic loci associated with the disorder. Genome-wide association studies have indicated that variants of the genes for two receptors of RANKL, RANK [2, 15, 17], and osteoprotegerin (OPG) [10, 21, 124] may influence the pathogenesis of PDB presumably through regulation of osteoclasts by NF-κB. The OPG variants appear mainly to affect females. More recently, genetic variants close to the colony-stimulating factor 1 (CSF 1) and optineurin (OPTN) genes also have been identified as potential risk factors [2, 15]. All of these genes except OPTN are known to play a role in the biology of osteoclasts, but more investigations are needed to define the exact role the genetic variants might play in the pathogenesis of PDB.

12.3.5 In Vitro and In Vivo Models of Paget's Disease

In vitro studies of bone marrow cultures from involved sites of PDB have shown that the osteoclasts formed express a "pagetic phenotype" that distinguishes them from normal osteoclasts (Table 12.1). The PDB osteoclasts may contain up to 100 nuclei/osteoclast compared to 3–10 nuclei/osteoclast from normal subjects. Osteoclastic precursors in PDB are hyperresponsive to RANKL, TNF-α, and 1,25 dihydroxyvitamin D_3 ($1,25(OH)_2D_3$) and form osteoclasts at physiologic concentrations of $1,25(OH)_2D_3$ (10^{-11} M) rather than the pharmaco-

Table 12.1 Osteoclast phenotype in Paget's disease

Increased osteoclast numbers
Increased nuclei/osteoclast
Increased bone resorption capacity/osteoclast
Increased 1,25-$(OH)_2D_3$ sensitivity
Increased TAF-12 expression
Increased RANKL and TNF sensitivity

logic 1,25$(OH)_2D_3$ concentrations (10^{-8} M) required for normal osteoclast formation in vitro [49, 53, 69]. The 1,25$(OH)_2D_3$ hyperresponsivity results from elevated levels of a novel VDR coactivator, TAF12 (formerly TAF_{II}-17), in osteoclasts from PDB patients [53]. Furthermore, osteoclasts secrete high levels of IL-6, which is detectable in marrow plasma and peripheral blood from PDB patients [97].

Of the numerous mutations found in the sequestosome 1/p62 gene, the $p62^{P392L}$ was the most common [56, 81, 88]. When the mutated protein was expressed in human osteoclast precursors in vitro, the cells expressing $p62^{P392L}$ did show hyperresponsiveness to RANKL, but not to 1,25 $(OH)_2D_3$, and the cells did not express high levels of IL-6 or TAF 12 [52]. Importantly, mice in which the $p62^{P394L}$ mutation (the mouse equivalent of $p62^{P392L}$) is knocked-in to replace the normal sequestosome 1/p62 gene do not develop bone lesions or osteoclasts characteristic of PDB [39].

As noted above, MV and other paramyxoviruses also have been implicated in the pathogenesis of PDB. In one study, osteoclasts from ~70% of PDB patients expressed the MVNP gene, and normal osteoclast precursors expressing MVNP formed osteoclasts that exhibit the "pagetic phenotype" [54]. Furthermore, 29% of transgenic mice with targeted expression of MVNP to osteoclasts (MVNP mice) developed osteoclasts and bone lesions characteristic of PDB [55] (Fig. 12.9).

To assess the relative contributions of MVNP and $p62^{P392L}$ in PDB bone marrow specimens from clinically involved and uninvolved bones of familial PDB patients with $p62^{P392L}$ or normal subjects were tested for MVNP expression, and the effects of antisense-MVNP (AS-MVNP) were tested on the osteoclasts that were formed [51]. AS-MVNP blocked the in vitro generation of osteoclasts with the pagetic phenotype in experiments utilizing osteoclast precursors from patients who expressed MVNP. In patients who did not express MVNP or normal subjects, the AS-MVP did not affect osteoclast formation. The patients who were MVNP negative but had the $p62^{P392L}$ were hyperresponsive to RANKL. To delineate the mechanism(s) responsible for the abnormal osteoclast activity and bone formation seen with coexpression of MVNP and mutant p62, $p62^{P394L}$ knock-in (p62KI) mice (the mouse equivalent of human $p62^{P392L}$) were bred to TRAP-MVNP transgenic mice to generate p62KI/MVNP mice [51]. These mice developed increased numbers of pagetic osteoclasts and more striking bone pathology when compared to MVNP mice. The bone lesions in p62KI/MVNP mice were strikingly similar to those seen in PDB. The $p62^{P392L}$ gene increased RANKL sensitivity of osteoclast precursors, while MVNP was responsible for osteoclast hypermultinucleation, increased TAF-12 expression, and IL-6 production through enhanced p38MAPK signaling induced by 1,25$(OH)_2D_3$. When MVNP mice were bred with IL-6 knock-out mice, the osteoclast precursors of the progeny did not form pagetic osteoclasts in vitro, and bone histomorphometry revealed that the mineralized perimeter and bone formation rate in the animals were lower than in the MVNP mice. The data suggest that IL-6 not only plays a role in osteoclast function but also is a factor in the increased osteoblastic activity seen in PDB. The results are consistent with the concept that the $p62^{P392L}$ mutation and possibly other genetic mutations linked to PDB increase osteoclast formation and activity, but MVNP is required to produce the characteristic lesions of PDB that include increased osteoblastic activity. Similar to studies with transgenic $p62^{P392L}$ mice, two recent studies have reported that transgenic mice expressing the mutant VCP gene linked to PDB also have increased osteoclast formation and develop progressive osteopenia but no osteoblastic lesions typical of PDB [3, 20].

Genetic mutations linked to PD appear to predispose patients to PDB but require coexpression of an environmental factor in osteoclast precursors for the development of a robust pagetic phenotype. In support of this conclusion, Gennari and colleagues recently reported that

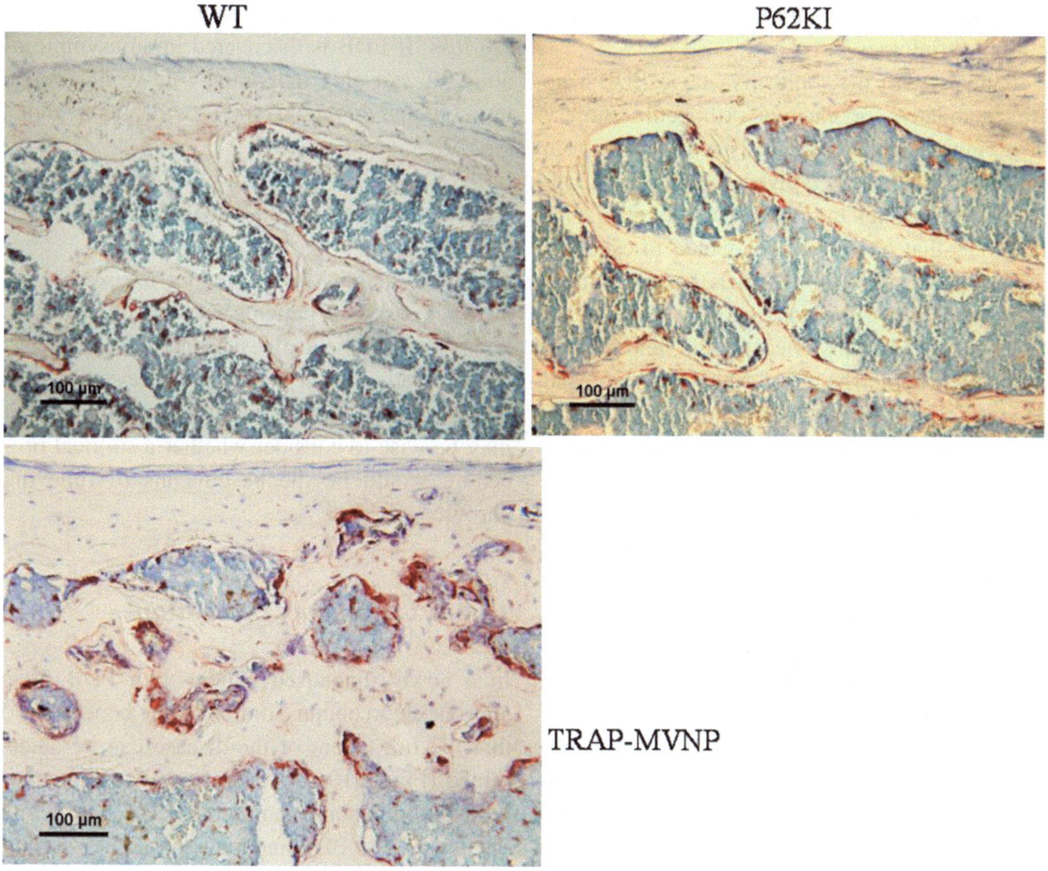

Fig. 12.9 Development of pagetic-like bone lesions and osteoclasts in TRAP-MVNP mice but not p62P392LKI or WT mice. Lumbar vertebral sections from WT, TRAP-MVNP, and p62P392LKI mice, 12–16 months of age, were TRAP stained. Only TRAP-MVNP developed pagetic-like osteoclasts and bone lesions (Courtesy of Dr. David W. Dempster and Hua Zhang, Regional Bone Center, Helen Hayes Hospital, West Haverstraw, NY)

there is a strong association between environmental factors and the development of severe PDB in patients with a genetic predisposition to PDB [30]. The observation that the incidence of PDB may be decreasing in a number of countries also is consistent with a change in the environment rather than a genetic influence [6, 87].

12.4 Treatment of Paget's Disease of Bone

12.4.1 Indications for Antiresorptive Therapy

Establishing a diagnosis of PDB does not automatically indicate the need for therapeutic intervention, particularly because the disease often is discovered by accident on an X-ray or because of elevated serum alkaline phosphatase activity on a chemistry panel. The location of the pagetic lesions, the presence of symptoms, and the age and expected duration of survival of the patient should be considered in deciding which, if any, treatment is likely to benefit the individual.

There is general agreement that bone pain, which is present in a minority of patients, is a clear indication for treatment. The degree of pain is generally mild to moderate, often is persistent, and is only slightly increased in weight-bearing bones by physical activity. Bone pain may be confused with arthritic or neurogenic pain in some patients. A therapeutic trial of a specific agent for PDB should reduce or relieve bone pain but not affect arthritic or neurogenic pain.

A partial response would suggest the pain has multiple etiologies.

Patients with metabolically active PDB who are candidates for elective orthopedic surgery involving a pagetic bone likely will benefit from antiresorptive therapy if given 2–3 months preoperatively. Although there are no randomized clinical trials that have been conducted to establish the benefit, it is known that such therapy reduces the vascularity of the bone and the surrounding soft tissue [123]. This effect should help prevent excessive hemorrhage during surgery and decrease the likelihood of the surgery to stimulate a marked increase in postoperative osteolytic activity, a finding that has been reported in untreated patients [47, 64].

Rarely, hypercalcemia may develop in a patient with PDB who is immobilized for any reason [82]. The absence of gravitational forces on the skeleton produces an increase in osteoclastic activity. Antiresorptive therapy can reverse the hypercalcemia [82].

In patients with extensive PDB of the skull, hearing loss is common [125]. Antiresorptive therapy has been reported to stabilize auditory acuity but not reverse the hearing loss [25].

In patients with deformities of weight-bearing bones, the degree of deformity often worsens over a period of years. There are no studies which indicate any benefit of antiresorptive therapy in preventing or delaying progression of deformities. This remains a theoretical possibility, and therapy might be considered in a patient with a long life expectancy.

The decision to treat a patient who is asymptomatic is more difficult to make because of the lack of very long-term clinical trials that would be needed to prove such a benefit. Because there is reasonable knowledge of the evolution of PDB, it is not inappropriate to consider treatment of some asymptomatic individuals. If an osteolytic lesion, particularly in a long bone of the lower extremity, the pelvis, the spine, or in the skull, is discovered in an individual who is 50 years old or younger, antiresorptive therapy could be used to reverse the lesion and presumably reduce the risk of future complications such as skeletal deformity, arthritic changes in an adjacent joint, neurogenic complications in the spine, and hearing loss. If PDB is discovered in an asymptomatic 90-year-old individual, it would seem unlikely that therapy would provide any benefit.

12.4.2 Nonspecific Therapy

Analgesic therapy should reduce the severity of all types of pain in patients with PDB. It is best to begin with simple analgesics and proceed to narcotic therapy only if pain remains severe. If narcotics are required to control pain chronically, it may be wise to consider whether a surgical procedure would be the best means of relieving chronic pain.

12.4.3 Laboratory Evaluation

In a newly diagnosed patient with PDB, it is appropriate to obtain a radioisotopic bone scan so that the full extent of the disease can be determined (Fig.12.10). X-rays of areas of increased radioisotope uptake can more specifically define the presence of PDB and may give some warning of impending problems such as degenerative joint disease.

The increased bone cell activity in PDB can produce numerous biochemical abnormalities measurable in serum and/or urine [102]. Increased osteoclastic activity is reflected by high serum levels or excretion of hydroxyproline, N-and C-telopeptides, deoxypyridinoline, tartrate resistant acid phosphatase, and RANK ligand. Increased bone formation is reflected by high serum levels of serum total alkaline phosphatase activity, bone specific alkaline phosphatase, and procollagen type 1 N-terminal propeptide. Serum osteocalcin, another protein synthesized by osteoblasts, has proven to be an inaccurate index of bone formation.

In clinical practice, the least expensive test, serum total alkaline phosphatase activity, has proven to be a reliable index of disease activity and remains the most widely used single test of disease activity. The other parameters are mainly used in clinical research studies.

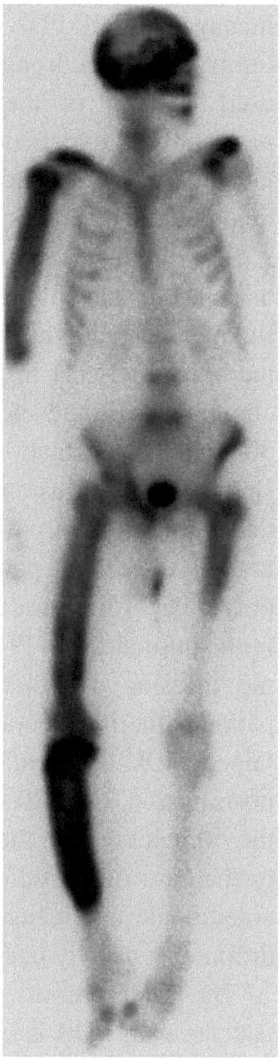

Fig. 12.10 Bone scan of 73-year-old man with polyostotic Paget's disease of bone

12.4.4 Antiresorptive Therapies for Paget's Disease of Bone

12.4.4.1 Calcitonin

Salmon calcitonin was the first effective treatment for PDB to achieve widespread use [112]. It was self-administered as a subcutaneous injection of 50–100 units daily or three times a week and inhibited osteoclast activity by binding to calcitonin receptors on the osteoclast cell membrane. Treatment caused an immediate decrease in bone resorption markers, and over 3–6 months maximal suppression of serum total alkaline phosphatase activity was about 50%. Relief of bone pain generally was noted during the first week of treatment. Osteolytic lesions, if present, often resolved after 1 year of treatment. Hearing loss was stabilized. Allergic reactions to this foreign protein were rare, although anti-salmon calcitonin antibodies could be detected in the serum of 50% or more of patients [105]. Resistance to salmon calcitonin therapy was manifested by a rise in biochemical markers of bone turnover despite continuing therapy in about 20% of patients. This fraction with resistance were usually the patients with the highest antibody titers. Such patients could be successfully treated by human calcitonin [104], but this option is no longer available. Side effects from the calcitonins included facial flushing and nausea, which sometimes resulted in termination of therapy. The use of calcitonin has decreased considerably since the development of more potent agents.

12.4.4.2 Bisphosphonates

The bisphosphonates are analogs of inorganic pyrophosphate, a factor involved in the mineralization of bone. Modification of the central P-O-P core of pyrophosphate to a P-C-P structure confers resistance to metabolic degradation and allows oral use of the drugs. These drugs bind to hydroxyapatite in bone, and the portion of the drug not taken up into the skeleton is excreted unchanged by the kidneys. The drugs inhibit osteoclast activity by different mechanisms of action than do calcitonin [96]. Etidronate and clodronate, the two earliest bisphosphonates, act by generating nonhydrolyzable analogs of adenosine trisphosphate, whereas all other bisphosphonates, which have one or more amino groups, inhibit farnesyl pyrophosphate synthase, an enzyme in the mevalonate pathway.

Etidronate, the first approved bisphosphonate, was widely used in a regimen of 400 mg daily given with water only for 6 months [45]. Like salmon calcitonin, it reduced markers of bone turnover by about 50%. Unlike salmon calcitonin, it sometimes increased bone pain during the early phase of treatment, but generally with time bone pain was reduced. Another drawback of etidronate treatment was that osteolytic lesions usually did not improve despite reduction in osteoclast activity. In such patients, calcitonin or more potent bisphosphonates could resolve the osteolytic lesions. When somewhat higher doses of etidronate were given, some patients developed osteomalacia as determined by bone biopsies [103]. A final negative aspect of etidronate therapy was the observation that prolonged intermittent use failed to suppress bone turnover to the same degree as the initial treatment [72].

A more potent agent, the aminobisphosphonate pamidronate, provided considerable improvement in the management of PDB. This was mainly given by intravenous infusions and was more effective in suppressing bone turnover. A single 60-mg infusion could reduce serum total alkaline phosphatase activity into the normal range for at least 1 year in patients with two-fold elevations of the enzyme activity [114]. Higher doses were required for patients with more severe disease. Unfortunately, there were no large clinical trials with pamidronate that could give good guidelines on treatment regimens for patients with more severe disease. Multiple doses, usually 90 mg each, could suppress disease activity back into the normal range in many patients, but in patients with markedly elevated serum total alkaline phosphatase activity, even infusions totaling as much as 2.5 g failed to normalize biochemical parameters [19]. In some patients treated intermittently for more than 3 years, some degree of biochemical resistance has been reported [116]. In general, the drug has been well tolerated, although an acute phase reaction producing a flu-like syndrome after the first infusion occurs in a significant number of patients and lasts several days . This reaction appears to be due to stimulation of gamma-delta T cells to release Il-6 and other cytokines [115].

Two more potent aminobisphosphonates became available after pamidronate, alendronate and risedronate. Alendronate was given as a 40-mg daily dose for 6 months before breakfast with water only [108], and risedronate was given as a 30-mg daily dose in a similar fashion but for only 2 months [109]. Both drugs produced good clinical results, with relief of bone pain and nearly equal suppression of bone turnover markers. No evidence of biochemical resistance with intermittent treatment of either drug has been reported. Some patients developed gastrointestinal side effects and stopped treatment.

Other oral bisphosphonates such as tiludronate, olpadronate, and neridronate were developed for clinical use, but the most impressive data in the management of PDB has come from trials of intravenous zoledronate [94]. Zoledronate was used initially in the management of cancer patients with hypercalcemia and/or bone metastases. Subsequently, it has been approved for the benign bone disorders, osteoporosis, and PDB.

The drug is the most potent of the bisphosphonates and has the highest affinity for hydroxyapatite. These features probably explain its remarkable therapeutic effects in patients with PDB. When compared with a 2-month course of risedronate, 30 mg daily, in a randomized, double-blind trial, a single 15-min infusion of 5 mg zoledronate produced a normal serum total alkaline phosphatase activity in 88% of patients by 90 days, whereas only 58% of the risedronate-treated patient were in the normal range [94]. Two years after the single infusion of zoledronate in nearly all the patients, the biochemical suppression was maintained [40]. In a preliminary report at 6 years postinfusion, only 20% of the patients exhibited their first loss of the therapeutic response [93]. As in the case of pamidronate, the first infusion of zoledronate may cause a fever and flu-like syndrome that usually occurs 8 h after the infusion.

The safety record of bisphosphonate use in patients with PDB is excellent. Allergic reactions are rare, usually manifesting as uveitis and/or scleritis, and most commonly occur with pamidronate [111]. Osteonecrosis of the jaw and atypical femoral fractures are extremely rare. Vitamin D deficiency should be ruled out and corrected before instituting therapy to prevent severe hypocalcemic reactions [122] and perhaps to reduce the severity of acute phase reactions after intravenous therapy [9]. Intravenous bisphosphonates should not be given to patients with an estimated creatinine clearance below 35 ml/min because high peak blood levels can produce renal damage. The drugs should be infused at the FDA recommended rate and that of other drug evaluation organizations.

12.4.5 Follow-up Evaluation and Retreatment

During the first year of treatment, measurement of serum total alkaline phosphatase activity approximately every 3 months should define the maximal response to the treatment. Depending on the potency and duration of action of the bisphosphonate, further tests should be performed every 3–12 months. Evaluation of osteolytic lesions would not generally be useful until 1 year after treatment has passed.

If the serum total alkaline phosphatase activity rises at least 25% above the nadir value, retreatment should be considered. If bone pain recurs, retreatment would be indicated.

12.4.6 Surgery

A small number of patients with PDB will require surgery for severe complications of the disorder. The most common procedures are probably hip [60, 66] and knee [29] joint replacement because of severe pain and limited mobility. Correction of spinal abnormalities [113], femoral fracture fixation [103], and straightening of lower extremity deformities [74] represent less frequent types of needed surgery, and surgery for hydrocephalus associated with marked cranial hypertrophy [98] would be rarely necessary. As previously mentioned, pretreatment with an antiresorptive agent 2–3 months before elective surgery will reduce blood flow in the affected bone and adjacent soft tissue and probably lessen perioperative hemorrhage without affecting bone healing. Surgeons who use autografts during a procedure should take care not to take the bone graft from a region of PDB because the disease can be transferred to previously normal bone [36].

References

1. Abe S, Ohno T, Park P, Higaki S, Unno K, Tateishi A. Viral behavior of paracrystalline inclusions in osteoclasts of Paget's disease of bone. Ultrastruct Pathol. 1995;19:455–61.
2. Albagha OM, Visconti MR, Alonso N, Langston AL, Cundy T, Dargie R, Dunlop MG, Fraser WD, Hooper MJ, Isaia G, Nicholson GC, del Pino MJ, Gonzalez-Sarmiento R, di Stefano M, Tenesa A, Walsh JP, Ralston SH. Genome-wide association study identifies variants at CSF1, OPTN and TNFRSF11A as genetic risk factors for Paget's disease of bone. Nat Genet. 2010;42:520–4.
3. Badadani M, Nalbandian A, Watts GD, Vesa J, Kitazawa M, Su H, Tanaja J, Dec E, Wallace DC, Mukherjee J, Caiozzo V, Warman M, Kimonis VE. VCP associated inclusion body myopathy and paget disease of bone knock-in mouse model exhibits tissue pathology typical of human disease. PLoS One. 2010;;5 .
4. Basle M, Rebel A, Pouplard A, Kouyoumdjian S, Filmon R, Lepatezour A. Demonstration of measles virus antigens in osteoclasts in Paget's disease of bone. C R Seances Acad Sci D. 1979;289:225–8.
5. Basle MF, Fournier JG, Rozenblatt S, Rebel A, Bouteille M. Measles virus RNA detected in Paget's disease bone tissue by in situ hybridization. J Gen Virol. 1986;67(Pt 5):907–13.
6. Bastin S, Bird H, Gamble G, Cundy T. Paget's disease of bone – becoming a rarity? Rheumatology (Oxford). 2009;48:1232–5.
7. Beclere M. Radiographie d'un cas de maladie de Paget. Bull Mem Soc Med Hop Paris. 1901;18: 929–31.
8. Beneton MN, Harris S, Kanis JA. Paramyxovirus-like inclusions in two cases of pycnodysostosis. Bone. 1987;8:211–7.
9. Bertoldo F, Pancheri S, Zenari S, Boldini S, Giovanazzi B, Zanatta M, Valenti MT, Dalle Carbonare L, Lo Cascio V. Serum 25-hydroxyvitamin D levels modulate the acute-phase response associated with the first nitrogen-containing bisphosphonate infusion. J Bone Miner Res. 2010;25:447–54.
10. Beyens G, Daroszewska A, de Freitas F, Fransen E, Vanhoenacker F, Verbruggen L, Zmierczak HG, Westhovens R, Van Offel J, Ralston SH, Devogelaer JP, Van Hul W. Identification of sex-specific associations between polymorphisms of the osteoprotegerin gene, TNFRSF11B, and Paget's disease of bone. J Bone Miner Res. 2007;22:1062–71.
11. Bianco P, Silvestrini G, Ballanti P, Bonucci E. Paramyxovirus-like nuclear inclusions identical to those of Paget's disease of bone detected in giant cells of primary oxalosis. Virchows Arch A Pathol Anat Histopathol. 1992;421:427–33.
12. Birch MA, Taylor W, Fraser WD, Ralston SH, Hart CA, Gallagher JA. Absence of paramyxovirus RNA in cultures of pagetic bone cells and in pagetic bone. J Bone Miner Res. 1994;9:11–6.
13. Brailsford JF. Paget's disease of bone, its frequency, diagnosis, and complications. Br J Radiol. 1938; 128:507.
14. Cartwright EJ, Gordon MT, Freemont AJ, Anderson DC, Sharpe PT. Paramyxoviruses and Paget's disease. J Med Virol. 1993;40:133–41.
15. Chung PY, Beyens G, Boonen S, Papapoulos S, Geusens P, Karperien M, Vanhoenacker F, Verbruggen L, Fransen E, Van Offel J, Goemaere S, Zmierczak HG, Westhovens R, Devogelaer JP, Van Hul W. The majority of the genetic risk for Paget's disease of bone is explained by genetic variants close to the CSF1, OPTN, TM7SF4, and TNFRSF11A genes. Hum Genet. 2010;128:615–26.
16. Chung PY, Beyens G, Guanabens N, Boonen S, Papapoulos S, Karperien M, Eekhoff M, Van Wesenbeeck L, Jennes K, Geusens P, Offeciers E, Van

Offel J, Westhovens R, Zmierczak H, Devogelaer JP, Van Hul W. Founder effect in different European countries for the recurrent P392L SQSTM1 mutation in Paget's disease of bone. Calcif Tissue Int. 2008;83:34–42.
17. Chung PY, Beyens G, Riches PL, Van Wesenbeeck L, de Freitas F, Jennes K, Daroszewska A, Fransen E, Boonen S, Geusens P, Vanhoenacker F, Verbruggen L, Van Offel J, Goemaere S, Zmierczak HG, Westhovens R, Karperien M, Papapoulos S, Ralston SH, Devogelaer JP, Van Hul W. Genetic variation in the TNFRSF11A gene encoding RANK is associated with susceptibility to Paget's disease of bone. J Bone Miner Res. 2010;25:2316–29.
18. Collet C, Michou L, Audran M, Chasseigneaux S, Hilliquin P, Bardin T, Lemaire I, Cornelis F, Launay JM, Orcel P, Laplanche JL. Paget's disease of bone in the French population: novel SQSTM1 mutations, functional analysis, and genotype-phenotype correlations. J Bone Miner Res. 2007;22:310–7.
19. Cundy T, Wattie D, King AR. High-dose pamidronate in the management of resistant Paget's disease. Calcif Tissue Int. 1996;58:6–8.
20. Custer SK, Neumann M, Lu H, Wright AC, Taylor JP. Transgenic mice expressing mutant forms VCP/p97 recapitulate the full spectrum of IBMPFD including degeneration in muscle, brain and bone. Hum Mol Genet. 2010;19:1741–55.
21. Daroszewska A, Hocking LJ, McGuigan FE, Langdahl B, Stone MD, Cundy T, Nicholson GC, Fraser WD, Ralston SH. Susceptibility to Paget's disease of bone is influenced by a common polymorphic variant of osteoprotegerin. J Bone Miner Res. 2004;19:1506–11.
22. Dickson GR, Shirodria PV, Kanis JA, Beneton MN, Carr KE, Mollan RA. Familial expansile osteolysis: a morphological, histomorphometric and serological study. Bone. 1991;12:331–8.
23. Edholm OG, Howarth S. Studies on the peripheral circulation in osteitis deformans. Clin Sci (Lond). 1953;12:277–91.
24. Eekhoff ME, van der Klift M, Kroon HM, Cooper C, Hofman A, Pols HA, Papapoulos SE. Paget's Disease of bone in the Netherlands: a population-based radiological and biochemical survey – the Rotterdam study. J Bone Miner Res. 2004;19:566–70.
25. el Sammaa M, Linthicum Jr FH, House HP, House JW. Calcitonin as treatment for hearing loss in Paget's disease. Am J Otol. 1986;7:241–3.
26. Erdheim J. Ueber die genese der Paget'schen knochenerkrankung. Beitr z path Anat u z allg Path. 1935;96:1–60.
27. Forman MS, Mackenzie IR, Cairns NJ, Swanson E, Boyer PJ, Drachman DA, Jhaveri BS, Karlawish JH, Pestronk A, Smith TW, Tu PH, Watts GD, Markesbery WR, Smith CD, Kimonis VE. Novel ubiquitin neuropathology in frontotemporal dementia with valosin-containing protein gene mutations. J Neuropathol Exp Neurol. 2006;65:571–81.
28. Franck WA, Bress NM, Singer FR, Krane SM. Rheumatic manifestations of Paget's disease of bone. Am J Med. 1974;56:592–603.
29. Gabel GT, Rand JA, Sim FH. Total knee arthroplasty for osteoarthrosis in patients who have Paget disease of bone at the knee. J Bone Joint Surg Am. 1991;73:739–44.
30. Gennari L, Gianfrancesco F, Di Stefano M, Rendina D, Merlotti D, Esposito T, Gallone S, Fusco P, Rainero I, Fenoglio P, Mancini M, Martini G, Bergui S, De Filippo G, Isaia G, Strazzullo P, Nuti R, Mossetti G. SQSTM1 gene analysis and gene-environment interaction in Paget's disease of bone. J Bone Miner Res. 2010;25:1375–84.
31. Gibbs CJ, Aaron JE, Peacock M. Osteomalacia in Paget's disease treated with short term, high dose sodium etidronate. Br Med J (Clin Res Ed). 1986;292:1227–9.
32. Goode A, Layfield R. Recent advances in understanding the molecular basis of Paget disease of bone. J Clin Pathol. 2010;63:199–203.
33. Gordon MT, Anderson DC, Sharpe PT. Canine distemper virus localised in bone cells of patients with Paget's disease. Bone. 1991;12:195–201.
34. Gordon MT, Mee AP, Anderson DC, Sharpe PT. Canine distemper virus transcripts sequenced from pagetic bone. Bone Miner. 1992;19:159–74.
35. Gutteridge DH, Ward LC, Stewart GO, Retallack RW, Will RK, Prince RL, Criddle A, Bhagat CI, Stuckey BG, Price RI, Kent GN, Faulkner DL, Geelhoed E, Gan SK, Vasikaran S. Paget's disease: acquired resistance to one aminobisphosphonate with retained response to another. J Bone Miner Res. 1999;14 Suppl 2: 79–84.
36. Hamadouche M, Mathieu M, Topouchian V, de Pinieux G, Courpied JP. Transfer of Paget's disease from one part of the skeleton to another as a result of autogenous bone-grafting: a case report. J Bone Joint Surg Am. 2002;84-A:2056–61.
37. Haworth S. Cardiac output in osteitis deformans. Clin Sci. 1953;12:271–5.
38. Helfrich MH, Hobson RP, Grabowski PS, Zurbriggen A, Cosby SL, Dickson GR, Fraser WD, Ooi CG, Selby PL, Crisp AJ, Wallace RG, Kahn S, Ralston SH. A negative search for a paramyxoviral etiology of Paget's disease of bone: molecular, immunological, and ultrastructural studies in UK patients. J Bone Miner Res. 2000;15:2315–29.
39. Hiruma Y, Kurihara N, Subler MA, Zhou H, Boykin CS, Zhang H, Ishizuka S, Dempster DW, Roodman GD, Windle JJ. A SQSTM1/p62 mutation linked to Paget's disease increases the osteoclastogenic potential of the bone microenvironment. Hum Mol Genet. 2008;17:3708–19.
40. Hosking D, Lyles K, Brown JP, Fraser WD, Miller P, Curiel MD, Devogelaer JP, Hooper M, Su G, Zelenakas K, Pak J, Fashola T, Saidi Y, Eriksen EF, Reid IR. Long-term control of bone turnover in Paget's disease with zoledronic acid and risedronate. J Bone Miner Res. 2007;22:142–8.

41. Howatson AF, Fornasier VL. Microfilaments associated with Paget's disease of bone: comparison with nucleocapsids of measles virus and respiratory syncytial virus. Intervirology. 1982;18:150–9.
42. Hoyland JA, Dixon JA, Berry JL, Davies M, Selby PL, Mee AP. A comparison of in situ hybridisation, reverse transcriptase-polymerase chain reaction (RT-PCR) and in situ-RT-PCR for the detection of canine distemper virus RNA in Paget's disease. J Virol Methods. 2003;109:253–9.
43. Hubbers CU, Clemen CS, Kesper K, Boddrich A, Hofmann A, Kamarainen O, Tolksdorf K, Stumpf M, Reichelt J, Roth U, Krause S, Watts G, Kimonis V, Wattjes MP, Reimann J, Thal DR, Biermann K, Evert BO, Lochmuller H, Wanker EE, Schoser BG, Noegel AA, Schroder R. Pathological consequences of VCP mutations on human striated muscle. Brain. 2007;130: 381–93.
44. Ju JS, Weihl CC. Inclusion body myopathy, Paget's disease of the bone and fronto-temporal dementia: a disorder of autophagy. Hum Mol Genet. 2010;19: R38–45.
45. Khairi MR, Altman RD, DeRosa GP, Zimmermann J, Schenk RK, Johnston CC. Sodium etidronate in the treatment of Paget's disease of bone. A study of long-term results. Ann Intern Med. 1977;87:656–63.
46. Khan SA, Brennan P, Newman J, Gray RE, McCloskey EV, Kanis JA. Paget's disease of bone and unvaccinated dogs. Bone. 1996;19:47–50.
47. Khurjekar KS, Vidyadhara S, Dheenadhayalan J, Rajasekaran S. Spontaneous rapid osteolysis in Paget's disease after internal fixation of subtrochanteric femoral fracture. Singapore Med J. 2006;47: 897–900.
48. Kimonis VE, Mehta SG, Fulchiero EC, Thomasova D, Pasquali M, Boycott K, Neilan EG, Kartashov A, Forman MS, Tucker S, Kimonis K, Mumm S, Whyte MP, Smith CD, Watts GD. Clinical studies in familial VCP myopathy associated with Paget disease of bone and frontotemporal dementia. Am J Med Genet A. 2008;146A:745–57.
49. Kukita A, Chenu C, McManus LM, Mundy GR, Roodman GD. Atypical multinucleated cells form in long-term marrow cultures from patients with Paget's disease. J Clin Invest. 1990;85:1280–6.
50. Kumar KR, Needham M, Mina K, Davis M, Brewer J, Staples C, Ng K, Sue CM, Mastaglia FL. Two Australian families with inclusion-body myopathy, Paget's disease of bone and frontotemporal dementia: novel clinical and genetic findings. Neuromuscul Disord. 2010;20:330–4.
51. Kurihara N, Hiruma Y, Yamana K, Michou L, Rousseau C, Morissette J, Galson DL, Teramachi J, Zhou H, Dempster DW, Windle JJ, Brown JP, Roodman GD. Contributions of the measles virus nucleocapsid gene and the SQSTM1/p62^{P392L} mutation to Paget's disease. Cell Metab. 2011;13:23–34.
52. Kurihara N, Hiruma Y, Zhou H, Subler MA, Dempster DW, Singer FR, Reddy SV, Gruber HE, Windle JJ, Roodman GD. Mutation of the sequestosome 1 (p62) gene increases osteoclastogenesis but does not induce Paget disease. J Clin Invest. 2007;117:133–42.
53. Kurihara N, Reddy SV, Araki N, Ishizuka S, Ozono K, Cornish J, Cundy T, Singer FR, Roodman GD. Role of TAFII-17, a VDR binding protein, in the increased osteoclast formation in Paget's disease. J Bone Miner Res. 2004;19:1154–64.
54. Kurihara N, Reddy SV, Menaa C, Anderson D, Roodman GD. Osteoclasts expressing the measles virus nucleocapsid gene display a pagetic phenotype. J Clin Invest. 2000;105:607–14.
55. Kurihara N, Zhou H, Reddy SV, Garcia Palacios V, Subler MA, Dempster DW, Windle JJ, Roodman GD. Expression of measles virus nucleocapsid protein in osteoclasts induces Paget's disease-like bone lesions in mice. J Bone Miner Res. 2006;21:446–55.
56. Laurin N, Brown JP, Morissette J, Raymond V. Recurrent mutation of the gene encoding sequestosome 1 (SQSTM1/p62) in Paget disease of bone. Am J Hum Genet. 2002;70:1582–8.
57. Leopold-Levi M, Londe A. Application des rayons de Roentgen a l'etude de la texture. N iconog de la Salpetriere. 1897;X:198–201.
58. Lucas GJ, Hocking LJ, Daroszewska A, Cundy T, Nicholson GC, Walsh JP, Fraser WD, Meier C, Hooper MJ, Ralston SH. Ubiquitin-associated domain mutations of SQSTM1 in Paget's disease of bone: evidence for a founder effect in patients of British descent. J Bone Miner Res. 2005;20:227–31.
59. Lucas GJ, Mehta SG, Hocking LJ, Stewart TL, Cundy T, Nicholson GC, Walsh JP, Fraser WD, Watts GD, Ralston SH, Kimonis VE. Evaluation of the role of valosin-containing protein in the pathogenesis of familial and sporadic Paget's disease of bone. Bone. 2006;38:280–5.
60. Lusty PJ, Walter WL, Walter WK, Zicat B. Cementless hip arthroplasty in Paget's disease at medium-term follow-up (average of 6.7 years). J Arthroplasty. 2007;22:692–6.
61. Mackenzie I, Young C, Fraser WD. Tinnitus and Paget's disease of bone. J Laryngol Otol. 2006;120: 899–902.
62. Maldague B, Malghem J. Dynamic radiologic patterns of Paget's disease of bone. Clin Orthop Relat Res. 1987;217:126–51.
63. Mangham DC, Davie MW, Grimer RJ. Sarcoma arising in Paget's disease of bone: declining incidence and increasing age at presentation. Bone. 2009;44: 431–6.
64. Marr DS, Rosenthal DI, Cohen GL, Tomford WW. Rapid postoperative osteolysis in Paget disease. A case report. J Bone Joint Surg Am. 1994;76:274–7.
65. Matthews BG, Afzal MA, Minor PD, Bava U, Callon KE, Pitto RP, Cundy T, Cornish J, Reid IR, Naot D. Failure to detect measles virus ribonucleic acid in bone cells from patients with Paget's disease. J Clin Endocrinol Metab. 2008;93:1398–401.
66. McDonald DJ, Sim FH. Total hip arthroplasty in Paget's disease. A follow-up note. J Bone Joint Surg Am. 1987;69:766–72.

67. Mee AP, Dixon JA, Hoyland JA, Davies M, Selby PL, Mawer EB. Detection of canine distemper virus in 100% of Paget's disease samples by in situ-reverse transcriptase-polymerase chain reaction. Bone. 1998; 23:171–5.
68. Mee AP, Hoyland JA, Baird P, Bennett D, Sharpe PT. Canine bone marrow cell cultures infected with canine distemper virus: an in vitro model of Paget's disease. Bone. 1995;17:461S–6.
69. Menaa C, Reddy SV, Kurihara N, Maeda H, Anderson D, Cundy T, Cornish J, Singer FR, Bruder JM, Roodman GD. Enhanced RANK ligand expression and responsivity of bone marrow cells in Paget's disease of bone. J Clin Invest. 2000;105:1833–8.
70. Merchant A, Smielewska M, Patel N, Akunowicz JD, Saria EA, Delaney JD, Leach RJ, Seton M, Hansen MF. Somatic mutations in SQSTM1 detected in affected tissues from patients with sporadic Paget's disease of bone. J Bone Miner Res. 2009;24:484–94.
71. Meunier P. La maladie osseuse de Paget – histologie quantitative, histopathogenie et perspectives therapeutiques. Lyon Med. 1975;233:839–53.
72. Meunier P, Ravault A. Treatment of Paget's disease with etidronate disodium. In: Singer FR, Wallach S, editors. Paget's Disease of bone, clinical assessment, present and future therapy. New York: Elsevier; 1991. p. 86–99.
73. Meunier PJ, Coindre JM, Edouard CM, Arlot ME. Bone histomorphometry in Paget's disease. Quantitative and dynamic analysis of pagetic and nonpagetic bone tissue. Arthritis Rheum. 1980;23: 1095–103.
74. Meyers MH, Singer FR. Osteotomy for tibia vara in Paget's disease under cover of calcitonin. J Bone Joint Surg Am. 1978;60:810–4.
75. Michou L, Morissette J, Gagnon ER, Marquis A, Dellabadia M, Brown JP, Siris ES. Novel SQSTM1 mutations in patients with Paget's disease of bone in an unrelated multiethnic American population. Bone. 2011;48:456–60. Epub 2010 Nov 10.
76. Mills BG, Singer FR. Nuclear inclusions in Paget's disease of bone. Science. 1976;194:201–2.
77. Mills BG, Singer FR, Weiner LP, Holst PA. Immunohistological demonstration of respiratory syncytial virus antigens in Paget disease of bone. Proc Natl Acad Sci USA. 1981;78:1209–13.
78. Mills BG, Singer FR, Weiner LP, Suffin SC, Stabile E, Holst P. Evidence for both respiratory syncytial virus and measles virus antigens in the osteoclasts of patients with Paget's disease of bone. Clin Orthop Relat Res. 1984;183:303–11.
79. Mills BG, Yabe H, Singer FR. Osteoclasts in human osteopetrosis contain viral-nucleocapsid-like nuclear inclusions. J Bone Miner Res. 1988;3:101–6.
80. Mirra JM, Brien EW, Tehranzadeh J. Paget's disease of bone: review with emphasis on radiologic features, part II. Skeletal Radiol. 1995;24:173–84.
81. Morissette J, Laurin N, Brown JP. Sequestosome 1: mutation frequencies, haplotypes, and phenotypes in familial Paget's disease of bone. J Bone Miner Res. 2006;21 Suppl 2:P38–44.
82. Nathan AW, Ludlam HA, Wilson DW, Dandona P. Hypercalcaemia due to immobilization of a patient with Paget's disease of bone. Postgrad Med J. 1982;58: 714–5.
83. Nuovo MA, Nuovo GJ, MacConnell P, Forde A, Steiner GC. In situ analysis of Paget's disease of bone for measles-specific PCR-amplified cDNA. Diagn Mol Pathol. 1992;1:256–65.
84. O'Driscoll JB, Anderson DC. Past pets and Paget's disease. Lancet. 1985;2:919–21.
85. Ooi CG, Walsh CA, Gallagher JA, Fraser WD. Absence of measles virus and canine distemper virus transcripts in long-term bone marrow cultures from patients with Paget's disease of bone. Bone. 2000;27: 417–21.
86. Paget J. On a form of chronic inflammation of bones (osteitis deformans). Med Chir Trans. 1877; 60(37–64):39.
87. Poor G, Donath J, Fornet B, Cooper C. Epidemiology of Paget's disease in Europe: the prevalence is decreasing. J Bone Miner Res. 2006;21:1545–9.
88. Ralston SH. Pathogenesis of Paget's disease of bone. Clin Rev Bone Miner Metab. 2002;1:109–14.
89. Rebel A, Basle M, Pouplard A, Kouyoumdjian S, Filmon R, Lepatezour A. Viral antigens in osteoclasts from Paget's disease of bone. Lancet. 1980;2:344–6.
90. Rebel A, Malkani K, Basle M. Nuclear anomalies in osteoclasts in Paget's bone disease. Nouv Presse Med. 1974;3:1299–301.
91. Reddy SV, Singer FR, Mallette L, Roodman GD. Detection of measles virus nucleocapsid transcripts in circulating blood cells from patients with Paget disease. J Bone Miner Res. 1996;11:1602–7.
92. Reddy SV, Singer FR, Roodman GD. Bone marrow mononuclear cells from patients with Paget's disease contain measles virus nucleocapsid messenger ribonucleic acid that has mutations in a specific region of the sequence. J Clin Endocrinol Metab. 1995;80: 2108–11.
93. Reid I, Lyles K, Su G, Brown J, Walsh J, Del Pino Montes J, Miller P, Fraser W, Gall M, Saidi Y, Bucci-Rechtweg C, Hosking D. Long-term efficacy of zoledronic acid compared with risedronate in Paget's disease. In: American Society for Bone and Mineral Research 31st annual meeting, Colorado Convention Center, Denver; 2009.
94. Reid IR, Miller P, Lyles K, Fraser W, Brown JP, Saidi Y, Mesenbrink P, Su G, Pak J, Zelenakas K, Luchi M, Richardson P, Hosking D. Comparison of a single infusion of zoledronic acid with risedronate for Paget's disease. N Engl J Med. 2005;353:898–908.
95. Rhodes EC, Johnson-Pais TL, Singer FR, Ankerst DP, Bruder JM, Wisdom J, Hoon DS, Lin E, Bone HG, Simcic KJ, Leach RJ. Sequestosome 1 (SQSTM1) mutations in Paget's disease of bone from the United States. Calcif Tissue Int. 2008;82:271–7.
96. Roelofs AJ, Thompson K, Ebetino FH, Rogers MJ, Coxon FP. Bisphosphonates: molecular mechanisms of action and effects on bone cells, monocytes and macrophages. Curr Pharm Des. 2010;16:2950–60.

97. Roodman GD, Kurihara N, Ohsaki Y, Kukita A, Hosking D, Demulder A, Smith JF, Singer FR. Interleukin 6. A potential autocrine/paracrine factor in Paget's disease of bone. J Clin Invest. 1992;89:46–52.
98. Roohi F, Mann D, Kula RW. Surgical management of hydrocephalic dementia in Paget's disease of bone: the 6-year outcome of ventriculo-peritoneal shunting. Clin Neurol Neurosurg. 2005;107:325–8.
99. Sauty A, Pecherstorfer M, Zimmer-Roth I, Fioroni P, Juillerat L, Markert M, Ludwig H, Leuenberger P, Burckhardt P, Thiebaud D. Interleukin-6 and tumor necrosis factor alpha levels after bisphosphonates treatment in vitro and in patients with malignancy. Bone. 1996;18:133–9.
100. Schuller A. Dysostosis hypophysaria. Br J Radiol. 1926;31:156–8.
101. Selby PL, Davies M, Mee AP. Canine distemper virus induces human osteoclastogenesis through NF-kappaB and sequestosome 1/P62 activation. J Bone Miner Res. 2006;21:1750–6.
102. Shankar S, Hosking DJ. Biochemical assessment of Paget's disease of bone. J Bone Miner Res. 2006;21 Suppl 2:P22–7.
103. Shardlow DL, Giannoudis PV, Matthews SJ, Smith RM. Stabilisation of acute femoral fractures in Paget's disease. Int Orthop. 1999;23:283–5.
104. Singer FR. Human calcitonin treatment of Paget's disease of bone. Clin Orthop Relat Res. 1977;127:86–93.
105. Singer FR, Fredericks RS, Minkin C. Salmon calcitonin therapy for Paget's disease of bone. The problem of acquired clinical resistance. Arthritis Rheum. 1980;23:1148–54.
106. Singer FR, Mills BG. Giant cell tumor arising in Paget's disease of bone. Recurrences after 36 years. Clin Orthop Relat Res. 1993;293:293–301.
107. Singer FR, Mills BG, Gruber HE, Windle JJ, Roodman GD. Ultrastructure of bone cells in Paget's disease of bone. J Bone Miner Res. 2006;21 Suppl 2:P51–4.
108. Siris E, Weinstein RS, Altman R, Conte JM, Favus M, Lombardi A, Lyles K, McIlwain H, Murphy Jr WA, Reda C, Rude R, Seton M, Tiegs R, Thompson D, Tucci JR, Yates AJ, Zimering M. Comparative study of alendronate versus etidronate for the treatment of Paget's disease of bone. J Clin Endocrinol Metab. 1996;81:961–7.
109. Siris ES, Chines AA, Altman RD, Brown JP, Johnston Jr CC, Lang R, McClung MR, Mallette LE, Miller PD, Ryan WG, Singer FR, Tucci JR, Eusebio RA, Bekker PJ. Risedronate in the treatment of Paget's disease of bone: an open label, multicenter study. J Bone Miner Res. 1998;13:1032–8.
110. Siris ES, Kelsey JL, Flaster E, Parker S. Paget's disease of bone and previous pet ownership in the United States: dogs exonerated. Int J Epidemiol. 1990;19:455–8.
111. Stack R, Tarr K. Drug-induced optic neuritis and uveitis secondary to bisphosphonates. N Z Med J. 2006;119:U1888.
112. Sturtridge WC, Harrison JE, Wilson DR. Long-term treatment of Paget's disease of bone with salmon calcitonin. Can Med Assoc J. 1977;117:1031–4.
113. Tancioni F, Di Ieva A, Levi D, Aimar E, Debernardi A, Colombo P, Gaetani P, Rodriguez YBR. Spinal decompression and vertebroplasty in Paget's disease of the spine. Surg Neurol. 2006;66:189–91; discussion 191.
114. Thiebaud D, Jaeger P, Gobelet C, Jacquet AF, Burckhardt P. A single infusion of the bisphosphonate AHPrBP (APD) as treatment of Paget's disease of bone. Am J Med. 1988;85:207–12.
115. Thompson K, Rogers Ms. Statins prevent bisphosphonate-induced gamma, delta-T-cell proliferation and activation in vitro.V Boneminer Res 2004;19:278–288.
116. Trombetti A, Arlot M, Thevenon S, Vebelhart B Meurler PS. Effect of mutiple intravenous pamidronat courses in Pagetis disease of bone. Rev Rhum Engl Ed. 1999;66:467–476.
117. Visconti MR, Langston AL, Alonso N, Goodman K, Selby PL, Fraser WD, Ralston SH. Mutations of SQSTM1 are associated with severity and clinical outcome in Paget disease of bone. J Bone Miner Res. 2010;25:2368–73.
118. Watts GD, Thomasova D, Ramdeen SK, Fulchiero EC, Mehta SG, Drachman DA, Weihl CC, Jamrozik Z, Kwiecinski H, Kaminska A, Kimonis VE. Novel VCP mutations in inclusion body myopathy associated with Paget disease of bone and frontotemporal dementia. Clin Genet. 2007;72:420–6.
119. Watts GD, Wymer J, Kovach MJ, Mehta SG, Mumm S, Darvish D, Pestronk A, Whyte MP, Kimonis VE. Inclusion body myopathy associated with Paget disease of bone and frontotemporal dementia is caused by mutant valosin-containing protein. Nat Genet. 2004;36:377–81.
120. Weihl CC, Pestronk A, Kimonis VE. Valosin-containing protein disease: inclusion body myopathy with Paget's disease of the bone and fronto-temporal dementia. Neuromuscul Disord. 2009;19:308–15.
121. Welsh RA, Meyer AT. Nuclear fragmentations and associated fibrils in giant cell tumor of bone. Lab Invest. 1970;22:63–72.
122. Whitson HE, Lobaugh B, Lyles KW. Severe hypocalcemia following bisphosphonate treatment in a patient with Paget's disease of bone. Bone. 2006;39:954–8.
123. Wootton R, Reeve J, Spellacy E, Tellez-Yudilevich M. Skeletal blood flow in Paget's disease of bone and its response to calcitonin therapy. Clin Sci Mol Med. 1978;54:69–74.
124. Wuyts W, Van Wesenbeeck L, Morales-Piga A, Ralston S, Hocking L, Vanhoenacker F, Westhovens R, Verbruggen L, Anderson D, Hughes A, Van Hul W. Evaluation of the role of RANK and OPG genes in Paget's disease of bone. Bone. 2001;28:104–7.
125. Young CA, Fraser WD, Mackenzie IJ. Detection of hearing impairment and handicap in Paget's disease of bone using a simple scoring system: a case control study. Bone. 2007;40:189–93.

13 Bone Loss in Space Flight and Countermeasures

Adrian D. LeBlanc, Elisabeth R. Spector, and Victor S. Schneider

Keywords
Space flight • Bone loss • Calcium balance • Gravitational effects on skeleton • Bone density

13.1 Introduction

Before manned space flight, it was known that immobilization of patients for extended periods, such as for fracture repair, to treat the paralysis of polio myelitis or paraplegia, often resulted in weakened and atrophic bones. Although the problems related to reduced gravitational forces on the musculoskeletal system were recognized, the full extent of the changes was not known. Therefore, studies were planned and conducted by the emerging American and Soviet space programs to determine the extent of, and potential harm associated with, bone loss that might occur during space flight.

The American human space flight program began in 1961 with the Mercury program which consisted of one-man capsules in low Earth orbit. A total of six Mercury flights took place, with the last ending in 1963. The Mercury program was followed by the Gemini program in 1965 and 1966 and consisted of 10 two-man flights. The Mercury flights were followed by the Apollo program that consisted of 11 three-man missions occurring between 1968 and 1972. In the final seven of these missions, two of the three crew members traveled and walked on the lunar surface, while the third remained in orbit around the moon. After the Apollo program, the National Aeronautics and Space Administration (NASA) launched the Skylab space station. Between 1973 and 1974, three 3-man crews occupied Skylab on missions lasting 28, 59, and 84 days. The Skylab missions focused extensively on life science investigations, including several studies related to the musculoskeletal system. In 1981, the Shuttle flight program began, with missions typically lasting approximately 1–2 weeks. The Shuttle program ended

A.D. LeBlanc, Ph.D. (✉)
Division of Space Life Sciences, Universities space Research Association, 3600 Bay Area Blvd, Houston, TX 77058, USA
e-mail: leblanc@dsls.usra.edu

E.R. Spector, B.S.
Bone and Mineral Lab, Wyle Laboratories, 1290 Hercules, Suite 120, Houston, TX 77058, USA

V.S. Schneider, M.D.
Office of the Chief Health and Medical Officer, NASA, 300 E Street SW, Washington, DC 20546, USA

F. Bronner et al. (eds.), *Bone-Metabolic Functions and Modulators*, Topics in Bone Biology,
DOI 10.1007/978-1-4471-2745-1_13,

Table 13.1 Manned space programs

National Programs					
USA		Russian		Chinese	
Mercury	1961–1963	Vostok	1961–1963		
Gemini	1965–1966	Voskhod	1964–1965		
Apollo	1968–1972	Soyuz	1967–1973		
Skylab	1973–1974	Soyuz/Salyut	1971–1985		
Shuttle	1981–2011	Mir	1986–2000	Shenzhou 5	2003
				Shenzhou 6	2005
				Shenzhou 7	2008
Joint International Programs					
Apollo–Soyuz		NASA/Russia		1975	
Shuttle/MIR		NASA/Russia		1995–1998	
ISS		Japan, Europe, Canada, Russia		1999–2020	
Commercial flight					
SpaceX				TBD	
Orbital Sciences				TBD	
Boeing Space Adventures				TBD	
Armadillo Aerospace				TBD	
Blue Origin				TBD	
Virgin Galactic				TBD	

in 2011 with the completion of the International Space Station (ISS).

The Russian program, while similar to the American program, placed greater emphasis on building large space stations, culminating with the completion of the Mir space station in 1986. The Mir space station was continuously occupied until 2000 when it was decommissioned and destroyed via a controlled reentry into the Earth's atmosphere. A period of US and Russian collaboration began in the early 1990s, including a series of visits to Mir by US astronauts using the Shuttle; these missions were referred to as the Shuttle/Mir Program. There were a total of seven missions, during which seven US astronauts and 14 Russian cosmonauts spent 4–9 months aboard the space station. From the musculoskeletal point of view, the Mir and Shuttle/Mir flights were important because they established that site-specific bone losses occurred in space. Bone mass was measured by dual X-ray absorptiometry (DXA). Current partners of the ISS are the USA, Russia, Canada, Japan, and members of the European Space Agency. Construction of the ISS began in 1999 and was completed in 2011. It is anticipated that the ISS will be used as a test bed for long-duration missions and as a model for international cooperation on future deep space missions to the planets and other destinations. Another development is the designation by the US Congress of the US portion of the ISS as a national laboratory; this is expected to increase financial support for research from commercial companies and other federal entities such as NIH, NSF, and USDA.

China is the third country to have launched humans into space. This program began with the launch of the Shenzhou 5 spacecraft, manned by a single crew member, in 2003. This launch was followed by a two-man flight in 2005 (Shenzhou 6) and a three-man flight in 2008 (Shenzhou 7). The USA, Russian, Chinese, and international manned space flight programs are summarized in Table 13.1. The future of US manned flight will be influenced heavily by commercial support for servicing the ISS and by other activities not yet envisioned at present. Table 13.1 lists some of the companies known to be developing commercial vehicles.

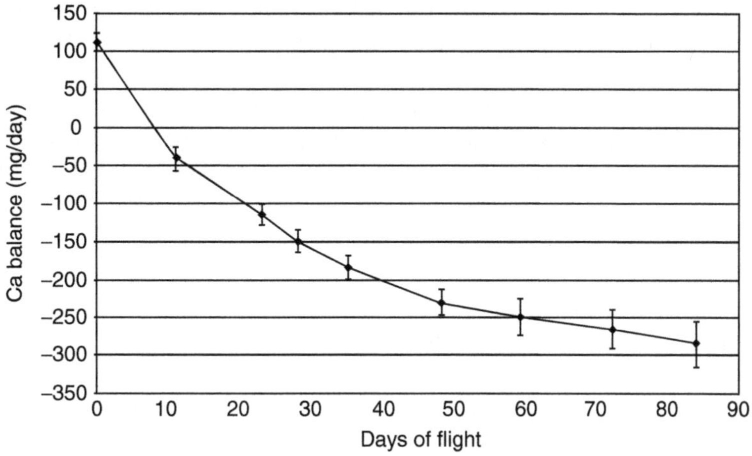

Fig. 13.1 Skylab calcium balance (Adapted from Rambaut and Johnston [31])

13.2 Bone Loss during Space Flight

During the early US space flight programs (Gemini, Apollo, and to some extent Skylab), there were no easy methods to measure changes in bone mass directly; hence, calcium (Ca) balance was used as an indirect measure of whole body bone loss. During the 14-day Gemini VII flight, an approximate metabolic balance study was attempted; the findings suggested a decrease in the Ca balance during space flight [23]. During the Apollo missions (Apollo 7–9, 11, 17), Ca balance was measured with varying levels of rigor; the findings pointed to significant Ca losses during space flight [4, 29]. In addition, regional bone density measurements were made with a new device designed and built for these missions [45]. The device was one of the first single-photon densitometers (SPA) used to measure bone density but was limited to the wrist and heel. Only small changes in bone density were observed, probably because of the short duration of these flights. Overall, the bone studies conducted during Apollo suggested that bone loss was not a major concern for missions that lasted only a few weeks.

Bone measurements were a focus of the three manned Skylab flights, which lasted 28, 59, and 84 days. These measurements included single-photon densitometry of the wrist and heel, urinary and fecal Ca output, and calculations of Ca balance. Urinary hydroxyproline was measured as an indicator of bone resorption. During all three flights, Ca balance was negative, averaging −200 mg/day for the 84-day Skylab IV flight [30, 31, 48]. The relationship between flight time and the average Ca balance for each flight is shown in Fig. 13.1.

In addition to the resulting negative calcium balances, urinary hydroxyproline levels were elevated above preflight levels in all three missions. This indicated a dramatic increase in bone resorption [31]. More recently, urine specimens that had been saved and frozen from the Skylab crew members were analyzed for NTX (N-telopeptide), a collagen breakdown product that is bone specific. In-flight increases in NTX approximated 100–150% above preflight levels, indicating elevated bone resorption similar to that suggested by hydroxyproline measurements in the 1970s [40]. Similar changes, although of lesser magnitude, have been documented during bed rest studies [14, 15, 37, 47, 50].

The single-photon densitometry device used during the Apollo program was also used during Skylab to measure pre- and postflight changes in the wrist and calcaneus (heel). No losses were seen in the wrist in any of the nine individuals of the Skylab crew, whereas three crew members showed losses (−7.4%, −4.5%, −7.9%) in the calcaneus [31]. These early experiments were important for several reasons. First, they provided clear evidence that bone loss might become a significant risk for long-duration space flight.

Secondly, these findings demonstrated that bone loss was not the same in all parts of the skeleton, for example, significant losses occurred in the calcaneus but not in the wrist. Thirdly, regional losses, on a percentage basis, were much greater than the total loss of bone mineral, as demonstrated by a comparison of the losses in the calcaneus with the total body losses calculated from the Ca balance.

In this same time frame, Soviet scientists were obtaining bone measurements comparable to those of the US program [3, 7]. Percentage losses of bone density in the calcaneus after missions lasting 75–184 days ranged from −0.9% to −19.8% [44]. The Soviets used computed tomography to estimate bone mineral density (BMD) changes in four cosmonauts after 5–7-month Salyut missions [26, 35]. Lumbar spine BMD values varied, with individual changes of 6.1%, −0.3%, −2.3%, and −0.8%.

In 1989, the American and Russian space agencies began a joint effort to obtain comprehensive measurements of BMD of cosmonauts before and after long-duration missions aboard the Mir spacecraft. The American space agency provided a Hologic 1,000 W dual energy X-ray absorptiometry scanner that was installed at the Cosmonaut Training Center in Star City, Russia, in January 1990. The testing protocol included individual scans of the whole body, lumbar spine, left hip, and left proximal tibia. The results from the first seven cosmonauts were published in 1992 [27]; those from the 18 cosmonauts were published in 2000 [16]. Table 13.2, from the latter publication, shows significant monthly BMD losses in the lumbar spine, femur neck, trochanter, pelvis, legs, and whole body of −1.1%, −1.2%, −1.6%, −1.4%, −0.3%, and −0.4%, respectively. The whole body BMD change (−0.4%/month) is comparable to the Ca losses noted during Skylab IV (average loss of −0.5%/month calculated from Ca balance) [31]. Although these flight changes are expressed as percent change per month in order to normalize for flight duration, it is likely that actual bone loss rates are not linear. This nonlinearity is evident from the Skylab Ca balance data (see Fig. 13.1) and from bed rest studies. A consistent finding of all disuse studies (both space flight and bed rest) has been the large variability in the loss of BMD in different subjects and from different bone sites in a given individual [17]. This is illustrated in Fig. 13.2, which shows the percentage losses in selected bone regions of crew members of the ISS and Mir missions normalized to 6 months in space; these data are derived assuming a linear relationship between time in space flight and change in bone mass. This large range in response to space flight means that it may be difficult to develop a simple prescription suitable for all crew members on long duration missions.

Table 13.2 BMD and body composition changes after 4–14.4 months of space flight (Mir)

Variable	*N*	%/month	SD
BMD lumbar spine	18	−1.06*	0.63
BMD femoral neck	18	−1.15*	0.84
BMD trochanter	18	−1.56*	0.99
BMD total body	17	−0.35*	0.25
BMD pelvis	17	−1.35*	0.54
BMD arm	17	−0.04	0.88
BMD leg	16	−0.34*	0.33

From LeBlanc et al. [16] *$p<0.05$

A review of Fig. 13.2 might give the impression that some crew members responded with only minor losses, and therefore, an analysis of these individuals could lead to countermeasures for others. Unfortunately, there is significant variability between bone sites as well as between individuals, inasmuch as 90% of the 64 astronauts and cosmonauts who flew on long-duration Mir or ISS missions (mean duration 174 ± 50 days) had at least a 5% BMD loss in one or more skeletal sites. Furthermore, more than 50% had a 10% or greater BMD loss in at least one site (see Fig. 13.3). If a crew member loses little to no bone in one region, he/she may well experience significant loss in one or more other regions. The changes in BMD occurred even though programs have employed exercise and dietary countermeasure regimens. The vast majority of long-duration space flight data obtained to date are from flights lasting approximately 4–6 months, with only a few flights extending near or just beyond the 1-year mark. Thus, the extent of ultimate bone loss on flights lasting years is unknown.

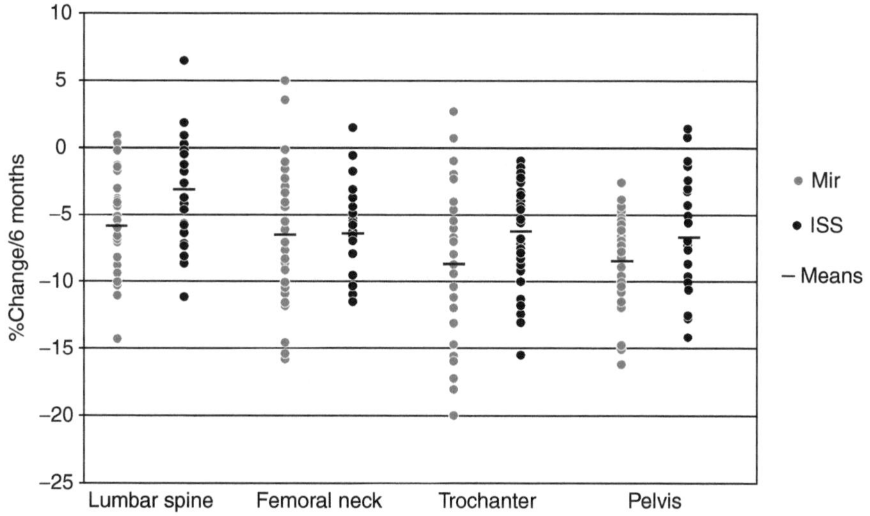

Fig. 13.2 DXA BMD loss in Mir and ISS crewmembers, normalized to 6 months of space flight (Mir – $n=33$; ISS – $n=33$)

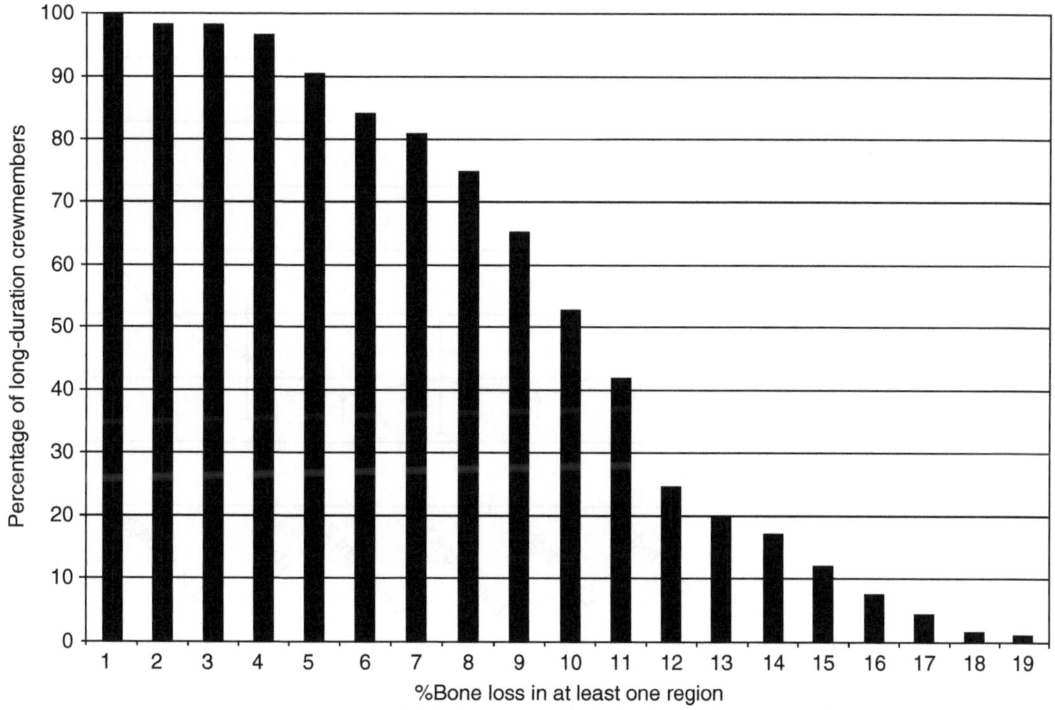

Fig. 13.3 DXA BMD loss in at least one region, Mir and ISS crewmembers ($n=64$) (Adapted from LeBlanc et al. [18])

In addition to the pre- and postflight DXA measurements, the Mir missions also included in-flight measures of blood and urinary bone markers. Figures 13.4 and 13.5 show published data from six male crew members who flew on missions lasting 4–6 months [41]. These data include measures of the bone resorption marker NTX and of the bone formation marker osteocalcin. Bone-specific alkaline phosphatase showed results similar to osteocalcin. Bone resorption was elevated,

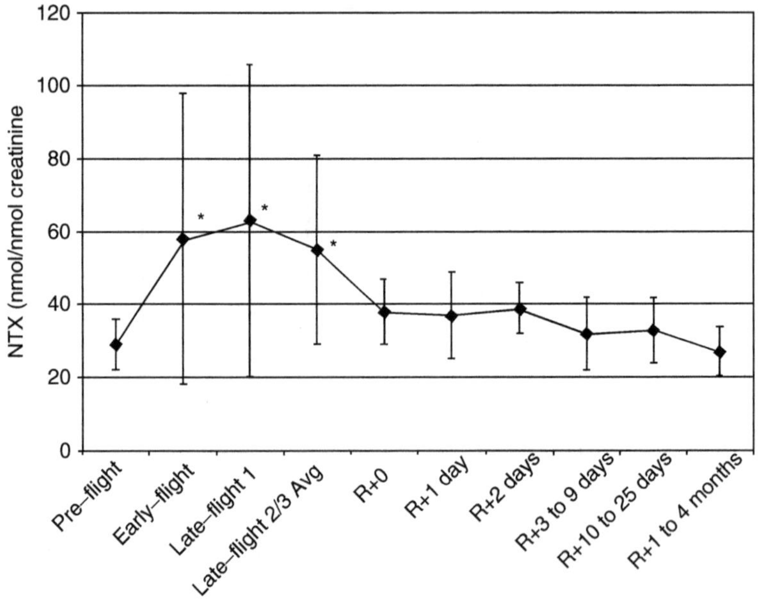

Fig. 13.4 N-telopeptide during and after Mir space flight (mean ± SD) (Adapted from Smith et al. [41], $*p<0.05$)

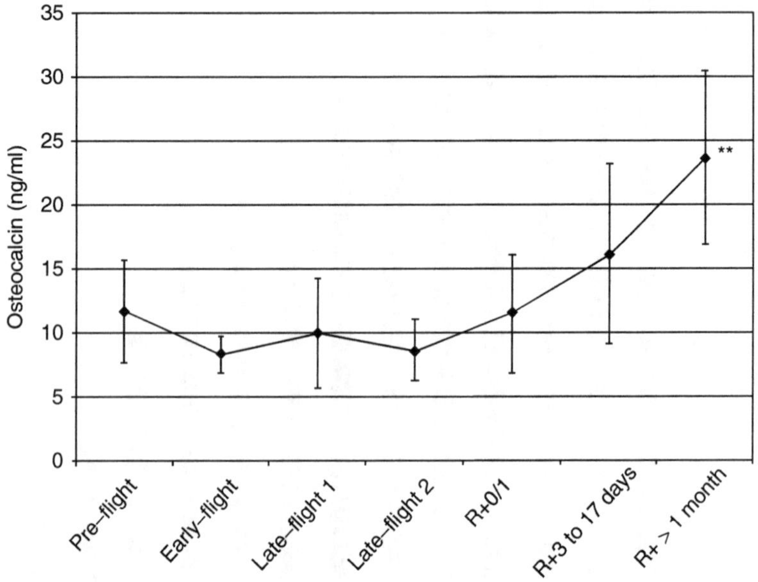

Fig. 13.5 Osteocalcin during and after Mir space flight (mean ± SD) (Adapted from Smith et al. [41], $**p<0.01$)

as seen in Skylab, with only minimal changes in bone formation. The bone formation data contradict results from early animal studies. This needs to be emphasized because many investigators are under the impression that suppressed bone formation is the major problem. However, in humans the problem appears to be a relative increase in bone resorption, caused either by an increase in the efficiency of osteoclast resorption, increased recruitment of osteoclasts, inhibition of osteoclast apoptosis, or a combination of all three mechanisms. This does not rule out the possibility that bone formation is depressed in some skeletal regions not reflected in the systemic marker data. Available data are consistent with increased remodeling and uncoupling of formation and resorption. This situation leads to rapid bone loss and possible architectural changes to bone.

In 2000, NASA funded a study to determine compartmental changes in bone mass and geometry with the aid of high-resolution quantitative computerized tomography (QCT) of the hip and spine. QCT scans were performed on 16 ISS crew members (both astronauts and cosmonauts) before and after ISS missions that lasted 4–6 months. Data were obtained in addition to the standard DXA measurements performed before and after each mission. The results on the first 14 subjects were published in 2004 [13]. Table 13.3 shows the trabecular as well as integral (combined cortical and trabecular) changes in volumetric bone mineral density (vBMD) of the spine and hip. The mean change in integral vBMD, comparable to areal (g/cm^2) DXA BMD, was –0.9%/month in the spine, similar to the mean –1%/month changes documented by DXA (see Table 13.2) [16]. As with the spine, DXA BMD changes in the hip were similar to integral vBMD measured by QCT (–1.4%/month) and similar also to published Mir results [16]. Unlike the spine, however, QCT of the hip revealed significant compartmental differences: –2.3%/month for trabecular bone loss of the total hip [13]. The QCT data also showed statistically significant decreases in cortical volume at the femoral neck, trochanter, and total femur (–1.2 to –1.3%/month). The changes suggest a reduction in femoral neck bending strength, with loss of cortical bone taking place from the endocortical side. The QCT results point to the value of high-resolution volumetric measurements of specific bone compartments to assess changes in bone strength. Bone strength is the variable that is ultimately of greatest interest when studying the effects of disuse. Biochemical measurements have no site specificity, and even standard DXA measurements do not offer a means of discerning compartmental or 3D geometric changes in bone. Figure 13.6 graphs the trabecular losses normalized to 6 months of flight in the 14 crew members from this study. A comparison of this graph with Fig. 13.2 demonstrates that the largest losses are in the trabecular bone in the hip. The findings also indicate the large intrasubject and regional variation in the changes in different bones. Any countermeasure must take into account this distribution, particularly the potential for large losses in some regions in some individuals. Designing a fully reliable countermeasure against bone loss will not be easy, and current knowledge suggests the need for a suite of countermeasures for long-duration flights to control this risk.

Table 13.3 QCT changes in BMD after long-duration space flight (ISS)

QCT changes in BMD in 14 ISS crewmembers (%/month ± SD)	
Lumbar spine, integral	–0.9±0.5**
Lumbar spine, trabecular	–0.7±0.6*
Total hip, integral	–1.4±0.8**
Total hip, trabecular	–2.3±0.8**
Femoral neck, integral	–1.2±0.7**
Femoral neck, trabecular	–2.7±1.9**

From Lang et al. [13] *$p<0.01$ **$p<0.001$

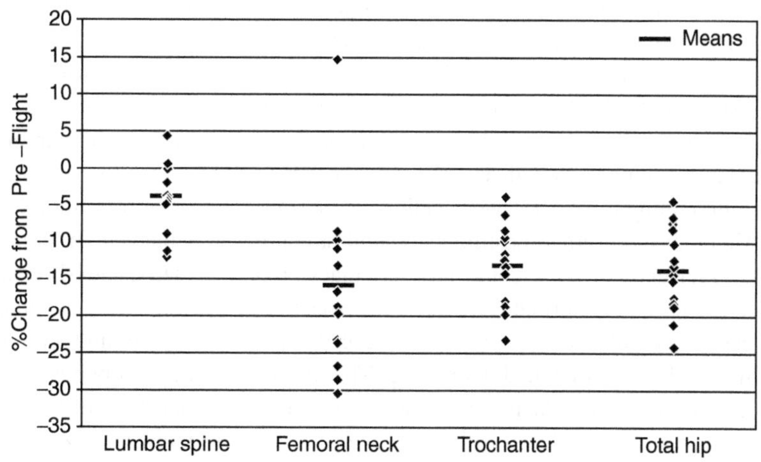

Fig. 13.6 Change in QCT trabecular BMD after long-duration ISS space flight ($n=14$)

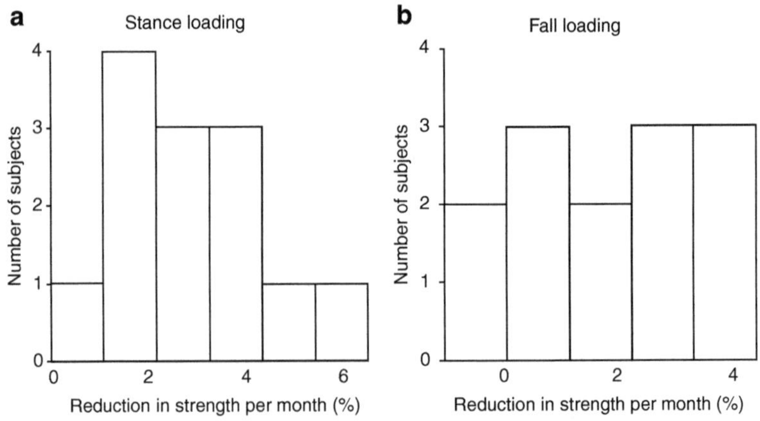

Fig. 13.7 Reduction in hip finite element-computed proximal femoral strength, percent per month (**a**) stance loading; (**b**) fall loading (Reprinted from Keyak et al. [12], Copyright 2009, with permission from Elsevier)

An important question is will this bone mass change increase the risk of bone fracture after return to one-G conditions on Earth or activity on distant planetary missions. Fracture risk is multifactorial and includes the manner and frequency of falling as well as bone strength. Although difficult to determine, the risk of falling is likely greater immediately after landing because of documented vestibular deficits following flight. Estimates of hip bone strength, however, were calculated using finite modeling techniques in the subjects from the QCT study described above [12]. Loading conditions representing either single-limb stance or a fall onto the posterolateral aspect of the greater trochanter were modeled, and finite element (FE) strength values were computed and expressed as multiples of crew member body weight. The mean strength decreased from 18.2 times body weight (BW) preflight to 15.6 BW postflight for stance loading and from 3.5 to 3.1 BW postflight for the fall loading condition. Normalized on a per-month basis, the changes were –2.6%/month (–0.6% to –5.0%) and –2.0%/month (–0.6% to –3.9%) for the two conditions. Figure 13.7 shows the individual crew member strength data as a percent change from preflight for the two loading conditions. Although the average postflight femoral strength was high enough to overcome the forces that would be due to falls or normal activities, the losses in at least some subjects were close to the estimated lifetime losses associated with aging. This means that in some individuals, their margin of safety was significantly reduced without recovery.

In addition to the fracture risk associated with weakened bones, another risk at least partially related to bone atrophy is high urinary Ca, which can increase the risk of renal stones. There have been 14 incidents of renal stone formation in 12 crew members reported in the US space program [28]. Most of these events occurred within the first 6 years after flight, with no events occurring during flight. In addition, multiple stone formation events have been reported in the Russian program, including one event during flight. In the latter case, the stone fortunately was "passed," avoiding the need to return the crew member to Earth in an emergency situation. Because we cannot currently predict which astronauts will develop renal stones, prophylactic reduction of risk factors, including excess urinary Ca output, becomes a key to enable long-term space flight. Any countermeasure that attenuates bone loss also should reduce the renal stone risk, at least for stones attributed to an increase in renal Ca excretion.

In summary, current knowledge regarding bone loss in humans in microgravity can be described as follows:

- Remodeling is elevated and uncoupled. Whole body bone marker measurements indicate that resorption is elevated (50–100%), whereas bone formation is little changed.
- Changes in bone mass measured by QCT, DXA, and SPA show bone losses in most skeletal sites; the magnitude of which are bone region and compartment specific, with the highest percentage rate in the trabecular compartment of the hip.
- Crew members are in negative Ca balance for as long as Ca balance has been measured in-flight (3 months), displaying an exponential shape and

implying a similar regional bone response. There is a need for additional information regarding the temporal relationship of in-flight bone loss. The resultant hypercalciuria during flight is frequently observed and is associated with increased risk for renal stone formation.

- Individual crew members show a wide variability of bone loss, as is also true for subjects in bed rest studies. Because the bed rest studies were conducted with healthy subjects under standardized conditions, a significant genetic component is suspected.
- Space flight-induced bone changes result in significant reductions in bone strength measured by FE modeling.
- Because of the inability to determine a priori the bone loss risk of an individual crew member and because of the potential that exercise equipment will fail, a robust suite of countermeasures is needed.

13.3 Recovery of Bone After Flight

Assuming that bone loss will always be a factor during long missions and that the development of an efficient and dependable set of countermeasures during flight will not materialize, it is crucial to know if bone loss is recovered in a reasonable time after the end of the flight. For example, will the activity of a returning astronaut need to be limited indefinitely or will recovery occur before the next scheduled space mission? There are at least four facets to these questions to consider: (1) recovery of bone mass at critical sites (e.g., spine, hip, and pelvis), (2) the differences in compartmental recovery (e.g., trabecular vs. cortical bone), (3) architectural and geometric changes (e.g., trabecular number, connectivity, cortical porosity, cortical thickness, and cross-sectional area), and (4) the effect of residual changes on bone strength under various terrestrial loading conditions.

A recent publication based on DXA measurements demonstrated that recovery occurs but does so slowly [39]. Available findings have come largely from a study that was not designed for investigating bone recovery and were obtained from individuals who flew a second mission after an initial flight, thus requiring a second baseline measurement. The data were fitted to an exponential function expressed as % change from the postflight BMD as a function of time after the first flight. Although there were limitations in this analysis, the results indicated that recovery may take 3–5 years following a 5–6-month space flight mission. Figure 13.8 shows a more limited set of data ($n = 27$) with individual crew members measured (DXA) sequentially immediately after flight and at 6 and 12 months postflight. While the postflight measurement time was less than in the preceding study, the data show a similar exponential response with up to several years required for full recovery. Another report on a subset of

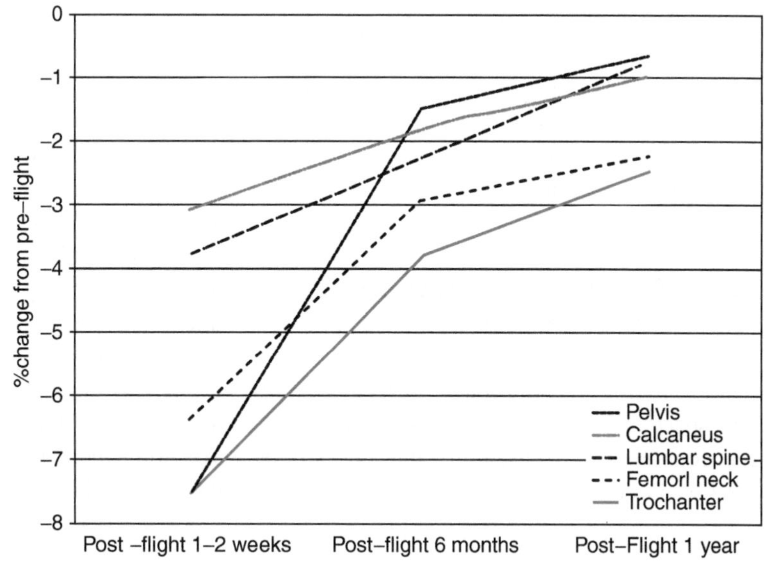

Fig. 13.8 DXA BMD recovery after long-duration Mir and ISS space flight ($n = 27$)

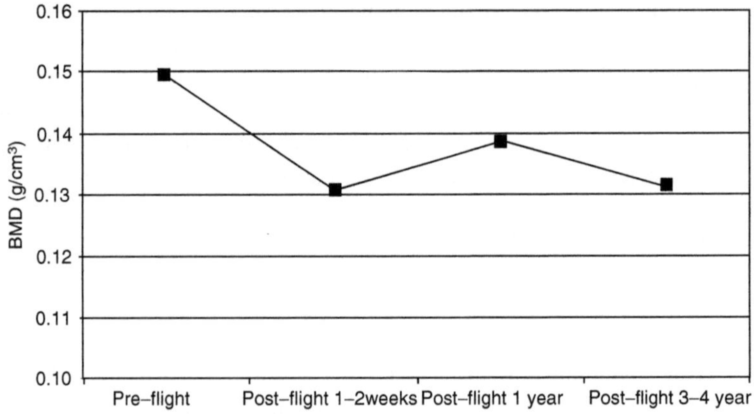

Fig. 13.9 Recovery of QCT trabecular BMD of the hip after long-duration ISS space flight ($n=8$)

the QCT data mentioned earlier demonstrated that postflight trabecular bone loss in the hip regions may not be complete 2.5–4 years after landing (see Fig. 13.9) [5]. Therefore, loss of bone mineral mass, as well as related architectural changes, may not be reversed after flights lasting 5–6 months. Data were insufficient to determine strength changes at the extended recovery time point.

These findings reinforce the need to develop effective countermeasure strategies and to implement bone measurements, such as QCT and peripheral QCT (pQCT), that can document compartmental changes in bone. Currently, QCT and pQCT are not routinely performed on crew members of long-duration flights.

In summary, integral bone mass, as measured by DXA, indicates that it takes several years to recover after flight. Recovery appears to be exponential, but QCT measurements during recovery have revealed compartmental differences that are masked by the integral measurements using DXA. The bone also undergoes geometrical cross-sectional changes that are not captured by routine DXA measurements.

Table 13.4 Potential countermeasures to space flight-induced bone loss

Artificial gravity	Short- or long-arm centrifuge
Exercise	Aerobic
	Bicycle ergometer
	Treadmill
	Resistive
	IRED
	ARED
Vibration	Low force
	High force
Nutrition	Vitamin D
	Na intake
	Omega 3
	Caloric sufficiency
Pharmacology	Antiresorptive
	Bisphosphonates
	OPG/RANK-L
	Anabolic
	PTH
	Antisclerostin

13.4 Countermeasures to Space Flight-Induced Bone Loss

Table 13.4 lists potential countermeasures to prevent space flight-induced bone loss. Past and current countermeasures listed in Table 13.4 will be discussed in the following sections.

13.4.1 Artificial Gravity (AG)

The most obvious countermeasure candidate against space flight-induced atrophy of bone, as well as for other physiological systems such as muscle, would be to create an artificial gravity (AG) environment that would replace normal Earth gravitational forces. This solution would mitigate the reduction in physical forces that the skeleton experiences during normal activity and the headward fluid shifts caused by microgravity.

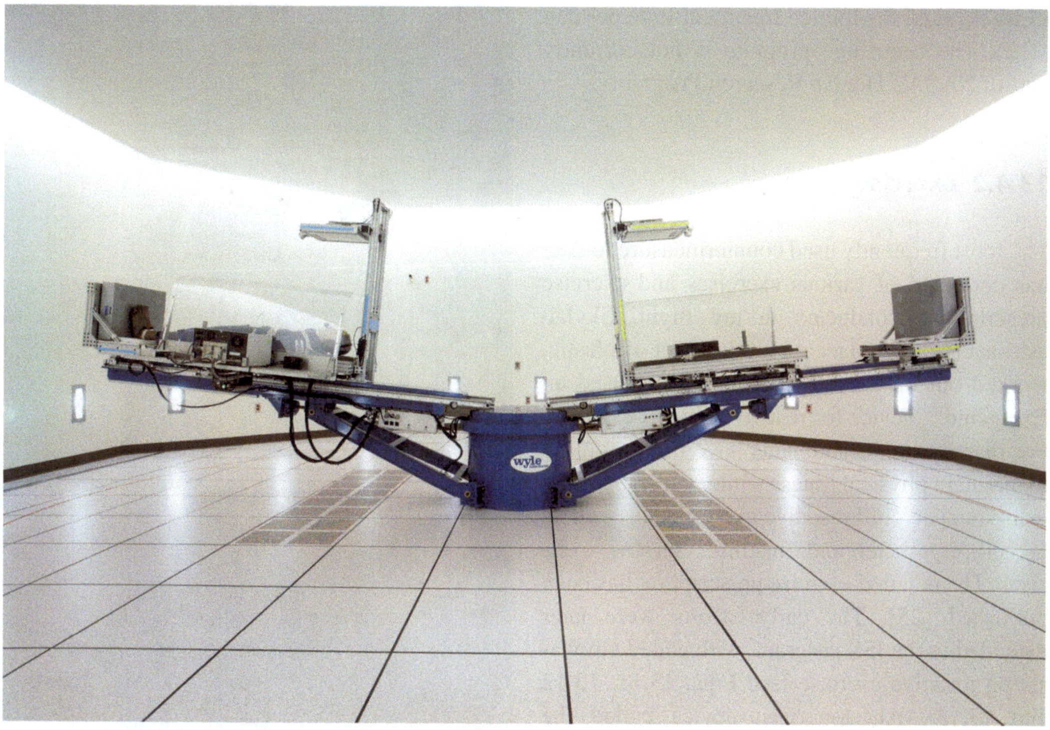

Fig. 13.10 NASA human centrifuge used to test artificial gravity countermeasure (Image courtesy of NASA)

One obvious way to do this would be to spin the spacecraft. The need for docking and sun/station alignment makes this a challenging and costly engineering task. Onboard short- or long-arm centrifugation, either continuous or intermittent, might be possible. A long-arm centrifuge, however, would have drawbacks in terms of size, mass, and cost. Therefore, one needs to know whether an onboard short-arm centrifuge providing noncontinuous centrifugation might be adequate. Using a short-arm centrifuge to create the g forces would likely have to overcome several potential negative side effects, including the Coriolis effects which are associated with motion sickness, dizziness, and possible effects on cognitive or motor function. NASA built a short-arm centrifuge to test if AG would serve this purpose with acceptable side effects (Fig. 13.10). NASA conducted a pilot study at the University of Texas Medical Branch (Galveston, Texas) to investigate this potential countermeasure. The study consisted of a 21-day period of 6° head-down-tilt (HDT) bed rest, with a 12-day period of data collection before bed rest and a 7-day data collection period after bed rest. The bed rest and AG protocols for this study have been described [2, 46]. In brief, 15 subjects were confined to strict 6° HDT bed rest. Eight of the subjects underwent 1 h of centrifugation to produce 2.5 g at the feet; the other seven were not centrifuged. Blood and urine samples were collected before, during, and after bed rest. Calcium balance was decreased during bed rest, but the difference between the two groups was not significant. Urinary excretion of resorption markers increased in the controls as expected but did not differ significantly from the centrifuged subjects. The same was true for measurements of serum C-telopeptide [42]. The centrifuge protocol was well tolerated, but the data did not demonstrate a potential benefit of AG exposure to prevent bone changes associated with disuse. The many shortcomings of this study, however, limited its usefulness to determine the potential of AG as a bone countermeasure. Not the least of these shortcomings was the relatively short period of bed rest

(3 weeks) and the limited treatment time per day (1 h). The centrifuge program is not currently part of NASA's Human Research Program.

13.4.2 Exercise

The most frequently used countermeasure to date has consisted of various exercises and exercise prescriptions conducted during flight. Skylab astronauts ran in place on a thin sheet of plastic, worked out on a cycle ergometer, and used an Exergenie™ device for resistive type of exercise. For many years, cosmonauts have been required to maintain physical fitness while in microgravity using bungee cord resistive exercises, as well as bicycle ergometer and treadmill aerobic exercises. The detailed exercise prescription has been published [25]. The early efforts were later extended to the ISS program, with added emphasis on resistive exercise (see Figs. 13.11, 13.12 and 13.13). An American device called the interim resistive exercise device (IRED) was placed aboard the ISS space station in 2001 to allow greater resistive exercise for crew members (see Fig. 13.12). The exercise programs have not been able to conclusively show that they attenuate bone loss. One reason for this uncertainty is that routine exercise is believed to be necessary, thus a nonexercising control group is not allowed. Rather, effectiveness or a lack thereof is based on the lack of significant improvement in bone loss from Skylab, Mir, and Shuttle/Mir to ISS despite the fact that the in-flight exercise program has been continually updated and improved. An important caveat to drawing conclusions concerning exercise countermeasure effectiveness is whether or not the exercise time available to crew members has been adequate because of the demands on crew time for other purposes. In addition, equipment failure has limited the amount of exercise performed during flight. Conceivably, bone loss would be even greater without exercise during flight. In any case, the data in Figs. 13.2 and 13.6 indicate that the current rate of bone loss is unacceptable for long-duration space flight. It is widely believed that if loading intensity can be increased sufficiently, the exercise countermeasure would have a more positive effect on bone, and crew time requirements could be shortened.

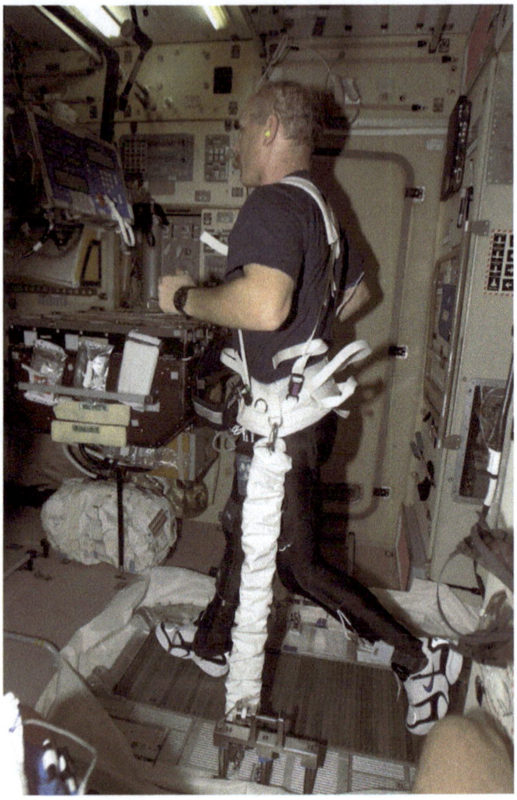

Fig. 13.11 Astronaut Kenneth Bowersox running on ISS treadmill (Image courtesy of NASA)

A new device called the ARED for advanced resistive exercise device was installed on ISS in 2008 to increase muscle and bone-loading forces (see Fig. 13.14). This device, compared to the IRED, has greater load bearing (600 vs. 300 lb), automatic recording of workload, and allows an increased number of exercises. Several long-duration ISS crew members have used the device for at least part of their mission. The data look favorable, but more studies are needed. High loading exercise in space may have potential disadvantages. A study published in 2009 documented the relatively large number of minor back injuries that have been experienced in the course of using exercise equipment on ISS. Most of the injuries involve muscle strains and are a reminder of the importance of proper equipment design

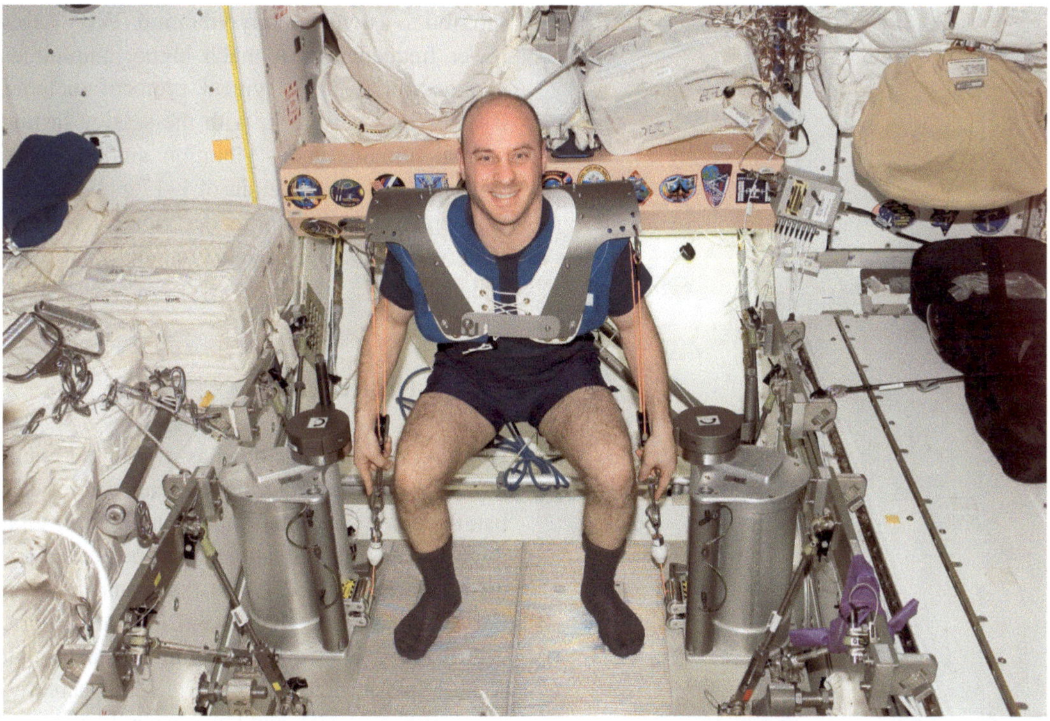

Fig. 13.12 Astronaut Garrett Reisman working out on the ISS interim resistive exercise device (Image courtesy of NASA)

and usage [6, 34]. Another concern with increasing loading during microgravity is increased risk for intervertebral disk damage or herniation. The postflight risk for disk herniation appears to be higher in astronauts [11]. As documented in bed rest studies [19], the intervertebral disks expand during disuse. Disk expansion likely occurs in space and can partly account for the change in astronaut height that has been measured during space flight. This expansion could increase the risk for disk herniation in flight with the sudden onset of high spinal-loading conditions using the ARED. Incorporating a scheme of gradual spine loading in the exercise protocol might reduce this potential risk.

13.4.3 Vibration

Rubin et al. [33] have studied the efficacy of mechanical vibration in preventing bone loss in 56 women who completed 1 year of 20 min/day treatment with either low-magnitude, high-frequency mechanical vibration or placebo [33]. The DXA results did not show changes in bone density based on intention-to-treat analysis, but postflight testing revealed protective effects in the quartile of subjects who had the highest level of compliance with treatment. A study to examine the efficacy of this treatment during 6° HDT bed rest was conducted in 2007. The study analyzed changes in bone, intervertebral disks, postural stability, muscle strength, and muscle volume in subjects subjected to 90 days of bed rest and compared to a bed rest control group who were untreated. The feet of the treated subjects were placed on the vibrating plate 10 min/day and loaded at 0.3–0.5 body weight with the aid of a body harness. The treated subjects showed some positive results [9], but QCT and DXA measures of the hip failed to show efficacy of the treatment. There are no NASA plans to test this mode of vibration as a countermeasure on ISS crews. A related technology generally

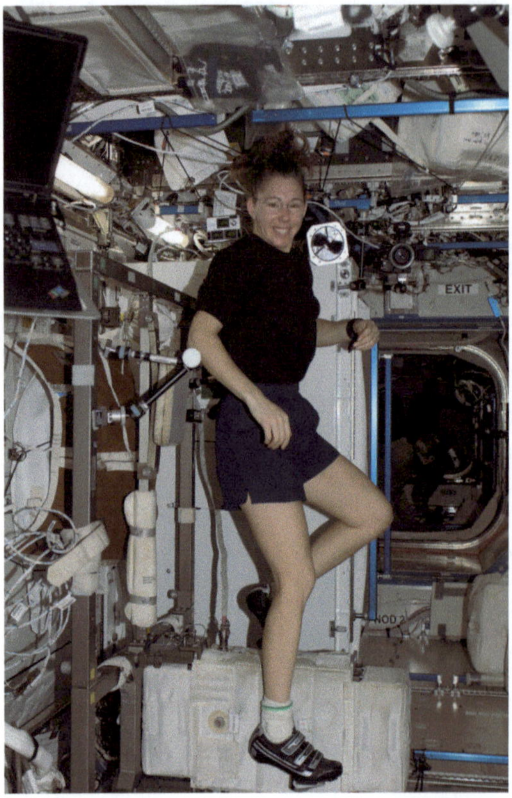

Fig. 13.13 Astronaut Sandra Magnus exercising on the ISS cycle ergometer (Image courtesy of NASA)

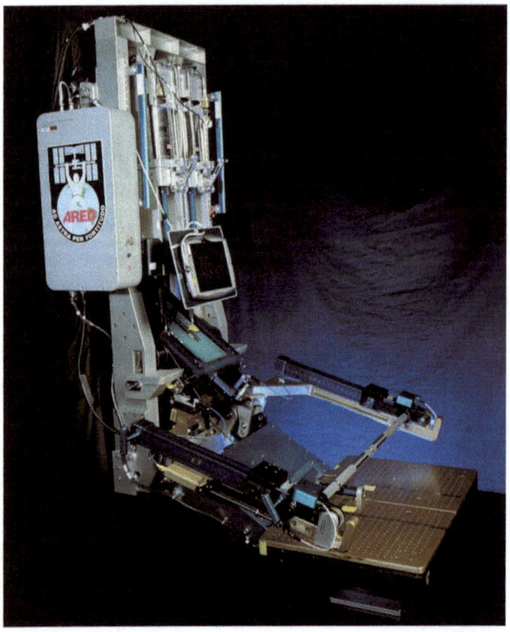

Fig. 13.14 Advanced resistive exercise device (ARED) currently being used on ISS (Image courtesy of NASA)

referred to as whole body vibration (WBV) uses lower frequencies but much higher amplitudes and accelerations; a typical protocol includes 2–3 sessions per week, with the session lasting several minutes using vibration amplitudes of 1–10 mm and accelerations of 1–17 g [10]. There are numerous publications describing this technology, but the clinical value remains controversial [1, 32].

13.4.4 Nutrition

Nutrition has been included as a potential countermeasure because diet deficiencies can exacerbate the bone loss problem; nutritional optimization might increase the effectiveness of other countermeasures. Nutritional issues that could have an impact on or exacerbate bone loss are caloric insufficiency, inadequate vitamin D intake, high sodium intake, high atmospheric CO_2 (increased respiratory acidosis), and low omega-3 levels.

NASA currently is funding studies to examine nutritional changes to the astronaut diet. The current diet has a very high salt content in order to preserve food for long periods without refrigeration. Most food on the ISS is repackaged from commercially available food. The average sodium content of the astronaut diet is about 5,000 mg/day compared with a recommended diet of 2,300 mg/day (FDA Daily Reference Values). The amount of sodium in the astronaut diet will probably be lowered in the coming years to reduce risk factors that are not directly related to bone health but may improve the Ca balance. Increasing the omega-3 fatty acids in the diet, i.e., increasing the amount of fish consumed during space flight may have a positive impact on bone loss [51]. Also, serum levels of 25-hydroxycholecalciferol have been suboptimal during flight. Current recommendations are to require 1,000 IU/day during flight. Astronauts tend to consume only about 80% of the recommended energy intake. As a result, they lose weight during flight, and this weight loss may contribute to bone loss during flight [43]. However, bone loss is also seen in flight and in bed rest studies when body weight has not decreased [17, 20]. In any case, correcting this dietary insufficiency could have a positive impact on bone loss as part of a comprehensive countermeasure strategy. One environmental factor that is not strictly nutritional is atmospheric carbon dioxide; the carbon dioxide content of the ISS atmosphere is 10-fold higher than found on Earth and may have a negative impact on Ca homeostasis [36, 49].

13.4.5 Pharmaceuticals

13.4.5.1 Antiresorptive Agents

Exercise is beneficial for multiple reasons including maintaining bone health and could be usefully supplemented with pharmaceutical countermeasures. A class of bone antiresorptive drugs seems most promising because the initiating event of space-induced bone loss appears to be an increase in bone resorption. Antiresorptive drugs called bisphosphonates have been developed to treat osteoporosis and other skeletal disorders and have been tested in ground-based studies for ameliorating disuse bone loss. Included in the tested bisphosphonates are alendronate, taken orally (10 mg/day); ibandronate, taken orally (150 mg/month); and zoledronic acid, administered as a single I.V. infusion of 5 mg every 12 months.

Alendronate has been tested in a 17-week bed rest study [15] with a daily oral dose of 10 mg. Efficacy was evaluated using DXA, urinary Ca, fecal Ca, Ca balance, bone formation and resorption markers, serum Ca, ionized Ca, parathyroid hormone (PTH), and vitamin D. The bisphosphonate prevented the increase in resorption and bone loss normally seen with bed rest.

A double-blind, placebo-controlled, randomized study of 15 spinal cord injury patients given either (a) zoledronic acid 4 or 5 mg as a single infusion or (b) placebo within 10 weeks of injury has been completed [38]. DXA scans of the hip and lumbar spine were performed at 0, 6, and 12 months. Compared to placebo, zoledronic acid had a protective effect on the hip. In a bed rest study, pamidronate was given intravenously to healthy male test subjects during 90 days of bed rest. Intravenous pamidronate administered 14 days before bed rest prevented bone loss.

NASA has approved a study "Bisphosphonates as a Countermeasure to Space Flight Induced Bone Loss" to test if bisphosphonates (either intravenously administered zoledronic acid 4 mg once before flight or oral alendronate 70 mg/week taken before and during flight) are effective in preventing space flight-induced bone loss. Based on the results of the ground-based studies described above, it is expected that both agents are likely to be effective. To date, seven crew members have taken oral alendronate (70 mg/week Fosamax^{R}) during long-duration missions on the ISS along with performing various amounts of exercise. The results look promising, with the study completion expected in 2012.

Another candidate drug for a bone loss countermeasure is denosumab, a newly approved drug for treatment of postmenopausal women who are at high risk for fractures [8]. Denosumab functions by reducing osteoclastic resorption, but unlike bisphosphonates, it is a monoclonal antibody that binds RANKL, a reaction that is important for the production, function, and survival of osteoclasts. Denosumab is an antibody that must be delivered by intramuscular injection every 6 months. Some testing has been done in animals flown on the shuttle, but bed rest analog testing in humans or flight studies have not yet been published. Denosumab may be a good alternative to bisphosphonates.

13.4.5.2 Anabolic Agents

Anabolic agents such as PTH have not been tested as countermeasures in space flight. The recombinant teriparatide, rhPTH, has been approved by the FDA for the treatment of osteoporosis. Teriparatide is a PTH fragment that increases vertebral BMD and reduces the risk of vertebral and nonvertebral fracture in osteoporotic women [21]. Teriparatide requires daily injection and has not been tested in bed rest studies. The drug may be useful for postflight treatment to accelerate bone recovery. A PTH-related peptide, PTHrP, also has an anabolic effect on bone formation [24].

Antisclerostin is another drug under development to increase bone formation [22]. Sclerostin is a naturally occurring protein that controls bone mass by inhibiting osteoblast activity. The investigational antisclerostin antibody targets a key inhibitor of bone-forming cells. From a theoretical standpoint, it is not clear if an anabolic compound is the best approach since in humans the underlying problem appears to be elevated bone resorption, not impaired formation. However, although bone formation markers are not decreased with space flight or bed rest, it is important to consider that there could be significant decreases in bone formation in some small but critical regions—for example, the proximal femur—that are not reflected in the serum concentration of formation markers. Also, if antisclerostin increases bone formation in the same regions of elevated resorption, coupling of remodeling might be restored but with an elevated remodeling rate. The use of anabolic agents may prove useful to stimulate/accelerate bone recovery after flight. More studies are needed to determine if stimulation of bone formation is a good approach.

13.5 Summary

Astronauts and cosmonauts who participated in long-duration flights aboard Mir and ISS have experienced consistent loss of regional bone mineral, with 90% experiencing a minimum 5% loss in at least one skeletal site and more than 50% experiencing a 10% or greater loss in at least one skeletal site. These losses occurred in spite of the crew members' participation in exercise and nutrition regimens aboard the space stations.

1. All data to date support the idea that the lack of mechanical forces on the skeleton in microgravity leads to increased bone resorption with little or no change in bone formation markers. Overall, the skeletal changes are manifested by elevated bone resorption markers, increased urinary Ca, negative Ca balance, reduced serum PTH, reduced 1,25 vitamin D, and reduced bone mass and strength. Bone loss is greatest in the lower limbs, i.e., pelvis, hips, and legs, with little loss in the upper skeleton. Trabecular loss in the hip is 50% greater than the combined trabecular + cortical loss. Although the percentage of trabecular bone loss is greater than cortical bone in some skeletal sites, the greatest loss on a mass basis is from cortical bone.
2. A consistent finding is the large variation in bone loss between bone sites and between individuals. These observations are seen in space flight and in bed rest studies. In the case of bed rest studies, physical activity, body weight, and diet are strictly controlled. Therefore, another untested variable, such as genetic variation, may play an important role.
3. As measured by DXA, bone recovers after bed rest or space flight, but the rate of recovery varies and ultimate recovery may take several years. In addition, QCT measurements suggest that structural changes to bone take place, i.e., geometric expansion, at the femur. Moreover, the trabecular bone mass in the hip may not completely return to preflight levels.
4. Most efforts to create an effective countermeasure to space-induced bone loss have involved in-flight exercise. The advantages of this countermeasure are that most crew members enjoy exercise, and exercise benefits the body as a whole. As yet, the optimum set of exercises has not been determined. The current NASA program is directed toward increasing resistive loading on the skeleton. Higher exercise loads however should be used with caution to minimize the risk of in-flight injuries [34].
5. Antiresorptive agents such as bisphosphonates have been shown to be effective in ground-based analog studies with testing in microgravity ongoing. Testing is expected to be complete in 2012. Some combination of exercise and drug therapy is likely to prove effective in preventing space flight-induced bone loss. Even with a successful exercise prescription, additional countermeasures will be needed to reduce risk on long missions, for example, if the equipment fails (as has been the case in the past), if a crew member

is injured, or if some other condition occurs that limits the ability of crew members to exercise.

6. An effective countermeasure would reduce urinary Ca output to decrease the risk of kidney stone formation and to prevent bone loss.
7. Attempts to test artificial gravity and high-frequency vibration in bed rest have not proved successful to date. Anabolic agents may have a use during postflight recovery for individuals whose bone loss during flight cannot be prevented.

References

1. Armbrecht G, Belavý DL, Gast U, Bongrazio M, Touby F, Beller G, Roth HJ, Perschel FH, Rittweger J, Felsenberg D. Resistive vibration exercise attenuates bone and muscle atrophy in 56 days of bed rest: biochemical markers of bone metabolism. Osteoporos Int. 2010;21(4):597–607.
2. Arya M, Paloski WH, Young LR. Centrifugation protocol for the NASA artificial gravity bed rest pilot study. J Gravit Physiol. 2007;14(1):P5–8.
3. Biriukov EN, Kraasnykh IG. Changes in the optical density of bone tissue and in the calcium metabolism of the astronauts. In: Nikivaev AG, Sevastianov VI, editors. Kosmicheskaia Biologiia I. Moscow: Meditsina; 1970. p. 42–45.
4. Brodzinski RL, Rancitelli LA, Haller WA, Dewey LS. Calcium, potassium, and iron loss by Apollo VII, VIII, IX, X and XI astronauts. Aerosp Med. 1971;42(6):621–6.
5. Carpenter RD, Leblanc AD, Evans H, Sibonga JD, Lang TF. Long-term changes in the density and structure of the human hip and spine after long-duration spaceflight. Acta Astronaut. 2010;67:71–81.
6. Frechette A, Evetts SN, Sundblad P. Human-in-the-loop on flight like hardware in representative environments as a prerequisite for development of new countermeasure equipment for human spaceflight. Aviat Space Environ Med. 2010;81(3):267.
7. Gazenko OG, Genin AM, Egorov AD. Summary of medical investigations in the U.S.S.R. Manned space missions. Acta Astronaut. 1981;8(9–10):907–17.
8. Han SL, Wan SL. Effect of teriparatide on bone mineral density and fracture in postmenopausal osteoporosis: meta-analysis of randomized controlled trials. Int J Clin Pract. 2012 Feb;66(2):199–209.
9. Holguin N, Muir J, Rubin C, Judex S. Short applications of very low-magnitude vibrations attenuate expansion of the intervertebral disc during extended bed rest. Spine. 2009;9:470–7.
10. Humphries B, Fenning A, Dugan E, Guinane J, MacRae K. Whole-body vibration effects on bone mineral density in women with or without resistance training. Aviat Space Environ Med. 2009;80(12):1025–31.
11. Johnston SL, Campbell MR, Scheuring R, Feiveson AH. Risk of herniated nucleus pulposus among US astronauts. Aviat Space Environ Med. 2010;81(6):566–74.
12. Keyak JH, Koyama AK, Leblanc A, Lu Y, Lang TF. Reduction in proximal femoral strength due to long-duration spaceflight. Bone. 2009;44(3):449–53.
13. Lang T, LeBlanc A, Evans H, Lu Y, Genant H, Yu A. Cortical and trabecular bone mineral loss from the spine and hip in long-duration spaceflight. J Bone Miner Res. 2004;19(6):1006–12.
14. LeBlanc A, Schneider V, Spector E, Evans H, Rowe R, Lane H, Demers L, Lipton A. Calcium absorption, endogenous excretion, and endocrine changes during and after long-term bed rest. Bone. 1995;16(4 Suppl):301S–4.
15. LeBlanc AD, Driscol TB, Shackelford LC, Evans HJ, Rianon NJ, Smith SM, Feeback DL, Lai D. Alendronate as an effective countermeasure to disuse induced bone loss. J Musculoskelet Neuronal Interact. 2002;2(4):335–43.
16. LeBlanc A, Schneider V, Shackelford L, West S, Oganov V, Bakulin A, Voronin L. Bone mineral and lean tissue loss after long duration space flight. J Musculoskelet Neuronal Interact. 2000;1(2):157–60.
17. LeBlanc AD, Schneider VS, Evans HG, Engelbretson DA, Krebs JM. Bone mineral loss and recovery after 17 weeks of bed rest. J Bone Miner Res. 1990;5(8):843–50.
18. LeBlanc AD, Spector ER, Evans HJ, Sibonga JD. Skeletal responses to space flight and the bed rest analog: a review. J Musculoskelet Neuronal Interact. 2007;7(1):33–47.
19. LeBlanc AD, Evans HJ, Schneider VS, Wendt III RE, Hedrick TD. Changes in intervertebral disc cross-sectional area with bed rest and space flight. Spine. 1994;19(7):812–7.
20. LeBlanc A, Lin C, Shackelford L, Sinitsyn V, Evans H, Belichenko O, Schenkman B, Kozlovskaya I, Oganov V, Bakulin A, Hedrick T, Feeback D. Muscle volume, MRI relaxation times (T2), and body composition after spaceflight. J Appl Physiol. 2000;89:2158–64.
21. Lewiecki EM. Safety and tolerability of denosumab for the treatment of postmenopausal osteoporosis. Drug Health Patient Saf. 2011;3:79–91.
22. Li X, Ominsky MS, Warmington KS, Morony S, Gong J, Cao J, Gao Y, Shalhoub V, Tipton B, Haldankar R, Chen Q, Winters A, Boone T, Geng Z, Niu QT, Ke HZ, Kostenuik PJ, Simonet WS, Lacey DL, Paszty C. Sclerostin antibody treatment increases bone formation, bone mass, and bone strength in a rat model of postmenopausal osteoporosis. J Bone Miner Res. 2009;24(4):578–88.
23. Lutwak L, Whedon GD, Lachance PA, Reid JM, Lipscomb HS. Mineral, electrolyte and nitrogen bal-

ance studies of the Gemini-VII fourteen-day orbital space flight. J Clin Endocrinol Metab. 1969;29(9): 1140–56.
24. Miao D, He B, Jiang Y, Kobayashi T, Soroceanu MA, Zhao J, Su H, Tong X, Amizuka N, Gupta A, Genant HK, Kronenberg HM, Goltzman D, Karaplis AC. Osteoblast-derived PTHrP is a potent endogenous bone anabolic agent that modifies the therapeutic efficacy of administered PTH 1–34. J Clin Invest. 2005;115:2402–11.
25. Nicogossian AE, Sawin CF, Grigoriev AI. Countermeasures to space deconditioning chapter 26. In: Nocogossian AE, Huntoon CL, Pool SL, editors. Space physiology and medicine. Philadelphia: Lea & Febiger; 1994. p. 447–67.
26. Oganov VS, Cann C, Rakhmanov AS, Ternovoi SK. Study of the musculoskeletal system of the spine in humans after long-term space flights by the method of computerized tomography. Kosmicheskaia Biologiia I Aviakosmicheskaia Meditsina. 1990;24(4):20–1.
27. Oganov VS, Grigoriev AI, Voronin LI, Rakhmanov AS, Bakulin AV, Schneider VS, LeBlanc AD. Bone mineral density in cosmonauts after flights lasting 4.5–6 months on the Mir orbital station. Aviakosm Ekolog Med. 1992;26(5–6):20–4.
28. Pietrzyk RA, Jones JA, Sams CF, Whitson PA. Renal stone formation among astronauts. Aviat Space Environ Med. 2007;78(4):A9–13.
29. Rambaut PC, Leach CS, Johnson PC. Calcium and phosphorus change of the Apollo 17 crew members. Nutr Metab. 1975;18(2):62–9.
30. Rambaut PC, Leach CS, Whedon GD. A study of metabolic balance in crew members of Skylab IV. Acta Astronaut. 1979;6(10):1313–22.
31. Rambaut PC, Johnston RS. Prolonged weightlessness and calcium loss in man. Acta Astronaut. 1979;6(9): 1113–22.
32. Rittweger J, Beller G, Armbrecht G, Mulder E, Buehring B, Gast U, Dimeo F, Schubert H, de Haan A, Stegeman DF, Schiessl H, Felsenberg D. Prevention of bone loss during 56 days of strict bed rest by side-alternating resistive vibration exercise. Prevention of bone loss during 56 days of strict bed rest by side-alternating resistive vibration exercise. Bone. 2010; 46(1):137–47.
33. Rubin C, Recker R, Cullen D, Ryaby J, McCabe J, McLeod K. Prevention of postmenopausal bone loss by a low-magnitude, high-frequency mechanical stimuli: a clinical trial assessing compliance, efficacy, and safety. J Bone Miner Res. 2004;19(3):343–51.
34. Scheuring RA, Mathers CH, Jones JA, Wear ML. Musculoskeletal injuries and minor trauma in space: incidence and injury mechanisms in U.S. Astronauts. Aviat Space Environ Med. 2009;80(2):117–24.
35. Schneider VS, LeBlanc AD, Taggart LC. Bone and mineral metabolism chapter 17. In: Nicogossian AE, Huntoon CL, Pool SL, editors. Space physiology and medicine. Philadelphia: Lea & Febiger; 1994. p. 327–33.
36. Sebastian A, Harris ST, Ottaway JH, Todd KM, Morris Jr RC. Improved mineral balance and skeletal metabolism in postmenopausal women treated with potassium bicarbonate. N Engl J Med. 1994;330(25): 1776–81.
37. Shackelford LC, LeBlanc AD, Driscoll TB, Evans HG, Rianon NG, Smith SM, Spector E, Feeback DL, Lai D. Resistance exercise as a countermeasure to disuse induced bone loss. J Appl Physiol. 2004;97(1): 119–29.
38. Shapiro J, Smith B, Beck T, Ballard P, Dapthary M, BrintzenhofeSzoc K, Caminis J. Treatment with zoledronic acid ameliorates negative geometric changes in the proximal femur following acute spinal cord injury. Calcif Tissue Int. 2007;80:316–22.
39. Sibonga JD, Evans HJ, Sung HG, Spector ER, Lang TF, Oganov VS, Bakulin AV, Shackelford LC, LeBlanc AD. Recovery of spaceflight-induced bone loss: bone mineral density after long-duration missions as fitted with an exponential function. Bone. 2007;41: 973–8.
40. Smith SM, Nillen JL, LeBlanc A, Lipton A, Demers LM, Lane HW, Leach CS. Collagen cross-link excretion during space flight and bed rest. J Clin Endocrinol Metab. 1998;83(10):3584–91.
41. Smith SM, Wastney ME, O'Brien KO, Morukov BV, Larina IM, Abrams SA, Davis-Street JE, Oganov V, Shackelford LC. Bone markers, calcium metabolism, and calcium kinetics during extended-duration space flight on the Mir space station. J Bone Miner Res. 2005;20(2):208–18.
42. Smith SM, Zwart SR, Heer MA, Baecker N, Evans HJ, Feiveson A, Shackelford LC, LeBlanc AD. Effects of artificial gravity during bed rest on bone metabolism in humans. J Appl Physiol. 2009;107:47–53.
43. Smith SM, Zwart SR, Block G, Rice BL, Davis-Street JE. The nutritional status of astronauts is altered after long-term space flight aboard the international space station. J Nutr. 2005;135:437–43.
44. Stupakov GP, Kazeikin VS, Kozlovskii AP, Korolev VV. Evaluation of the changes in the bone structures of the human axial skeleton in prolonged space flight. Kosm Biol Aviakosm Med. 1984;18(2):33–7.
45. Vogel JM, Anderson JT. Rectilinear transmission scanning of irregular bones for quantification of mineral content. J Nucl Med. 1972;13(1):13–8.
46. Warren LE, Reinertson RC, Camacho ME, Paloski WH. Implementation of the NASA artificial gravity bed rest pilot study. J Gravit Physiol. 2007;14(1): P1–4.
47. Watanabe Y, Ohshima H, Mizuno K, Sekiguchi C, Fukunaga M, Kohri K, Rittweger J, Felsenberg D, Matsumoto T, Nakamura T. Intravenous pamidronate prevents femoral bone loss and renal stone formation during 90-day bed rest. J Bone Miner Res. 2004; 19(11):1771–8.
48. Whedon GD, Lutwak L, Rambaut PC, Whittle MW, Smith MC, Reid J, Leach CS, Stadler CR, Sanford DD. Mineral and nitrogen metabolic studies, experiment

M071. In: Johnson RS, Dietlein LE, editors. Biomedical results from Skylab NASA SP-377. Washington, DC: NASA; 1977. p. 164–74.
49. Wynn E, Krieg MA, Lanham-New SA, Burckhardt P. Postgraduate symposium: positive influence of nutritional alkalinity on bone health. Proc Nutr Soc. 2010;69(1):166–73.
50. Zerwekh JE, Ruml LA, Gottschalk F, Pak CY. The effects of twelve weeks of bed rest on bone histology, biochemical markers of bone turnover, and calcium homeostasis in eleven normal subjects. J Bone Miner Res. 1998;13(10):1594–601.
51. Zwart SR, Pierson D, Mehta S, Gonda S, Smith SM. Capacity of omega-3 fatty acids or eicosapentaenoic acid to counteract weightlessness-induced bone loss by inhibiting NF-KB activation: from cells to bed rest to astronauts. J Bone Miner Res. 2010;25(5):1049–57.

Osteoimmunology: Relation to Disease and Therapy

14

M. Neale Weitzmann and Roberto Pacifici

Keywords
Bone • Estrogen • PTH • T cells • B cells • Osteoimmunology

14.1 Introduction

The association between inflammation and bone loss long has been recognized, leading to speculation that cells of the immune system participate in the control of bone remodeling. The discovery that the receptor activator of NF-κB (ligand) RANKL/RANK system plays a pivotal role in both adaptive immunity and osteoclastogenesis has provided molecular evidence firmly linking the immune system and bone. Although studies from our laboratory and from others have shown that activated T cells secrete RANKL, it was Kong et al. [38] who demonstrated that T cell–derived RANKL plays a pivotal role in an experimental bone loss model. It now is clear that T cells regulate bone homeostasis by causing bone marrow (BM) stromal cells (SCs) and osteoblasts (OBs) to release osteoclastogenic cytokines and Wnt ligands and to drive bone turnover in inflammatory states. Under physiological conditions, B cells are also critical for the regulation of bone turnover as they are a significant source of OPG in the BM microenvironment [44]. Consequently, lymphocytes play critical roles in the stabilization of bone homeostasis. Pathological disruption of immune function as occurs during HIV-1 infection contributes to bone destruction though an imbalance in the RANKL/OPG ratio.

In this chapter, we focus on the role of T cells in the mechanism by which parathyroid hormone, PTH, regulates bone, the role of B cells and T cells in maintaining basal bone homeostasis, and how immunological disruption drives bone loss during HIV-1 infection.

14.2 Effects of PTH on Bone

PTH plays a critical regulatory role in calcium metabolism. Secreted in response to small drops in serum ionized calcium levels, PTH defends against hypocalcemia, in part, by stimulating bone resorption and releasing calcium from the skeleton. PTH regulates serum calcium, but sustained overproduction or continuous infusion of PTH (cPTH) is a cause of bone disease. Secondary hyperparathyroidism has been implicated in the pathogenesis of senile osteoporosis [69] and

M.N. Weitzmann, Ph.D. • R. Pacifici, M.D. (✉)
Division of Endocrinology, Metabolism and Lipids, Department of Medicine, Emory University, 101 Woodruff Circle, WMRB 1307, Atlanta, GA 30322, USA
e-mail: roberto.pacifici@emory.edu

F. Bronner et al. (eds.), *Bone-Metabolic Functions and Modulators*, *Topics in Bone Biology*,
DOI 10.1007/978-1-4471-2745-1_14, © Springer-Verlag London 2012

primary hyperparathyroidism and is associated with accelerated bone loss and osteopenia [60]. When injected daily at a low dose, a regimen known as intermittent PTH (iPTH) treatment, the hormone stimulates trabecular and cortical bone formation and increases bone volume and strength. Attesting to its potency, iPTH decreases fracture risk in humans. It is an FDA-approved treatment modality for postmenopausal women and men with osteoporosis [12].

Of the three receptors for PTH, the one that mediates the effects of PTH in bone is the PTH/PTHrP receptor (PPR or PTHR1), one of a seven-member transmembrane-spanning domain receptor family, the G protein–coupled receptors [11, 41, 63]. An alternative PTH receptor is PTHR2, a protein expressed primarily in the central nervous and the cardiovascular systems, which is not known to play a role in bone [22, 30, 75]. Ligand binding to PPR activates the cyclic AMP–dependent protein kinase A and calcium-dependent protein kinase C signaling pathways. Mice in which the PPR has been ablated by homologous recombination develop decreased trabecular bone and increased thickness of cortical bone during fetal development [41]. Conversely, osteoblastic expression of the constitutively active PPR increases osteoblastic function in the trabecular and endosteal compartments and decreases OB activity in the periosteum [11]. The net effect is a substantial increase in trabecular bone volume and a decrease in long bone thickness [11]. Transgenic mice expressing a constitutively active PTH receptor in osteocytes also exhibit increased bone mass and bone remodeling [54]. Their expression of sclerostin, the osteocyte-derived Wnt antagonist, is decreased and Wnt signaling is increased, as is the number of osteoblasts (OB) and osteoclasts. Osteoblast apoptosis is decreased. PTH receptor signaling in osteocytes increases bone mass and bone remodeling via LRP5-dependent and LRP5-independent mechanisms, respectively.

PTH promotes bone formation by increasing the number of osteoblasts [45, 47]. This is achieved through activation of quiescent osteoblastic lining cells [20], an increase in proliferation [58] and differentiation [48] of osteoblasts, attenuation of pre-OB and OB apoptosis [8, 31], and increase in signaling in osteocytes [54]. The relative contributions of each of these mechanisms to the overall anabolic activity of PTH remain controversial.

Wnts are signaling proteins that modulate diverse developmental processes and initiate a canonical signaling cascade by binding to receptors of the frizzled family together with coreceptors. Coreceptors are members of the low-density lipoprotein receptor-related protein (LRP) family, LRP5 and LRP6, molecules that stabilize cytosolic β-catenin. LRP4, a new member of this receptor family, has been identified in OBs and implicated in the mechanism of action of PTH [15]. LRP4 binds Dkk1 and sclerostin in vitro [15]. A nuclear complex of β-catenin and the T cell factor/lymphoid enhancer factor (TCF/LEF) interacts with DNA to regulate the transcription of Wnt target genes [6]. Wnt proteins also signal through noncanonical pathways that involve the Src/ERK and Pi3K/Akt cascades [2].

PTH is a canonical Wnt signaling agonist that increases β-catenin levels in osteoblastic cells [39]. PTH, once bound to PPR, forms a complex with LRP6 that increases LRP6 signaling and activates β-catenin [77]. PTH activates Wnt signaling in osteoblastic cells through both Wnt ligand–dependent and Wnt ligand–independent mechanisms. Moreover, PTH downregulates the production of sclerostin. Recently, convincing evidence has emerged showing that PTH receptor signaling occurs in osteocytes and that the resulting direct regulation of sclerostin production plays a significant role in the anabolic activity of PTH [54]. PTH also regulates Dickkopf-1, a soluble LRP5 and LRP6 signaling inhibitor [39], and Sfrp-4, a factor that binds Wnt proteins and antagonizes canonical and noncanonical Wnt signaling [62]. Uncertainty remains with regard to the identity and source of Wnt ligands that activate Wnt signaling in response to PTH treatment.

14.3 T Cells and PTH-Induced Bone Loss

T lymphocytes express functional PPR [73], respond to PTH [71], and stimulate OB differentiation [67]. T cells, therefore, may play a role in the proresorptive effect of cPTH treatment. As predicted, studies revealed that continuous PTH (cPTH) treatment fails to induce osteoclast formation, bone resorption, or cortical bone loss in mice lacking T cells [23]. By contrast, continuous PTH stimulates bone formation in T cell–replete and T cell–deficient mice. Hence, T cells are required for PTH to exert its effect in bone, but it is uncertain whether cPTH action on bone is mediated directly via T cells. To address these issues, PPR receptors in T cells were silenced by disruption of the PPR gene by means of targeted deletion of exon E1 of PPR with the aid of Cre-LoxP technology [34]. Crossing mice expressing an exon E1-floxed PPR allele [37] with mice that express Cre recombinase under the control of the T cell–specific promoter Lck [42] generated mice with disrupted PPR genes in T cells ($PPR^{T\ cells-/-}$ mice), but with normal PPR expression in other cell types [35]. It, therefore, was possible to determine if PTH activation of PPR in T cells is required for cPTH to exert its catabolic activity in bone.

Mice at 6 weeks of age lack PPR signaling in T cells, have a normal bone phenotype, and have normal serum levels of calcium, phosphate, and PTH, indicating that PPR signaling in T cells does not play a major role in baseline bone modeling. However, at 18 weeks of age, mice lacking functional PPR in T cells displayed lower bone volume than $PPR^{fl/fl}$ mice, suggesting that PPR signaling in T cells contributes to the anabolic activity of endogenous PTH in bone. Moreover, $PPR^{T\ cells-/-}$ mice have a normal number of T cells with a degree of activation and proliferation similar to that of control T cells. However, when challenged with cPTH, $PPR^{T\ cells-/-}$ mice are protected against the loss of cortical and trabecular bone observed in the control mice. The resistance to cPTH-induced bone loss in $PPR^{T\ cells-/-}$ mice can be explained by the reduced capacity of cPTH to stimulate bone resorption and expand the pool of resorbing OCs. Silencing of PPR signaling in T cells modifies the effects of cPTH from a net trabecular bone loss in the controls to bone gain in the $PPR^{T\ cells-/-}$ mice. This bone gain can be attributed to the ability of cPTH to stimulate bone formation.

Initial studies have revealed the existence of cross talk between T cells and SCs, mediated by the CD40L/CD40 signaling system. CD40L is a surface costimulatory molecule expressed primarily, but not exclusively, in $CD4^{+}$ cells. CD40L, also known as CD154, exerts its effects by binding to CD40 [64] and several integrins [4, 43, 61, 84]. CD40 is expressed on antigen (Ag) presenting cells [26], SCs and OBs [1]. The CD40/CD40L system is crucial for T cell activation and many additional functions of the immune system. It promotes macrophage activation and differentiation and antibody isotype switching and is involved in the organization of immunologic memory in B cells [28]. Binding to the integrins $\alpha_{IIb}\beta_3$ [4, 61], Mac-1 [84], and $\alpha_5\beta_1$, all of which are widely expressed in the BM, accounts for additional inflammatory effects of CD40L [43].

T cells provide proliferative and survival cues to SCs and sensitize SCs to PTH through CD40L. An important element of this regulatory loop is PTH's ability to upregulate the expression of CD40 in SC from T cell–replete mice, but not from T cell–deficient mice [23]. Thus, T cells contribute to the CD40L/CD40-mediated exchange of information between T cells and SCs by providing CD40L and by upregulating the expression of CD40 on SCs. As a result, mice lacking T cells or T cell–expressed CD40L have fewer SCs. Furthermore, these SCs produce less RANKL and their OPG secretion is less suppressed in response to PTH. Therefore, SCs from T cell–deficient mice have a lower capacity to support OC formation in vivo and in vitro. The alteration in SC function is the ultimate reason why deletion of T cells or T cell–expressed CD40L blunts the bone catabolic activity of PTH [23].

Interestingly, cPTH regulates the CD40L/CD40 mediated cross talk between T cells and SCs, not by regulating CD40L expression in T cells, but by increasing the expression of CD40 in SCs. The stimulation by cPTH on SC CD40 expression is silenced in T cell–deficient mice; this indicates that cPTH regulates the expression of CD40 in SCs via a T cell–dependent mechanism that is yet to be discovered [23]. Importantly, while cPTH treatment increases

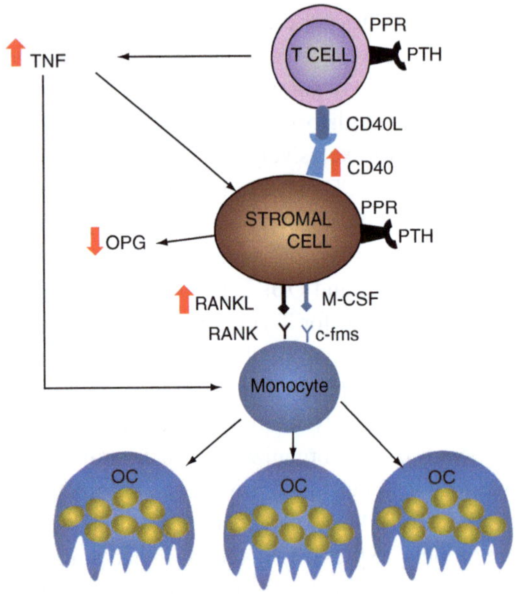

Fig. 14.1 Schematic representation of the role of T cells in the mechanism by which continuous PTH stimulates OC formation and induces bone loss. PTH binding to PPR in T cells stimulates the production of TNF. This cytokine increases CD40 expression by SCs. Binding of CD40 by T cell–expressed CD40L increases SC sensitivity to PTH, resulting in enhanced SC production of RANKL and diminished secretion of OPG in response to PTH. T cell–produced TNF further stimulates OC formation through its direct effects on maturing OC precursors. The *red arrows* represent the main modifications induced by activation of PPR signaling in T cells

CD40 expression in SCs derived from the BM of control mice, it fails to do so in SC from $PPR^{T\ cells-/-}$ mice. Furthermore, similar to SCs from mice lacking T cells, CD40L, or CD40 [23], the SCs from $PPR^{T\ cells-/-}$ mice exhibit altered RANKL/OPG production and their osteoclastogenic response to cPTH is blunted. These findings indicate that T cell–expressed PPR mediates the osteoclastogenic response of SCs to cPTH by upregulating CD40 expression, thereby facilitating CD40L/CD40 signaling

Studies have revealed the existence of a second regulatory effect of PTH that is mediated by T cells. PTH activation of the T cell PPR stimulates $CD4^+$ cells and $CD8^+$ T cell production of the osteoclastogenic cytokine tumor necrosis factor, TNF (Fig. 14.1). This cytokine is a potent osteoclastogenic factor that plays a pivotal role in the bone loss induced by inflammation, periodontal bone disease, and estrogen deficiency [80]. Importantly, cPTH fails to induce bone loss or stimulate bone resorption in $TNF^{-/-}$ or nude mice adoptively transferred with $TNF^{-/-}$ T cells. The effects of cPTH are, however, restored by adoptive transfer of wild type (WT) T cells. T cell–produced TNF plays a key role in cPTH-induced bone loss. The diminished cPTH-induced TNF production by T cells from $PPR^{T\ cells-/-}$ mice establishes TNF production by T cells as a downstream effector of cPTH stimulation of PPR in T cells. These findings may help explain increased levels of circulating TNF found in patients with primary hyperparathyroidism [29].

Additional progress in the understanding of the role of T cells in the mechanism of action of PTH has come from the finding that, similar to the silencing of PPR, deletion of TNF in T cells blocks cPTH from upregulating CD40 expression or from increasing the RANKL/OPG ratio in SCs. PPR signaling in T cells, thus, mediates cPTH-induced CD40 expression in SCs by controlling TNF production by T cells. It should be mentioned that TNF stimulates bone resorption and increases bone loss by additional mechanisms, such as by potentiating the osteoclastogenic activity of RANKL produced in the BM microenvironment [13, 40] or increasing the production of RANKL by SCs and OBs [34].

Even though PTH acts directly on T cells, it does not increase Ag presentation and T cell activation. However, because the expression of CD40L is a feature of activated T cells, it is likely that baseline Ag presentation, which leads to spontaneous activation of T cells in the BM, may be required for PTH to induce its catabolic effect. Indeed the BM contains a relatively large number of memory T cells that have increased reactivity to self-peptides and foreign Ags. T cell activation takes place in the presence of several signals. The first is the presentation to the T cell receptor (TCR) of Ag-derived peptides bound to MHC molecules that are expressed on the surface of Ag-presenting cells (APCs). A second set of signals is provided by the interaction of the costimulatory molecules on APCs with the ligands expressed by T cells including CD28 and CD40L. A pharmacological approach to test the role of costimulation is provided by abatacept, an agent approved for the treatment of rheumatoid arthritis that also blocks the bone loss induced by ovariectomy [27]. Bone loss due to PTH is prevented with the aid of this inhibitor of costimulation. Arrest of Ag presentation through silencing of class I and class II MHC-TCR interactions prevents cPTH from inducing cortical bone loss [49]. These findings provide further evidence of a novel regulatory link between the immune system and the mechanism of action of PTH.

In summary, the effects of cPTH on bone are the result of a mechanism that involves PPR activation and TNF production in T cells. TNF produced by T cells stimulates bone resorption directly by potentiating the sensitivity of maturing OCs to RANKL. In addition, TNF enhances CD40L/CD40 signaling from T cells to SCs by upregulating CD40 expression, an effect attributed to the increased capacity of SCs to support OC formation. Thus, complex cross talk between T cells and the osteoclastogenic machinery of the BM is central to the bone catabolic activity of cPTH.

14.4 Role of T Cells in the Anabolic Activity of Intermittent PTH Treatment

The increasing evidence in favor of a pivotal role of T cells in the mechanism of action of cPTH prompted us to investigate if T cells mediate the anabolic activity of iPTH. Studies conducted in four strains of T cell–deficient mice (TCRβ$^{-/-}$, RAG2$^{-/-}$, class I and II MHC double knockout (KO) mice, and nude mice) revealed that mice lacking T cells exhibit a blunted response to iPTH with respect to the increase in bone formation and trabecular bone volume [73]. Furthermore, adoptive transfer of T cells into T cell–deficient mice restored a normal response to iPTH. T cells augmented the capacity of iPTH to improve architecture in trabecular, but not in cortical, bone. Although the reason for this bone tissue selectivity is unknown, lack of access of T cells at cortical surfaces is not a likely explanation, as T cells reach the endosteal and periosteal bone surfaces through blood vessels and recirculate in and out of the BM [19].

The effects of iPTH on bone volume and the indices of bone strength are blunted, but not abolished, in the absence of T cells. By contrast, direct measurement of bone strength by four-point bending has revealed that the capacity of iPTH to improve bone strength depends completely on the presence of T cells. The reason for this is not known, but T cells may be required to improve the material property of bone. Even though PTH stimulation of bone formation is severely blunted in T cell–deficient mice, T cells inexplicably do not improve cPTH stimulation of bone formation. Regarding the mechanism by which T cells potentiate the anabolic activity of iPTH, it has been shown in bone that in the absence of T cells, iPTH does not commit SCs to the osteoblastic lineage, cannot induce OB proliferation or differentiation, and does not mitigate OB apoptosis. All of these actions of PTH hinge on T cells activating Wnt signaling in osteoblasts [73], yet little information is available on the nature and source of the Wnt ligands that activate Wnt signaling. PTH stimulates BM CD8^{+} T cells to produce large amounts of Wnt10b [73], a protein that activates Wnt signaling in SCs and OBs, thus increasing OB proliferation, differentiation, and life span. Treatment with iPTH slightly increases production of Wnt10b by BM CD4^{+} cells. This, in turn, is associated with a diminished anabolic response in class II MHC$^{-/-}$ mice. In other words, production of Wnt10b by CD4^{+} cells contributes, in small part, to the anabolic activity of iPTH. The relevance of CD8^{+} cells can be inferred from the inability of iPTH to promote bone anabolism in class I MHC$^{-/-}$ mice, a strain that lacks CD8^{+} cells [73]. Additional studies revealed that iPTH does not improve bone architecture in T cell–deficient mice reconstituted with CD4^{+} cells, but does do so in mice adoptively transferred with CD8^{+} cells [73]. The pivotal role of T cells produced by Wnt10b can be deduced from the subdued effect of iPTH on bone volume in TCRβ$^{-/-}$ mice reconstituted with T cells from Wnt10b$^{-/-}$ mice. It is likely that iPTH directly targets CD8^{+} T cells and stimulates their production of Wnt10b. This hypothesis is supported by the

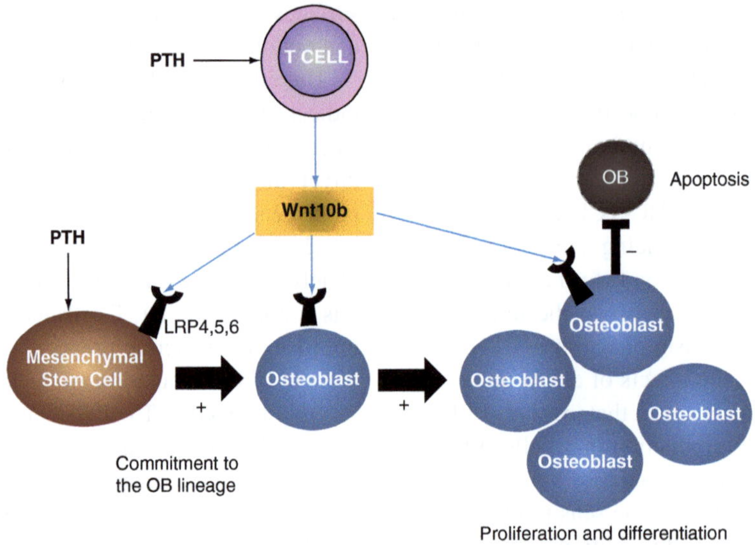

Fig. 14.2 Schematic representation of the role of T cells in the mechanism by which intermittent PTH treatment stimulates bone formation. PTH stimulates T cells to secrete Wnt10b, a Wnt ligand required to activate Wnt signaling in SCs and OBs. In the presence of T cell–produced Wnt10b, stimulation of osteoblastic cells by PTH activates the Wnt signaling pathway. This event leads to increased commitment of mesenchymal stem cells to the osteoblastic lineage, increased OB proliferation and differentiation, and decreased OB apoptosis (Reprinted from Bone, Pacifici [57], Copyright 2010, with permission from Elsevier)

strong expression of PPR in $CD8^+$ T cells and the finding that PTH treatment promotes cAMP production and Wnt10b expression in $CD8^+$ murine and human lymphocyte cell cultures. However, detailed studies using mice lacking a functional PPR receptor in T cells remain to be conducted.

Together, the data indicate that $CD8^+$ T cells potentiate the anabolic activity of PTH by providing Wnt10b, a critical Wnt ligand necessary to activate Wnt signaling in osteoblasts. Therefore, in the absence of $CD8^+$ cells, stimulation of osteoblasts by PTH does not elicit maximum Wnt activation because of the lack of a critical Wnt ligand (Fig. 14.2). The residual bone anabolic activity of PTH observed in T cell–deficient mice presumably is explained by ligand-independent activation of LRP6 [77] and by suppressed production of sclerostin [7, 33, 54].

PTH treatment increased Wnt10b production by all cultured T cells, but iPTH upregulated Wnt10b production only in T cells from BM. This difference may be attributed to differences in the dose and time of exposure to PTH. However, inasmuch as adoptive transfer of spleen T cells into $TCR\beta^{-/-}$ mice is followed by a restoration of a full response to iPTH, the ability of T cells to upregulate their production of Wnt10b in response to iPTH may not be intrinsic to the T cells but may be due to environmental cues.

The anabolic activity of iPTH is not the same in all strains of T cell–deficient mice. In fact, some strains do not increase bone volume in response to PTH, whereas other strains exhibit a blunted, but measurable, response. Osteoblasts produce several bone anabolic Wnt ligands, including Wnt10b, Wnt7a, and Wnt3b [46, 65] that are likely to contribute to the anabolic activity of iPTH that is independent of T cells. Differential responses to these factors may contribute to the quantitative differences in osteoblast production that are observed, accounting, in part, for the strain-dependent variability in the response to iPTH. Furthermore, the magnitude of the anabolic response to iPTH in T cell–null mice may relate to a strain- and age-dependent capacity of iPTH to inhibit bone production of Wnt inhibitors such as sclerostin [7, 33], Dickkopf-1 [39], and Sfrp-4 [62], all of which contribute to the anabolic activity of iPTH through T cell–independent mechanisms. The enhancement of bone formation induced by iPTH is accompanied by increased bone resorption driven by increased production of RANKL and decreased release of OPG in the bone microenvironment. The direct effects of PTH on RANKL/OPG production are mediated, in part, by the iPTH-induced activation of β-catenin in OBs, as this transcriptional regulator stimulates production of OPG [25] and represses expression of RANKL [70]. The latter effect is one of the mechanisms that prevent bone resorption from offsetting the entire anabolic activity of iPTH.

In contrast to their counterparts from T cell–deficient mice, osteoblastic cells cultured from WT mice treated with iPTH exhibit increased commitment to proliferate and differentiate into mature osteoblasts and to increase their life span. Thus, T cells, like PTH, affect all aspects of the OB life cycle. Remarkably, the differences between OBs from T cell–replete and T cell–deficient mice were demonstrated in OBs purified from BM cultured for 7 days without the addition of PTH. This suggests that the hormone regulates early commitment of SCs in vivo and affects their osteoblastic progeny through T cell–produced Wnt10b. These steps are not reversed by the absence of PTH and T cells in vitro. This model is consistent with the ability of Wnt signaling to direct cell behavior [52]. A similar paradigm has been described in ovariectomized mice, in which estrogen withdrawal forms SCs that increase osteoclastogenesis in vitro over 4 weeks [35].

It should be noted that our work is not the first to report an association between T cells and the anabolic activity of PTH. In fact, Pettway et al. [59] investigated the effects of daily injections of PTH for up to 7 weeks on the growth of ectopic "ossicles" implanted in nude mice and found that iPTH increased the bone content of the implanted WT ossicles, a structure that contains normal BM. However, iPTH failed to induce vertebral bone growth in host nude mice, a strain devoid of T cells [59].

Remarkable progress has been made in understanding how T cells participate in the regulation of bone remodeling in both health and disease. In parallel with exciting discoveries about molecular and signaling pathways by which T cells and their products control OC and OB development and function, there has been the recognition of the specialized function of distinct T cell populations such as Tregs and Th17. Progress has been made in recognizing that T cells play an unexpected role in the actions of the major calciotropic and reproductive hormones including PTH and estrogen, as well as in common and clinically relevant forms of bone loss such as occur in postmenopausal osteoporosis and hyperparathyroidism. Much remains to be done to translate observations made in experimental animals into human clinical studies. Strategies to utilize T cell interactions with bone cells as the basis of new therapies also remain to be developed.

14.5 Role of Lymphocytes in the Regulation of Skeletal Integrity

The depth of the integration of the immunoskeletal interface only now is beginning to be appreciated. Pathological T cell and B cell activation is central to the pathogenesis of multiple disorders associated with bone loss, including postmenopausal osteoporosis [18, 21, 78–80], rheumatoid arthritis [17, 38, 68], periodontitis [32, 36, 72], cancer-induced bone loss [24], and hyperparathyroidism [5, 23]. In contrast to the pro-osteoclastogenic roles of B cells and T cells under inflammatory conditions, where the predominance of RANKL production over that of OPG drives osteoclastogenesis and bone resorption, the immune and skeletal systems together afford skeletal protection through vigorous defense of bone homeostasis. We recently demonstrated that in animals, lymphocytes contribute to the maintenance of skeletal integrity through the regulation of OPG production. Although many cell types can make OPG, mature B cells account for up to 45% of total OPG concentration in the bone microenvironment. Consequently, under basal conditions, mature B cells provide significant protection to the skeleton. These findings are consistent with previous studies demonstrating that ablation of B cells intensifies periodontal bone loss [36] and, when combined with our earlier report, demonstrate that human B cells exhibit antiosteoclastic activity [72]. Interestingly, because these studies

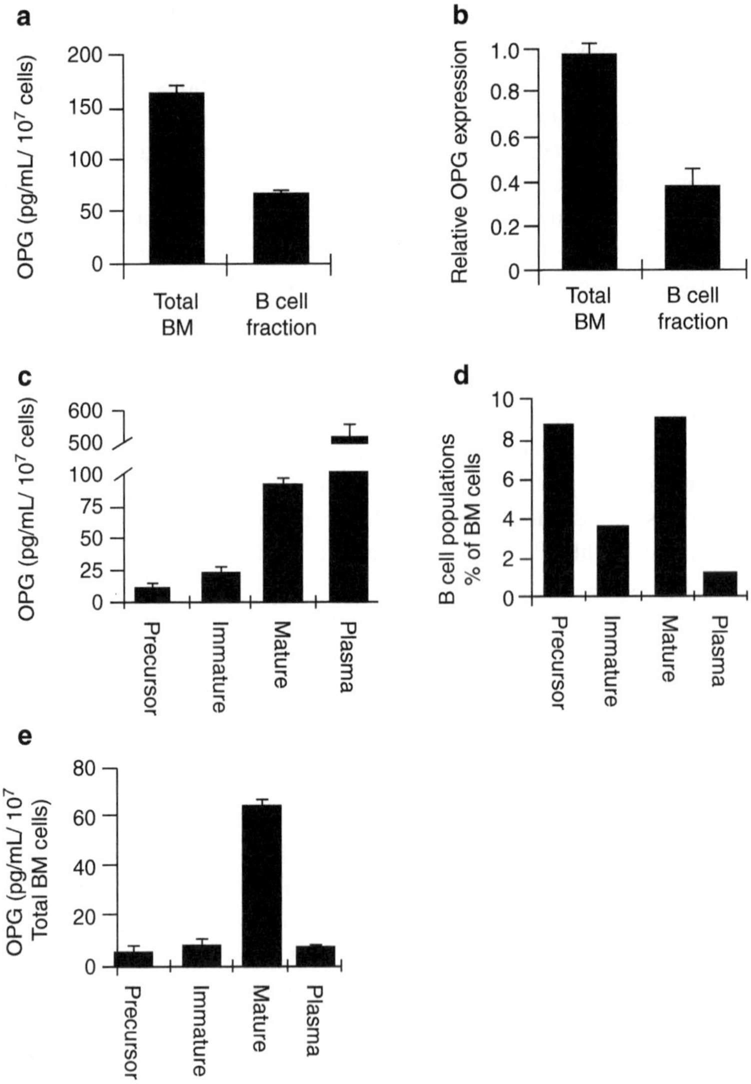

Fig. 14.3 B-lineage cells are a major source of OPG production. (**a**) OPG secretion by total bone marrow nucleated cells or the B cell fraction contained therein was quantitated by ELISA. Mean ± SD of triplicates. Data are representative of more than six independent experiments. (**b**) Relative OPG transcription was quantitated by RT-PCR in total BM nucleated cells or B cell fraction contained therein. Data are presented as mean ± SD of three independent mice per group. (**c**) OPG production by equivalent numbers (1×10^7 cells) of purified BM B cell precursors, immature B cells, mature B cells, and plasma cells. (**d**) B-lineage cell composition as a percentage of total nucleated BM cells. (**e**) Actual concentration of OPG secreted by specific B-lineage cells per 10^7 total nucleated BM cells. The total OPG production was 134±26.1 pg/mL/10^7 total nucleated BM cells (This research was originally published in Li et al. [44]. © the American Society of Hematology)

were undertaken before the identification of OPG, the antiosteoclastogenic effects of OPG were attributed to overproduction of TGF-β, a cytokine that promotes OPG production, but the observations remain the same.

Although mature B cells are the dominant B-lineage that produces OPG in the bone microenvironment, B cell precursors and terminally differentiated plasma cells further contribute a small amount of OPG such that the entire B cell lineage accounts for 64% of total bone marrow–related OPG production (Fig. 14.3). Attesting to the role of B cells in maintaining skeletal integrity under physiological conditions, μMT KO mice, a strain that is characterized by the absence of mature B and plasma cells, progressively lost bone mineral density (BMD) and bone volume, reaching significant levels by 16 weeks of age. Development of bone loss in B cell KO mice was rescued by adoptive transfer with B cells, a result that highlights the importance of B cells for skeletal protection (Fig. 14.4).

OPG is critical to protect vertebrate bone. Compelling evidence comes from experiments in which ablation of the OPG genes in mice led to a severe osteoporotic phenotype [10, 49], with evidence of bone fractures that had occurred within 1 month of birth in some animals [10]. Mature

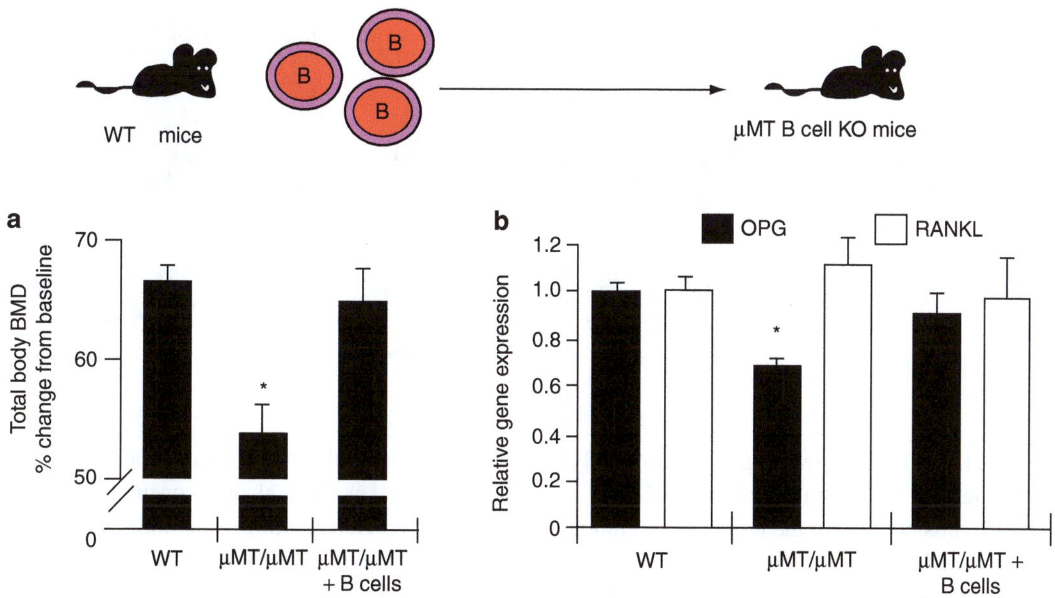

Fig. 14.4 B cell KO mice display decreased baseline BMD and increase bone resorption, concurrent with decreased BM OPG concentrations. (**a**) B cell reconstitution of μMT/μMT B cell KO rescues loss of BMD (*$P<.01$ vs. WT) and (**b**) OPG production (*$P<.05$ vs. WT). Mice were reconstituted at 4 weeks of age, and BMD and RT-PCR studies preformed at 12 weeks of age (This research was originally published in Blood. Li et al. [44]. © the American Society of Hematology)

B cells contribute approximately half of total bone marrow OPG. The μMT KO mouse is best compared to the heterozygous OPG KO mouse in which loss of a single OPG allele leads to an initially normal phenotype whose progressive loss of bone mass is significant by 6 months of age [10]. Similarly, B cell KO mice are born with normal bone mass, with significant loss of BMD and bone volume by 4 months of age.

B cells interact with and are regulated through interactions with T cells. Consistent with this notion of the role of T cells, B cells either may stimulate or inhibit osteoclastogenesis in the context by which they have been acted on by cytokines produced by T cells. Furthermore, B cell OPG production can be upregulated by activation of the CD40 costimulatory receptor on human B cells in culture. CD40L [83], the counterpart of CD40, is expressed predominantly by activated T cells. T cells subject to CD40/CD40L costimulation regulate B cell OPG production in vivo. The basal BMD in T cell–deficient nude mice is reduced significantly [74], an unexpected finding given the pro-osteoclastogenic roles of T cells. Subsequent analysis correlated BMD loss with an OPG deficiency in the bone microenvironment. This deficit is a consequence of diminished B cell function. The importance of the CD40/CD40L costimulatory loop in this response is seen in CD40 and CD40L KO mice, in which a diminished BMD and volume is seen, and whose B cell and OPG production are impaired [44].

14.6 Disruption of the Immunoskeletal Interface Leads to Bone Loss in HIV/AIDS

The importance of T cells and B cells to pathological bone turnover long has been appreciated in autoimmune and inflammatory conditions such as rheumatoid arthritis and periodontitis. Another condition characterized by massive disruption of immune function is the acquired immune deficiency syndrome (AIDS), a consequence of infection by the human immunodeficiency virus-1

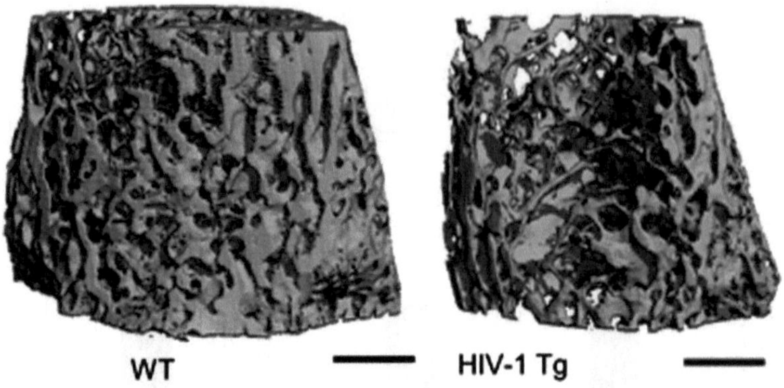

Fig. 14.5 Microcomputed tomography reconctructions of trabecular bone in WT and HIV-1 Tg rats. Longitudinal trabecular (12 μm) 3D reconstructions of femurs from WT and HIV-1 Tg rats were generated by μCT (This research was originally published in Vikulina et al. [76])

(HIV-1). AIDS disease progression not only is characterized by a dramatic decline in CD4 T and CD8 T cells but also in the numbers and function of the B cell population [50] and in the number of active monocytes/macrophages [16]. A constellation of alterations impair B cells, severely reducing humoral immunity. The changes that occur include an enhanced frequency of activation, exhausted memory, an increase in immature/transitional B cells, and a decline in resting memory B cells [50, 51].

Given the role of lymphocytes in the regulation of bone homeostasis, bone turnover would predictably be seriously disrupted in patients infected with HIV-1. Osteoporosis and osteopenia have been documented in AIDS patients [83], and almost two of three patients with HIV-1 infection have reduced BMD [9]. A recent meta-analysis of bone-related studies in AIDS- and HIV-1-infected patients concludes that the overall prevalence of osteoporosis is 15%, and of osteopenia is 52% [56]. The high rate of diminished BMD has raised fears of a future epidemic of fractures in this population [3]. Moreover, with a rapidly aging AIDS patient population, the combination of AIDS and age-associated decline in BMD is likely to exacerbate skeletal deterioration and to increase fracture risk. Furthermore, exacerbated skeletal deterioration in postmenopausal women with HIV-1 infection has been confirmed [82].

The causes of bone loss in the AIDS population remain highly controversial. Explanations include direct virus-related effects on bone cells, as well as traditional osteoporosis risk factors that are prevalent in the AIDS population, including, for example, smoking, alcohol consumption, vitamin D deficiency [53, 81], indirect AIDS-associated pathologies (muscle wasting, kidney disease, and hypogonadism), and the hotly debated direct and indirect roles of pharmaceuticals utilized in active antiretroviral therapy (HAART) formulations (reviewed in [55]). In reality, many if not all of these factors likely play a role in the high rates of aberrant bone turnover observed in these patients. Identifying and investigating the contribution of specific causes of bone loss in this high risk population are extremely challenging.

In order to investigate the role of the immunoskeletal interface in the bone loss associated with AIDS, we turned to a simplified yet powerful animal model of chronic HIV-1 infection, the HIV-1 transgenic (Tg) rat. This noninfectious small animal model expresses a constitutively active gag-pol-deleted HIV-1 provirus and develops numerous immunological and metabolic pathologies synonymous with human AIDS [66]. The confounding influence of lifestyle factors, antiretroviral drugs, and other agents used for the prophylaxis of AIDS complications such as glucocorticoids can be controlled in this model. We examined the role of direct adaptive immune disruption in the skeletal pathology. As in humans who have AIDS, the HIV-1 Tg rats exhibited a significant skeletal degeneration and a dramatic loss of BMD in bone volume (Fig. 14.5). Osteoclastic bone resorption was upregulated [76], and OPG expression was significantly diminished, both observations concurrent with a severe decline in B cell OPG expression. These observations are consistent with a published study that reported diminished serum OPG concentrations in AIDS patients [14].

Interestingly, the deficit in OPG was exacerbated by a significant elevation in B cell RANKL production, suggestive of an activated B cell phenotype. The elevation in the RANKL/OPG ratio was accompanied by a dramatic increase in the concentration of osteoclast precursors in the BM [76]. Taken together, these findings suggest that with all other contributing factors put aside, a severely disrupted immune compartment is a likely driving force for the creation of conditions favorable to osteoclastic bone loss in HIV/AIDS patients.

Studies are currently under way to translate these observations for the treatment of AIDS patients and to investigate the specific B cell subsets that are responsible for diminished OPG and enhanced RANKL production in this group. Understanding the mechanisms involved may facilitate the development of better screening techniques in viewing parameters to predict the extent of bone loss that may occur in individual AIDS patients. Strong emphasis on diagnosis and early therapeutic intervention are important to avoid a significant new health threat in the aging HIV/AIDS community.

Acknowledgments The authors gratefully acknowledge the financial support from NIAMS (AR059364, AR053607 and AR056090) and the Biomedical Laboratory Research & Development Service of the VA Office of Research and Development (5I01BX000105) to MNW and by NIAMS and NIA(AR49659 and AG28278) to RP.

References

1. Ahuja SS, Zhao S, Bellido T, Plotkin LI, Jimenez F, Bonewald LF. CD40 ligand blocks apoptosis induced by tumor necrosis factor alpha, glucocorticoids, and etoposide in osteoblasts and the osteocyte-like cell line murine long bone osteocyte-Y4. Endocrinology. 2003;144:1761–9.
2. Almeida M, Han L, Bellido T, Manolagas SC, Kousteni S. Wnt proteins prevent apoptosis of both uncommitted osteoblast progenitors and differentiated osteoblasts by beta-catenin-dependent and -independent signaling cascades involving Src/ERK and phosphatidylinositol 3-kinase/AKT. J Biol Chem. 2005;280: 41342–51.
3. Amorosa V, Tebas P. Bone disease and HIV infection. Clin Infect Dis. 2006;42:108–14.
4. Andre P, Prasad KS, Denis CV, He M, Papalia JM, Hynes RO, et al. CD40L stabilizes arterial thrombi by a beta3 integrin–dependent mechanism. Nat Med. 2002;8:247–52.
5. Bedi B, Li JY, Grassi F, Tawfeek H, Weitzmann MN, Pacifici R. Inhibition of antigen presentation and T cell costimulation blocks PTH-induced bone loss. Ann N Y Acad Sci. 2010;1192:215–21.
6. Behrens J, von Kries JP, Kuhl M, Bruhn L, Wedlich D, Grosschedl R, et al. Functional interaction of beta-catenin with the transcription factor LEF-1. Nature. 1996;382:638–42.
7. Bellido T, Ali AA, Gubrij I, Plotkin LI, Fu Q, O'Brien CA, et al. Chronic elevation of parathyroid hormone in mice reduces expression of sclerostin by osteocytes: a novel mechanism for hormonal control of osteoblastogenesis. Endocrinology. 2005;146: 4577–83.
8. Bellido T, Ali AA, Plotkin LI, Fu Q, Gubrij I, Roberson PK, et al. Proteasomal degradation of Runx2 shortens parathyroid hormone-induced anti-apoptotic signaling in osteoblasts. A putative explanation for why intermittent administration is needed for bone anabolism. J Biol Chem. 2003;278:50259–72.
9. Brown TT, Qaqish RB. Antiretroviral therapy and the prevalence of osteopenia and osteoporosis: a meta-analytic review. AIDS. 2006;20:2165–74.
10. Bucay N, Sarosi I, Dunstan CR, Morony S, Tarpley J, Capparelli C, et al. Osteoprotegerin-deficient mice develop early onset osteoporosis and arterial calcification. Genes Dev. 1998;12:1260–8.
11. Calvi LM, Sims NA, Hunzelman JL, Knight MC, Giovannetti A, Saxton JM, et al. Activated parathyroid hormone/parathyroid hormone-related protein receptor in osteoblastic cells differentially affects cortical and trabecular bone. J Clin Invest. 2001;107:277–86.
12. Canalis E, Giustina A, Bilezikian JP. Mechanisms of anabolic therapies for osteoporosis. N Engl J Med. 2007;357:905–16.
13. Cenci S, Weitzmann MN, Roggia C, Namba N, Novack D, Woodring J, et al. Estrogen deficiency induces bone loss by enhancing T-cell production of TNF-alpha. J Clin Invest. 2000;106:1229–37.
14. Chakravarti A, Marceau AA, Flamand L, Poubelle PE. Normal human primary CD4+ T lymphocytes synthesize and release functional osteoprotegerin in vitro. Lab Invest. 2008;88:171–84.
15. Choi HY, Dieckmann M, Herz J, Niemeier A. Lrp4, a novel receptor for Dickkopf 1 and sclerostin, is expressed by osteoblasts and regulates bone growth and turnover in vivo. PLoS One. 2009;4:e7930.
16. Coleman CM, Wu L. HIV interactions with monocytes and dendritic cells: viral latency and reservoirs. Retrovirology. 2009;6:51.
17. Colucci S, Brunetti G, Cantatore F, Oranger A, Mori G, Quarta L, et al. Lymphocytes and synovial fluid fibroblasts support osteoclastogenesis through RANKL, TNFalpha, and IL-7 in an in vitro model

derived from human psoriatic arthritis. J Pathol. 2007;212:47–55.
18. D'Amelio P, Grimaldi A, Di Bella S, Brianza SZ, Cristofaro MA, Tamone C, et al. Estrogen deficiency increases osteoclastogenesis up-regulating T cells activity: a key mechanism in osteoporosis. Bone. 2008;43:92–100.
19. Di Rosa F. T-lymphocyte interaction with stromal, bone and hematopoietic cells in the bone marrow. Immunol Cell Biol. 2008;87:20–9.
20. Dobnig H, Turner RT. Evidence that intermittent treatment with parathyroid hormone increases bone formation in adult rats by activation of bone lining cells. Endocrinology. 1995;136:3632–8.
21. Eghbali-Fatourechi G, Khosla S, Sanyal A, Boyle WJ, Lacey DL, Riggs BL. Role of RANK ligand in mediating increased bone resorption in early postmenopausal women. J Clin Invest. 2003;111:1221–30.
22. Eichinger A, Fiaschi-Taesch N, Massfelder T, Fritsch S, Barthelmebs M, Helwig JJ. Transcript expression of the tuberoinfundibular peptide (TIP)39/PTH2 receptor system and non-PTH1 receptor-mediated tonic effects of TIP39 and other PTH2 receptor ligands in renal vessels. Endocrinology. 2002;143:3036–43.
23. Gao Y, Wu X, Terauchi M, Li JY, Grassi F, Galley S, et al. T cells potentiate PTH-induced cortical bone loss through CD40L signaling. Cell Metab. 2008;8:132–45.
24. Giuliani N, Colla S, Sala R, Moroni M, Lazzaretti M, La Monica S, et al. Human myeloma cells stimulate the receptor activator of nuclear factor-kappa B ligand (RANKL) in T lymphocytes: a potential role in multiple myeloma bone disease. Blood. 2002;100: 4615–21.
25. Glass 2nd DA, Bialek P, Ahn JD, Starbuck M, Patel MS, Clevers H, et al. Canonical Wnt signaling in differentiated osteoblasts controls osteoclast differentiation. Dev Cell. 2005;8:751–64.
26. Grammer AC, Lipsky PE. CD40-mediated regulation of immune responses by TRAF-dependent and TRAF-independent signaling mechanisms. Adv Immunol. 2000;76:61–178.
27. Grassi F, Tell G, Robbie-Ryan M, Gao Y, Terauchi M, Yang X, et al. Oxidative stress causes bone loss in estrogen-deficient mice through enhanced bone marrow dendritic cell activation. Proc Natl Acad Sci USA. 2007;104:15087–92.
28. Grewal IS, Flavell RA. The role of CD40 ligand in costimulation and T-cell activation. Immunol Rev. 1996;153:85–106.
29. Grey A, Mitnick MA, Shapses S, Ellison A, Gundeberg C, Insogna K. Circulating levels of intreleukin-6 and tumor necrosis factor α are elevated in primary hyperparathyroidism and correlate with markers of bone resorption. J Clin Endocrinol Metab. 1996;81:3450–68.
30. Hoare SR, Clark JA, Usdin TB. Molecular determinants of tuberoinfundibular peptide of 39 residues (TIP39) selectivity for the parathyroid hormone-2 (PTH2) receptor. N-terminal truncation of TIP39 reverses PTH2 receptor/PTH1 receptor binding selectivity. J Biol Chem. 2000;275:27274–83.
31. Jilka RL, Weinstein RS, Bellido T, Roberson P, Parfitt AM, Manolagas SC. Increased bone formation by prevention of osteoblast apoptosis with parathyroid hormone. J Clin Invest. 1999;104:439–46.
32. Kawai T, Matsuyama T, Hosokawa Y, Makihira S, Seki M, Karimbux NY, et al. B and T lymphocytes are the primary sources of RANKL in the bone resorptive lesion of periodontal disease. Am J Pathol. 2006;169: 987–98.
33. Keller H, Kneissel M. SOST is a target gene for PTH in bone. Bone. 2005;37:148–58.
34. Khosla S. Minireview: the OPG/RANKL/RANK system. Endocrinology. 2001;142:5050–5.
35. Kimble RB, Srivastava S, Ross FP, Matayoshi A, Pacifici R. Estrogen deficiency increases the ability of stromal cells to support murine osteoclastogenesis via an interleukin-1and tumor necrosis factor-mediated stimulation of macrophage colony-stimulating factor production. J Biol Chem. 1996;271:28890–7.
36. Klausen B, Hougen HP, Fiehn NE. Increased periodontal bone loss in temporarily B lymphocyte-deficient rats. J Periodontal Res. 1989;24:384–90.
37. Kobayashi T, Chung UI, Schipani E, Starbuck M, Karsenty G, Katagiri T, et al. PTHrP and Indian hedgehog control differentiation of growth plate chondrocytes at multiple steps. Development. 2002;129:2977–86.
38. Kong YY, Feige U, Sarosi I, Bolon B, Tafuri A, Morony S, et al. Activated T cells regulate bone loss and joint destruction in adjuvant arthritis through osteoprotegerin ligand. Nature. 1999;402:304–9.
39. Kulkarni NH, Halladay DL, Miles RR, Gilbert LM, Frolik CA, Galvin RJ, et al. Effects of parathyroid hormone on Wnt signaling pathway in bone. J Cell Biochem. 2005;95:1178–90.
40. Lam J, Takeshita S, Barker JE, Kanagawa O, Ross FP, Teitelbaum SL. TNF-alpha induces osteoclastogenesis by direct stimulation of macrophages exposed to permissive levels of RANK ligand. J Clin Invest. 2000;106:1481–8.
41. Lanske B, Amling M, Neff L, Guiducci J, Baron R, Kronenberg HM. Ablation of the PTHrP gene or the PTH/PTHrP receptor gene leads to distinct abnormalities in bone development. J Clin Invest. 1999;104:399–407.
42. Lee PP, Fitzpatrick DR, Beard C, Jessup HK, Lehar S, Makar KW, et al. A critical role for Dnmt1 and DNA methylation in T cell development, function, and survival. Immunity. 2001;15:763–74.
43. Leveille C, Bouillon M, Guo W, Bolduc J, Sharif-Askari E, El-Fakhry Y, et al. CD40 ligand binds to alpha5beta1 integrin and triggers cell signaling. J Biol Chem. 2007;282:5143–51.
44. Li Y, Toraldo G, Li A, Yang X, Zhang H, Qian WP, et al. B cells and T cells are critical for the preservation of bone homeostasis and attainment of peak bone mass in vivo. Blood. 2007;109:3839–48.

45. Lindsay R, Cosman F, Zhou H, Bostrom MP, Shen VW, Cruz JD, et al. A novel tetracycline labeling schedule for longitudinal evaluation of the short-term effects of anabolic therapy with a single iliac crest bone biopsy: early actions of teriparatide. J Bone Miner Res. 2006;21:366–73.
46. Luo Q, Kang Q, Si W, Jiang W, Park JK, Peng Y, et al. Connective tissue growth factor (CTGF) is regulated by Wnt and bone morphogenetic proteins signaling in osteoblast differentiation of mesenchymal stem cells. J Biol Chem. 2004;279:55958–68.
47. Ma YL, Zeng Q, Donley DW, Ste-Marie LG, Gallagher JC, Dalsky GP, et al. Teriparatide increases bone formation in modeling and remodeling osteons and enhances IGF-II immunoreactivity in postmenopausal women with osteoporosis. J Bone Miner Res. 2006;21:855–64.
48. Meng XW, Liang XG, Birchman R, Wu DD, Dempster DW, Lindsay R, et al. Temporal expression of the anabolic action of PTH in cancellous bone of ovariectomized rats. J Bone Miner Res. 1996;11:421–9.
49. Mizuno A, Amizuka N, Irie K, Murakami A, Fujise N, Kanno T, et al. Severe osteoporosis in mice lacking osteoclastogenesis inhibitory factor/osteoprotegerin. Biochem Biophys Res Commun. 1998;247:610–5.
50. Moir S, Fauci AS. B cells in HIV infection and disease. Nat Rev Immunol. 2009;9:235–45.
51. Moir S, Ho J, Malaspina A, Wang W, DiPoto AC, O'Shea MA, et al. Evidence for HIV-associated B cell exhaustion in a dysfunctional memory B cell compartment in HIV-infected viremic individuals. J Exp Med. 2008;205:1797–805.
52. Moon RT, Bowerman B, Boutros M, Perrimon N. The promise and perils of Wnt signaling through beta-catenin. Science. 2002;296:1644–6.
53. Mueller NJ, Fux CA, Ledergerber B, Elzi L, Schmid P, Dang T, et al. High prevalence of severe vitamin D deficiency in combined antiretroviral therapy-naive and successfully treated swiss HIV patients. AIDS. 2010;24:1127–34.
54. O'Brien CA, Plotkin LI, Galli C, Goellner JJ, Gortazar AR, Allen MR, et al. Control of bone mass and remodeling by PTH receptor signaling in osteocytes. PLoS One. 2008;3:e2942.
55. Ofotokun I, Weitzmann MN. HIV-1 infection and antiretroviral therapies: risk factors for osteoporosis and bone fracture. Curr Opin Endocrinol Diabetes Obes. 2010;17:523–9.
56. Paccou J, Viget N, Legrout-Gerot I, Yazdanpanah Y, Cortet B. Bone loss in patients with HIV infection. Joint Bone Spine. 2009;76:637–41.
57. Pacifici R. T cells: critical bone regulators in health and disease. Bone. 2010;47(3):461–71.
58. Pettway GJ, Meganck JA, Koh AJ, Keller ET, Goldstein SA, McCauley LK. Parathyroid hormone mediates bone growth through the regulation of osteoblast proliferation and differentiation. Bone. 2007;42:806–18.
59. Pettway GJ, Schneider A, Koh AJ, Widjaja E, Morris MD, Meganck JA, et al. Anabolic actions of PTH (1–34): use of a novel tissue engineering model to investigate temporal effects on bone. Bone. 2005;36:959–70.
60. Potts J. Primary hyperparathyroidism. In: Avioli LV, Krane S, editors. Metabolic bone diseases. San Diego: Academic; 1998. p. 411–42.
61. Prasad KS, Andre P, He M, Bao M, Manganello J, Phillips DR. Soluble CD40 ligand induces beta3 integrin tyrosine phosphorylation and triggers platelet activation by outside-in signaling. Proc Natl Acad Sci USA. 2003;100:12367–71.
62. Qin L, Qiu P, Wang L, Li X, Swarthout JT, Soteropoulos P, et al. Gene expression profiles and transcription factors involved in parathyroid hormone signaling in osteoblasts revealed by microarray and bioinformatics. J Biol Chem. 2003;278:19723–31.
63. Qin L, Raggatt LJ, Partridge NC. Parathyroid hormone: a double-edged sword for bone metabolism. Trends Endocrinol Metab. 2004;15:60–5.
64. Quezada SA, Jarvinen LZ, Lind EF, Noelle RJ. CD40/CD154 interactions at the interface of tolerance and immunity. Annu Rev Immunol. 2004;22:307–28.
65. Rawadi G, Vayssiere B, Dunn F, Baron R, Roman-Roman S. BMP-2 controls alkaline phosphatase expression and osteoblast mineralization by a Wnt autocrine loop. J Bone Miner Res. 2003;18:1842–53.
66. Reid W, Sadowska M, Denaro F, Rao S, Foulke Jr J, Hayes N, et al. An HIV-1 transgenic rat that develops HIV-related pathology and immunologic dysfunction. Proc Natl Acad Sci USA. 2001;98:9271–6.
67. Rifas L. T-cell cytokine induction of BMP-2 regulates human mesenchymal stromal cell differentiation and mineralization. J Cell Biochem. 2006;98:706–14.
68. Rifas L, Weitzmann MN. A novel T cell cytokine, secreted osteoclastogenic factor of activated T cells, induces osteoclast formation in a RANKL-independent manner. Arthritis Rheum. 2009;60:3324–35.
69. Riggs BL, Melton LJ. Medical progress: involutional osteoporosis. N Eng J Med. 1986;314:1676–84.
70. Spencer GJ, Utting JC, Etheridge SL, Arnett TR, Genever PG. Wnt signalling in osteoblasts regulates expression of the receptor activator of NFkappaB ligand and inhibits osteoclastogenesis in vitro. J Cell Sci. 2006;119:1283–96.
71. Stojceva-Taneva O, Fadda GZ, Smogorzewski M, Massry SG. Parathyroid hormone increases cytosolic calcium of thymocytes. Nephron. 1993;64:592–9.
72. Taubman MA, Kawai T. Involvement of T-lymphocytes in periodontal disease and in direct and indirect induction of bone resorption. Crit Rev Oral Biol Med. 2001;12:125–35.
73. Terauchi M, Li JY, Bedi B, Baek KH, Tawfeek H, Galley S, et al. T lymphocytes amplify the anabolic activity of parathyroid hormone through Wnt10b signaling. Cell Metab. 2009;10:229–40.
74. Toraldo G, Roggia C, Qian W-P, Pacifici R, Weitzmann MN. IL-7 induces bone loss in vivo by induction of

receptor activator of nuclear factor kappa B ligand and tumor necrosis factor alpha from T cells. Proc Natl Acad Sci USA. 2003;100:125–30.
75. Usdin TB, Hoare SR, Wang T, Mezey E, Kowalak JA. TIP39: a new neuropeptide and PTH2-receptor agonist from hypothalamus. Nat Neurosci. 1999;2:941–3.
76. Vikulina T, Fan X, Yamaguchi M, Roser-Page S, Zayzafoon M, Guidot DM, et al. Alterations in the immuno-skeletal interface drive bone destruction in HIV-1 transgenic rats. Proc Natl Acad Sci USA. 2010;107:13848–53.
77. Wan M, Yang C, Li J, Wu X, Yuan H, Ma H, et al. Parathyroid hormone signaling through low-density lipoprotein-related protein 6. Genes Dev. 2008;22: 2968–79.
78. Weitzmann MN, Pacifici R. The role of T lymphocytes in bone metabolism. Immunol Rev. 2005;208: 154–68.
79. Weitzmann MN, Pacifici R. Role of the immune system in postmenopausal bone loss. Curr Osteoporos Rep. 2005;3:92–7.
80. Weitzmann MN, Pacifici R. Estrogen deficiency and bone loss: an inflammatory tale. J Clin Invest. 2006;116:1186–94.
81. Yin MT, Lu D, Cremers S, Tien PC, Cohen MH, Shi Q, et al. Short-term bone loss in HIV-infected premenopausal women. J Acquir Immune Defic Syndr. 2010;53:202–8.
82. Yin MT, McMahon DJ, Ferris DC, Zhang CA, Shu A, Staron R, et al. Low bone mass and high bone turnover in postmenopausal human immunodeficiency virus-infected women. J Clin Endocrinol Metab. 2010;95:620–9.
83. Yun TJ, Chaudhary PM, Shu GL, Frazer JK, Ewings MK, Schwartz SM, et al. OPG/FDCR-1, a TNF receptor family member, is expressed in lymphoid cells and is up-regulated by ligating CD40. J Immunol. 1998;161:6113–21.
84. Zirlik A, Maier C, Gerdes N, MacFarlane L, Soosairajah J, Bavendiek U, et al. CD40 ligand mediates inflammation independently of CD40 by interaction with Mac-1. Circulation. 2007;115:1571–80.

15 Bone and the Ear

Kathleen C. Horner

Keywords
Bones in ear • Hearing • Ossicles • Vestibular function • Otoconia • Bone conduction

15.1 Introduction

This chapter describes how balanced bone metabolism assures not only a healthy skeletal structure but also optimal hearing and vestibular functions. Hearing function is assured by the sequential collaboration of three different parts of the ear – the outer ear that captures the acoustic signal, the middle ear ossicles that transmit an amplified signal to the cochlea, and the inner ear that harbors the sensory cells. The inner ear, consisting of the cochlea and the vestibular receptors, is concealed in a multilayered bony structure.

The membranous cochlea is coiled around an axial bony cylinder containing the nerve trunk. This assembly is imprisoned within the bony labyrinth (otic capsule), which in turn is held within a bony case (temporal bone), located bilaterally within the skull (Fig. 15.1a). The membranous vestibular organs, located toward the base of each cochlea, are likewise surrounded by bone (Fig. 15.1c). There are five different vestibular epithelia on each side of the skull. There are detectors of head rotation (three cristae within the ampullae of the semicircular canals) (Fig. 15.1b) and detectors of gravity and linear acceleration (two otoconial organs, namely, the sacculus and the utriculus) (Fig. 15.1d). Otoconia are sometimes referred to as "ear stones". They consist of conglomerations of calcium carbonate crystals. Although they are not bones, events that affect normal bone and calcium metabolism can affect the otoconia, and so they will be considered here as well.

While the bony armor serves to protect the sensory organ, mechanical trauma can result in cracks or fissures to the bone with possible irremediable damage to the sensory organ. Furthermore, disturbed bone metabolism can have repercussions on the middle ear and labyrinthine bone and so can affect hearing and/or vestibular function.

The entire membranous labyrinth reaches its adult size in utero and becomes ossified before birth – thereafter there is no further growth. The whole organ is miniature with the human cochlea being only about the size of a small pea (around 5-mm diameter). Hearing begins in

K.C. Horner, Ph.D.
Faculté des Sciences et Techniques,
INSERM, CRN2M, Université Paul Cézanne,
Avenue Escadrille Normandie-Niémen,
Marseille, Cedex 20 13397, France
e-mail: kathleen.horner@univ-cezanne.fr

F. Bronner et al. (eds.), *Bone-Metabolic Functions and Modulators*, Topics in Bone Biology,
DOI 10.1007/978-1-4471-2745-1_15, © Springer-Verlag London 2012

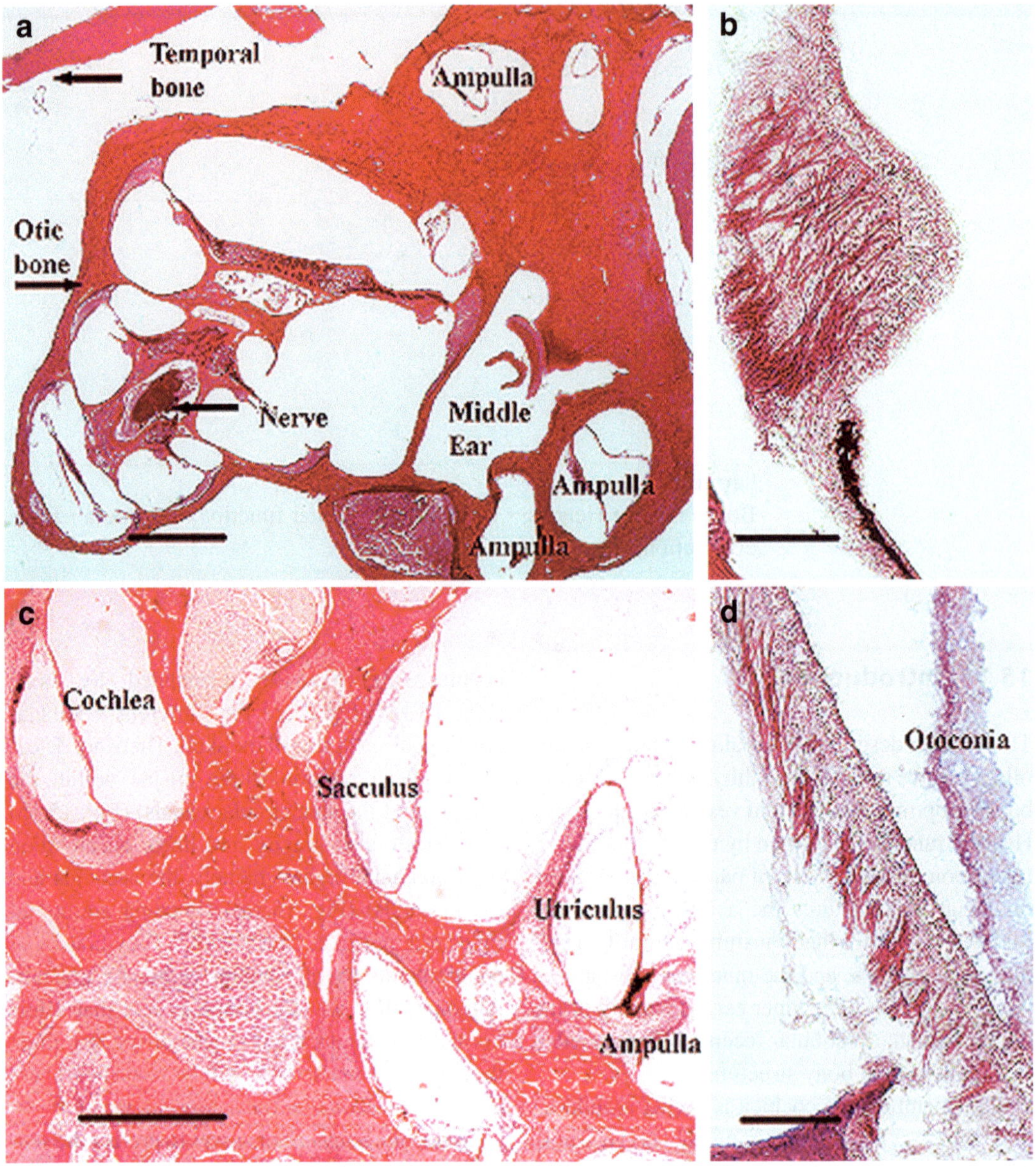

Fig. 15.1 Cryostat section of a guinea pig temporal bone, stained histologically with Periodic Acid Schiff. (**a**) An overview of the cochlea and vestibule. (**b**) An ampulla. (**c**) The vestibular organs located toward the base of the cochlea. (**d**) An otolithic organ showing the otoconial mass lying over the sensory epithelium. Scale bar 1 mm (**a**, **c**); 100 μm (**b**, **d**)

utero, in the third trimester of pregnancy, where sounds are transmitted by bone conduction to the cochlea. Stable structure of all bone depends on the regular housekeeping tasks of remodeling – resorption and rebuilding – under neural and hormonal control. Abnormal bone mineralization in development or change in bone metabolism with aging or during periods of intense hormonal changes can affect cochlear/vestibular function. This chapter will explore several hormones known to affect the skeleton as well as the ear. Finally, prospects of new clinical treatment of temporal bone pathologies will be considered.

15.2 Ossification of the Developing Labyrinth

The human temporal bone is made up of four different bones, originating from two types of ossification [133, 148]. The squamous and tympanic bones originate from intramembranous ossification derived from mesenchyme cell activity. In contrast, the petrous and styloid bones originate from endochondral ossification of embryonic cartilage from fourteen and two ossification centers, respectively. The inner ear lies within the petrous part of the temporal bone.

Ossification of the inner ear begins at the base of the cochlea, when the membranous labyrinth has reached its adult dimensions, at around week 15. At 23 weeks, the ossified cochlea has reached its "impressive" adult height of close to 5 mm [122]. The last part to ossify, overlying the posterior semicircular canal, is not complete until about week 24 [133]. Incomplete ossification at this time can underlie some auditory/vestibular anomalies that are detected in later life (see Sect. 15.4). Recently, 3D-microcomputed tomography has confirmed that different parts of the labyrinth reach adult size at different times – the cochlea and round window at 23 weeks, the superior semicircular canal at 24 weeks, the posterior and lateral (horizontal) canals at 25 weeks of gestation, the oval window at 35 weeks, and vestibular aqueduct after birth [122].

The bone of the otic capsule is made up of three layers – two periosteal layers that sandwich an endochondral layer. The outermost periosteal layer has slow bone turnover, but it can undergo some remodeling following insults. The middle endochondral layer ossifies in isolated sites, known as *globuli ossei*, but with some cartilage persisting after birth. The inner periosteal layer contacts the inner ear soft tissues and remains quite inert throughout life – due at least in part to inhibitory influences from the perilymph (see Sect. 15.8.1).

The middle ear ossicles – malleus, incus, and stapes – are the smallest bones in the body (around 4–7 μm). Vibrations of the tympanic membrane are transmitted via this ossicular chain, which carries out the impedance matching between air and liquid, to the fluid-filled compartments of the inner ear. A coupling pulley system together with a difference in surface area between the tympanic membrane and the oval window ensures that the signal is amplified. The bones of the middle ear develop embryologically from the branchial arches. Most of the body of the malleus and the incus develops from the first branchial arch, Merkel's cartilage, while the stapes develops from the second branchial arch, Reichert's cartilage [98]. The malleus/incus and stapes begin to ossify from their cartilaginous origins around week 16 and 18, respectively. By 20 weeks, the malleus and incus have reached adult positions and by 26 weeks bone remodeling begins. The stapes footplate resembles the endochondral layer of the otic capsule, in that after birth it maintains viable chondrocytes and does not heal well after injury.

The complete encapsulation by bone of the middle and inner ear in utero provides a certain protection for this otherwise fragile membranous structure. On the other hand, the bony armor remains shock sensitive and is slow to repair because of low bone turnover.

15.3 Hearing via Bone Conduction In Utero

Although the first studies of human hearing in utero were carried out over 60 years ago [5], testing paradigms have been and are still restricted by obvious ethical concerns. Many studies have therefore been carried out in the laboratory on animal models. Studies on in utero hearing have often employed guinea pigs or sheep since in those animals, the auditory system begins to function already in utero – unlike other small laboratory mammals where the maturation continues after birth. The injection of 14 C-deoxyglucose in awake pregnant guinea pigs, exposure to loud pure tones, and subsequent autoradiography have demonstrated tonotopic activation of the central auditory nuclei in late-term fetuses [62]. Furthermore, excessive exposure to low-pass noise induced temporary threshold shifts [65] and resulted in sensory hair cell loss in the upper part of the cochlea of sheep in utero [39]. Intrauterine recordings, via a miniature hydrophone, of the acoustic environment within the amniotic sac of pregnant ewes showed that the mother's vocalizations are a prominent part of the normal sound environment [2]. The level of sound necessary to evoke auditory responses in sheep fetuses in utero was elevated when a sound-attenuating hood was placed over the head of the fetus. Those data indicated that sounds reach the ear in utero by bone conduction through the skull [38].

In humans, pneumatization of the middle ear begins as early as around 12 weeks and is complete around week 24 [170]. Embryonic connective tissue within the middle ear decreases with fetal development giving way to the middle ear cavity at the end of gestation [79]. Middle ear impedance in newborns 2–24 h old is similar to those at 36–150 h [103], indicating that the middle ear can function to some extent already in utero. The recording of changes in heartbeat and motor responses to external sounds has been largely employed for detection of human fetal hearing. Responses begin around 24 weeks and are consistently evoked at 28 weeks [17]. Ultrasound imaging of the auropalpebral reflex (blink response) of the human fetus to a specific vibroacoustic stimulus can also be recorded [8]. Intrauterine recordings from women at the beginning of labor and after amniotomy have shown that external sounds at the air-abdomen interface in humans are attenuated negligibly below 250 Hz, by about 20 dB at 1,000 Hz and not beyond 30 dB at higher frequencies [118]. Not only does hearing occur in utero but the last trimester of pregnancy is considered rather as a period of enriched acoustic environment with long-term effects on the baby. Newborns prefer their mother's voice to other voices including that of the father – indicating that prenatal auditory experience may be important for bonding [26]. On the other hand, overexposure to noise is a potential hazard, and exposure to occupational noise during pregnancy can increase the risk of hearing loss in children [86].

15.4 Consequences of Incomplete Ossification

The semicircular canals are the last part of the inner ear to ossify. Incomplete ossification of the semicircular canals, known as dehiscence, can give rise to sound-induced vestibular and/or auditory anomalies. Incomplete ossification results in the equivalent of a third window (the other two being the oval and round windows) in the bone and rerouting of sound signals away from the cochlea toward the vestibule. Tullio was first to demonstrate, in pigeons and then in rabbits and dogs, that following fenestration of a semicircular canal, sound stimulation caused eye and head movement toward the affected side – the Tullio phenomenon [67, 167]. It is intriguing that for almost 70 years, those observations had little impact on the management of idiopathic auditory/vestibular dysfunctions. Interest in this area was renewed in 1998 following the description, by Minor and colleagues, of vertigo in patients induced by sound or change in middle ear or intracranial pressure. That study employed high-resolution computed tomography and showed a correlation between the vertigo and dehiscence of the bone overlying a semicircular canal. Furthermore, the symptoms were relieved after plugging the dehiscence [109]. Those data provided a fine explanation for the early observations that change in pressure within the external ear canal could produce vertigo in some patients – Hennebert sign [51].

Dehiscence in various sites of the labyrinth can give rise not only to vestibular but also cochlear anomalies. The cochlear anomalies are associated with a difference between air and bone-conduction hearing thresholds – known as an air-bone gap. It has been hypothesized that in the case of a third window, some acoustic energy is diverted from the cochlea into the vestibule resulting in a hearing loss by air conduction. In contrast, a third window would increase the difference between the impedance of the scala vestibuli and scala tympani side of the cochlear partition, and so render the cochlea hypersensitive to bone conduction [105] (Fig. 15.2).

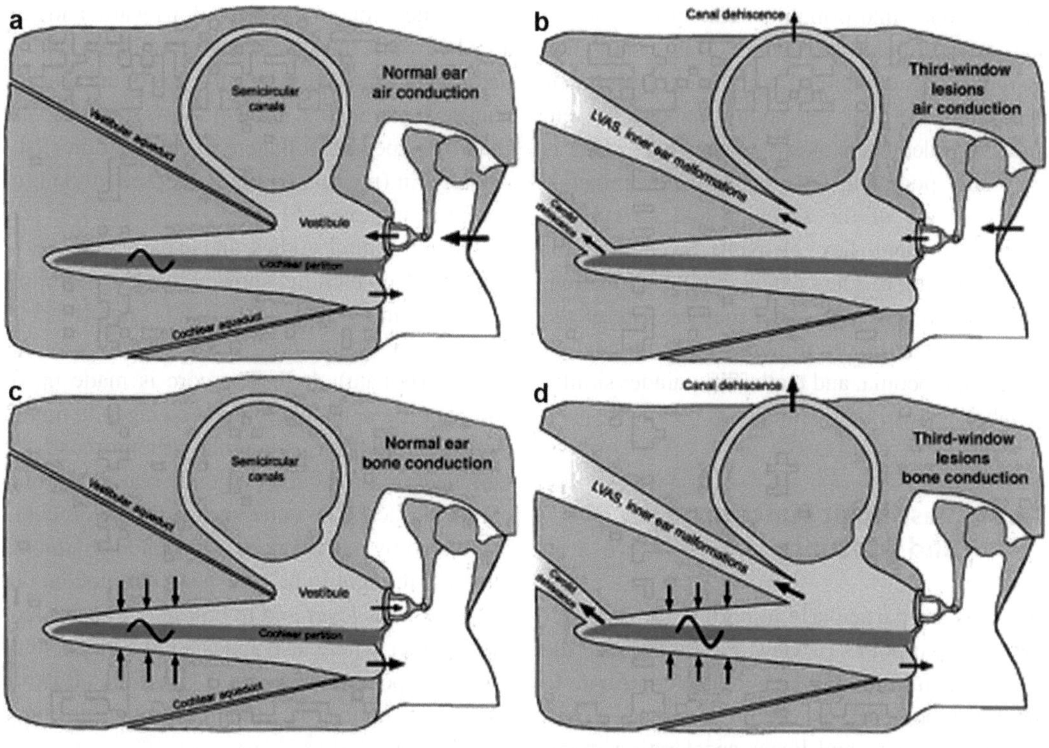

Fig. 15.2 Schematic representations of mechanism of air-bone gap in third-window lesions. (**a**) Normal ear, air conduction. Air-conducted sound stimuli enter the vestibule through motion of the stapes. There is a pressure difference between the scala vestibuli and the scala tympani, resulting in motion of the cochlear partition. The volume velocities of the oval and round windows are equal in magnitude but opposite in phase. (**b**) Third-window lesions, air conduction. It is hypothesized that a third window (in one of the canals, the vestibule or the scala vestibuli) allows a portion of the acoustic energy entering the vestibule through motion of the stapes to be shunted away from the cochlea. The shunting occurs primarily at low frequencies, resulting in a hearing loss by air conduction. (**c**) Normal ear, bone conduction. Compression of inner ear fluid by bone-conducted sound results in a hearing percept because of an inequality in the impedance between the scala vestibuli side and the scala tympani side of the cochlear partition. This inequality is primarily due to a difference in the impedance between the oval and windows. As a result, there is a pressure difference across the cochlear partition, resulting in motion of the basilar membrane that leads to perception of bone-conducted sound. (**d**) Third-window lesions, bone conduction. A third window increases the difference between the impedance on the scala vestibuli side and the scala tympani side of the cochlear partition by lowering the impedance on the vestibuli side, thereby improving the cochlear response to bone conduction (With kind permission from the Editor and the authors Merchant and Rosowski [105])

The hearing anomalies in humans include reduced sensitivity to air-conducted sounds – especially at low frequencies – hypersensitivity to bone-conducted sounds, and an air-bone gap which is not improved by stapedectomy [108].

Experimental fenestration of the superior semicircular canal in chinchilla resulted in cochlear low-frequency sensitivity loss which was canceled when the dehiscence was mended [145]. Furthermore, the otolith organs – sacculus and utriculus – in mammals can respond to air-borne and especially bone-conducted sounds [47], while the ampullae are normally insensitive to air-conducted sounds. Following fenestration, the vestibular afferent responses, including those from the ampullae, showed increase in firing [18, 106]. The vestibular responses to sounds, in the case of dehiscence, might therefore interfere with and partially mask the already perturbed cochlear response.

Dehiscence within the vestibular part of the labyrinth represents one situation of pathology where bone malformation can give rise to auditory/vestibular anomalies. But even when ossification is completed without mishaps, optimal functioning of the audiovestibular system relies on adequate upkeep of the bone. This is especially poignant with regard to the mineralized otoconia of the sacculus and utriculus – which represent key elements necessary for vestibular and, to a less extent, auditory function. Otoconia are not bones, but they are one of the three tissues normally mineralized in the body – skeleton, otoconia, and teeth [78] – under similar metabolic constraints as bone.

15.5 Vestibular Function and Otoconia

Otoconia are particularly important for the inner ear from two points of view. First, they play the role of calcium ion reserves and so contribute to the ionic homeostasis of the inner ear [127]. Secondly, gravity and linear acceleration monitoring in higher mammals is achieved by otoconia within the statoconial vestibular organs – the sacculus and utriculus. Otoconia are conglomeration (2–3 mm long) of thousands of calcium carbonate crystals (0.1–30 μm length). When stimulated by vibration, movement, or sound, the heavy mass of the otoconia introduces an inertial lag relative to the soft tissue below which leads to deflection of the stereocilia, stimulation of the vestibular sensory cells, and transduction of the signal. In this way, the vestibular organs can sense gravity and linear acceleration as well as low-frequency sounds. In nonplacental jawed vertebrates, there is an additional third statoconial organ – the lagena [126]. In those vertebrates, the otoconial crystal masses are represented by otoliths – taking the form of a single entity of calcium carbonate – that grow continuously throughout life. In fish, the bilateral set of three otoliths are oriented in such a way that they can detect particle vibration in three orthogonal directions and so help with sound localization [49].

The otoconial mass lies on a gelatinous otoconial membrane made up of two layers. The upper is composed of a dense network of filaments into which the otoconia project downward and are attached while the lower layer resembles a columnar network through which the tips of the sensory hair-cell stereocilia project upward [70, 91]. Inner-ear-specific collagens such as otolin (fish) or otogelin (mammals) bind otoconia to the otoconial membrane [96].

Ultrastructural studies, and in particular quick-freezing deep etching, showed that the morphology of the individual otoconium is complex [93]. There is an organic core and a mineralized (calcium carbonate) shell. The core is made up of compact filaments likely to be collagen in nature [96]. The shell has a laminar structure, and the lamellae are orientated perpendicular to the otoconial surface. The outer surface of the otoconia is covered by a network of collagenous filaments which is thought to help suspend the otoconia in the gelatinous layer and to link individual otoconia together. There also appears to be a system of pores that penetrates the shell – possibly allowing some communication with the surrounding endolymph [93].

The mechanisms controlling the seeding and the growth of the otoconia are not fully known [95]. It may involve a two-step procedure with otoconia crystals being seeded at the periphery of the sensory epithelium "macula," and then they grow centrally [96]. But the endolymph has a low Ca^{++} concentration, and one outstanding question is how calcium carbonate concentrations can be raised locally in order for otoconia seeding to be triggered. It is thought that seeding is achieved by the sequestering of Ca^{++} by otoconia-specific proteins produced by nonsensory cells [162]. The growth of otoconia may be facilitated by Ca^{++} extruded from sensory cells and then sequestered by several matrix proteins [96, 183]. Supporting this idea is the fact that the core matrix is formed before the deposition of calcium carbonate, and this matrix is essential for the determination of size and shape of the calcium carbonate crystals [183]. The matrix proteins are the same as or belong to the same family of bone matrix proteins [96, 182, 183]. The core is composed principally of glycoproteins – called otoconins, and the particular otoconin is species specific [116]. The major protein in mammals is otoconin-90 that represents 90% of the core protein [116, 174]. Otoconin-90 is essential for the formation of the core matrix by specifically recruiting other proteins including the minor protein otolin. Otoconin-90 deletion results in absence of the otoconial core matrix, formation of giant crystallites, and reduction in overall otoconial weight by 50% leading to vestibular deficits. Furthermore, the principal scaffold protein, otolin1, is drastically reduced [183].

Another minor protein present in otoconia – osteopontin – is not affected in the otoconin-90 null mice [130, 159]. In osteopontin knockout mice, the otoconia have normal morphology, protein, and calcium content. Furthermore, vestibular evoked potentials and a battery of behavioral tests failed to show dysfunction of the vestibular system [182]. On the other hand, osteopontin might function to limit the size of otoconia, as does fetuin [96, 161], because it limits bone crystal size [137] as well as being an in vivo inhibitor of ectopic calcification in aortic valve [154].

15.6 Consequences of Pathological Otoconia

The fate of otoconia has been investigated on cadavers from fetuses through to aged individuals. Otoconia are formed during development of the embryo [1] and reach full size soon after birth in mammals. Fetuses, who died of sudden death syndrome, show abnormal otoconia that are often dislodged [91]. Mature otoconia are not thought to grow, but there may be calcium turnover [77, 117, 160], and they are sensitive to different factors. Ototoxic drug treatment can result in giant otoconia crystals [91]. Ovariectomy in rat results in decreased number of otoconia together with an increase in size [172]. With aging, the otoconia crystals can decrease in number and size – especially in the sacculus – and those that remain take on a hollowed out appearance [125]. Dislodged otoconia particles from the utriculus can be carried off, in the majority of cases, into the posterior or lateral (horizontal) canal (canalithiasis) and in less than 5% of cases

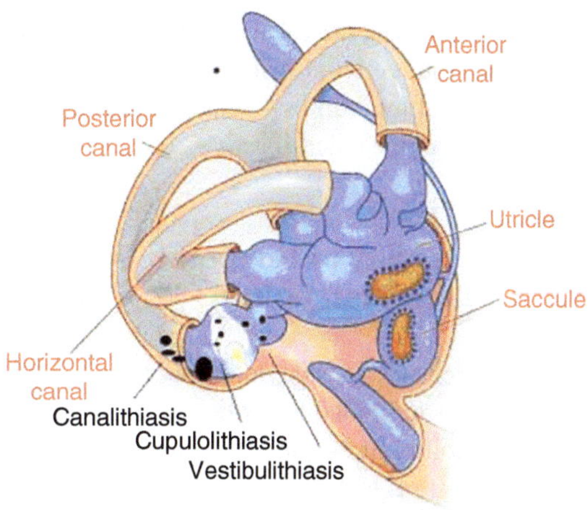

Fig. 15.3 Schematic representation of different vestibular anomalies resulting from displaced otoconia (From http://www.dizziness-and-hearing.com/disorders/bppv/bppv.html. With kind permission from Timothy Hain)

onto a cupula (cupulolithiasis) or into the vestibular side of the labyrinth (vestibulolithiasis) [46] (Fig. 15.3).

Displaced otoconia can result in benign paroxysmal positional vertigo (BPPV) which is considered the most common vestibular anomalie [46, 112]. The phenomenon was first characterized and defined in 1952 by Dix and Hallpike [27]. While the symptoms often resolve spontaneously, a particle reposition maneuver – the Dix and Hallpike maneuver – can be performed, in which the head is rotated in such a way as to return loose particles to the correct place within the vestibule [46]. According to a report by the American Academy of Otolaryngology – Head and Neck Surgery Foundation [6], dizziness accounts for 5.6 million visits in the United States per year, and between 17% and 42% of the patients with vertigo will be diagnosed with age-related BPPV. Epidemiological studies have shown that BPPV affects more women than men [131], suggesting that sex hormones may intervene. Some patients with osteoporosis may also have BPPV [171]. Furthermore, a statistical significant negative association was found between treated osteoporosis patients and BPPV, suggesting that the treatment for osteoporosis might prevent BPPV [107]. Indeed, these recent data provide further evidence that metabolism of bone and otoconia are related. Adequate maintenance of the skeleton with aging might help maintain healthy otoliths – with overall reduced risk of falls in the elderly.

15.7 Stability of Temporal Bone Metabolism

The calcified otic capsule does not grow, but evidence points to limited turnover and some limited repair capability after injury. The external periosteal bone can start making new lamellar bone in response to injury or inflammation. Studies with bone-seeking fluorochromes have shown in rabbits [146, 147] and dogs [35] that there is a centrifugal gradient for turnover that increases toward the exterior – suggesting that there is perilymphatic influence which restricts bone resorption [147] as nicely illustrated by Sorensen and colleagues (Fig. 15.4). Indeed bone turnover, in dog, has been estimated to be around 0.13% per year for the innermost zone toward the perilymph and up to about 10% per year at the periphery [35].

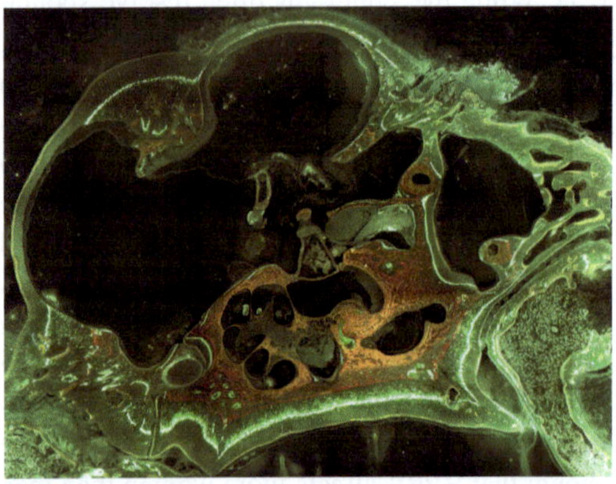

Fig. 15.4 Inhibition of otic capsule remodeling. Undecalcified section of temporal bone from 6-week-old rabbit. Demeclocycline (*orange*) was administered 7 days before birth, which was followed by postnatal injections of alizarin complexone (*red*) at 2.5 weeks and calcein green (*green*) at 5.5 weeks. The persistent orange labeling of the otic capsule indicates lack of remodeling. The bony walls have taken up the calcein (*green*) indicating remodeling (With kind permission from Springer Science+Business Media: and the authors Sorensen et al. [147])

15.8 Some Key Actors Involved in Temporal Bone Metabolism

15.8.1 OPG/RANKL/RANK

The last 20 years have seen the discovery and description of the key cytokines, and members of the tumor necrosis factor family, involved in control of bone metabolism [144]. Bone marrow mesenchymal stem cells, in the presence of different factors, differentiate into chondrocytes, osteoblasts, and adipocytes. Bone marrow hematopoietic stem cells give rise to blood cells, immune cells, and osteoclast precursor cells. The maturation of osteoclasts is under the control of osteoblasts. The development of osteoclasts occurs after stimulation from macrophage colony-stimulating factor and when the receptor activator of nuclear-factor kappa B (NF-κB) ligand (RANKL), produced on osteoblast precursor cells, binds to its receptor RANK on osteoclast precursors. Osteoprotegerin (OPG), which is also produced by osteoblast precursor cells, is a decoy receptor for RANKL. OPG binds to RANKL, and so prevents its binding to its receptor RANK on osteoclast precursors – hence blocking the differentiation and activation of osteoclasts. Deficiency in either RANKL [82] or RANK [28, 90] as well as overexpression of OPG [144] results in osteopetrosis. In contrast, deficiency in OPG results in osteoporosis in mice [15, 110]. The final OPG/RANKL ratio, therefore, becomes critical for determining bone turnover [54].

Recent evidence suggests that the temporal bone might be under similar controlling mechanisms. OPG is expressed in the spiral ligament of the cochlea and is found at high concentrations in the perilymph [152, 179]. In OPG knockout mice, there is abnormal bone remodeling of the otic capsule [178] as well as resorption of the middle ear ossicles and hearing loss [72]. It seems likely that the OPG/RANKL/RANK system, under the influence of neural and hormonal activities, plays a central role in the management of temporal bone metabolism [100].

15.8.2 Sympathetic Activity

Sympathetic influence on bone metabolism was first suggested over 60 years ago [32]. Bone receives a rich supply of sympathetic and sensory fibers. Both osteoblasts and osteoclasts express receptors for noradrenalin and neuropeptides, both of which play important roles in bone metabolism [165]. Stress, via the hypothalamus-pituitary-adrenal axis and the autonomic nervous system, results in skeletal bone loss in mice [177]. A considerable body of experimental evidence indicates that stress also affects audiovestibular function [57, 58, 99]. This is particularly the case with regard to idiopathic clinical disorders such as Ménière's disease where symptoms are often triggered by situations of stress.

First conclusive evidence for sympathetic innervations of the inner ear came from Spoendlin and colleagues [149, 150]. Two systems were described. First is a blood vessel-independent system which arises from the ipsilateral superior cervical ganglion. This system is identified within the modiolus and the osseous spiral lamina, but the fibers have not been seen to go beyond the habenula – they do not enter the organ of Corti [149, 150]. Some data suggest that this system modulates the sensitivity of the cochlea to sounds [40, 60], although this is debated [97]. The endolymphatic sac is also innervated by this system [7]. In addition, a rich sympathetic innervation of the middle ear periosteum originates in the ipsilateral superior cervical ganglion [69]. The second system is a blood vessel-dependent system which arises from ipsi- and contralateral stellate ganglia [149, 150]. The blood vessel-dependent system innervates the otic capsule [13] and helps regulates cochlear blood supply [87].

The first observations of the effects of sympathectomy on the temporal bone were carried out by Chole and colleagues. Bone remodeling was increased 1 week after unilateral surgical ablation of the superior cervical ganglion [140], or 2 weeks after pharmacological sympathectomy, by subcutaneous injection of guanethidine sulfate [139], or 1 week after chemical sympathectomy, by intraperitoneal injection of 6-hydroxydopamine [138], in the cochlear bulla of gerbil. Those data were partially in accord with earlier observations on 4-week-old rat, where bone loss occurred in the mandible 1 week after superior cervical ganglionectomy. However, in the latter study, the bone returned to normal at week two and three [132]. Bone remodeling was also reported after treatment of neonatal rats with guanethidine [52]. On the other hand, guanethidine treatment for 21 days in adult rats resulted in reduction in number of osteoclasts and reduction in bone resorption in the mandible [21]. These conflicting reports are likely to be linked to release of neuropeptides [83] including substance P [180] and difference in postsympathectomy delay before observation. Indeed, administration of capsaicin, which depletes substance P-containing fibers, blocked bone resorption in gerbil cochlear bulla, usually observed 1 week after 6-hydroxydopamine injection [141]. In vitro substance P stimulates osteoblast precursors and enhances mineralization in differentiated bone marrow stroma cells, but also facilitates osteoclastogenesis and bone absorption [173]. The overall effect of sympathectomy on the temporal bone is likely to depend on drug concentrations and on postsympathectomy delay.

In vivo studies have indicated that sympathetic signaling through β adrenergic receptors on osteoblasts stimulates bone resorption [111, 158]. The sympathetic system inhibits osteoblast proliferation via the molecular clock mechanism [36] and regulates RANKL expression in osteoblasts [30] promoting bone resorption. β-blockers prevent the development of bone loss in rats after ovariectomy [9]. Low sympathetic tone in mutant mice results in heavy bones [157]. These interesting data from laboratory studies suggested that β-blockers might reduce risk of bone fracture in humans too. While some positive effects of β-blockers on bone conservation have been reported [10], a recent review has pointed out that the data are variable with both positive and negative effects. In particular, the limitations of published studies are outlined, and the author has concluded that available evidence does not support the use of β-blockers as a treatment for osteoporosis [121]. The possible effect of β-blockers on temporal bone pathologies is not known, although some isolated reports have indicated that treatment with β-blockers has been linked to sudden-onset hearing loss. In the future, this type of data might be retrievable from studies aimed at investigating the effects of β-blockers on osteoporosis.

15.8.3 Leptin

Since its discovery in 1994 [181], the hormone leptin has been acknowledged as a major anorexigenic factor. It is mostly produced by white adipose tissue, many peripheral organs, the brain [168], and bone marrow adipocytes [85]. The association between high bone mass, low sympathetic activity, and absence of leptin in the obese mouse mutant (ob/ob) led Karsenty and colleagues to discover that leptin has a powerful central control over bone metabolism [29]. Indeed, intracerebroventricular injection of leptin in ob/ob mice restored normal bone mass by inhibition of osteoblast function [29, 30]. The central effect of leptin on bone remodeling occurs via the sympathetic system, and this can occur independent of leptin's effect on energy metabolism [143]. The sympathetic control of bone remodeling is achieved by two complimentary modes: one acting upon bone resorption and the other on bone formation [30, 158].

There is, in addition, some evidence for a direct peripheral mechanism whereby leptin promotes bone conservation. Leptin receptors have been demonstrated in bone of mice fetuses [55], osteoblasts of rat [25, 88], and human marrow stromal cells [163]. Leptin stimulates human osteoblastic cell proliferation and mineralization [41] and inhibits osteoclast generation in vitro [56]. Furthermore, leptin increases OPG and decreases the expression of RANKL in human marrow stromal cells in vitro [16]. Intraperitoneal injection of leptin increases bone strength in mouse [25], stimulates bone growth in ob/ob mice [48, 155], and reduces ovariectomy-induced bone loss in rats [16].

As discussed above, the temporal bone has a substantial sympathetic innervation, and the OPG/RANKL/RANK system affects bone of the otic capsule. But evidence that leptin affects the temporal bone metabolism is scarce and indirect. Hearing/vestibular dysfunction can be associated with metabolic disorders and hyperlipidemia in particular [129, 166]. One report described combined hyperlipidemia and otosclerosis in four generations of a single family [89]. Leptin receptor mRNA has been detected over the cochlear duct of fetal mice [55], indicating that leptin might affect, at least during development, the labyrinth. Leptin receptor expression has been observed in the cochlear nucleus of rat [43] and in the cochlear-vestibular nerve of guinea pig [64], although the functional significance is obscure. Interestingly, long-term estrogen-induced anorexia in the guinea pig induced hearing loss together with otic capsule bone remodeling [59, 63]. The new bone cells presented immunolabeling for leptin receptors [64] – suggesting that leptin might be involved in the limited remodeling of the otic capsule.

15.8.4 Glucocorticoids

Glucocorticoids provoke bone loss and increased risk of fracture in humans independent of age and gender [169] by inducing apoptosis of osteoblasts [175] and stimulating osteoclast generation by increasing RANKL/OPG ratio [53]. Because the OPG/RANKL/RANK system might prove to be a key regulator of bone remodeling in the temporal bone, it is of interest to take into consideration the possible effects of glucocorticoids on the temporal bone. The literature shows that glucocorticoids are generously prescribed by otolaryngologists for a wide spectrum of conditions including cancer, Bell's palsy, sinusitis, tonsillectomy, adenoidal hypertrophy, allergic rhinitis, otitis externa, sudden sensorineural hearing loss, acoustic trauma, tinnitus, and Ménière's disease, as well as otosclerosis. While the efficiency regarding the short-term goals seems to be established, the possible long-term effects have rarely been investigated. Considering that intratympanic delivery of drugs to the inner ear is an expanding therapeutic approach in otolaryngology, the possible detrimental effects of glucocorticoids on the temporal bone metabolism ought to be considered.

15.8.5 Estrogen

There is no doubt regarding the association between estrogen deficiency and osteoporosis, in women and men alike [123, 124]. Estrogen protects from bone loss because it stimulates OPG expression in osteoblasts [11], decreases osteoclast precursor responsiveness to RANKL [151], decreases RANKL-induced osteoclast differentiation [142], and induces apoptosis of osteoclasts [71]. In estrogen deficiency, the cumulative action of various proinflammatory cytokines leads to bone absorption [113] and in aging women and men estrogen deficiency leads to bone loss [123, 124]. But the risk of a clinical vertebral fracture is about three times higher in white women than men [104]. Age-related hearing loss is also gender dependent. While women hear better than men at higher frequencies, men are more sensitive at low frequencies [37, 114], but hearing declines substantially in men already above the age of 20, while loss in women is lesser [42]. In a gerontological population, there was a predominant high-frequency hearing loss in both men and women at 70 years old, but men had an average 10 dB greater loss at 8 kHz than women. Hearing further deteriorated in men between the ages of 70 and 81, while the hearing loss in women did not evolve between the ages of 79 and 81 [115]. Already in 1948, Fowler hypothesized that estrogen might be involved in otosclerosis – a form of osteoporosis of the middle ear bones and/or the otic capsule [34]. Otosclerotic foci can be found in temporal bones of females twice as often as in those of males [3]. Interestingly, cell cultures of stapes and external auditory canal from patients with otosclerosis expressed predominantly ERα [68] which have been implicated in the regulation of OPG/RANKL and preservation of bone in mice [92].

Age-related hearing loss is often sensorineural, although it would seem logical that part of the sensitivity loss would be conductive. Indeed, CT scans of the temporal bone have revealed a positive correlation between cochlear bone density loss and bone conduction hearing loss [66]. However, only few data are available which support the thesis that age-related osteoporosis is accompanied by temporal bone remodeling. On one hand, bone mineral density (BMD) of the lower hip or heal was found to be only moderately associated with conductive hearing loss in elderly men but not in women [50]. In contrast, there was a consistent inverse association between femoral neck bone mass and age-related hearing loss in women between 60 and 85 years [22]. A significant clinical association was observed between diagnosed osteoporosis and confirmed otosclerosis in postmenopausal women [23]. Interestingly, a significantly high association has been reported between otosclerosis or osteoporosis and polymorphic markers within the COL1A1 (collagen 1A1) gene, suggesting a shared genetic etiology between otosclerosis and osteoporosis [101].

15.8.6 Prolactin

Prolactin is an important regulator of intestinal calcium transport [19]. The effect of prolactin on bone in vivo is likely to be age dependent since daily injection of prolactin to rats enhanced turnover of bone in adults but increased calcium deposit in young rats [84]. Exposure of osteoblasts derived from tibia of adult rat [20] or osteoblast-like MG-63 cells [136] to prolactin resulted in reduced expression of RANKL as well as OPG [20] or increased the expression ratio RANKL/OPG [136] indicating prolactin-induced increase in bone resorption. In contrast, prolactin decreased the expression ratio of RANKL/OPG in human fetal osteoblast cells, indicating a favor for bone gain [135].

Hyperprolactinemia is the most common endocrine disorder of the hypothalamic-pituitary axis. Notably, neuroleptic drug treatment results in hyperprolactinemia, which is accompanied by a decrease in bone mineral density [80]. Estrogen is a potent activator of prolactin release [120], and long-term hormonal contraceptive or hormone replacement therapy [81] as well as pregnancy and breastfeeding [74] can result in hyperprolactinemia and transitory bone resorption. Interestingly, pregnancy, and more particularly multiple pregnancies, has often been associated with the onset or aggravation of otosclerosis. In one study of 94 women who had undergone stapedectomy, half the women had had children, and the other half were without. That study found no difference in hearing loss between the two groups and so no effect of pregnancies [94]. On the other hand, a retrospective study on a sample of 479 women with otosclerosis showed that according to a mathematical model, the chance for subjective hearing deterioration with bilateral otosclerosis increased from 33% after one pregnancy to 63% after six pregnancies [44].

However, few studies have specifically dealt with the possible effect of hyperprolactinemia on the temporal bone. Hyperprolactinemia was remarked in some patients presenting hearing loss, tinnitus, and vertigo [31, 61], although the possible contribution of temporal bone pathology was not investigated. Similarly, laboratory studies are scarce. Prolactin receptors have been identified in fetal rat cochlear duct [128], which might indicate that prolactin has a role at least during the developmental phase of the labyrinth. Mutant mice lacking the prolactin receptor gene have hyperprolactinemia with impaired ossification in neonates, and decrease in bone mineral density in adults [24], but the effects on the temporal bone have not been described. Experimental hyperprolactinemia, induced by chronic administration of estrogen in guinea pig, resulted in hearing loss and notably bone dysmorphology of the otic capsule [59, 63]. According to that particular experimental protocol, it is likely that high prolactin and/or estrogen contributed to temporal bone changes. On the other hand, prolactin stimulates leptin secretion by white adipose tissue in rat [45], and leptin increases prolactin action of milk production in bovine mammary gland [33] so that leptin may possibly have contributed to the changes in temporal bone [64]. These preliminary data provide some limited evidence that the effect of hyperprolactinemia on bone metabolism might extend to that of the temporal bone.

15.9 Pathologies of the Temporal Bone and Treatment Prospects

A substantial body of literature is available regarding clinical aspects of the many temporal bone pathologies including several excellent recent reviews [4, 76, 102, 153]. Bone pathologies can arise from abnormal mineralization and/or change in bone mineral density. *Osteogenesis imperfecta* or brittle bone disorder is caused by mutations in COL1A1 or COL1A2 genes. Mutation results in a defect in the synthesis of collagenous matrix necessary for mineralization. The disorder can be associated with middle ear bone disorders combined or not with otosclerosis as well as sensorineural deficits. *Otosclerosis* is a bone disorder specific to the temporal bone. Otosclerosis is typified by an abnormal increase in bone turnover in particular foci and often seen around the oval window with fixation of the stapedial footplate. Otosclerosis appears to be affected by genetic [164], hormonal (see Sect. 15.8), and viral [75, 76] influences. *Osteopetrosis* is a bone disorder due to reduced activity of osteoclasts with resultant increased bone density and overgrowth of bone. When osteopetrosis affects the temporal bone, there can be bone compression of the auditory nerve. *Paget's disease* is a skeletal disorder characterized by marked increase in bone turnover affecting osteoclasts and osteoblasts and affects bone structure. The onset of the disorder is age related and is usually detected after 50 years old. Environmental factors such as paramyxovirus infection are hypothesized to trigger the disorder, although the available data are conflictual [119]. The disease can affect any bone, and when it affects the skull, one major consequence of the disorder is deafness due to overgrowth of bone and nerve compression.

In the 1960s, it was shown that drinking water that contained fluorides was associated with a low prevalence of otosclerosis. Since that time, fluorides have been employed safely for the management of otosclerosis [153, 156]. In the 1990s, some preliminary studies of bisphosphonate treatment for otosclerosis have been carried out and considered helpful [14], although other studies reported a rather negative effect on hearing [12, 176]. Bisphosphonate treatment of OPG knockout mice has been reported to stop bone loss in ossicles and improve hearing [73]. However, bisphosphonates administered either intravenously or orally over the long-term to patients with skeletal disorders can give rise to necrosis of the jaw bone. The occurrence of jaw necrosis, although rare, has given the alert as to possible undesired effects of bisphosphonates. From around the year 2000, given the novelty of OPG-RANKL-RANK mechanisms in bone metabolism, attention has turned toward the possibility of anti-RANKL therapy for osteoporosis. The side effects and the long-term effects of anti-RANKL therapy are still under review in the context of bone metabolism studies [134], although it has been suggested that short-term treatment might prove useful in early stages of otosclerosis [75].

Conclusion

This chapter shows how the bony armor of the ear is terminated around the time of birth. The final size of the otic capsule is determined at that stage – undergoing only slow and limited bone turnover afterward. A body of literature indicates that factors that affect skeletal bone metabolism can possibly also affect the temporal bone and so hearing/vestibular function. Recently, research has brought to light some molecular mechanisms common to both bony sites which opens the way toward an alternative approach to prevention and therapy of temporal bone pathologies.

Acknowledgments The author is indebted to J Schacht for his encouragement and insightful comments. Grateful thanks also to KM Stankovic, AD Hawkins, and the editors for their helpful suggestions.

References

1. Anniko M. Development of otoconia. Am J Otolaryngol. 1980;1:400–10.
2. Armitage SE, Baldwin BA, Vince MA. The fetal sound environment of sheep. Science. 1980;208:1173–4.
3. Arnold W, Niedermeyer HP, Altermatt HJ, Neubert WJ. Pathogenesis of otosclerosis. "State of the art". HNO. 1996;44:121–9.
4. Arnold W, Hausler R, editors. Otosclerosis and stapes surgery. Advances in oto-rhino-laryngology. Basel: Karger; 2007.
5. Bernard J, Sontag L. Fetal reactivity to tonal stimulation: a preliminary report. J Genet Psychol. 1947;70:205–10.
6. Bhattacharyya N, Baugh RF, Orvidas L, Barrs D, Bronston LJ, Cass S, Chalian AA, Desmond AL, Earll JM, Fife TD, Fuller DC, Judge JO, Mann NR, Rosenfeld RM, Schuring LT, Steiner RW, Whitney SL, Haidari J. Clinical practice guideline: benign paroxysmal positional vertigo. Otolaryngol Head Neck Surg. 2008;139:S47–81.
7. Birgersson L, Friberg U, Rask-Andersen H, Erwall C, Widenfalk B. Origin of sympathetic and sensory innervation of the endolymphatic sac. A retrograde axonal tracing study in the guinea pig. ORL J Otorhinolaryngol Relat Spec. 1992;54:188–90.
8. Birnholz JC, Benacerraf BR. The development of human fetal hearing. Science. 1983;222:516–8.
9. Bonnet N, Beaupied H, Vico L, Dolleans E, Laroche N, Courteix D, Benhamou CL. Combined effects of exercise and propranolol on bone tissue in ovariectomized rats. J Bone Miner Res. 2007;22:578–88.
10. Bonnet N, Gadois C, McCloskey E, Lemineur G, Lespessailles E, Courteix D, Benhamou CL. Protective effect of beta blockers in postmenopausal women: influence on fractures, bone density, micro and macroarchitecture. Bone. 2007;40:1209–16.
11. Bord S, Ireland DC, Beavan SR, Compston JE. The effects of estrogen on osteoprotegerin, RANKL, and estrogen receptor expression in human osteoblasts. Bone. 2003;32:136–41.
12. Boumans LJ, Poublon RM. The detrimental effect of aminohydroxypropylidene bisphosphonate (APD) in otospongiosis. Eur Arch Otorhinolaryngol. 1991;248:218–21.
13. Brechtelsbauer PB, Prazma J, Garrett CG, Carrasco VN, Pillsbury 3rd HC. Student Research Award 1990. Catecholaminergic innervation of the inner ear. Otolaryngol Head Neck Surg. 1990;103:566–74.
14. Brookler KH, Tanyeri H. Etidronate for the neurotologic symptoms of otosclerosis: preliminary study. Ear Nose Throat J. 1997;76:371–6, 379–81.
15. Bucay N, Sarosi I, Dunstan CR, Morony S, Tarpley J, Capparelli C, Scully S, Tan HL, Xu W, Lacey DL, Boyle WJ, Simonet WS. Osteoprotegerin-deficient mice develop early onset osteoporosis and arterial calcification. Genes Dev. 1998;12:1260–8.
16. Burguera B, Hofbauer LC, Thomas T, Gori F, Evans GL, Khosla S, Riggs BL, Turner RT. Leptin reduces ovariectomy-induced bone loss in rats. Endocrinology. 2001;142:3546–53.
17. Busnel MC, Granier-Deferre C, Lecanuet JP. Fetal audition. Ann N Y Acad Sci. 1992;662:118–34.
18. Carey JP, Hirvonen TP, Hullar TE, Minor LB. Acoustic responses of vestibular afferents in a model of superior canal dehiscence. Otol Neurotol. 2004;25:345–52.
19. Charoenphandhu N, Krishnamra N. Prolactin is an important regulator of intestinal calcium transport. Can J Physiol Pharmacol. 2007;85:569–81.

20. Charoenphandhu N, Teerapornpuntakit J, Methawasin M, Wongdee K, Thongchote K, Krishnamra N. Prolactin decreases expression of Runx2, osteoprotegerin, and RANKL in primary osteoblasts derived from tibiae of adult female rats. Can J Physiol Pharmacol. 2008;86:240–8.
21. Cherruau M, Facchinetti P, Baroukh B, Saffar JL. Chemical sympathectomy impairs bone resorption in rats: a role for the sympathetic system on bone metabolism. Bone. 1999;25:545–51.
22. Clark K, Sowers MR, Wallace RB, Jannausch ML, Lemke J, Anderson CV. Age-related hearing loss and bone mass in a population of rural women aged 60 to 85 years. Ann Epidemiol. 1995;5:8–14.
23. Clayton AE, Mikulec AA, Mikulec KH, Merchant SN, McKenna MJ. Association between osteoporosis and otosclerosis in women. J Laryngol Otol. 2004;118:617–21.
24. Clement-Lacroix P, Ormandy C, Lepescheux L, Ammann P, Damotte D, Goffin V, Bouchard B, Amling M, Gaillard-Kelly M, Binart N, Baron R, Kelly PA. Osteoblasts are a new target for prolactin: analysis of bone formation in prolactin receptor knockout mice. Endocrinology. 1999;140:96–105.
25. Cornish J, Callon KE, Bava U, Lin C, Naot D, Hill BL, Grey AB, Broom N, Myers DE, Nicholson GC, Reid IR. Leptin directly regulates bone cell function in vitro and reduces bone fragility in vivo. J Endocrinol. 2002;175:405–15.
26. DeCasper AJ, Fifer WP. Of human bonding: newborns prefer their mothers' voices. Science. 1980;208:1174–6.
27. Dix MR, Hallpike CS. The pathology, symptomatology and diagnosis of certain common disorders of the vestibular system. Ann Otol Rhinol Laryngol. 1952;61:987–1016.
28. Dougall WC, Glaccum M, Charrier K, Rohrbach K, Brasel K, De Smedt T, Daro E, Smith J, Tometsko ME, Maliszewski CR, Armstrong A, Shen V, Bain S, Cosman D, Anderson D, Morrissey PJ, Peschon JJ, Schuh J. RANK is essential for osteoclast and lymph node development. Genes Dev. 1999;13:2412–24.
29. Ducy P, Amling M, Takeda S, Priemel M, Schilling AF, Beil FT, Shen J, Vinson C, Rueger JM, Karsenty G. Leptin inhibits bone formation through a hypothalamic relay: a central control of bone mass. Cell. 2000;100:197–207.
30. Elefteriou F, Ahn JD, Takeda S, Starbuck M, Yang X, Liu X, Kondo H, Richards WG, Bannon TW, Noda M, Clement K, Vaisse C, Karsenty G. Leptin regulation of bone resorption by the sympathetic nervous system and CART. Nature. 2005;434:514–20.
31. Falkenius-Schmidt K, Rydmarker S, Horner KC. Hyperprolactinemia in some meniere patients even in the absence of incapacitating vertigo. Hear Res. 2005;203:154–8.
32. Fell WA. The effect of sympathectomy on the size of haversian canals in the cat. J Anat. 1949;83:67.
33. Feuermann Y, Shamay A, Mabjeesh SJ. Leptin upregulates the lactogenic effect of prolactin in the bovine mammary gland in vitro. J Dairy Sci. 2008;91:4183–9.
34. Fowler EP. Estrogen, bone metabolism and otosclerosis. Arch Otolaryngol Head Neck Surg. 1948;48: 637–44.
35. Frisch T, Sorensen MS, Overgaard S, Bretlau P. Estimation of volume referent bone turnover in the otic capsule after sequential point labeling. Ann Otol Rhinol Laryngol. 2000;109:33–9.
36. Fu L, Patel MS, Bradley A, Wagner EF, Karsenty G. The molecular clock mediates leptin-regulated bone formation. Cell. 2005;122:803–15.
37. Gates GA, Cooper Jr JC, Kannel WB, Miller NJ. Hearing in the elderly: the Framingham cohort, 1983–1985. Part I. Basic audiometric test results. Ear Hear. 1990;11:247–56.
38. Gerhardt KJ, Huang X, Arrington KE, Meixner K, Abrams RM, Antonelli PJ. Fetal sheep in utero hear through bone conduction. Am J Otolaryngol. 1996;17:374–9.
39. Gerhardt KJ, Pierson LL, Huang X, Abrams RM, Rarey KE. Effects of intense noise exposure on fetal sheep auditory brain stem response and inner ear histology. Ear Hear. 1999;20:21–32.
40. Giraudet F, Horner KC, Cazals Y. Similar half-octave TTS protection of the cochlea by xylazine/ketamine or sympathectomy. Hear Res. 2002;174:239–48.
41. Gordeladze JO, Drevon CA, Syversen U, Reseland JE. Leptin stimulates human osteoblastic cell proliferation, de novo collagen synthesis, and mineralization: impact on differentiation markers, apoptosis, and osteoclastic signaling. J Cell Biochem. 2002;85: 825–36.
42. Gordon-Salant S. Hearing loss and aging: new research findings and clinical implications. J Rehabil Res Dev. 2005;42:9–24.
43. Grill HJ, Schwartz MW, Kaplan JM, Foxhall JS, Breininger J, Baskin DG. Evidence that the caudal brainstem is a target for the inhibitory effect of leptin on food intake. Endocrinology. 2002;143:239–46.
44. Gristwood RE, Venables WN. Pregnancy and otosclerosis. Clin Otolaryngol Allied Sci. 1983;8:205–10.
45. Gualillo O, Lago F, Garcia M, Menendez C, Senaris R, Casanueva FF, Dieguez C. Prolactin stimulates leptin secretion by rat white adipose tissue. Endocrinology. 1999;140:5149–53.
46. Hain TC. Atypical BPPV. 2011. http://www.dizziness-and-hearing.com/disorders/bppv/bppv.html. 12 May 2011.
47. Halmagyi GM, Curthoys IS, Colebatch JG, Aw ST. Vestibular responses to sound. Ann N Y Acad Sci. 2005;1039:54–67.
48. Hamrick MW, Della-Fera MA, Choi YH, Pennington C, Hartzell D, Baile CA. Leptin treatment induces loss of bone marrow adipocytes and increases bone formation in leptin-deficient ob/ob mice. J Bone Miner Res. 2005;20:994–1001.
49. Hawkins AD, Horner K. Directional characteristics of primary auditory neurons from the cod ear. In: Tawolga WN, Popper AN, Fay RR, editors. Hearing and sound communication in fishes. New York: Springer; 1981. p. 311–27.

50. Helzner EP, Cauley JA, Pratt SR, Wisniewski SR, Talbott EO, Zmuda JM, Harris TB, Rubin SM, Taaffe DR, Tylavsky FA, Newman AB. Hearing sensitivity and bone mineral density in older adults: the health, aging and body composition study. Osteoporos Int. 2005;16:1675–82.
51. Hennebert C. A new syndrome in hereditary syphilis of the labyrinth. Presse Med Belg Brux. 1911;63:467.
52. Hill EL, Turner R, Elde R. Effects of neonatal sympathectomy and capsaicin treatment on bone remodeling in rats. Neuroscience. 1991;44:747–55.
53. Hofbauer LC, Gori F, Riggs BL, Lacey DL, Dunstan CR, Spelsberg TC, Khosla S. Stimulation of osteoprotegerin ligand and inhibition of osteoprotegerin production by glucocorticoids in human osteoblastic lineage cells: potential paracrine mechanisms of glucocorticoid-induced osteoporosis. Endocrinology. 1999;140: 4382–9.
54. Hofbauer LC, Khosla S, Dunstan CR, Lacey DL, Boyle WJ, Riggs BL. The roles of osteoprotegerin and osteoprotegerin ligand in the paracrine regulation of bone resorption. J Bone Miner Res. 2000; 15:2–12.
55. Hoggard N, Mercer JG, Rayner DV, Moar K, Trayhurn P, Williams LM. Localization of leptin receptor mRNA splice variants in murine peripheral tissues by RT-PCR and in situ hybridization. Biochem Biophys Res Commun. 1997;232:383–7.
56. Holloway WR, Collier FM, Aitken CJ, Myers DE, Hodge JM, Malakellis M, Gough TJ, Collier GR, Nicholson GC. Leptin inhibits osteoclast generation. J Bone Miner Res. 2002;17:200–9.
57. Horner KC. The emotional ear in stress. Neurosci Biobehav Rev. 2003;27:437–46.
58. Horner KC, Cazals Y. Stress in hearing and balance in Meniere's disease. Noise Health. 2003;5:29–34.
59. Horner KC, Cazals Y, Guieu R, Lenoir M, Sauze N. Experimental estrogen-induced hyperprolactinemia results in bone-related hearing loss in the guinea pig. Am J Physiol Endocrinol Metab. 2007;293: E1224–32.
60. Horner KC, Giraudet F, Lucciano M, Cazals Y. Sympathectomy improves the ear's resistance to acoustic trauma–could stress render the ear more sensitive? Eur J Neurosci. 2001;13:405–8.
61. Horner KC, Guieu R, Magnan J, Chays A, Cazals Y. Prolactinoma in some Meniere's patients–is stress involved? Neuropsychopharmacology. 2002;26:135–8.
62. Horner KC, Serviere J, Granier-Deferre C. Deoxyglucose demonstration of in-utero hearing in the guinea pig foetus. Hear Res. 1987;26:327–33.
63. Horner KC, Troadec JD, Dallaporta M, Pio J. Effect of chronic estradiol administration on vimentin and GFAP immunohistochemistry within the inner ear. Neurobiol Dis. 2009;35:201–8.
64. Horner KC, Troadec J-D, Blanchard M-P, Dallaporta M, Pio J. Receptors for leptin in the otic labyrinth and the cochlear-vestibular nerve of guinea pig are modified in hormone-induced anorexia. Hear Res. 2010;270: 48–55.
65. Huang X, Gerhardt KJ, Abrams RM, Antonelli PJ. Temporary threshold shifts induced by low-pass and high-pass filtered noises in fetal sheep in utero. Hear Res. 1997;113:173–81.
66. Huizing EH, de Groot JA. Densitometry of the cochlear capsule and correlation between bone density loss and bone conduction hearing loss in otosclerosis. Acta Otolaryngol. 1987;103:464–8.
67. Huizinga E. On the sound reaction of tullio in the pigeon and the fenestration operation in man. Acta Otolaryngol Suppl. 1952;100:174–80.
68. Imauchi Y, Laine P, Sterkers O, Ferrary E, Bozorg Grayeli A. Effect of 17 beta-estradiol on diastrophic dysplasia sulfate transporter activity in otosclerotic bone cell cultures and SaOS-2 cells. Acta Otolaryngol. 2004;124:890–5.
69. Ito J, Oyagi S, Honjo I. Autonomic innervations in the middle ear and pharynx. Acta Otolaryngol Suppl. 1993;506:90–3.
70. Kachar B, Parakkal M, Fex J. Structural basis for mechanical transduction in the frog vestibular sensory apparatus: I. The otolithic membrane. Hear Res. 1990;45:179–90.
71. Kameda T, Mano H, Yuasa T, Mori Y, Miyazawa K, Shiokawa M, Nakamaru Y, Hiroi E, Hiura K, Kameda A, Yang NN, Hakeda Y, Kumegawa M. Estrogen inhibits bone resorption by directly inducing apoptosis of the bone-resorbing osteoclasts. J Exp Med. 1997;186:489–95.
72. Kanzaki S, Ito M, Takada Y, Ogawa K, Matsuo K. Resorption of auditory ossicles and hearing loss in mice lacking osteoprotegerin. Bone. 2006; 39:414–9.
73. Kanzaki S, Takada Y, Ogawa K, Matsuo K. Bisphosphonate therapy ameliorates hearing loss in mice lacking osteoprotegerin. J Bone Miner Res. 2009;24:43–9.
74. Karlsson C, Obrant KJ, Karlsson M. Pregnancy and lactation confer reversible bone loss in humans. Osteoporos Int. 2001;12:828–34.
75. Karosi T, Konya J, Szabo LZ, Pytel J, Jori J, Szalmas A, Sziklai I. Codetection of measles virus and tumor necrosis factor-alpha mRNA in otosclerotic stapes footplates. Laryngoscope. 2005;115:1291–7.
76. Karosi T, Sziklai I. Etiopathogenesis of otosclerosis. Eur Arch Otorhinolaryngol. 2010;267:1337–49.
77. Kawamata S, Igarashi Y. Growth and turnover of rat otoconia as revealed by labeling with tetracycline. Anat Rec. 1995;242:259–66.
78. Kawasaki K, Buchanan AV, Weiss KM. Biomineralization in humans: making the hard choices in life. Annu Rev Genet. 2009;43:119–42.
79. Keith RW. Middle ear function in neonates. Arch Otolaryngol. 1975;101:376–9.
80. Kishimoto T, Watanabe K, Shimada N, Makita K, Yagi G, Kashima H. Antipsychotic-induced hyperprolactinemia inhibits the hypothalamo-pituitary-gonadal axis and reduces bone mineral density in male patients with schizophrenia. J Clin Psychiatry. 2008;69: 385–91.

81. Klibanski A, Neer RM, Beitins IZ, Ridgway EC, Zervas NT, McArthur JW. Decreased bone density in hyperprolactinemic women. N Engl J Med. 1980;303:1511–4.
82. Kong YY, Yoshida H, Sarosi I, Tan HL, Timms E, Capparelli C, Morony S, Oliveira-dos-Santos AJ, Van G, Itie A, Khoo W, Wakeham A, Dunstan CR, Lacey DL, Mak TW, Boyle WJ, Penninger JM. OPGL is a key regulator of osteoclastogenesis, lymphocyte development and lymph-node organogenesis. Nature. 1999;397:315–23.
83. Konttinen Y, Imai S, Suda A. Neuropeptides and the puzzle of bone remodeling. State of the art. Acta Orthop Scand. 1996;67:632–9.
84. Krishnamra N, Seemoung J. Effects of acute and long-term administration of prolactin on bone 45Ca uptake, calcium deposit, and calcium resorption in weaned, young, and mature rats. Can J Physiol Pharmacol. 1996;74:1157–65.
85. Laharrague P, Larrouy D, Fontanilles AM, Truel N, Campfield A, Tenenbaum R, Galitzky J, Corberand JX, Penicaud L, Casteilla L. High expression of leptin by human bone marrow adipocytes in primary culture. FASEB J. 1998;12:747–52.
86. Lalande NM, Hetu R, Lambert J. Is occupational noise exposure during pregnancy a risk factor of damage to the auditory system of the fetus? Am J Ind Med. 1986;10:427–35.
87. Laurikainen EA, Kim D, Didier A, Ren T, Miller JM, Quirk WS, Nuttall AL. Stellate ganglion drives sympathetic regulation of cochlear blood flow. Hear Res. 1993;64:199–204.
88. Lee YJ, Park JH, Ju SK, You KH, Ko JS, Kim HM. Leptin receptor isoform expression in rat osteoblasts and their functional analysis. FEBS Lett. 2002;528: 43–7.
89. Levy Y, da Silva M, Eliachar I, Glick-Avraham Z, Viskoper RJ, Brook JG. Familial combined hyperlipidemia and otosclerosis–the occurrence in a large kindred. Am J Med Sci. 1985;289:107–9.
90. Li J, Sarosi I, Yan XQ, Morony S, Capparelli C, Tan HL, McCabe S, Elliott R, Scully S, Van G, Kaufman S, Juan SC, Sun Y, Tarpley J, Martin L, Christensen K, McCabe J, Kostenuik P, Hsu H, Fletcher F, Dunstan CR, Lacey DL, Boyle WJ. RANK is the intrinsic hematopoietic cell surface receptor that controls osteoclastogenesis and regulation of bone mass and calcium metabolism. Proc Natl Acad Sci U S A. 2000;97:1566–71.
91. Lim DJ. The development and structure of the otoconia. In: Friedmann I, Ballantyne J, editors. Ultrastructural atlas of the inner ear. London: Butterworths & Co; 1984.
92. Lindberg MK, Erlandsson M, Alatalo SL, Windahl S, Andersson G, Halleen JM, Carlsten H, Gustafsson JA, Ohlsson C. Estrogen receptor alpha, but not estrogen receptor beta, is involved in the regulation of the OPG/RANKL (osteoprotegerin/receptor activator of NF-kappa B ligand) ratio and serum interleukin-6 in male mice. J Endocrinol. 2001;171:425–33.
93. Lins U, Farina M, Kurc M, Riordan G, Thalmann R, Thalmann I, Kachar B. The otoconia of the guinea pig utricle: internal structure, surface exposure, and interactions with the filament matrix. J Struct Biol. 2000;131:67–78.
94. Lippy WH, Berenholz LP, Schuring AG, Burkey JM. Does pregnancy affect otosclerosis? Laryngoscope. 2005;115:1833–6.
95. Lu W, Zhou D, Freeman JJ, Thalmann I, Ornitz DM, Thalmann R. In vitro effects of recombinant otoconin 90 upon calcite crystal growth. Significance of tertiary structure. Hear Res. 2010;268:172–83.
96. Lundberg YW, Zhao X, Yamoah EN. Assembly of the otoconia complex to the macular sensory epithelium of the vestibule. Brain Res. 2006;1091:47–57.
97. Maison SF, Le M, Larsen E, Lee SK, Rosowski JJ, Thomas SA, Liberman MC. Mice lacking adrenergic signaling have normal cochlear responses and normal resistance to acoustic injury but enhanced susceptibility to middle-ear infection. J Assoc Res Otolaryngol. 2010;11(3):449–61.
98. Mallo M. Embryological and genetic aspects of middle ear development. Int J Dev Biol. 1998;42: 11–22.
99. Mazurek B, Stover T, Haupt H, Klapp BF, Adli M, Gross J, Szczepek AJ. The significance of stress: its role in the auditory system and the pathogenesis of tinnitus. HNO. 2010;58:162–72.
100. McKenna MJ, Kristiansen AG. Molecular biology of otosclerosis. Adv Otorhinolaryngol. 2007;65:68–74.
101. McKenna MJ, Nguyen-Huynh AT, Kristiansen AG. Association of otosclerosis with Sp1 binding site polymorphism in COL1A1 gene: evidence for a shared genetic etiology with osteoporosis. Otol Neurotol. 2004;25:447–50.
102. McKenna MJ, Merchant SN. Disorders of bone. In: Schuknecht HF, Merchant SN, Nadol JB, editors. Schuknecht's pathology of the ear. Shelton: People's Medical Publishing House-USA; 2010. p. 716–75.
103. McLellan MS, Brown JR, Rondeau H, Shoughro E, Johnson RA, Hale AR. Embryonal connective tissue and exudate in ear. A histological study of ear sections of fetuses and infants. Am J Dis Child. 1964;108:164–70.
104. Melton 3rd LJ, Chrischilles EA, Cooper C, Lane AW, Riggs BL. Perspective. How many women have osteoporosis? J Bone Miner Res. 1992;7:1005–10.
105. Merchant SN, Rosowski JJ. Conductive hearing loss caused by third-window lesions of the inner ear. Otol Neurotol. 2008;29:282–9.
106. Mikaelian D. Vestibular response to sound: single unit recording from the vestibular nerve in fenestrated deaf mice (Df/Df). Acta Otolaryngol. 1964;58:409–22.
107. Mikulec AA, Kowalczyk KA, Pfitzinger ME, Harris DA, Jackson LE. Negative association between treated osteoporosis and benign paroxysmal positional vertigo in women. J Laryngol Otol. 2010;124(4):374–6. Epub 2009 Nov 25.

108. Mikulec AA, McKenna MJ, Ramsey MJ, Rosowski JJ, Herrmann BS, Rauch SD, Curtin HD, Merchant SN. Superior semicircular canal dehiscence presenting as conductive hearing loss without vertigo. Otol Neurotol. 2004;25:121–9.
109. Minor LB, Solomon D, Zinreich JS, Zee DS. Sound- and/or pressure-induced vertigo due to bone dehiscence of the superior semicircular canal. Arch Otolaryngol Head Neck Surg. 1998;124:249–58.
110. Mizuno A, Amizuka N, Irie K, Murakami A, Fujise N, Kanno T, Sato Y, Nakagawa N, Yasuda H, Mochizuki S, Gomibuchi T, Yano K, Shima N, Washida N, Tsuda E, Morinaga T, Higashio K, Ozawa H. Severe osteoporosis in mice lacking osteoclastogenesis inhibitory factor/osteoprotegerin. Biochem Biophys Res Commun. 1998;247:610–5.
111. Moore RE, Smith 2nd CK, Bailey CS, Voelkel EF, Tashjian Jr AH. Characterization of beta-adrenergic receptors on rat and human osteoblast-like cells and demonstration that beta-receptor agonists can stimulate bone resorption in organ culture. Bone Miner. 1993;23:301–15.
112. Oghalai JS, Manolidis S, Barth JL, Stewart MG, Jenkins HA. Unrecognized benign paroxysmal positional vertigo in elderly patients. Otolaryngol Head Neck Surg. 2000;122:630–4.
113. Pacifici R. Estrogen, cytokines, and pathogenesis of postmenopausal osteoporosis. J Bone Miner Res. 1996;11:1043–51.
114. Pearson JD, Morrell CH, Gordon-Salant S, Brant LJ, Metter EJ, Klein LL, Fozard JL. Gender differences in a longitudinal study of age-associated hearing loss. J Acoust Soc Am. 1995;97:1196–205.
115. Pedersen KE, Rosenhall U, Moller MB. Changes in pure-tone thresholds in individuals aged 70–81: results from a longitudinal study. Audiology. 1989;28:194–204.
116. Pote KG, Ross MD. Each otoconia polymorph has a protein unique to that polymorph. Comp Biochem Physiol B. 1991;98:287–95.
117. Preston RE, Johnsson LG, Hill JH, Schacht J. Incorporation of radioactive calcium into otolithic membranes and middle ear ossicles of the gerbil. Acta Otolaryngol. 1975;80:269–75.
118. Querleu D, Renard X, Boutteville C, Crepin G. Hearing by the human fetus? Semin Perinatol. 1989;13:409–20.
119. Ralston SH, Langston AL, Reid IR. Pathogenesis and management of Paget's disease of bone. Lancet. 2008;372:155–63.
120. Raymond V, Beaulieu M, Labrie F, Boissier J. Potent antidopaminergic activity of estradiol at the pituitary level on prolactin release. Science. 1978;200:1173–5.
121. Reid IR. Effects of beta-blockers on fracture risk. J Musculoskelet Neuronal Interact. 2008;8:105–10.
122. Richard C, Laroche N, Malaval L, Dumollard JM, Martin C, Peoch M, Vico L, Prades JM. New insight into the bony labyrinth: a microcomputed tomography study. Auris Nasus Larynx. 2010;37:155–61.
123. Riggs BL, Khosla S, Melton 3rd LJ. Sex steroids and the construction and conservation of the adult skeleton. Endocr Rev. 2002;23:279–302.
124. Riggs BL, Khosla S, Melton 3rd LJ. A unitary model for involutional osteoporosis: estrogen deficiency causes both type I and type II osteoporosis in postmenopausal women and contributes to bone loss in aging men. J Bone Miner Res. 1998;13:763–73.
125. Ross MD, Peacor D, Johnsson LG, Allard LF. Observations on normal and degenerating human otoconia. Ann Otol Rhinol Laryngol. 1976;85:310–26.
126. Ross MD, Pote KG. Some properties of otoconia. Philos Trans R Soc Lond B Biol Sci. 1984;304: 445–52.
127. Ross MD, Williams TJ. Otoconial complexes as ion reservoirs in endolymph. Physiologist. 1979;22: S63–4.
128. Royster M, Driscoll P, Kelly PA, Freemark M. The prolactin receptor in the fetal rat: cellular localization of messenger ribonucleic acid, immunoreactive protein, and ligand-binding activity and induction of expression in late gestation. Endocrinology. 1995;136:3892–900.
129. Rybak LP. Metabolic disorders of the vestibular system. Otolaryngol Head Neck Surg. 1995;112: 128–32.
130. Sakagami M. Role of osteopontin in the rodent inner ear as revealed by in situ hybridization. Med Electron Microsc. 2000;33:3–10.
131. Salvinelli F, Firrisi L, Casale M, Trivelli M, D'Ascanio L, Lamanna F, Greco F, Costantino S. Benign paroxysmal positional vertigo: diagnosis and treatment. Clin Ter. 2004;155:395–400.
132. Sandhu HS, Herskovits MS, Singh IJ. Effect of surgical sympathectomy on bone remodeling at rat incisor and molar root sockets. Anat Rec. 1987;219:32–8.
133. Schuknecht HF, Gulya AJ. The anatomy of the temporal bone with surgical implications. Philadelphia: Lea & Febiger; 1986.
134. Schwarz EM, Ritchlin CT. Clinical development of anti-RANKL therapy. Arthritis Res Ther. 2007;9 Suppl 1:S7.
135. Seriwatanachai D, Charoenphandhu N, Suthiphongchai T, Krishnamra N. Prolactin decreases the expression ratio of receptor activator of nuclear factor kappaB ligand/osteoprotegerin in human fetal osteoblast cells. Cell Biol Int. 2008;32:1126–35.
136. Seriwatanachai D, Thongchote K, Charoenphandhu N, Pandaranandaka J, Tudpor K, Teerapornpuntakit J, Suthiphongchai T, Krishnamra N. Prolactin directly enhances bone turnover by raising osteoblast-expressed receptor activator of nuclear factor kappaB ligand/osteoprotegerin ratio. Bone. 2008;42:535–46.
137. Shapses SA, Cifuentes M, Spevak L, Chowdhury H, Brittingham J, Boskey AL, Denhardt DT. Osteopontin facilitates bone resorption, decreasing bone mineral crystallinity and content during calcium deficiency. Calcif Tissue Int. 2003;73:86–92.

138. Sherman BE, Chole RA. Effect of chemical sympathectomy with 6-hydroxydopamine on osteoclast activity in the gerbilline middle ear bulla. Otol Neurotol. 2001;22:237–41.
139. Sherman BE, Chole RA. Effect of pharmacological sympathectomy on osteoclastic activity in the gerbilline auditory bulla in vivo. Ann Otol Rhinol Laryngol. 1999;108:1078–87.
140. Sherman BE, Chole RA. In vivo effects of surgical sympathectomy on intramembranous bone resorption. Am J Otol. 1996;17:343–6.
141. Sherman BE, Chole RA. A mechanism for sympathectomy-induced bone resorption in the middle ear. Otolaryngol Head Neck Surg. 1995;113:569–81.
142. Shevde NK, Bendixen AC, Dienger KM, Pike JW. Estrogens suppress RANK ligand-induced osteoclast differentiation via a stromal cell independent mechanism involving c-Jun repression. Proc Natl Acad Sci U S A. 2000;97:7829–34.
143. Shi Y, Yadav VK, Suda N, Liu XS, Guo XE, Myers Jr MG, Karsenty G. Dissociation of the neuronal regulation of bone mass and energy metabolism by leptin in vivo. Proc Natl Acad Sci U S A. 2008;105:20529–33.
144. Simonet WS, Lacey DL, Dunstan CR, Kelley M, Chang MS, Luthy R, Nguyen HQ, Wooden S, Bennett L, Boone T, Shimamoto G, DeRose M, Elliott R, Colombero A, Tan HL, Trail G, Sullivan J, Davy E, Bucay N, Renshaw-Gegg L, Hughes TM, Hill D, Pattison W, Campbell P, Sander S, Van G, Tarpley J, Derby P, Lee R, Boyle WJ. Osteoprotegerin: a novel secreted protein involved in the regulation of bone density. Cell. 1997;89:309–19.
145. Songer JE, Rosowski JJ. The effect of superior canal dehiscence on cochlear potential in response to air-conducted stimuli in chinchilla. Hear Res. 2005;210:53–62.
146. Sorensen MS, Jorgensen MB, Bretlau P. Distribution of bone remodeling units in the otic capsule of the rabbit. A semiquantitative morphometric study. Acta Otolaryngol. 1992;112:462–9.
147. Sorensen MS, Jorgensen MB, Bretlau P. Drift barriers in the postcartilaginous development of the mammalian otic capsule. Eur Arch Otorhinolaryngol. 1992;249:56–61.
148. Sperber G. Craniofacial development. London: BC Decker INC; 2001.
149. Spoendlin H. Autonomic innervation of the inner ear. Adv Otorhinolaryngol. 1981;27:1–13.
150. Spoendlin H, Lichtensteiger W. The adrenergic innervation of the labyrinth. Acta Otolaryngol. 1966;61:423–34.
151. Srivastava S, Toraldo G, Weitzmann MN, Cenci S, Ross FP, Pacifici R. Estrogen decreases osteoclast formation by down-regulating receptor activator of NF-kappa B ligand (RANKL)-induced JNK activation. J Biol Chem. 2001;276:8836–40.
152. Stankovic KM, Adachi O, Tsuji K, Kristiansen AG, Adams JC, Rosen V, McKenna MJ. Differences in gene expression between the otic capsule and other bones. Hear Res. 2010;265(1-2):83–9.
153. Stankovic KM, McKenna MJ. Current research in otosclerosis. Curr Opin Otolaryngol Head Neck Surg. 2006;14:347–51.
154. Steitz SA, Speer MY, McKee MD, Liaw L, Almeida M, Yang H, Giachelli CM. Osteopontin inhibits mineral deposition and promotes regression of ectopic calcification. Am J Pathol. 2002;161:2035–46.
155. Steppan CM, Crawford DT, Chidsey-Frink KL, Ke H, Swick AG. Leptin is a potent stimulator of bone growth in ob/ob mice. Regul Pept. 2000;92:73–8.
156. Szekanecz Z, Szekanecz E, Morvai K, Racz T, Szegedi G, Sziklai I. Current aspects of the pathogenesis and clinical characteristics of otosclerosis: possibilities of drug therapy. Orv Hetil. 1999;140:2435–40.
157. Takeda S, Elefteriou F, Levasseur R, Liu X, Zhao L, Parker KL, Armstrong D, Ducy P, Karsenty G. Leptin regulates bone formation via the sympathetic nervous system. Cell. 2002;111:305–17.
158. Takeda S, Karsenty G. Molecular bases of the sympathetic regulation of bone mass. Bone. 2008;42:837–40.
159. Takemura T, Sakagami M, Nakase T, Kubo T, Kitamura Y, Nomura S. Localization of osteopontin in the otoconial organs of adult rats. Hear Res. 1994;79:99–104.
160. Takumida M, Zhang DM, Yajin K, Harada Y. Polychromatic labeling of otoconia for the investigation of calcium turnover. ORL J Otorhinolaryngol Relat Spec. 1997;59:4–9.
161. Thalmann I, Hughes I, Tong BD, Ornitz DM, Thalmann R. Microscale analysis of proteins in inner ear tissues and fluids with emphasis on endolymphatic sac, otoconia, and organ of corti. Electrophoresis. 2006;27:1598–608.
162. Thalmann R, Ignatova E, Kachar B, Ornitz DM, Thalmann I. Development and maintenance of otoconia: biochemical considerations. Ann N Y Acad Sci. 2001;942:162–78.
163. Thomas T, Gori F, Khosla S, Jensen MD, Burguera B, Riggs BL. Leptin acts on human marrow stromal cells to enhance differentiation to osteoblasts and to inhibit differentiation to adipocytes. Endocrinology. 1999;140:1630–8.
164. Thys M, Van Camp G. Genetics of otosclerosis. Otol Neurotol. 2009;30:1021–32.
165. Togari A. Adrenergic regulation of bone metabolism: possible involvement of sympathetic innervation of osteoblastic and osteoclastic cells. Microsc Res Tech. 2002;58:77–84.
166. Torossian F, Laredo C. Cochleovestibular disorders and hyperlipidemia. A controlled trial with fenofibrate. Monogr Atheroscler. 1986;14:222–9.
167. Tullio P. Das Ohr und die Entstehung der Sprache und Schrift. Berlin: Urban & Schwarzenberg; 1929.
168. Ur E. Neuroendocrinology of leptin. Frontiers of Hormone Research. London: Karger; 2000.
169. van Staa TP. The pathogenesis, epidemiology and management of glucocorticoid-induced osteoporosis. Calcif Tissue Int. 2006;79:129–37.

170. Vasiliu DI. Contributions to the morphophysiological study of the auditory apparatus. When does the pneumatization of cephalic cavities appear? When does hearing appear in humans? Rev Roum Physiol. 1969;6:159–67.
171. Vibert D, Kompis M, Hausler R. Benign paroxysmal positional vertigo in older women may be related to osteoporosis and osteopenia. Ann Otol Rhinol Laryngol. 2003;112:885–9.
172. Vibert D, Sans A, Kompis M, Travo C, Muhlbauer RC, Tschudi I, Boukhaddaoui H, Hausler R. Ultrastructural changes in otoconia of osteoporotic rats. Audiol Neurootol. 2008;13:293–301.
173. Wang L, Zhao R, Shi X, Wei T, Halloran BP, Clark DJ, Jacobs CR, Kingery WS. Substance P stimulates bone marrow stromal cell osteogenic activity, osteoclast differentiation, and resorption activity in vitro. Bone. 2009;45:309–20.
174. Wang Y, Kowalski PE, Thalmann I, Ornitz DM, Mager DL, Thalmann R. Otoconin-90, the mammalian otoconial matrix protein, contains two domains of homology to secretory phospholipase A2. Proc Natl Acad Sci U S A. 1998;95:15345–50.
175. Weinstein RS, Jilka RL, Parfitt AM, Manolagas SC. Inhibition of osteoblastogenesis and promotion of apoptosis of osteoblasts and osteocytes by glucocorticoids. Potential mechanisms of their deleterious effects on bone. J Clin Invest. 1998;102:274–82.
176. Yasil S, Comlekci A, Guneri A. Further hearing loss during osteoporosis treatment with etidronate. Postgrad Med J. 1998;74:363–4.
177. Yirmiya R, Goshen I, Bajayo A, Kreisel T, Feldman S, Tam J, Trembovler V, Csernus V, Shohami E, Bab I. Depression induces bone loss through stimulation of the sympathetic nervous system. Proc Natl Acad Sci U S A. 2006;103:16876–81.
178. Zehnder AF, Kristiansen AG, Adams JC, Kujawa SG, Merchant SN, McKenna MJ. Osteoprotegrin knockout mice demonstrate abnormal remodeling of the otic capsule and progressive hearing loss. Laryngoscope. 2006;116:201–6.
179. Zehnder AF, Kristiansen AG, Adams JC, Merchant SN, McKenna MJ. Osteoprotegerin in the inner ear may inhibit bone remodeling in the otic capsule. Laryngoscope. 2005;115:172–7.
180. Zhang SQ, Terenghi G, Unger WG, Ennis KW, Polak J. Changes in substance P- and neuropeptide Y-immunoreactive fibres in rat and guinea-pig irides following unilateral sympathectomy. Exp Eye Res. 1984;39:365–72.
181. Zhang Y, Proenca R, Maffei M, Barone M, Leopold L, Friedman JM. Positional cloning of the mouse obese gene and its human homologue. Nature. 1994;372: 425–32.
182. Zhao X, Jones SM, Thoreson WB, Lundberg YW. Osteopontin is not critical for otoconia formation or balance function. J Assoc Res Otolaryngol. 2008;9: 191–201.
183. Zhao X, Yang H, Yamoah EN, Lundberg YW. Gene targeting reveals the role of Oc90 as the essential organizer of the otoconial organic matrix. Dev Biol. 2007;304:508–24.

Bone and the cAMP Signaling Pathway: Emerging Therapeutics

16

Paul M. Epstein

Keywords

Cyclic nucleotide phosphodiesterases • G proteins • Rho GTPases • Cyclic AMP signaling pathways • Bone formation • Osteoporosis

16.1 Introduction

This chapter will review the evidence that stimulation of cAMP signaling through inhibition of cyclic nucleotide phosphodiesterases (PDEs) may provide a novel means to build bone and thus form the basis of a new therapeutic treatment for osteoporosis. The maintenance of normal bone mass depends on a balance between osteoblastic bone formation and osteoclastic bone destruction [8, 10, 24]. Osteoclasts are highly motile cells, and bone resorption involves active motility of osteoclasts on bone surfaces to be resorbed [13]. Hence, agents that inhibit osteoclast motility should inhibit bone resorption. Rho GTPases, small GTP-binding proteins that belong to the Ras superfamily, represent a group of proteins that play a pivotal role in regulating cell motility and migration [69]. RhoA, a major isoform of Rho, promotes stress fiber formation in cells through activation of a downstream kinase effector termed ROCK (Rho-associated kinase). Once activated by RhoA, ROCK promotes phosphorylation of myosin light chain (MLC), producing increased contractility and stress fiber formation, necessary for motility [25]. In osteoclasts, RhoA is activated by engagement of the αV/β3 integrin receptor and the hyaluronan receptor, CD44, by osteopontin, and this activation of RhoA in osteoclasts is critical for its motility and function [13–15, 58]. RhoA can be directly phosphorylated and inactivated by cAMP-dependent protein kinase (PKA) [25, 45]. Hence, agents that stimulate the cAMP signaling pathway should inactivate RhoA, inhibit osteoclast motility, and inhibit bone resorption. Inhibitors of cyclic nucleotide phosphodiesterases (PDEs), the enzymes that normally degrade cAMP, would be excellent candidates for increasing cAMP and inhibiting motility in osteoclasts. PDEs are encoded by 21 different genes grouped into 11 different gene families based on sequence similarity, mode of regulation, and specificity for cAMP or cGMP as substrate [17]. With alternative splicing as well as the existence of multiple transcription initiation sites, at least 100 different forms of PDE have been cloned and many are expressed in a cell and tissue selective manner.

P.M. Epstein, Ph.D.
Department of Cell Biology,
University of Connecticut Health Center,
263 Farmington Avenue, Farmington, CT 06030, USA
e-mail: epstein@nso1.uchc.edu

F. Bronner et al. (eds.), *Bone-Metabolic Functions and Modulators*, Topics in Bone Biology,
DOI 10.1007/978-1-4471-2745-1_16,

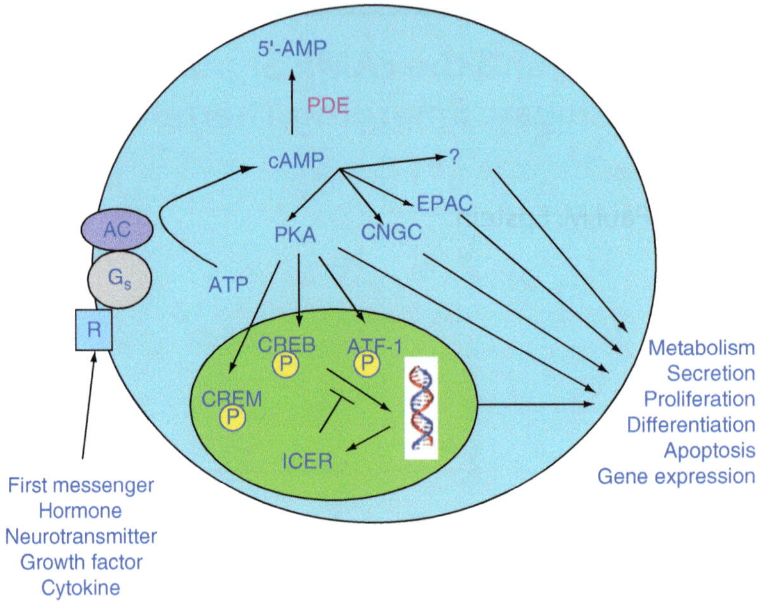

Fig. 16.1 Role of PDEs in regulation of signal transduction. In the model of the second messenger concept originally put forth by Sutherland and colleagues, first messengers, such as hormones, neurotransmitters, cytokines, and growth factors, upon interacting with receptors on the cell surface, generate the production of a "second messenger" such as cAMP, which then redirects the machinery of the cell, affecting many physiological processes. PDEs by controlling the steady-state levels and temporal and spatial components of cAMP are central to controlling and regulating this signal transduction (This figure was originally published in Lerner and Epstein [48], © the Biochemical Society)

As depicted in Fig. 16.1, PDEs play a central role in controlling cAMP signaling in that they regulate the steady-state levels of cAMP as well as the temporal and spatial components of cAMP within the cell, thus affecting a host of cell processes through both posttranslational modification of proteins, as well as changes in gene transcription. Pharmacological inhibitors of PDEs are under intense development and are rapidly becoming available for clinical use. Moreover, recent studies have shown that inhibitors of the fourth gene family of PDE (PDE4) profoundly inhibit the migration of several types of cells, including fibroblasts [25, 92], endothelial cells [60], leukocytes [21, 34], and several types of cancer cells [23, 57, 62, 80]. Little work has been done on modulation of RhoA activity in osteoclasts, by PDE inhibitors and the cAMP signaling pathway, but studies have demonstrated effects of PDE4 inhibitors to increase bone density. Although the mechanism(s) by which PDE4 inhibitors achieve this is still not known, we hypothesize that they may act in part through inhibition of RhoA, to inhibit osteoclast motility and function, thus inhibiting bone resorption and increasing bone density. Additionally, PDE inhibitors appear to have direct effects on osteoblasts, as well, to stimulate bone formation [37–39, 44, 53, 93, 97, 100]. This chapter will examine current evidence that PDE inhibitors may be beneficial as therapeutic agents to build bone density and treat osteoporosis.

16.2 cAMP Signaling and Bone Resorption

The maintenance of normal bone mass depends on a balance between osteoblastic bone formation and osteoclastic bone destruction. Bone resorption is carried out primarily by osteoclasts. The overall rate of osteoclastic bone resorption is regulated at two main levels: (1) determining the number of osteoclasts through the regulation of the osteoclast precursor pool and their rate of differentiation, i.e., regulating osteoclastogenesis; and (2) determining the bone-resorbing activity of individual osteoclasts through the regulation of their key functional features. In both cases, it is now apparent that activation of RANK (receptor activator of nuclear factor kappa B) signaling by its extracellular ligand RANKL (RANK ligand; also known as TNF-related activation-induced cytokine or TRANCE, osteoprotegerin ligand or OPGL, and osteoclast differentiation factor, or ODF) plays a central role, as does osteoprotegerin (OPG), a soluble decoy receptor for RANKL [8, 10, 24]. While RANKL and macrophage colony-stimulating factor (M-CSF) promote osteoblast differentiation, OPG, by acting as a decoy receptor for RANKL, inhibits this process [8, 24]. Indeed, underscoring the importance of RANKL in this process, in June 2010, the US Food and Drug Administration approved the use of denosumab (Prolia), a monoclonal antibody targeted to RANKL, for treatment of osteoporosis in postmenopausal women with high risk for fracture [19, 95]. Additionally, osteoclasts are highly motile cells, and bone resorption involves active motility of osteoclasts on bone surfaces to be resorbed [13]. Hence, agents that inhibit bone resorption may act through inhibiting the recruitment and differentiation of osteoclasts, inhibiting their activity, or inhibiting their motility.

One of the key signaling pathways by which osteoclast differentiation and function may be regulated is the cAMP signaling pathway. For example, PTH, when given continuously, induces the expression of RANKL in neighboring osteoblast and stromal cells inhibits the expression of OPG, predominantly through this pathway [26, 46]. cAMP levels are controlled by their rate of synthesis by adenylyl cyclase and by their rate of degradation by cyclic nucleotide phosphodiesterases (PDEs). A number of studies have shown PDE inhibitors to promote bone formation through a mechanism(s) not yet known. Some of the effects of PDE inhibitors to increase bone formation may result from an inhibition of bone resorption through inhibition of osteoclastogenesis [54, 61, 65, 104, 106] or through promotion of osteoblast formation [37–39, 44, 53, 93, 97, 100], either directly or through potentiation of other effectors such as PGE_2, PTH, and bone morphogenic protein (BMP).

Osteoclasts are highly motile cells, and inhibition of their motility inhibits bone resorption [24]. Cell motility and migration involves the extension of a leading edge protrusions or lamellipodia, the establishment of new adhesion sites at the front, cell body contraction, and detachment of adhesions at the rear. All these steps involve the assembly, the disassembly, or the reorganization of the actin cytoskeleton. Recently, Rho GTPases are a group of proteins that clearly has been shown to play a pivotal role in regulating motility and migration [69]. Rho GTPases are small GTP-binding proteins that belong to the Ras superfamily and include Rho, Rac, and Cdc42. Rho promotes formation of stress fibers, Rac induces formation of lamellipodia, and Cdc42 induces formation of filopodia. Rho GTPases are activated by many different stimuli, with integrin clustering or engagement being a main stimulus. Rho GTPases oscillate between an active GTP-bound state and an inactive GDP-bound state, as regulated by two other classes of proteins: GAPs – GTPase-activating proteins, which promote hydrolysis of bound GTP forming the inactive state – and GEFs – guanine nucleotide exchange factors, which promote the exchange of GTP for GDP and thereby promote the activated GTP-bound form of Rho. In resting cells, inactive GDP-bound Rho is complexed with guanine nucleotide dissociation inhibitors (RhoGDIs) in the cytosol. Upon activation, Rho dissociates from GDIs allowing GEF to exchange GTP for GDP. For localization to the cell membrane, which is critical for its function, Rho is posttranslationally modified by prenylation, followed by carboxymethylation of its C-terminus. It was found that alendronate, a bisphosphonate widely used clinically to inhibit bone resorption, inhibits the prenylation of Rho, thereby disrupting its localization and inhibiting its function which may account in part for its inhibition of bone resorption through the resultant inhibition of osteoclast motility [18, 77].

One of the principal functions of RhoA is to promote the formation of stress fibers in the cell.

Stress fiber formation is regulated by the state of myosin light chain (MLC) phosphorylation. Phosphorylation of MLC allows myosin to interact with actin to produce contractility. Phosphorylation of MLC is regulated both by the Ca^{2+}-calmodulin-dependent myosin light chain kinase and by the downstream effector of RhoA, ROCK. Additionally, ROCK also phosphorylates and inactivates MLC phosphatase, preventing MLC dephosphorylation. RhoA can be phosphorylated and inhibited by PKA [45]. A study showed that PDE4 inhibitors profoundly inhibited the migration of fibroblasts through inhibition of RhoA, which prevented the activation of ROCK and stress fiber formation [25]. In osteoclasts, RhoA is activated by engagement of the $\alpha V/\beta 3$ integrin receptor and the hyaluronan receptor, CD44, by osteopontin, and this activation of RhoA in osteoclasts is critical for its motility and function [13–15, 58]. It is quite possible, therefore, that PDE inhibitors, acting through inhibition of RhoA, will inhibit osteoclast motility and function and inhibit bone resorption. Yet, surprisingly, modulation of RhoA activity in osteoclasts, by PDE inhibitors and the cAMP signaling pathway, has not yet been examined.

16.3 Regulation of Osteoblast Differentiation

Osteoblasts arise from immature mesenchymal cells, and the signals that lead to their differentiation into a mature phenotype expressing characteristic osteoblast marker proteins such as osteocalcin, alkaline phosphatase, and type I collagen are complex and involve a host of different transcription factors [10, 105]. One transcription factor that is clearly central to osteoblast differentiation is core-binding factor alpha 1 (Cbfa1), also called Runx2 [10, 105]. Cbfa1 is absolutely essential for osteoblast development, as targeted inactivation of Cbfa1 in mice, generated animals that have no osteoblasts [105]. Cbfa1 also has been shown to play a critical role in cell cycle entry and exit in osteoblasts. Calvarial cells from Cbfa1-deficient mice exhibited increased cell growth rates, and reintroduction of Cbfa1 restored the stringent growth control of these cells [68]. Other factors that play a large role in osteoblastic differentiation are the bone morphogenic proteins (BMPs). BMPs are members of the transforming growth factor-ß (beta) superfamily of proteins that act as morphogens in bone formation. They are believed to control the commitment of mesenchymal pluripotent cells to the osteoblast phenotype and were shown to induce ectopic bone formation in vivo [10]. The molecular signaling of BMPs is through heterotrimeric complexes of transmembrane Ser/Thr kinase receptors that then propagate signals to Smad proteins, which mediate BMP-induced signals from the cell surface to the nucleus [10, 63, 85]. Overexpression of BMP-2 was shown to markedly inhibit proliferation of UMR-106 rat osteosarcoma cells and stimulate the expression of osteocalcin and alkaline phosphatase, indicating a role for BMP in osteoblastic differentiation [42].

16.4 Influence of Agents Acting Through the Cyclic Nucleotide Pathways on Osteoblast Differentiation

The cyclic nucleotides, cAMP and cGMP, have dramatic effects on osteoblasts. cGMP has been shown to regulate the proliferation and differentiation of osteoblasts [9, 31, 35, 43, 103], to reduce PTH- and prostaglandin E_2 (PGE_2)-induced resorption of bone [84, 99] and to mediate the osteoblast anabolic response to mechanical stimulation [70]. The importance of cGMP for bone growth also is seen in the phenotypes of mice with disruptions in the cGMP signaling pathway. Cn/cn mice, which exhibit a dwarfism phenotype, contain a missense mutation in the natriuretic peptide receptor 2 (NPR2) gene, also called the guanylyl cyclase-B (GC-B) gene, which disrupts its guanylyl cyclase activity, rendering it insensitive to C-type natriuretic peptide (CNP), which is normally responsible for positively regulating longitudinal bone growth [96]. Similarly, Prkg2 (–/–) mice, deficient in type II cGMP-dependent protein kinase (PKG), also develop dwarfism as a result of impaired endochondral ossification [55].

cAMP can inhibit osteoblast proliferation through attenuation of MAP kinase pathways [12] and through effects on Cbfa1 and BMP signaling pathways [72]. The effects of agents that act via the cAMP pathway on osteoblast differentiation can, however, be complex. Parathyroid hormone (PTH), acting primarily through a cAMP-PKA pathway, can have either anabolic [94] or catabolic [107] effects, depending on the cell line used, the stage of differentiation, culture conditions, and treatment duration [47]. When PTH is given continuously, its stimulation of osteoclasts and bone resorption predominates and it becomes catabolic; when given intermittently, its stimulation of osteoblastic activity predominates, promoting anabolic formation of bone [20, 87]. Currently, an amino-terminal PTH peptide (amino acids 1–34 of the 84-amino acid full-length PTH protein), referred to as teriparatide, is FDA-approved and has been marketed in the United States since 2002 under the name. Forteo is the only approved anabolic treatment for osteoporosis in the United States [11, 36]. A full-length recombinant form of PTH, Preos, is marketed by Nycomed GmbH in Europe. PTH and its active amino-terminal peptide acting through the PTH receptor 1 (PTHR1) signal through several pathways, including the Ca^{2+}-PKC, and the cAMP-PKA pathways [2, 20, 59]. Numerous studies have shown that the cAMP-PKA pathway mediates many of the therapeutic actions of PTH [2, 59]. PTH working through the cAMP pathway stimulates expression of Cbfa1-regulated osteoblast-specific genes such as osteopontin, type I collagen, bone sialoprotein, and osteocalcin [72]. Direct effects of PKA on Cbfa1 were demonstrated in a study wherein Cbfa1 was shown to be a substrate for phosphorylation by PKA, and PTH induced a PKA-dependent transactivation of Cbfa1 [79]. Cbfa1 also is phosphorylated by PKG and appears also to be important in mediating the effects of NO-cGMP-PKG signaling on extracellular matrix remodeling and osteogenesis [109]. Indirect effects of PKA on Cbfa1 have been reported in the mouse osteoblast MC3T3-E1 cell line via effects of cAMP on the ubiquitin/proteasome pathway [90]. Thus, it appears that cAMP can have multiple effects on Cbfa1, both direct and indirect, with the resultant outcome dependent on the cell type and state of differentiation of the cell(s) being studied. With respect to BMPs, results show that cAMP potentiates their effects on promoting osteoblast differentiation and new bone formation. In particular, studies with inhibitors of PDEs used to activate the cAMP signaling pathway have shown that BMP-stimulated osteoblast differentiation and new bone formation can be potentiated both by the nonspecific PDE inhibitor pentoxifylline [38] and by the PDE4-selective inhibitors, rolipram [39, 100] and denbufylline [54]. Additionally, type I PKG was shown to interact with and phosphorylate the BMP-2 receptor, dissociate from the receptor upon stimulation, associate with activated Smads and undergo nuclear translocation, whereupon it enhanced the transcriptional activation of BMP target genes [78]. Another PDE4-selective inhibitor, XT-611, was shown to act synergistically with PGE_2 to inhibit osteoclastogenesis [104] and stimulate the differentiation of osteoblast progenitor cells [53]. In addition to effects on cell differentiation, cAMP signaling is crucial in regulating cell adhesion [98], and a recent study has shown that cAMP acting through the PKA pathway enhances adhesion of MC3T3-E1 osteoblastic cells to biomaterials [49]. Although PDEs were not examined in this study, based on these observations, PDE inhibitors may prove to be important agents for promoting successful implants in bone regeneration technologies. Further research on a role for PDEs in this process is certainly warranted. Studies have also shown that PDEs play a role in chondrocyte function and that inhibition of PDEs, particularly PDE4, may have chondroprotective effects and may be excellent candidates for treatment of osteoarthritis [89].

16.5 Metabolism of Cyclic Nucleotides in Osteoblast Cells

The PDEs are the enzymes that hydrolyze the cyclic nucleotides, cAMP and cGMP, to their corresponding 5′-nucleotides and are therefore responsible, to a large degree, for controlling the levels of these key second messengers in the cell.

To date, 21 different genes encoding different PDEs have been identified. With expression of splice variants of these genes and multiple transcription initiation sites, more than 100 different forms of PDE have been identified and cloned [17]. These PDEs differ with respect to substrate specificity (preference for cAMP vs. cGMP), mode of regulation, tissue expression, and subcellular distribution. This extreme diversity of expression, tissue selectivity, and subcellular localization of these different PDEs allow for very fine control of second messenger concentrations in specific cells and subcellular locales. The 21 genes encoding PDEs have been grouped into 11 different gene families (PDE1–11) based on similarity in structure and regulatory properties and selective pharmacological inhibitors for these gene families continue to be developed. Of the 11 different PDE gene families, PDEs 4, 7, and 8 are specific for cAMP; PDEs 5, 6, and 9 are specific for cGMP; and PDEs 1, 2, 3, 10, and 11 hydrolyze both cyclic nucleotides [48]. Inhibitors of specific PDEs have now been developed that can very selectively modulate cAMP levels in a particular cell and subcellular compartment expressing that form of PDE, with few effects elsewhere. These PDE inhibitors thus may provide a new means to treat osteoporosis by inhibiting osteoclast motility and bone resorption and also by stimulating osteoblast formation. There is particular interest of late in the development of inhibitors of PDE4 because of the potential of PDE4 as a therapeutic target in a wide range of disorders, including depression, asthma, rheumatoid arthritis, multiple sclerosis, inflammatory bowel disease, psoriasis, Alzheimer's disease, and several lymphoid and myeloid malignancies [7, 41, 48, 50]. In bone, most studies to date have implicated PDE4 as an important target for increasing bone density. Consistent with this, a recent genetic study showed an association between single-nucleotide polymorphic variants in the gene encoding PDE4D and resultant bone mineral density in humans [71]. A highly selective PDE4 inhibitor, roflumilast (Daxas), developed by Nycomed GmbH, was approved for clinical use by the European Commission in July 2010, for the indication of chronic obstructive pulmonary disease (COPD), and is currently under review for approval by the US Food and Drug Administration [28, 32]. Hence, there is now at least one PDE4-selective inhibitor already in clinical use.

Surprisingly, despite the observations that PDE inhibitors increase bone density in numerous experimental systems, few studies have yet characterized PDEs in bone-derived cells. Limited studies have been reported on the expression of PDE isoforms in osteoblastic cells and cell lines and in osteosarcoma cells [3–6, 61, 67, 100], but analysis of PDE expression has not yet been reported in osteoclastic cells. Of note, based on these studies reported so far, it appears that the expression of PDEs in these cells varies considerably, depending on the species and cell type examined and the transformation state of the cells. Ahlstrom and Lamberg-Allardt examined both the cAMP PDE [4] and cGMP PDE [3] activities in mouse UMR-106 osteoblastic-like osteosarcoma cells by regulatory and inhibitor sensitivity analysis of the peaks of activity separated by Q-Sepharose chromatography. Based on this analysis, they found that 85% of the total cAMP-hydrolyzing activity in these cells could be attributed to PDE4, a little less than 4% to PDE2, and a slightly less than 2% to PDE1. The remaining 9–10% of cAMP PDE activity could not be defined using the available tools at the time but would be contributed by one or more cAMP PDEs other than PDEs 1, 2, and 4, notably PDEs 3, 7, 8, 10, and 11. Inasmuch as the undefined peak of cAMP PDE activity had a Km of 13 μM for cAMP, this would be most consistent with this representing PDE11, which has reported Kms somewhat close to this (1–6 μM), whereas the Kms of PDEs 3, 7, 8, and 10 are all at least 2–3 orders of magnitude lower [48]. The cGMP hydrolytic activity in UMR-106 cells could be accounted for almost entirely by PDE1, PDE2, and PDE5 [3]. Using the same technique of Q-Sepharose chromatography followed by analysis of the separated peaks of activity, Ahlstrom et al. analyzed the PDE activity in the human nontransformed osteoblast cell line, NHOst, and the human osteosarcoma cell line, SaOS-2 [5]. All of the cAMP PDE hydrolytic activity was separated into three peaks in both of these cell lines, although the characteristics of the activity peaks were not exactly the same between the two cell lines. The NHOst cells exhibited peaks of activity consistent with PDE1, PDE3, and an undefined activity peak that was insensitive to inhibitors of PDE1, PDE3, or PDE4 but sensitive to the nonspecific PDE inhibitor, 3-isobutyl-1-methyl-xanthine (IBMX). There was no evidence by activity analysis of the expression of PDE4 in these cells. In contrast, the SaOS-2 cell line exhibited peaks of activity consistent with PDE1 and PDE4 and the same undefined activity peak insensitive to inhibitors of PDE1, PDE3, or PDE4, but sensitive to IBMX, with no evidence by activity analysis of the expression of PDE3 in these cells. The cGMP PDE activity in both of these cell lines was accounted for entirely by PDE1. Further analysis of mRNA expression in these cell lines was performed by RT-PCR, using primers specific for PDEs 1–7 and their subtypes. By this analysis, NHOst expressed mRNA transcripts for PDEs 1A, 1C, 3A, 4A, 4B, 7A, and 7B and SaOS-2 expressed mRNA transcripts for PDEs 1C, 3A, 4A, 4B, 7A, and 7B. Based on the appearance of mRNA for PDE7 in these cells, Ahlstrom et al. ascribed the undefined, IBMX-sensitive cAMP PDE activity peak to PDE7; however, based on this limited analysis, it could just as easily represent PDEs 10 or 11. Inasmuch as this peak was sensitive to IBMX, it excludes PDE8, since PDE8 is insensitive to IBMX [21, 48]. Interestingly, these cell lines both express mRNA for PDEs 3A, 4A, and 4B; yet, by activity analysis, NHOst cells do not express measurable PDE4 activity and the SaOS-2 cells express no measurable PDE3 activity. It is noteworthy that in the mouse osteosarcoma cell line, UMR-106, and the human osteosarcoma cell line, SaOS-2, PDE4 is expressed as a major form, whereas the human nontransformed human cell line, NHOst, appears not to express measurable PDE4 activity at all. Where examined, expression of a wider range of PDEs at the mRNA transcript level than by activity analysis is commonly seen for these bone-derived cells, suggesting that many of these mRNA transcripts may be expressed in trace amounts or absent at the protein level or that analysis of protein expression of PDEs by activity analysis is simply not sensitive enough to detect expression of PDE isoforms expressed at low levels in these cells. Expression of PDE transcripts 1–9 was examined by RT-PCR in the mouse osteoblastic cell line, MC3T3-E1, and the mouse stromal cell line, ST2 [100], and by this analysis, both cell lines expressed a wide range of PDE mRNAs. MC3T3-E1 cells expressed mRNA for PDEs 1A, 1B, 2A, 3A, 4A, 4D, 7A, 8A, and 9A, and ST2 cells expressed mRNA for PDEs 1B, 2A, 3A, 4A, 4D, 7A, 8A, and 9A. PDE expression at the protein level was not examined in this study, but, as with other bone-derived cell lines, very likely many of these PDE mRNAs are not expressed to any appreciable degree at the protein level. For example, in a further study, Ahlstrom et al. compared cAMP PDE expression at the mRNA transcript level for PDEs 1–11, with expression at the protein level by activity analysis, in the two human osteosarcoma cell lines, MG-63 and SaOS-2 [6]. The investigators also found that both cell lines expressed a wide range of cAMP PDEs at the mRNA level, including PDEs 1A, 1C, 2A, 3A, 4A, 4B, 4C, 4D, 7A, 7B, 8A, 10A, and 11A. In contrast, by activity analysis, the vast majority of the cAMP PDE activity in these two cell lines could be accounted for by PDEs 1 and 4. The cAMP PDE activity in MG-63 cells was calculated to be 32% PDE1 and 63% PDE4, and that in SaOS-2 cells to be 56% PDE1 and 21% PDE4. Hence, from the limited analyses of osteoblast-like cells so far, it appears (1) that a wide range of PDEs are expressed at the mRNA transcript level, but only a very limited expression of PDEs occurs at the protein level; (2) that where investigated, the PDE activities expressed in osteoblastic cells appear primarily to be PDEs 1, 3, and 4; and (3) osteosarcoma cell lines appear to express PDE4 as a prominent form, whereas the one nontransformed osteoblast cell line examined so far, NHOst, does not express appreciable PDE4 activity.

Pekkinen et al. estimated the contributions of PDE4 and PDE7 to the overall cAMP hydrolytic activity of osteoblasts differentiated from human mesenchymal stem cells [67]. The cAMP hydrolytic activity was inhibited about 10% by the selective PDE4 inhibitor, rolipram, about 10% by the selective PDE7 inhibitor, BRL-50481, and about 90% by the nonspecific PDE inhibitor, IBMX, suggesting that cAMP PDE activity in these cells is composed of about 10% PDE4, 10% PDE7, and 10% PDE8 (the IBMX-insensitive activity), with the remaining 70% contributed by other cAMP PDEs. The PDE7 activity, although only comprising 10%, was shown to be important in controlling cAMP levels in these cells in that silencing of PDE7 expression by siRNA increased forskolin-stimulated cAMP levels in these cells by greater than threefold. Functionally, these cells differed in response to silencing of PDE7A/B expression by siRNA, as compared to silencing of PDE8A by siRNA. Silencing of PDE7 increased the expression of several osteogenic genes, whereas silencing of PDE8A did not. Similarly, silencing of PDE7 increased alkaline phosphatase activity and mineralization in these cells, whereas silencing of PDE8A did not. These studies suggest that in addition to PDE4, PDE7 may be an important target for increasing bone density in humans. Noh et al. examined mRNA expression of PDEs 3 and 4 in mouse primary calvarial osteoblasts and in the mouse osteoblast UAMS-32 cell line [61]. By RT-PCR, transcripts encoding PDEs 3A, 3B, 4A, 4B, and 4D were expressed in both of these cell types, while those for PDE4C were not. The PDE3-selective inhibitor, milrinone, and the PDE4-selective inhibitor, rolipram, each increased PGE_2-stimulated RANKL mRNA expression and osteoclast formation, whereas the PDE2-selective inhibitor, EHNA, and the PDE1-selective inhibitor, vinpocetine, did not. Dipyridamole, a nonselective PDE inhibitor capable of inhibiting PDE8 [21], also increased RANKL mRNA expression but did not increase osteoclast formation. These studies indicate that in addition to PDE4, targeting PDE3 may also modulate PGE_2 effects on bone homeostasis. It is noteworthy that in some other systems, such as for inducing apoptosis of some types of leukemic cells, it is necessary to inhibit PDE3 and/or PDE7 in addition to PDE4 in order to see a full effect [22, 56], and it has been suggested that dual PDE inhibitors targeting PDE 3/4 or PDE 4/7 may be better anti-inflammatory mediators than PDE4-selective inhibitors alone [27, 83], and combinations of PDE inhibitors also may prove to be more effective in treating bone diseases.

16.6 Effects of PDE Inhibitors on Bone Resorption and Bone Formation

PDE inhibitors have been shown, in several animal models, to both inhibit bone resorption as well as stimulate bone formation. One such animal model tested is that of Walker 256/S carcinoma-bearing rats, which develop an osteoporosis-like phenotype within 2 weeks. These rats given daily administration of denbufylline (1,3-di-*n*-butyl-7-(2′-oxopropyl)-xanthine), an alkylxanthine inhibitor with selectivity for PDE4, for 13 days, showed significantly less decrease in femur bone mineral density (BMD) compared to those not treated with denbufylline [54]. Denbufylline had no effect on the BMD of healthy rats in this study. Additionally, the number of osteoclasts on the bone surface was increased about twofold and the number of osteoblasts decreased about fivefold in the tumor-bearing rats, and denbufylline largely prevented this change in these cell numbers. In the same study, using an in vitro bone marrow culture system, denbufylline, another PDE4-selective inhibitor, RO 20-1724, and the nonselective PDE inhibitor, IBMX, all produced an increase in mineralized nodules and a decrease in tartrate-resistant acid phosphatase (TRAP)-positive multinucleated cells, whereas the PDE3-selective inhibitor, milrinone, and the PDE5-selective inhibitor, zaprinast, were without effect [54]. Another alkylxanthine PDE4-selective inhibitor, XT-44 (1-*n*-butyl-3-*n*-propylxanthine), also increased femoral BMD in this Walker 256/S carcinoma-bearing osteopenia rat model as well as in two other osteopenia models, sciatic neurectomized rats and ovariectomized rats [101]. A study using normal mice compared responses to the nonselective PDE inhibitor, pentoxifylline (1-(5-oxohexyl)-3, 7-dimethylxanthine), the PDE4-selective inhibitor, rolipram, or saline once per day for 5 weeks. Based on microdensitometry and histomorphometry analyses, the pentoxifylline- and rolipram-treated mice showed significantly increased cortical and cancellous bone mass relative to saline controls, and this appeared to be due mainly to accelerated bone formation during bone remodeling [44].

In addition to directly stimulating bone formation, PDE inhibitors also enhance the effects of BMP on this process. In a model system in which mice were implanted with porous collagen discs impregnated with recombinant BMP-2, and then injected once per day for 3 weeks with PDE inhibitors, it was found that both pentoxifylline [38] and rolipram [39] significantly enhanced BMP-2-induced ectopic bone formation, as determined by radiological and histological analyses showing increased calcified mass and increased BMD. In addition, in a related study, when mice implanted with BMP-2-impregnated discs were treated with pentoxifylline, PTH, or both pentoxifylline and PTH together, it was found that the combination of pentoxifylline and PTH together produced a greater effect than either pentoxifylline or PTH alone, in terms of increased ossicle size, calcium content, and higher BMD [37]. The PDE inhibitor IBMX also potentiated the effects of PTH and BMP-2 on maintenance of high intracellular concentrations of cAMP and expression of mRNAs for alkaline phosphatase, osteocalcin, and Smad6 in osteoblastic MC3T3-E1 cells [59]. Inasmuch as the PDE4-selective inhibitor, rolipram, produces significant side effects of nausea and emesis in humans, a study was performed to examine the effectiveness of a local delivery system, rather than systemic application of rolipram, on BMP-2-induced ectopic bone formation, wherein the rolipram was impregnated in the implanted collagen disc along with the recombinant BMP-2, and it was found in this system that rolipram enhanced the capacity of BMP-2 to induce bone formation by 1.5-fold [93]. In further examination of the ability of PDE inhibitors to enhance the effects of BMP on bone formation, these same investigators confirmed a direct anabolic enhancing effect of pentoxifylline to enhance BMP-4-induced chondro-/osteogenic differentiation of undifferentiated mesenchymal C3H10T1/2 cells and bone marrow stromal ST2 cells [97]. Studies with the PDE4-selective inhibitor, XT-611 (3,4-dipropyl-4,5,7,8-tetrahydro-3*H*-imidazo[1,2-*i*]-purin-5-one), also showed an anabolic effect of this inhibitor on bone marrow cells in culture [53]. When isolated bone marrow cells from either rat or mouse placed in culture were pulse treated with XT-611, wherein they were exposed to this inhibitor for 24 h from day 3–4 of a 10-day culture period, mineralized nodule formation in the cultures was greatly increased. Inasmuch as this effect of XT-611 was blocked by COX-2 inhibitors and EP4 receptor antagonists, the authors concluded that PGE_2 stimulates differentiation of osteoblast progenitor cells through the EP4 receptor in an autocrine fashion and that XT-611 potentiates the effects of PGE_2 on this differentiation.

In addition to the anabolic effects of PDE inhibitors that stimulate bone formation directly, effects on osteoclastogenesis occur as well. XT-611 not only acts synergistically with PGE_2 to mediate an anabolic effect on osteoblast progenitor cells [53] but it also acts synergistically with PGE_2 to inhibit osteoclastogenesis [104]. When examined in three different mouse bone marrow cell culture systems: direct cultured bone marrow cells (BMCs), coculture of ST2 cells and adherent cell-depleted (ACD) BMCs, and primary culture of ACD-BMCs, XT-611 directly inhibited osteoclastogenesis in BMCs and in the cocultured cells and inhibited it in conjunction with PGE_2 in the ACD-BMCs, as evidenced by a significant decrease in the formation of TRAP-positive multinucleated cells. In ACD-BMCs, intracellular cAMP concentration was only slightly increased by XT-611 or PGE_2 alone but greatly increased by the combined presence of both of these agents. Inasmuch as XT-611 did not change the expression levels of RANK, RANKL, OPG or c-fms, the receptor for M-CSF, the authors concluded that the actions of XT-611 to inhibit osteoclastogenesis are not based upon a decrease in the RANK/RANKL-dependent cell-cell interaction, changes in OPG, or M-CSF signaling. They suggest rather that XT-611 inhibits osteoclast multinucleation or maturation by acting synergistically on osteoclast progenitors with PGE_2 secreted from stromal cells and not by influencing cell-cell interaction between stromal cells and osteoclast progenitors. The PDE4 inhibitor rolipram also was shown to act synergistically with PGE_2 to inhibit osteoclastogenesis in a mouse bone marrow cell-derived osteoclastogenesis model, and this effect appeared to be due to a synergistic action of rolipram and PGE_2 to reduce osteoclast progenitor cell viability [65]. In a study of ovariectomized rats in which bone resorption exceeded bone formation, rolipram both prevented and restored ovariectomy-induced cancellous and cortical bone loss in the tibia, femur, and lumbar vertebra and reduced bone turnover at the trabecular and endocortical bone surfaces [106]. The effects of rolipram on prevention of further bone loss were comparable to those of the bisphosphonate alendronate. Paradoxically, in contrast to these studies, studies from the laboratory of Mijung Yim reported that the PDE inhibitors rolipram, pentoxifylline, and IBMX stimulate osteoclast formation [16, 86]. Subsequent studies by this laboratory, however, indicate that rolipram acts in a manner very similar to PTH on osteoblasts, including effects on induction of COX-2 expression, increased PGE_2 production, and an increase in the RANKL/OPG mRNA ratio, and they suggest that, like PTH, the ultimate effects of PDE inhibitors on osteoclast formation may depend on the manner in which the PDE inhibitor is given, i.e., if it is given continuously or by periodic intermittent application [64, 66].

In sum, it appears from both animal and cell culture studies that PDE inhibitors are very effective anabolic agents acting both directly and through potentiation of the effects of BMP and PGE_2 to increase bone formation, and also possibly acting synergistically with PGE_2, to decrease osteoclastogenesis and thereby inhibit bone resorption.

16.7 A Potential Role for PDE Inhibitors in the Treatment of Glucocorticoid-Induced Osteoporosis

Glucocorticoid-induced osteoporosis is the second most common cause of osteoporosis after menopause [75, 88]. It is estimated that over 50% of chronic glucocorticoid users will develop bone loss leading to fractures [51], and fracture risk is clearly increased after only 3 months of glucocorticoid treatment [1, 30]. Inasmuch as 0.2–0.5% of the population, or greater than one million people, are on glucocorticoid therapy, this constitutes a common medical problem for which there is urgent need for more effective therapeutic option [30, 75]. The nature of glucocorticoid-induced osteoporosis differs substantially from other forms of osteoporosis, in that glucocorticoids primarily affect osteoblasts, both inhibiting their function and reducing their viability [88]. Estrogen deficiency typically leads to a high-turnover form of osteoporosis in which both formation and resorption are accelerated but the relative activity of the osteoclast is greater than that of the osteoblast. In contrast, glucocorticoids lead to a low-turnover form of the disease in which both formation and resorption are suppressed but the former more so than the latter [88]. Currently, bisphosphonates are the most widely prescribed agents for treatment of all forms of osteoporosis, including that induced by glucocorticoids. However, bisphosphonates, which inhibit resorption, are far more effective in preventing bone loss in states of high rather than low turnover and thus are not ideal for the treatment of glucocorticoid-induced osteoporosis, which would be far better treated by anabolic agents that act on osteoblasts to promote bone formation. Hence, PDE inhibitors, which can act both to promote bone formation as well as inhibit bone resorption, would potentially be far better agents for treating glucocorticoid-induced osteoporosis and would thus fill a critical need in this area.

The mechanism(s) by which glucocorticoids inhibit osteoblast function is not fully understood. It is well known that there is considerable interplay between the cAMP and glucocorticoid signaling pathways [48, 91], and it is possible that some of the effects of glucocorticoids may result from their effects on cAMP signaling. In 1984, we reported, for example, that long-term (0.5–3 days) treatment of ROS 17/2.8 rat osteosarcoma cells with dexamethasone dramatically potentiated the increase in cAMP levels induced by PTH in these cells [73]. This appeared not to result from any change in low Km cAMP PDE activity (measured at 1 μM substrate), although a significant reduction of 15–20% was seen in high Km cAMP PDE activity (measured at 100 μM substrate), following exposure to dexamethasone, which could in part account for this observation. Our further evidence suggested that this phenomenon may result largely from increased hormone receptor-adenylyl cyclase coupling [73], and a subsequent study showed an increase in abundance of Gs in these cells following exposure to dexamethasone [74]. Interestingly, in late-passage cultures of ROS 17/2.8 cells, although PTH readily increases cAMP levels in these cells, surprisingly, it fails to activate PKA activity; however, after exposure of the cells to hydrocortisone or dexamethasone, PTH treatment now results in activation of PKA [108]. It is now well accepted that cAMP can exist in discrete microdomains or compartments within the cell maintained in large part by specific subcellular distribution of PDEs [40], and it is probable that dexamethasone alters these subcellular compartments such that the cAMP generated by PTH can now gain access to and activate PKA. Significant downregulation of PDE activity following long-term treatment with dexamethasone has been reported in a number of different cell systems. PDE activity in cultured hepatoma cells treated long-term with dexamethasone was reduced 25–40%, leading to marked enhancement of the elevation of cAMP in the cells in response to epinephrine and theophylline [52]. Subsequent studies with cultured rat hepatocytes showed that dexamethasone selectively reduced the expression of PDE4D mRNA [33]. In the human osteosarcoma cell line, MG-63, long-term dexamethasone treatment decreased PDE activity by 50%, and this was shown to be accompanied by a selective 50–70% reduction in the mRNA expression for PDE4A4 and PDE4B1 [6]. Thus, glucocorticoids can alter cAMP signaling through effects on PDEs, at least PDE4 subtypes, and possibly others as well, and this may ultimately affect osteoblast function and/or viability, through the many ways in which cAMP signaling regulates these critical processes in osteoblasts. To better understand this and take full advantage of this knowledge for the treatment of glucocorticoid-induced osteoporosis, it is important that the full expression profiles of PDEs in osteoblasts and osteoblast progenitor cells, and the effect of glucocorticoids on these PDEs, be analyzed.

16.8 Conclusions/Perspectives

Osteoporosis is a very prevalent disease that is estimated to afflict eight million women and two million men in the United States [11]. Since the approval of alendronate (Fosamax) by the US Food and Drug Administration in 1995, bisphosphonates have become the dominant therapy for this disease and are in widespread clinical use. Although bisphosphonates have exhibited appreciable clinical efficacy in reducing incidence of fractures [82], inasmuch as they only inhibit bone resorption and have no effect on bone formation, they are not ideal therapeutic agents for patients with very low bone mass. Glucocorticoid-induced osteoporosis in particular, which is a low-turnover form of osteoporosis, primarily affecting osteoblasts, is poorly treated by bisphosphonates. Moreover, although a rare complication of their clinical use long term bisphosphonates may compromise bone quality and resulting in increased skeletal microdamage and reduced bone toughness [88]. Additionally, perhaps as a result of this, with widespread, long-term use of bisphosphonates, a number of serious side effects have begun to appear in patients treated with these agents, including osteonecrosis of the jaw [102], a possible twofold increase in the risk of esophageal cancer [29], and the appearance of atypical femoral fractures [81, 102]. Teriparatide (Forteo), the 34-amino acid amino-terminal fragment of PTH, is the only approved treatment for osteoporosis in the United States that acts to stimulate bone anabolism and indeed, in comparative clinical trials, teriparatide was superior to alendronate in the treatment of glucocorticoid-induced osteoporosis [76]; however, the high cost and necessity for daily subcutaneous injection have limited the use of teriparatide [1]. For this reason, bisphosphonates, despite their relative ineffectiveness and recent reports of concenerning side effects, still are more commonly prescribed for all forms of osteoporosis, including that induced by glucocorticoids. Hence, there exists a clearly urgent need for better agents for the treatment of osteoporosis. PDE inhibitors, with their ability to both inhibit bone resorption and stimulate anabolic bone formation, are candidates that exhibit excellent promise as novel, highly effective agents for treatment of osteoporosis.

To take full advantage of the development of PDE inhibitors for osteoporosis treatment, more work needs to be performed to fully understand the ways in which PDEs and the cAMP signaling pathway act to regulate the many facets of bone cell formation and function. The whole area of targeting the cAMP signaling pathway with PDE inhibitors to block osteoclast cell migration, and thus bone resorption, remains completely unexplored and is ripe for investigation. Similarly, there only has been limited analysis of PDE expression in bone cells both at the mRNA and protein level, and no examination of the subcellular distribution of PDE isoforms or their association with the many partner or chaperone proteins with which they interact [40]. Similarly, the effects of disruption of this targeting. This is an area clearly in need of more work. PDE expression in osteoclasts has not been investigated at all, and analysis in other bone cell types is quite limited. Although much work, based on the use of PDE inhibitors in cell-free systems as well as in in vivo animal studies, supports and validates the concept that PDE inhibitors may be excellent targets for treating osteoporosis and point to PDE4 as the important PDE gene family to target, the contribution of other PDEs, particularly the more recently discovered PDE genes, PDEs 7–11, to regulation of bone function and importance as targets for stimulating bone formation, remain largely unexplored. Although clinical trials in humans with PDE inhibitors to treat osteoporosis have not yet been undertaken, the recent approval of roflumilast (Daxas), a PDE4 inhibitor, for treatment of chronic obstructive pulmonary disease, may facilitate such trials. Moreover, it is noteworthy that when 25,000 single-nucleotide polymorphisms located within 16,000 different genes were examined for association with BMD in 138 women with low and 138 women with high lumbar spine BMD, PDE4D stood out as the gene with the highest association among the 16,000 genes examined [71], which further underscores the importance of PDE4 in determining BMD in humans. Based on the evidence reviewed in this chapter, PDEs are potentially excellent targets for building bone, by both inhibiting resorption and at the same time stimulating anabolic bone formation, and thus may well provide the type of agent needed to more adequately treat osteoporosis. In order to fulfill the promise that PDE inhibitors hold for a novel, more effective treatment of osteoporosis, it is important that more research be conducted to fill in the gaps in our knowledge that are highlighted in this chapter.

Acknowledgments First and foremost, I would like to thank my dear friend and colleague, Dr. Felix Bronner, for encouraging me to write this chapter and for his many stimulating discussions on this and a host of other topics over the 32 years that we have known each other. I would also like to dedicate this article to my two late colleagues, Dr. Gideon Rodan (1934–2006) and Dr. Lawrence Raisz (1925–2010), both of whom devoted their lives to developing treatments for osteoporosis, and in so doing, became renowned in the bone biology field. I am particularly grateful to Drs. Gideon and Sevgi Rodan for befriending me when I first came to the University of Connecticut Health Center in 1979 and inviting me to join their weekly signaling discussion groups at their home in West Hartford, where I first came to appreciate the importance of cAMP signaling in the regulation of bone development and function. And I especially dedicate this article to my beautiful, sweet, shining star of a daughter, Serena Rae Epstein (1984–2011), who has been my inspiration for everything I have done for the 27 years that she was alive. I thank Dr. Karl Insogna for his critical reading of this manuscript. I also thank Mary Smart and the Smart Family Foundation for their continued support of my research that enabled me to write this chapter. Serena Rae Epstein (1984–2011) The PDE4-selective inhibitor roflumilast has now been approved by the US FDA and is marketed under the name Daliresp.

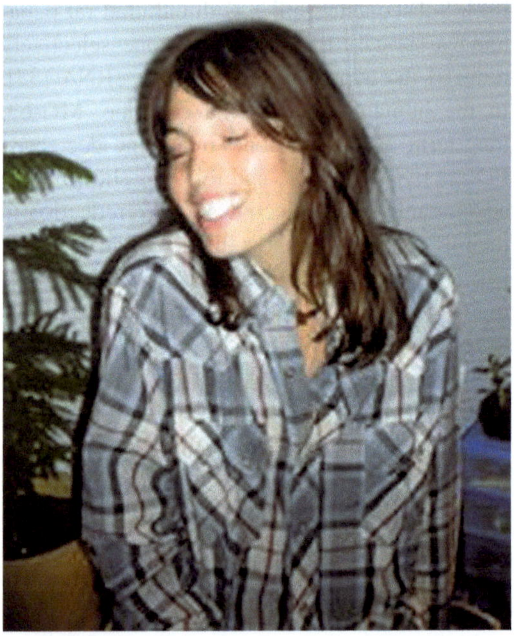

References

1. Adler RA. Glucocorticoid-induced osteoporosis: management update. Curr Osteoporos Rep. 2010; 8:10–4.
2. Aghaloo TL, Pirih FQ, Shi A, Bezouglaia O, Tetradis S. Parathyroid hormone induces mitogen-activated kinase phosphatase 1 in murine osteoblasts primarily through cAMP-protein kinase A signaling. J Periodontol. 2006;77:21–30.
3. Ahlstrom M, Lamberg-Allardt C. Inactivation of atrial natriuretic factor-stimulated cyclic guanosine 3′,5′-monophosphate (cGMP) in UMR-106 osteoblast-like cells. Biochem Pharmacol. 2000;59:1133–9.
4. Ahlstrom M, Lamberg-Allardt C. Regulation of adenosine 3′,5′-cyclic monophosphate (cAMP) accumulation in UMR-106 osteoblast-like cells: role of cAMP-phosphodiesterase and cAMP efflux. Biochem Pharmacol. 1999;58:1335–40.
5. Ahlstrom M, Pekkinen M, Huttunen M, Lamberg-Allardt C. Cyclic nucleotide phosphodiesterases (PDEs) in human osteoblastic cells; the effect of PDE inhibition on cAMP accumulation. Cell Mol Biol Lett. 2005;10:305–19.
6. Ahlstrom M, Pekkinen M, Huttunen M, Lamberg-Allardt C. Dexamethasone down-regulates cAMP-phosphodiesterase in human osteosarcoma cells. Biochem Pharmacol. 2005;69:267–75.
7. Bender AT, Beavo JA. Cyclic nucleotide phosphodiesterases: molecular regulation to clinical use. Pharmacol Rev. 2006;58:488–520.
8. Boyle WJ, Simonet WS, Lacey DL. Osteoclast differentiation and activation. Nature. 2003;423:337–42.
9. Broderick KE, Zhang T, Rangaswami H, Zeng Y, Zhao X, Boss GR, Pilz RB. Guanosine 3′,5′-cyclic monophosphate (cGMP)/cGMP-dependent protein kinase induce interleukin-6 transcription in osteoblasts. Mol Endocrinol. 2007;21:1148–62.
10. Bukka P, McKee MD, Karaplis AC. Molecular regulation of osteoblast differentiation. In: Bronner F, Farach-Carson MC, editors. Bone formation. New York: Springer; 2004. p. 1–17.
11. Canalis E. Update in new anabolic therapies for osteoporosis. J Clin Endocrinol Metab. 2010;95: 1496–504.
12. Chaudhary LR, Avioli LV. Identification and activation of mitogen-activated protein (MAP) kinase in normal human osteoblastic and bone marrow stromal cells: attenuation of MAP kinase activation by cAMP, parathyroid hormone and forskolin. Mol Cell Biochem. 1998;178:59–68.
13. Chellaiah MA, Biswas RS, Rittling SR, Denhardt DT, Hruska KA. Rho-dependent Rho kinase activation increases CD44 surface expression and bone resorption in osteoclasts. J Biol Chem. 2003;278:29086–97.
14. Chellaiah MA, Hruska KA. The integrin alpha(v)beta(3) and CD44 regulate the actions of osteopontin on osteoclast motility. Calcif Tissue Int. 2003;72:197–205.
15. Chellaiah MA, Soga N, Swanson S, McAllister S, Alvarez U, Wang D, Dowdy SF, Hruska KA. Rho-A is critical for osteoclast podosome organization, motility, and bone resorption. J Biol Chem. 2000;275: 11993–2002.
16. Cho ES, Yu JH, Kim MS, Yim M. Rolipram, a phosphodiesterase 4 inhibitor, stimulates osteoclast formation by inducing TRANCE expression in mouse calvarial cells. Arch Pharm Res. 2004;27:1258–62.
17. Conti M, Beavo J. Biochemistry and physiology of cyclic nucleotide phosphodiesterases: essential components in cyclic nucleotide signaling. Annu Rev Biochem. 2007;76:481–511.
18. Coxon FP, Rogers MJ. The role of prenylated small GTP-binding proteins in the regulation of osteoclast function. Calcif Tissue Int. 2003;72:80–4.
19. Cummings SR, San Martin J, McClung MR, Siris ES, Eastell R, Reid IR, Delmas P, Zoog HB, Austin M, Wang A, Kutilek S, Adami S, Zanchetta J, Libanati C, Siddhanti S, Christiansen C. Denosumab for prevention of fractures in postmenopausal women with osteoporosis. N Engl J Med. 2009;361:756–65.
20. Datta NS, Abou-Samra AB. PTH and PTHrP signaling in osteoblasts. Cell Signal. 2009;21:1245–54.
21. Dong H, Osmanova V, Epstein PM, Brocke S. Phosphodiesterase 8 (PDE8) regulates chemotaxis of activated lymphocytes. Biochem Biophys Res Commun. 2006;345:713–9.
22. Dong H, Zitt C, Auriga C, Hatzelmann A, Epstein PM. Inhibition of PDE3, PDE4 and PDE7 potentiates glucocorticoid-induced apoptosis and overcomes glucocorticoid resistance in CEM T leukemic cells. Biochem Pharmacol. 2010;79:321–9.
23. Dua P, Gude RP. Pentoxifylline impedes migration in B16F10 melanoma by modulating Rho GTPase activity and actin organisation. Eur J Cancer. 2008;44: 1587–95.
24. Duong LT, Rodan GA. Regulation of osteoclast formation and function. Rev Endocr Metab Disord. 2001;2:95–104.
25. Fleming YM, Frame MC, Houslay MD. PDE4-Regulated cAMP degradation controls the assembly of integrin-dependent actin adhesion structures and REF52 cell migration. J Cell Sci. 2004;117:2377–88.
26. Fu Q, Jilka RL, Manolagas SC, O'Brien CA. Parathyroid hormone stimulates receptor activator of NFkappa B ligand and inhibits osteoprotegerin expression via protein kinase A activation of cAMP-response element-binding protein. J Biol Chem. 2002;277: 48868–75.
27. Giembycz MA. Can the anti-inflammatory potential of PDE4 inhibitors be realized: guarded optimism or wishful thinking? Br J Pharmacol. 2008;155:288–90.
28. Giembycz MA, Field SK. Roflumilast: first phosphodiesterase 4 inhibitor approved for treatment of COPD. Drug Des Devel Ther. 2010;4:147–58.
29. Green J, Czanner G, Reeves G, Watson J, Wise L, Beral V. Oral bisphosphonates and risk of cancer of oesophagus, stomach, and colorectum: case–control analysis within a UK primary care cohort. BMJ. 2010; 341:c4444.
30. Grossman JM, Gordon R, Ranganath VK, Deal C, Caplan L, Chen W, Curtis JR, Furst DE, McMahon M, Patkar NM, Volkmann E, Saag KG. American College

of Rheumatology 2010 recommendations for the prevention and treatment of glucocorticoid-induced osteoporosis. Arthritis Care Res (Hoboken). 2010;62: 1515–26.
31. Hagiwara H, Inoue A, Yamaguchi A, Yokose S, Furuya M, Tanaka S, Hirose S. cGMP produced in response to ANP and CNP regulates proliferation and differentiation of osteoblastic cells. Am J Physiol. 1996;270:C1311–8.
32. Hatzelmann A, Morcillo EJ, Lungarella G, Adnot S, Sanjar S, Beume R, Schudt C, Tenor H. The preclinical pharmacology of roflumilast – a selective, oral phosphodiesterase 4 inhibitor in development for chronic obstructive pulmonary disease. Pulm Pharmacol Ther. 2010;23:235–56.
33. Hermsdorf T, Richter W, Dettmer D. Effects of dexamethosone and glucagon after long-term exposure on cyclic AMP phosphodiesterase 4 in cultured rat hepatocytes. Cell Signal. 1999;11:685–90.
34. Hidi R, Timmermans S, Liu E, Schudt C, Dent G, Holgate ST, Djukanovic R. Phosphodiesterase and cyclic adenosine monophosphate-dependent inhibition of T-lymphocyte chemotaxis. Eur Respir J. 2000;15:342–9.
35. Hikiji H, Shin WS, Oida S, Takato T, Koizumi T, Toyo-oka T. Direct action of nitric oxide on osteoblastic differentiation. FEBS Lett. 1997;410:238–42.
36. Hodsman AB, Bauer DC, Dempster DW, Dian L, Hanley DA, Harris ST, Kendler DL, McClung MR, Miller PD, Olszynski WP, Orwoll E, Yuen CK. Parathyroid hormone and teriparatide for the treatment of osteoporosis: a review of the evidence and suggested guidelines for its use. Endocr Rev. 2005;26: 688–703.
37. Horiuchi H, Saito N, Kinoshita T, Wakabayashi S, Tsutsumimoto T, Otsuru S, Takaoka K. Enhancement of recombinant human bone morphogenetic protein-2 (rhBMP-2)-induced new bone formation by concurrent treatment with parathyroid hormone and a phosphodiesterase inhibitor, pentoxifylline. J Bone Miner Metab. 2004;22:329–34.
38. Horiuchi H, Saito N, Kinoshita T, Wakabayashi S, Tsutsumimoto T, Takaoka K. Enhancement of bone morphogenetic protein-2-induced new bone formation in mice by the phosphodiesterase inhibitor pentoxifylline. Bone. 2001;28:290–4.
39. Horiuchi H, Saito N, Kinoshita T, Wakabayashi S, Yotsumoto N, Takaoka K. Effect of phosphodiesterase inhibitor-4, rolipram, on new bone formations by recombinant human bone morphogenetic protein-2. Bone. 2002;30:589–93.
40. Houslay MD. Underpinning compartmentalised cAMP signalling through targeted cAMP breakdown. Trends Biochem Sci. 2010;35:91–100.
41. Houslay MD, Schafer P, Zhang KY. Keynote review: phosphodiesterase-4 as a therapeutic target. Drug Discov Today. 2005;10:1503–19.
42. Huang W, Rudkin GH, Carlsen B, Ishida K, Ghasri P, Anvar B, Yamaguchi DT, Miller TA. Overexpression of BMP-2 modulates morphology, growth, and gene expression in osteoblastic cells. Exp Cell Res. 2002;274:226–34.
43. Inoue A, Hiruma Y, Hirose S, Yamaguchi A, Furuya M, Tanaka S, Hagiwara H. Stimulation by C-type natriuretic peptide of the differentiation of clonal osteoblastic MC3T3-E1 cells. Biochem Biophys Res Commun. 1996;221:703–7.
44. Kinoshita T, Kobayashi S, Ebara S, Yoshimura Y, Horiuchi H, Tsutsumimoto T, Wakabayashi S, Takaoka K. Phosphodiesterase inhibitors, pentoxifylline and rolipram, increase bone mass mainly by promoting bone formation in normal mice. Bone. 2000; 27:811–7.
45. Lang P, Gesbert F, Delespine-Carmagnat M, Stancou R, Pouchelet M, Bertoglio J. Protein kinase A phosphorylation of RhoA mediates the morphological and functional effects of cyclic AMP in cytotoxic lymphocytes. EMBO J. 1996;15:510–9.
46. Lee SK, Lorenzo JA. Regulation of receptor activator of nuclear factor-kappa B ligand and osteoprotegerin mRNA expression by parathyroid hormone is predominantly mediated by the protein kinase a pathway in murine bone marrow cultures. Bone. 2002; 31:252–9.
47. Leis HJ, Hulla W, Gruber R, Huber E, Zach D, Gleispach H, Windischhofer W. Phenotypic heterogeneity of osteoblast-like MC3T3-E1 cells: changes of bradykinin-induced prostaglandin E2 production during osteoblast maturation. J Bone Miner Res. 1997;12: 541–51.
48. Lerner A, Epstein PM. Cyclic nucleotide phosphodiesterases as targets for treatment of haematological malignancies. Biochem J. 2006;393:21–41.
49. Lo KW, Ashe KM, Kan HM, Lee DA, Laurencin CT. Activation of cyclic amp/protein kinase: a signaling pathway enhances osteoblast cell adhesion on biomaterials for regenerative Engineering. J Orthop Res. 2011;29:602–8.
50. Lugnier C. Cyclic nucleotide phosphodiesterase (PDE) superfamily: a new target for the development of specific therapeutic agents. Pharmacol Ther. 2006; 109:366–98.
51. Lukert BP, Raisz LG. Glucocorticoid-induced osteoporosis: pathogenesis and management. Ann Intern Med. 1990;112:352–64.
52. Manganiello V, Vaughan M. An effect of dexamethasone on adenosine 3′,5′-monophosphate content and adenosine 3′,5′-monophosphate phosphodiesterase activity of cultured hepatoma cells. J Clin Invest. 1972;51:2763–7.
53. Miyamoto K, Suzuki H, Yamamoto S, Saitoh Y, Ochiai E, Moritani S, Yokogawa K, Waki Y, Kasugai S, Sawanishi H, Yamagami H. Prostaglandin E2-mediated anabolic effect of a novel inhibitor of phosphodiesterase 4, XT-611, in the in vitro bone marrow culture. J Bone Miner Res. 2003;18:1471–7.
54. Miyamoto K, Waki Y, Horita T, Kasugai S, Ohya K. Reduction of bone loss by denbufylline, an inhibitor of phosphodiesterase 4. Biochem Pharmacol. 1997; 54:613–7.

55. Miyazawa T, Ogawa Y, Chusho H, Yasoda A, Tamura N, Komatsu Y, Pfeifer A, Hofmann F, Nakao K. Cyclic GMP-dependent protein kinase II plays a critical role in C-type natriuretic peptide-mediated endochondral ossification. Endocrinology. 2002;143:3604–10.
56. Moon E, Lee R, Near R, Weintraub L, Wolda S, Lerner A. Inhibition of PDE3B augments PDE4 inhibitor-induced apoptosis in a subset of patients with chronic lymphocytic leukemia. Clin Cancer Res. 2002;8:589–95.
57. Murata K, Sudo T, Kameyama M, Fukuoka H, Muka M, Doki Y, Sasaki Y, Ishikawa O, Kimura Y, Imaoka S. Cyclic AMP specific phosphodiesterase activity and colon cancer cell motility. Clin Exp Metastasis. 2000;18:599–604.
58. Nakamura I, le Duong T, Rodan SB, Rodan GA. Involvement of alpha(v)beta3 integrins in osteoclast function. J Bone Miner Metab. 2007;25:337–44.
59. Nakao Y, Koike T, Ohta Y, Manaka T, Imai Y, Takaoka K. Parathyroid hormone enhances bone morphogenetic protein activity by increasing intracellular 3′, 5′-cyclic adenosine monophosphate accumulation in osteoblastic MC3T3-E1 cells. Bone. 2009;44:872–7.
60. Netherton SJ, Maurice DH. Vascular endothelial cell cyclic nucleotide phosphodiesterases and regulated cell migration: implications in angiogenesis. Mol Pharmacol. 2005;67:263–72.
61. Noh AL, Yang M, Lee JM, Park H, Lee DS, Yim M. Phosphodiesterase 3 and 4 negatively regulate receptor activator of nuclear factor-kappaB ligand-mediated osteoclast formation by prostaglandin E2. Biol Pharm Bull. 2009;32:1844–8.
62. O'Connor KL, Nguyen BK, Mercurio AM. RhoA function in lamellae formation and migration is regulated by the alpha6beta4 integrin and cAMP metabolism. J Cell Biol. 2000;148:253–8.
63. Ohta Y, Nakagawa K, Imai Y, Katagiri T, Koike T, Takaoka K. Cyclic AMP enhances Smad-mediated BMP signaling through PKA-CREB pathway. J Bone Miner Metab. 2008;26:478–84.
64. Park H, No AL, Lee JM, Chen L, Lee SY, Lee DS, Yim M. PDE4 inhibitor upregulates PTH-induced osteoclast formation via CRE-mediated COX-2 expression in osteoblasts. FEBS Lett. 2010;584:173–80.
65. Park H, Yim M. Rolipram, a phosphodiesterase 4 inhibitor, suppresses PGE2-induced osteoclast formation by lowering osteoclast progenitor cell viability. Arch Pharm Res. 2007;30:486–92.
66. Park H, Young Lee S, Lee DS, Yim M. Phosphodiesterase 4 inhibitor regulates the TRANCE/OPG ratio via COX-2 expression in a manner similar to PTH in osteoblasts. Biochem Biophys Res Commun. 2007;354:178–83.
67. Pekkinen M, Ahlstrom ME, Riehle U, Huttunen MM, Lamberg-Allardt CJ. Effects of phosphodiesterase 7 inhibition by RNA interference on the gene expression and differentiation of human mesenchymal stem cell-derived osteoblasts. Bone. 2008;43:84–91.
68. Pratap J, Galindo M, Zaidi SK, Vradii D, Bhat BM, Robinson JA, Choi JY, Komori T, Stein JL, Lian JB, Stein GS, van Wijnen AJ. Cell growth regulatory role of Runx2 during proliferative expansion of preosteoblasts. Cancer Res. 2003;63:5357–62.
69. Raftopoulou M, Hall A. Cell migration: Rho GTPases lead the way. Dev Biol. 2004;265:23–32.
70. Rangaswami H, Marathe N, Zhuang S, Chen Y, Yeh JC, Frangos JA, Boss GR, Pilz RB. Type II cGMP-dependent protein kinase mediates osteoblast mechanotransduction. J Biol Chem. 2009;284:14796–808.
71. Reneland RH, Mah S, Kammerer S, Hoyal CR, Marnellos G, Wilson SG, Sambrook PN, Spector TD, Nelson MR, Braun A. Association between a variation in the phosphodiesterase 4D gene and bone mineral density. BMC Med Genet. 2005;6:9.
72. Rodan GA, Noda M. Gene expression in osteoblastic cells. Crit Rev Eukaryot Gene Expr. 1991;1:85–98.
73. Rodan SB, Fischer MK, Egan JJ, Epstein PM, Rodan GA. The effect of dexamethasone on parathyroid hormone stimulation of adenylate cyclase in ROS 17/2.8 cells. Endocrinology. 1984;115:951–8.
74. Rodan SB, Rodan GA. Dexamethasone effects on beta-adrenergic receptors and adenylate cyclase regulatory proteins Gs and Gi in ROS 17/2.8 cells. Endocrinology. 1986;118:2510–8.
75. Saag KG. Glucocorticoid-induced osteoporosis. Endocrinol Metab Clin North Am. 2003;32:135–57, vii.
76. Saag KG, Shane E, Boonen S, Marin F, Donley DW, Taylor KA, Dalsky GP, Marcus R. Teriparatide or alendronate in glucocorticoid-induced osteoporosis. N Engl J Med. 2007;357:2028–39.
77. Sawada K, Morishige K, Tahara M, Kawagishi R, Ikebuchi Y, Tasaka K, Murata Y. Alendronate inhibits lysophosphatidic acid-induced migration of human ovarian cancer cells by attenuating the activation of rho. Cancer Res. 2002;62:6015–20.
78. Schwappacher R, Weiske J, Heining E, Ezerski V, Marom B, Henis YI, Huber O, Knaus P. Novel crosstalk to BMP signalling: cGMP-dependent kinase I modulates BMP receptor and Smad activity. EMBO J. 2009;28:1537–50.
79. Selvamurugan N, Pulumati MR, Tyson DR, Partridge NC. Parathyroid hormone regulation of the rat collagenase-3 promoter by protein kinase A-dependent transactivation of core binding factor alpha1. J Biol Chem. 2000;275:5037–42.
80. Serrels B, Sandilands E, Serrels A, Baillie G, Houslay MD, Brunton VG, Canel M, Machesky LM, Anderson KI, Frame MC. A complex between FAK, RACK1, and PDE4D5 controls spreading initiation and cancer cell polarity. Curr Biol. 2010;20:1086–92.
81. Shane E, Burr D, Ebeling PR, Abrahamsen B, Adler RA, Brown TD, Cheung AM, Cosman F, Curtis JR, Dell R, Dempster D, Einhorn TA, Genant HK, Geusens P, Klaushofer K, Koval K, Lane JM, McKiernan F, McKinney R, Ng A, Nieves J, O'Keefe R, Papapoulos S, Sen HT, van der Meulen MC, Weinstein RS, Whyte M. Atypical subtrochanteric and diaphyseal femoral fractures: report of a task force of the American Society for Bone and Mineral Research. J Bone Miner Res. 2010;25:2267–94.

82. Siris ES, Pasquale MK, Wang Y, Watts NB. Estimating bisphosphonate use and fracture reduction among U.S. women age 45 and older, 2001–2008. J Bone Miner Res. 2010;26:3–11.
83. Spina D. PDE4 inhibitors: current status. Br J Pharmacol. 2008;155:308–15.
84. Stern PH, Diamond J. Sodium nitroprusside increases cyclic GMP in fetal rat bone cells and inhibits resorption of fetal rat limb bones. Res Commun Chem Pathol Pharmacol. 1992;75:19–28.
85. Sugama R, Koike T, Imai Y, Nomura-Furuwatari C, Takaoka K. Bone morphogenetic protein activities are enhanced by 3′,5′-cyclic adenosine monophosphate through suppression of Smad6 expression in osteoprogenitor cells. Bone. 2006;38:206–14.
86. Takami M, Cho ES, Lee SY, Kamijo R, Yim M. Phosphodiesterase inhibitors stimulate osteoclast formation via TRANCE/RANKL expression in osteoblasts: possible involvement of ERK and p38 MAPK pathways. FEBS Lett. 2005;579:832–8.
87. Tam CS, Heersche JN, Murray TM, Parsons JA. Parathyroid hormone stimulates the bone apposition rate independently of its resorptive action: differential effects of intermittent and continuous administration. Endocrinology. 1982;110:506–12.
88. Teitelbaum SL, Seton MP, Saag KG. Should bisphosphonates be used for long-term treatment of glucocorticoid-induced osteoporosis? Arthritis Rheum. 2011;63:325–8.
89. Tenor H, Hedbom E, Hauselmann HJ, Schudt C, Hatzelmann A. Phosphodiesterase isoenzyme families in human osteoarthritis chondrocytes–functional importance of phosphodiesterase 4. Br J Pharmacol. 2002;135:609–18.
90. Tintut Y, Parhami F, Le V, Karsenty G, Demer LL. Inhibition of osteoblast-specific transcription factor Cbfa1 by the cAMP pathway in osteoblastic cells. Ubiquitin/proteasome-dependent regulation. J Biol Chem. 1999;274:28875–9.
91. Tiwari S, Dong H, Kim EJ, Weintraub L, Epstein PM, Lerner A. Type 4 cAMP phosphodiesterase (PDE4) inhibitors augment glucocorticoid-mediated apoptosis in B cell chronic lymphocytic leukemia (B-CLL) in the absence of exogenous adenylyl cyclase stimulation. Biochem Pharmacol. 2005;69:473–83.
92. Togo S, Liu X, Wang X, Sugiura H, Kamio K, Kawasaki S, Kobayashi T, Ertl RF, Ahn Y, Holz O, Magnussen H, Fredriksson K, Skold CM, Rennard SI. PDE4 inhibitors roflumilast and rolipram augment PGE2 inhibition of TGF-{beta}1-stimulated fibroblasts. Am J Physiol Lung Cell Mol Physiol. 2009;296:L959–69.
93. Tokuhara Y, Wakitani S, Imai Y, Nomura C, Hoshino M, Yano K, Taguchi S, Kim M, Kadoya Y, Takaoka K. Local delivery of rolipram, a phosphodiesterase-4-specific inhibitor, augments bone morphogenetic protein-induced bone formation. J Bone Miner Metab. 2010;28:17–24.
94. Towler DA, Rodan GA. Identification of a rat osteocalcin promoter 3′,5′-cyclic adenosine monophosphate response region containing two PuGGTCA steroid hormone receptor binding motifs. Endocrinology. 1995;136:1089–96.
95. Traynor K. Osteoporosis drug licensed for women with high fracture risk. Am J Health Syst Pharm. 2010;67:1046.
96. Tsuji T, Kunieda T. A loss-of-function mutation in natriuretic peptide receptor 2 (Npr2) gene is responsible for disproportionate dwarfism in cn/cn mouse. J Biol Chem. 2005;280:14288–92.
97. Tsutsumimoto T, Wakabayashi S, Kinoshita T, Horiuchi H, Takaoka K. A phosphodiesterase inhibitor, pentoxifylline, enhances the bone morphogenetic protein-4 (BMP-4)-dependent differentiation of osteoprogenitor cells. Bone. 2002;31:396–401.
98. Vang AG, Ben-Sasson SZ, Dong H, Kream B, DeNinno MP, Claffey MM, Housley W, Clark RB, Epstein PM, Brocke S. PDE8 regulates rapid Teff cell adhesion and proliferation independent of ICER. PLoS One. 2010;5:e12011.
99. Vargas SJ, Holden SN, Fall PM, Raisz LG. Effects of atrial natriuretic factor on cyclic nucleotides, bone resorption, collagen and deoxyribonucleic acid synthesis, and prostaglandin E2 production in fetal rat bone cultures. Endocrinology. 1989;125:2527–31.
100. Wakabayashi S, Tsutsumimoto T, Kawasaki S, Kinoshita T, Horiuchi H, Takaoka K. Involvement of phosphodiesterase isozymes in osteoblastic differentiation. J Bone Miner Res. 2002;17:249–56.
101. Waki Y, Horita T, Miyamoto K, Ohya K, Kasugai S. Effects of XT-44, a phosphodiesterase 4 inhibitor, in osteoblastgenesis and osteoclastgenesis in culture and its therapeutic effects in rat osteopenia models. Jpn J Pharmacol. 1999;79:477–83.
102. Watts NB, Diab DL. Long-term use of bisphosphonates in osteoporosis. J Clin Endocrinol Metab. 2010;95:1555–65.
103. Wimalawansa SJ. Nitric oxide: novel therapy for osteoporosis. Expert Opin Pharmacother. 2008;9:3025–44.
104. Yamagami H, Nishioka T, Ochiai E, Fukushima K, Nomura M, Kasugai S, Moritani S, Yokogawa K, Miyamoto K. Inhibition of osteoclastogenesis by a phosphodiesterase 4 inhibitor XT-611 through synergistic action with endogenous prostaglandin E2. Biochem Pharmacol. 2003;66:801–7.
105. Yang X, Karsenty G. Transcription factors in bone: developmental and pathological aspects. Trends Mol Med. 2002;8:340–5.
106. Yao W, Tian XY, Chen J, Setterberg RB, Lundy MW, Chmielzwski P, Froman CA, Jee WS. Rolipram, a phosphodiesterase 4 inhibitor, prevented cancellous and cortical bone loss by inhibiting endosteal bone resorption and maintaining the elevated periosteal bone formation in adult ovariectomized rats. J Musculoskelet Neuronal Interact. 2007;7:119–30.
107. Yohay DA, Zhang J, Thrailkill KM, Arthur JM, Quarles LD. Role of serum in the developmental

expression of alkaline phosphatase in MC3T3-E1 osteoblasts. J Cell Physiol. 1994;158:467–75.

108. Zajac JD, Livesey SA, Michelangeli VP, Rodan SB, Rodan GA, Martin TJ. Glucocorticoid treatment facilitates cyclic adenosine 3′,5′-monophosphate-dependent protein kinase response in parathyroid hormone-responsive osteogenic sarcoma cells. Endocrinology. 1986;118:2059–64.

109. Zaragoza C, Lopez-Rivera E, Garcia-Rama C, Saura M, Martinez-Ruiz A, Lizarbe TR, Martin-de-Lara F, Lamas S. Cbfa-1 mediates nitric oxide regulation of MMP-13 in osteoblasts. J Cell Sci. 2006;119:1896–902.

Nervous System Diseases, Disorders, and Bone: Emerging Therapeutics and Treatment Options

17

Mary F. Barbe and Steven N. Popoff

Keywords
Bone • Bone innervation • Neuropeptides • Glutamate signaling • Leptin
Spinal cord injury • Traumatic brain injury

17.1 Introduction

Clinical literature and experimental data support a link between neurological disorders and bone metabolism. Because bone tissue has a rich nerve supply, as discussed in this chapter, it has long been speculated that nerve input has an active role in bone metabolism. Despite the limitations of conventional histological techniques that limited a full exploration of this question for decades, clinical observations of bone changes in patients with neurological disorders, such as spinal cord injury, in which patients have localized osteopenia, increased lower extremity fractures, and increased sites of pathological ossification have fueled researchers in their studies of the relationships between the nervous and bone systems. It is now known that bone metabolism and growth are regulated not only by mechanical loading, humoral factors (such as hormones), and local factors (such as cytokines released by osteoclasts), but also by neuronal signals released from the peripheral and central nervous systems. This has created a new field of neuroskeletal biology from which key findings are covered in this chapter.

17.2 Innervation of Bone: Where and What Types of Nerve Fibers?

Knowing the extent of the innervation of bone by peripheral nerves is essential for understanding the interactions between the nervous system and bone. For example, bone resorption after peripheral nerve injury, stroke, or in association with cerebral palsy may not be just a consequence of disuse (as a result of reduced loading from muscles or weight bearing) as much of the clinical literature suggests but may also be the consequence of bone denervation.

A large number of papers, beginning in 1846 [59], have identified sympathetic and sensory peripheral nerve endings in periosteal, cancellous, and cortical bone regions (see reviews of the early literature by Calvo [23], Thurston [139],

M.F. Barbe, Ph.D. (✉) • S.N. Popoff, Ph.D.
Department of Anatomy and Cell Biology,
Temple School of Medicine,
3500 N. Broad Street, Philadelphia,
PA 19140, USA
e-mail: mbarbe@temple.edu

F. Bronner et al. (eds.), *Bone-Metabolic Functions and Modulators*, Topics in Bone Biology,
DOI 10.1007/978-1-4471-2745-1_17, © Springer-Verlag London 2012

and Sherman [130]; see also [40, 65, 96, 129]). The sensory innervation is most commonly used to explain the phenomenon of bone pain, while the sympathetic motor innervation is commonly used to explain the central nervous system control of bone formation and resorption [5, 28, 113, 135].

Cancellous bone and periosteum are richly innervated, particularly in epiphyseal regions (Fig. 17.1). In the periosteum, most nerve fibers are thin, unmyelinated fibers. In cancellous bone, nerve fibers innervate trabeculae facing the growth plates. Many types of nerve fibers are in the vicinity of osteoblasts, osteoclasts, hematopoietic cells, and bone lining cells (see Sects. 17.2.1 and 17.2.2 below and in Table 17.1). Interestingly, mineralized bone regions subject to the greatest mechanical load have high densities of nerve fibers, particularly peptidergic nerve fibers [27, 96], suggesting neural innervation is involved in "sensing" mechanical stress on bone.

Nerve fibers also run within the Haversian and Volkmann's canals in cortical bone. Furthermore, intraosseous blood vessels are heavily supplied by both sensory and sympathetic nerves, which follow nutrient arteries into bones as part of the fine network of nerve fibers that accompany vessels (*nervi vasorum*) [40, 129]. The association of nerve fibers with blood vessels provides a structural basis for a role of the autonomic nervous system in regulating bone blood flow and metabolism [40, 62].

17.2.1 Bone Is Richly Innervated by Intraosseous Sympathetic Nerves

Normal bone is supplied by sympathetic nerve fibers that are immunoreactive for several neuropeptides: vasoactive intestinal peptide (*VIP*): neuropeptide Y (*NPY*); the rate-limiting enzyme in catecholamine synthesis, tyrosine hydroxylase (*TH*); and dopamine beta-hydroxylase (*DβH*) (Table 17.1) [62, 65]. VIP-immunoreactive (-IR) fibers are frequent in epiphyseal, but sparse in diaphyseal regions [65, 129]. These fibers are localized to periosteum, on the trabeculae of subcortical bone, and associated with periosteal vascular elements and hematopoietic cells. In contrast, TH-IR and NPY-IR fibers have more diaphyseal and epiphyseal distribution compared to VIP-IR nerve fibers, and are found in cancellous and cortical bone, bone marrow, periosteum, and on blood vessels. Like VIP fibers, TH-IR nerve fibers have been identified in contact with hematopoietic cells [129] (Table 17.1). DβH-IR fibers are associated primarily with blood vessels [62].

VIP-IR nerve fibers originate from sympathetic ganglia [65]. This has been as shown by injecting fast blue into rib periosteum. Thoracic sympathetic ganglia, but not sensory dorsal root ganglia, were labeled in a retrograde fashion. Chemical sympathectomy using guanethidine monosulfate treatment (an adrenergic neuronal blocking agent) reduced VIP-, NPY-, and DβH-immunoreactivity in periosteum of treated animals compared to controls. These findings, further verify their sympathetic origin [62].

17.2.2 Bone Is Highly Innervated by Sensory Intraosseous Nerves

Immunohistochemical analysis of frozen-sectioned bones that are not demineralized, so as to preserve neurotransmitter antigenicity, has revealed several types of afferent nerve fibers in bone, including substance P, calcitonin gene-related peptide (*CGRP*), and glutaminergic (*Glu*) fibers. Substance P is a peptidergic neurotransmitter localized primarily in fine caliber, unmyelinated C fibers, the sensory neurons that carry the sensation of pain to the spinal cord and brain. Substance P is the key excitatory neurotransmitter that is responsible for the mediation of pain sensation after its release from terminal endings on the C fibers and then binding to neurokinin receptors on postsynaptic neurons. CGRP is a 37-amino-acid peptide generated by the calcitonin gene by means of alternative RNA splicing [55]. CGRP belongs to the calcitonin (*CT*) family of peptides, which also includes CT, amylin, and adrenomedullin, as well as the recently described intermedin and calcitonin-receptor-stimulating

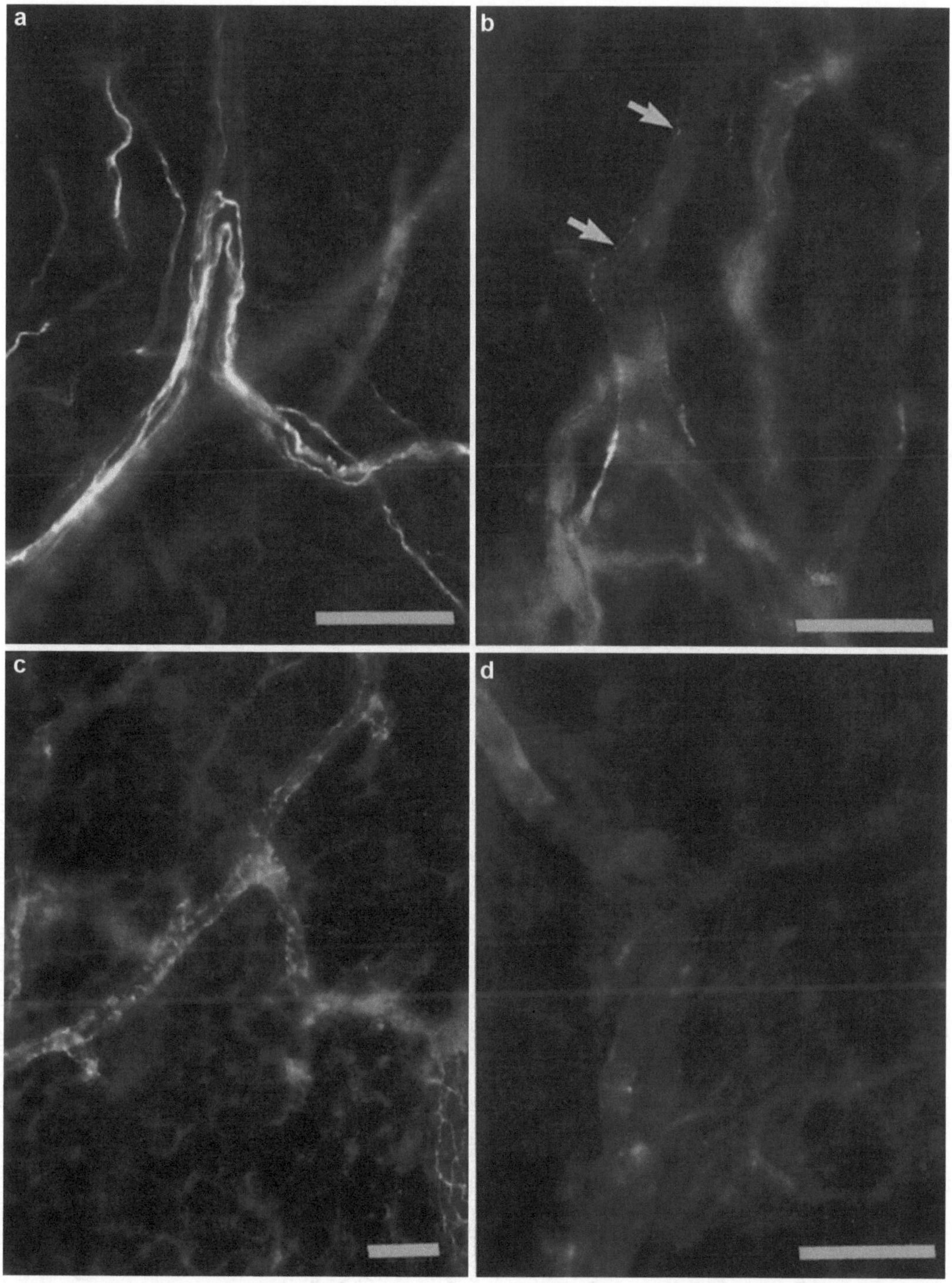

Fig. 17.1 Effects of denervations in periosteum from calvaria. (**a**) CGRP immunoreactivity in control rat is intense and widely distributed; (**b**) CGRP immunoreactivity is largely eliminated in neonatally capsaicin-treated animals, although a few immunoreactive fibers (*arrows*) are still present; (**c**) NPY immunoreactivity is present on blood vessels in control animal; and (**d**) NPY immunoreactivity largely eliminated in calvarial periosteum from guanethidine-treated animals. *Bars* 100 micrometer (or μm) (With kind permission from Springer Science + Business Media: Hill and Elde [62]. Springer-Verlag)

Table 17.1 The relationship of key neurotransmitters and their receptors with bone cells

Neurotransmitters in nerve fibers innervating bone			
Neurotransmitters on nerves	Bone cells in the vicinity of these nerve fibers	Receptor	Bone cell expressing receptor
Bradykinin	Osteoblasts		
Calcitonin gene-related peptide (CGRP)	Osteoclasts Endothelium	Calcitonin receptor (CTR) Calcitonin receptor-like receptor (CRLR)	Bone-marrow-derived macrophages; osteoblasts
Dopamine beta-hydroxylase (DβH)			
Glutamate (Glu)	Osteoblasts	*N*-methyl-D-aspartate acid receptors[a] (NMDAR); kainic acid receptors[a] (GluR567) AMPA receptors[a] (GluR2/3, GluR4)	Osteoblasts; preosteoblasts; osteoclasts; osteocytes; bone lining cells
Neuropeptide Y (NPY)	Bone lining cells	Y2 receptor	
Serotonin (5-HT)	Osteoblasts	5-HT_{2B} receptor[a] (5-HT_{2B}R)	Osteoblasts
Substance P		Neurokinin-1 receptor (NK1R)	Osteoclasts > osteoblasts and osteocytes
Tyrosine hydroxylase (TH) (a rate-limiting enzyme for 5-HT synthesis)	Preosteoblasts; osteoblasts and osteocytes cell lines Hematopoietic cells		
Vasoactive intestinal peptide (VIP) Pituitary adenylate cyclase-activating peptide (PACAP; a VIP analog)	Hematopoietic cells; epiphyseal cartilage canals; osteoclasts	VIP-1R[a]; VIP-2R[a]; PACAP-R	Osteoclasts; osteoblasts
Neuropeptides produced by hypothalamus that affect bone			
Neurotransmitters/neuropeptides	Bone cells affected	Neurotransmitter receptor	Bone cell expression of these receptors
Leptin	Osteoblasts indirectly via sympathetic nervous system (SNS)[b]	Leptin receptor in hypothalamus Leptin acts on SNS to stimulate adrb2 on osteoblasts	None[b]
Noradrenaline	Osteoblasts; osteoclasts	Adrenergic beta-2 receptor (adrb2) (stimulated by catecholamine release by sympathetic nervous system)	Osteoblasts[a]; osteoclasts[c]
Neuromedin U (NMU)	Osteoblasts' molecular clock indirectly by unknown mechanism[b]	NMU receptor in hypothalamus	Unknown link to osteoblasts

[a]Indicates a functional receptor
[b]Leptin and neuromedin U regulate bone metabolism by central mechanisms only
[c]adrb2 not functional in osteoclasts

peptide ([75, 91]; see also Chap. 6). Like substance P with which it frequently colocalizes, CGRP is associated with the mediation of pain sensation. CGRP is also present on autonomic nerves [55, 75, 79, 80]. Both substance P and CGRP are released from nerve terminals after stimulation or sensitization and have been identified as potent vasodilators and as playing neurotrophic effector roles [63, 66, 73, 90].

Nerve fibers that are immunoreactive for both substance P and CGRP densely innervate trabeculae on the epiphyseal side of growth plates. They are found also in the periosteum and are associated with blood vessels, but are less frequent in diaphyseal and metaphyseal regions [17, 57, 58, 62, 73]. Each is sparse in cortical bone. Substance P nerve fibers usually enter the medullary space with blood vessels but then branch off and terminate as unmyelinated fine caliber axons in the marrow cavity [70–72]. CGRP-IR fibers are also located in the marrow space in close contact with osteoclasts [61] (Table 17.1). Retrograde labeling with fast blue and Fluorogold from the periosteum to sensory ganglia established substance P- and CGRP-IR fibers as bone afferents [63]. Capsaicin (a sensory nerve specific neurotoxin) treatment chemically denervates sensory fibers and reduces these nerve fibers in periosteum [62]. Bone fracture and even a light touch to the periosteum elicit intense pain. Therefore, the occurrence of substance P and CGRP nerve endings in bone may be of clinical importance.

Glutamate (Glu) is the primary excitatory neurotransmitter of the peripheral and central nervous systems, known for transduction of touch, pressure, and mechanical stimulation. Elevation of glutamate in skin, muscles, and tendons is associated with chronic pain conditions, presumably due to nociceptor sensitization, although this effect has not been studied with regard to bone pain. A dense network of thin Glu-IR nerve fibers is present along bone blood vessels and in close proximity to osteoblastic cells located on endosteal surfaces [129] (Table 17.1). A neuronal glutamate transporter, VGLUT-1 (one of the vesicular glutamate transporters), is present in bone. Also, osteoclasts and osteoblasts express several different subtypes of Glu receptors (GluR; Table 17.1). Changes in bone mass due to mechanical loading have been linked to changes in expression of glutamate signalling components in bone (see Sect. 17.3.1).

17.3 Bone Cells Have Functional Receptors for Neurotransmitters

While no typical synapses have been observed between axons and bone cells, direct contact has been demonstrated [29]. More importantly, most bone cells express a variety of functional neurotransmitter receptors ([57, 60, 129, 132, 134, 135]; see Table 17.1). The presence of functional receptors in the network that innervate bone tissue suggests a neural component to the regulation of bone metabolism. Alternatively, bone cells may simply use a similar signaling system to regulate bone homeostasis.

17.3.1 Evidence for Glutamate Receptors and Glutamate Signaling in Bone

Glutaminergic signaling is not restricted to the central nervous system (CNS), but is also involved in the regulation of bone homeostasis [104, 113, 132, 135]. Glutamate works through two main classes of glutamate receptors: metabotropic receptors that signal through diacylglycerol, IP3 and cyclic AMP (e.g., the metabotropic glutamate receptor type 8, mGluR-8), and ionotropic receptors that can alter membrane permeability to cations, for example, *N*-methyl-D-aspartic acid (NMDA) receptors and non-NMDA receptors (AMPA and kainate). There are also glutamate transporters in plasma membranes (e.g., GLAST, GLT-1) and in vesicles (VGLUT isoforms 1–3). These transporters have key roles in regulating extracellular glutamate concentrations. VGLUT1 is involved in glutamate osteoclast signaling to regulate the balance between bone resorption and formation [104, 105]. When osteoclasts degrade bone, they endocytose the degradation fragments, which are packed into transcytotic vesicles.

VLUT1 is localized with the transcytotic vesicles along with the degraded bone products and serves to accumulate L-glutamate, which therefore is also colocalized in the transcytotic vesicles. L-glutamate and the degraded bone products are cosecreted in a calcium-dependent manner upon stimulation with KCL or ATP and exocytose through membranes of osteoclast basolateral origin. The released L-glutamate suppresses further transcytosis through an mGLUR-8-mediated inhibitory cyclic AMP cascade. Osteoclasts from VLUT1-knockout mice ($VGLUT1^{-/-}$) lack the KCL- or ATP-dependent secretion of L-glutamate, have enhanced bone digestive activity, and develop osteoporosis [104]. NMDA, AMPA, and kainic acid receptor antagonists inhibit osteoclast resorptive abilities [134]. Thus osteoclasts use glutamate signalling as a type of negative feedback reporting system.

NMDA receptors and several of the GluR receptors are present on the surfaces of rat osteoblasts and osteoclasts, but not those of osteocytes [60, 134]. Glutamate NMDA receptors detect activation and membrane depolarization in the CNS and appear to have similar functions in osteoblasts. Mechanical loading of forelimb and hindlimb bones leads to a loss of immunoexpression of GluR2/3, GluR4, GluR567, and NMDAR2A on osteoclasts and of NMDAR2A, NMDAR2B, GluR2/3, and GluR4 in bone lining cells, compared to contralaterally unloaded limbs [134]. Because rat osteoblasts express these receptors, and because mechanical loading modulates glutamate receptor subunit levels in bone, the NMDA receptors may serve as a rapid sensing/signaling system in bone [132]. Osteoblasts have a functional NMDA receptor with a classical voltage-sensitive Mg^{2+} regulatory block [60]. In other words, these receptors function like neuronal NMDA receptors to detect both receptor activation and membrane depolarization. Osteoblasts, like osteoclasts, also release glutamate by vesicular exocytosis [132]. Binding of glutamate to AMPA and NMDA receptors initiates signaling cascades that autoregulate further glutamate exocytosis. Thus, both osteoblasts and osteoclasts use paracrine/autocrine glutamate signaling as a type of activity reporting system, but perhaps also as a between (juxtacrine) cell type signaling system to regulate the balance of bone resorption and formation for the maintenance of bone mass.

17.3.2 Evidence for Cannabinoid Receptors and the Endocannabinoid System in Bone

The endocannabinoid system plays an important role in regulating processes like pain perception, appetite, energy balance, and immune responses. Recent studies have shown that endocannabinoids and their G-protein-coupled cannabinoid receptors type 1 (CB1) and type 2 (CB2) are in the skeleton. Knockout mice in which either the CB1 or CB2 receptor has been deleted exhibit abnormalities in bone mass [10, 20]. Even though it is evident that the endocannabinoid system regulates the differentiation and function of bone cells, the precise mechanisms of action are only beginning to be understood.

Both the CB1 and CB2 receptors are expressed in bone cells. CB2 receptors are expressed in a wide variety of cells within the bone microenvironment, including osteoblasts and osteoclasts [68, 110]. CB2 expression increases when bone marrow stromal cells are grown in osteogenic medium, in parallel to the expression of osteoblastic marker genes, such as tissue-nonspecific alkaline phosphatase (*TNSALP*), parathyroid hormone receptor (*PTHRc1*), and the osteoblastic master regulatory gene RUNX2 [110]. The presence of functional CB1 receptors in bone cells is more controversial, but CB1 receptors have been reported in osteoblasts and osteoclasts at levels that are lower than those that are for CB2 receptors in these same cells [68, 69, 110]. CB1 receptors have been detected in sympathetic nerve processes innervating bone. CB1 may therefore regulate bone turnover by a neural mechanism [137, 138], as opposed to the local production of CB1 receptor ligands by bone cells.

There is now also evidence that indicates that the main endocannabinoids, 2-arachidonoylglycerol (2-AG) and anandamide, are produced locally in the bone microenvironment. The levels of these endocannabinoids in bone are high and comparable to levels in the brain [9, 138]. Inasmuch as blood levels of 2-AG and anandamide are much lower than in brain and bone, the endocannabinoids found in bone are likely produced locally [9]. In fact, both ligands are produced by osteoblasts and osteoclasts in culture [121, 138]. In addition, the 2-AG synthesizing enzymes, diacylglycerol α and β, are also expressed in bone cells [138]. These findings implicate the occurrence of a functional skeletal endocannabinoid system.

Recognition that the endocannabinoid system regulates bone metabolism is only beginning. Future studies will have to elucidate the precise mechanisms that activate CB receptors in bone cells and identify the signaling pathways that are activated, the regulation of how the endocannabinoids bring about receptor expression in bone cells, and how CB receptor agonists and antagonists affect bone cell differentiation and function. Another critical area research must focus is on the relative importance of central versus peripheral mechanisms in regulating bone metabolism. These types of studies have the potential to lead to the development of novel anabolic therapeutic strategies for the treatment of various forms of osteopenia (e.g., postmenopausal and age-related osteoporosis) and to accelerate bone formation in situations (e.g., fracture healing, distraction osteogenesis) where such intervention would have a favorable clinical outcome.

17.4 Neuro-osteogenic Networks Modulate Bone Remodeling

Nerves innervating bone have a variety of neuropeptide receptors, including noradrenaline, serotonin, and glutamate. Receptors for most of these neural mediators have been identified (see Table 17.1). Administration of these neurotransmitters affects activities of osteoblasts and osteoclasts (for reviews, see [42, 58, 92, 113]). CGRP is made by cells of the central and peripheral nervous system and is secreted by nerve terminals. CGRP secretion provokes intracellular cyclic AMP signaling events in osteoblasts and stimulates their proliferation and the synthesis of the insulin-like growth factors (IGF-1 and IGF-2), interleukin-6, and collagen [42], most likely by acting through a receptor shared with amylin [17, 73]. Injection of CGRP protects rats partially against gonadectomy-induced bone loss, and *Cgrp*-deficient mice are mildly osteopenic. CGRP also acts directly on osteoclasts through cyclic AMP signaling to inhibit bone resorption by inhibiting osteoclast motility [147].

The concept that neurotransmitters contribute to the regulation of bone mass derives support from the reduction in bone mineral density (BMD) that follows the systemic administration of an antagonist against the main receptor for substance P, the NK1 receptor (LY303870). For more discussion, see Sect. 17.5.1). Application of the NMDA receptor antagonist, MK801, and the AMPA/kainic acid receptor antagonist, NBQX, to osteoclast cultures inhibited their resorptive function. This finding suggests that the receptor function of the NMDA and the kainic acid receptors is required for normal osteoclast function [134]. For a discussion of glutamate signaling in bone loading, see Sect. 17.3.2. The role played by serotonin in osteoblast function has been discussed by Collet et al. [33]. These authors point out that the serotonin receptor expression of 5-HT_{2B}R increases in vivtro as osteoblasts differentiate. Primary osteoblast cultures that are depleted of this receptor have reduced proliferation. Knockout mice for this receptor ($5\text{-}HT_{2B}R^{-/-}$) display reduced bone density and osteopenia due to decreased bone formation [33]. Thus, bone turnover can be regulated by the local effects of neurotransmitters on osteoblasts and osteoclasts.

Evidence of central nervous system (CNS) regulation of bone formation and resorption has been reviewed [5, 28, 113, 135]. The most striking evidence for this higher neural regulatory system comes from studies that show that leptin regulates bone remodeling through the hypothalamus. Leptin, a 16-kDa peptide hormone synthesized by adipocytes, affects appetite and energy metabolism by binding to leptin receptors in the hypothalamus. The signaling mechanisms between adipocytes and the hypothalamus are not yet known. It is known, however, that the hypothalamic relay nuclei for leptin are the arcuate in the ventromedial (VMH) and paraventricular (PVN) hypothalamus. It is also known that functional VMH neurons are required for leptin-dependent central regulation of bone mass. Whether leptin acts directly or indirectly on VMH nuclei to modulate sympathetic activity is not yet known. In human obesity, bone mass is increased, and reduced leptin signaling leads to a diminished bone mass. Leptin-deficient mice (*ob/ob*) and *db/db* mice that lack functional leptin receptors (Y2 receptors) are obese and sterile due to hypogonadism, a condition that is commonly associated with osteoporosis in humans. Interestingly, their bone mass is not reduced, but rather increased. The *ob/ob* mice have high bone mass even when fed diets intended to make them lean. Mice with lipodystrophy have low body weight, low serum leptin, and high bone mass [38]. Their high bone mass phenotype is rescued by transgenic expression of leptin [42]. Even humans with lipodystrophy as a result of a mutation in the leptin gene have high bone mass.

Leptin's control of bone remodeling is not humoral, but is mediated by the sympathetic nervous system (*SNS*) [37, 42, 113, 125, 135]. Intracerebroventricular infusion of leptin into *ob/ob* mice at a dose that does not leak into the peripheral circulation normalizes their bone formation parameters and bone mass. This indicates that leptin acts through the central nervous system [38]. Fusing two *ob/ob* by parabiosis and then infusing one of the mice intracerebroventricularly with leptin leads to a decrease in bone mass in the infused mouse, but to no change in bone mass in the contralateral mouse [32, 132, 136]. Evidence that the sympathetic nervous system is the mediator of leptin comes from studies that show the sympathetic tone of *ob/ob* mice to be low. Sympathectomy eliminates the effect of leptin, with leptin infusion increasing catecholamine secretion. This, in turn, increases osteoblast proliferation and differentiation through beta 2 adrenergic receptors. Leptin infusion also increases bone resorption. A clear central neuronal circuit has been identified from the spinal cord and brainstem to the hypothalamus using recombinant pseudorabies virus labeling [125]. Osteoblasts have been identified as located next to sympathetic nerve fibers in bone osteoblasts and also express beta 2 adrenergic receptors (*adrb2*). Mice treated with a general beta-blocker (isoproterenol) undergo a decrease in bone mass, and mice lacking the dopamine beta-hydroxylase enzyme necessary for production of norepinephrine and epinephrine have a high bone mass phenotype and exhibit an increase in bone formation parameters. Several studies have shown that beta-blockers constitute effective treatment for patients with osteoporosis who have bone loss due to altered sympathetic function, such as in patients with complex complicated regional pain syndrome. Because of the signaling pathways that are involved, beta agonists may be candidates for the treatment of bone disorders that arise from nervous system disorders.

17.5 Peripheral Nerve and Spinal Cord Injuries and Disorders Affecting Lower Motor Neurons and Sensory Afferents: Are the Effects on Bone the Result of Disuse, Denervation, or Both?

Loss of the local nerve regulatory system is postulated to contribute to negative bone balance in denervated bone. Studies in animals and humans have investigated the peripheral changes in models of disuse, such as spaceflight, bed rest, hindlimb immobilization, tetrodotoxin, spinal cord transection, or denervation. However, studies that involve peripheral nerve transection, nerve crush, or nerve compression should also be considered as models of bone denervation.

Clinical correlates of full or partial peripheral nerve injury in animals include nerve crush, compression, stretch, or traction injuries, as in brachial plexus injuries, carpal or tarsal tunnel syndromes, flaccid paralysis associated with spinal cord injury, and hypotonic cerebral palsy. Bone loss as a result of flaccid paralysis is quite severe [14]. While spinal cord injury is also associated with spastic paralysis due to loss of supraspinal inhibitory control of spinal cord motor neurons (see below), if the cell bodies of motor neurons located in the ventral horns of spinal cord segment are lesioned, then flaccid paralysis occurs due to loss of the lower motor neurons. This is associated with segmental muscle weakness, hypotonia and atrophy. Furthermore, a severe thoracic spinal cord lesion in the ventral horn would usually include a loss of the sympathetic motor neuronal cell bodies from the adjacent intermediate horn of the spinal cord and resulting loss of sympathetic neuronal signaling to bone. Hemisection or complete lesions of the spinal cord also affect the dorsal horns, dorsal root ganglia and sensory nerve signaling. Clinical problems that involve bone pain as a consequence of fracture, Charcot neuropathies, and complex regional pain syndrome should each be re-evaluated in light of the neuroosseous axis [78], inasmuch as each is also associated with bone loss.

17.5.1 Effects of Peripheral Nerve Transection (Neurectomy) and Bone Injuries in Animal Models

Findings from experimental studies support a role for peripheral neurons in the modulation of bone turnover. These experiments include sciatic neurectomy and other types of experimentally induced peripheral nerve injuries, chemical sensory denervation, and chemical sympathectomy. Clinical correlates include peripheral neuropathies from diabetes and chemotherapy, as well as nerve compression and crush injuries. Reduced bone mineral density (BMD) is often a characteristic of these clinical conditions.

Sciatic neurectomy is a standard model of disuse osteopenia, as atrophy of muscles from the denervation leads to reduced movement and less bone loading. For example, unilateral sciatic neurectomy leads to disuse with associated muscle atrophy, accelerated bone resorption, and bone loss. It is also associated with a total ipsilateral loss of the sympathetic nervi vasorum in nutrient vessels to the ipsilateral, denervated hindlimb [40]. Likewise, surgical sympathectomy via unilateral selective ganglionectomy also results in an ipsilateral loss of the sympathetic nervi vasorum in nutrient vessels supplied by the removed ganglia [40]. Chemical sympathectomy of adult rats using guanethidine (a specific sympathetic neurotoxin) decreases TH and VIP fibers (but not CGRP or substance P fibers). At the same time, the number of osteoclasts is reduced, as are their progenitors in the denervated bone [30, 62]. These findings give support to a crucial role by sympathetic nerve fibers in the local regulation of bone metabolism.

Sciatic neurectomy also reduces substance P and CGRP-IR content of nerves in bone [61, 83]. Osteoclasts show increased TRACPase activity and increased cement formation at sites of reduced CGRP-IR nerves. This indicates site-specific increases in increased osteoclastic bone resorption after nerve section [61]. Chemical sensory denervation of adult rats using capsaicin reduces CGRP- and substance P-IR nerve fibers in bone and decreases osteoclast recruitment and attachment [1]. This is a further confirmation of the sensory origin of these nerve fibers. Substance P stimulates formation of bone colonies in cultured bone marrow cells and stimulates bone formation in primary cultures of osteoblasts [3, 131]. Release of substance P by nerves in bone may therefore directly stimulate osteoblastic bone formation through NK1 receptors. Reduction in the levels of substance P after nerve transection contributes to bone loss.

Sciatic nerve section also leads to bone loss in the contralateral intact hindlimb (albeit to a lesser extent than in the ipsilateral denervated hindlimb) despite the lack of apparent disuse of that limb [83]. Results of ex vivo cultures of bone marrow from the neurectomized limbs show not only reduced osteoblastic activity but also increased osteoclast precursor differentiation and osteoclastogenesis, as compared to cultures from intact limbs [123]. Either of the two changes – increased osteoclastogenesis and decreased osteoblast activity – may contribute to the contralateral loss in bone density. Studies have also shown that alterations in contralateral nerve anatomy and function and neurotransmitter expression occur typically after neurectomy [83]. The reduction in substance P in the ipsilateral denervated limb noted above also occurs in the contralateral intact bone [83], and use of a NK1 receptor antagonist, LY303870, enhances this bone loss even further. This suggests that residual substance P signaling has contributed to residual bone integrity bilaterally.

Studies from the field of neuroscience may also help explain the contralateral changes. The presence of "mirror allodynia" (contralateral pain) in cases of unilateral chronic constriction nerve injury, where there is a contralateral spread of symptoms to the uninjured limb, provides evidence that dorsal root ganglia and the spinal cord exhibit plasticity after nerve injury [26, 36, 53, 67, 101, 144]. These changes have been termed "central sensitization." Not only is there an increase in cytokines and neurotransmitters, such as substance P, at the site of ipsilateral nerve injury, but there are also central changes in neuronal structure, protein production, function, and survival, as well as biochemical alterations in the responses by dorsal root ganglia, afferent terminals, spinal cord neurons and glia [145]. For example, proinflammatory cytokines, TNFα (alpha) and IL-1β (beta), are significantly increased in spinal cord neurons and microglia in models of peripheral neuropathy, chronic constriction, and cryoneurolysis [36, 43–46]. The released neuromodulators spread to nearby nerve terminals, affecting other nerves and postsynaptic sensory processing, in turn leading to remote and contralateral effects [26].

In a study by Sample et al. [124], neuronal signaling between upper extremity bones and the spinal cord was blocked by means of a transient perineural anesthesia of the brachial plexus. The blockade of neuronal signaling during ulna loading significantly reduced bone formation when compared to bones loaded without anesthetic blockade. There were persistent increases in bone substance P levels after a single loading, compared to the unloaded contralateral ulna. Perineural anesthesia of the brachial plexus produced even higher levels of substance P in the loaded bones. These results are controversial [132], but provide further support that bone innervation modulates the function of bone.

17.5.2 Effects of Peripheral Nerve Injuries on Bone in Patient Populations

In addition to the brachial plexus injury study discussed above [124], carpal tunnel syndrome (CTS) is a type of peripheral nerve injury. CTS is a slow constriction nerve injury that affects the median nerve as it passes through the carpal tunnel of the wrist. Erselcan et al. [47] examined 33 premenopausal women with electrophysiologically diagnosed CTS for bone density modifications in the forearm (radius and ulna) and the metacarpal bones. Bone mineral density (BMD) was decreased 7% in the distal radius and ulna and 18% in metacarpal bones in subjects with thenar muscle atrophy; disease duration (mean duration 3.2 ± 2.7 years) was significantly correlated with the decrease in metacarpal bone density. These findings suggest the need for further studies to assess the clinical significance and morbidity of this pathology, especially in patients with thenar muscle atrophy. It is not unexpected that thenar atrophy might reduce skeletal loading of the metacarpal bones and lead to reduced BMD. However, few studies have examined the role of the confounding variables that may change bone mass and integrity in patients with nerve compression injuries.

17.5.3 Neural Pain from Bone Tissues in Patients with Complex Regional Pain Syndrome

Complex regional syndrome disorder, the current nomenclature for reflex sympathetic dystrophy (RSD) [100], is a neurological disease characterized by local sympathetic activation, osteopenia, and increased bone fractures. The term complex regional pain syndrome type I (CRPS-I) replaced RSD for patients with no known nerve injuries. CRPS-II replaced causalgia or patients with known nerve injuries, although few of the 90% of patients diagnosed with CRPS-I have undergone a full neuromuscular consultation [109]. CRPS-I is a human disease characterized by hyperadrenergic activity and a 31% incidence in distal tibial fracture. Many CRPS patients experience chronic pain. Newer ultrastructural studies indicate that small-fiber (type C, or nociceptive, fibers) losses predominant in the axonal degeneration that is present in patients with CRPS-I [4, 108, 109]. The neuropathic pain present in these patients is most likely due to ectopic firing from surviving small caliber fibers termed irritable nociceptors

[146] or from changes in the central terminals of the damaged neurons with subsequent central glial activation that then sensitize nearby glia and postsynaptic neurons, as described earlier in Sect. 17.5.1.

Many patients with CRPS-I complain of deep pain in their affected bones, which can show evidence of bone marrow edema, hyperperfusion, endosteal and intracortical excavations, and trabecular bone demineralization or resorption. The affected bones take up more tracer in the last phase of bone scintigraphy [86, 87]. The increased tracer uptake reflects an increase in osteoclast activity, which may explain why bisphosphonates, β(beta)-blockers, and other inhibitors of bone resorption can reduce CRPS pain [2, 113]. The bone changes are postulated to be a result of the observed small-fiber axonal degeneration, with associated reductions in the secretion of neuromodulators, such as substance P and CGRP, from these nerve terminals into bone [3, 61, 71, 83, 111].

17.5.4 Treatments for Denervation-Induced Bone Loss

The effects of denervation on muscle atrophy and bone loss can be partly prevented in animal models and in patients with the aid of whole body vibration, exercise, androgenic steroids, and low-frequency ultrasound therapy. Capacitively delivered low-frequency electric fields suppress osteoclast-like cell activity in vitro and reverse the osteoporosis caused by denervation of the rat tibia [19].

Testosterone replacement therapy increases BMD in hypogonadic men with idiopathic osteoporosis. Treatment with testosterone and nandrolone is effective in blocking immobilization-induced decreases in BMD in a rat model of hindlimb unloading. Nandrolone has also been used to treat denervation-induced bone loss in a rat model of sciatic neurectomy [24]. In that study, nandrolone, if administered for 28 days beginning at 20 days post neurectomy, preserved 80% and 60% of BMD in the tibia and femur (which had 12% and 7% losses at 56 days after denervation), respectively. Nandrolone treatment also increased BMD of the sham-transected hindlimb tibia and femur. The time of administration of nandrolone was chosen on the basis of an earlier study [148]. Nandrolone may therefore constitute effective therapy for low BMD due to severe disuse and denervation. Complex regional pain disorder has been treated with β(beta)-blockers for pain and to halt the bone destruction associated with this disorder [113].

Intraperitoneal administration of anti-NGF antibody has been tested for its ability to reduce pain in a rat fracture model of CRPS because nerve growth factor (*NGF*) administration leads to nociceptive sensitization in rodents [6, 7, 15, 122]. CGRP and substance P levels increase post-fracture, each a known sensitizer of nociceptors; anti-NGF treatment significantly decreased their levels at 4 weeks postfracture. Also, anti-NGF treatment reduced the development of mechanical allodynia and inhibited fracture-induced bone loss, but did not abrogate postfracture edema or enhanced cytokine levels [7]. The differential effects of NGF underscore the complexity of this condition. Anti-NGF treatment may prove useful in treating CRPS. In another rat model of CRPS, the effectiveness of a cytokine inhibitor, pentoxifylline, was tested because cytokines are both nociceptor sensitizers and induce osteoclast activity. Pentoxifylline reduced cytokine levels, attenuated nociceptive sensitization, and decreased hindpaw temperature, but was not effective in reducing fracture-induced edema or bone loss [143]. These findings support the generally held belief that CRPS is a syndrome that involves multiple pathophysiological mechanisms that will require blockade of more than one target molecule.

17.6 Brain and Spinal Cord Injuries: Are the Effects on Bone the Result of Increased Loading from Spasticity, Disuse, Altered Neuromodulation, or a Combination?

Spastic paralysis is the result of injury to descending (upper) motor pathways in the brain or spinal cord. It is defined as velocity-dependent increases in tonic stretch reflexes (which increase muscle tone), peak muscle torque, and coactivations of muscles around a joint that results from hyperexcitability of stretch reflexes [88, 116, 117]. Each of these factors can increase strain and traction from the muscles on bones. Since the response of bone is osteogenic, this leads to secondary bone malformation such as joint valgus, varus, and rotational changes. The combination of immobilization and disuse plus changes in neural input lead to the reduced bone mineral content (BMC) and the underdeveloped bone structure observed in children with cerebral palsy, and the osteoporsosis observed in patients with spinal cord injury.

17.6.1 Effects of Spinal Cord Injury on Bone

Patients with spinal cord injury (SCI) have localized osteopenia, an increase in bone fragility, and in the incidence of lower extremity fractures. Healing of these fractures is also reduced, and sites of pathological ossification are increased [94].The most common explanation for the bone loss with SCI is immobilization or disuse due to nonloading of the bone. However, approximately 40% of all patients with SCI report problematic spastic paralysis which would result in an increase in loading on involved bones [93]. The degree of spasticity has been reported to reduce the risk of osteoporosis and the decline in BMD in individuals with SCI [94]. Unfortunately, the increase in bone fragility and reduction in fracture healing are not spared by the presence of spastic paralysis. The underlying mechanisms of this increase in bone fragility are still under investigation. Interestingly, a rat study [74] showed SCI caused more damage to bone mass, structure, and metabolism than sciatic neurectomy. Jiang et al. [74] have proposed three mechanisms for the pathogenesis of the osteopenia in SCI compared to neurectomy. One is metabolic changes including impaired renal function, loss of gonadal function, and depressed hormone and insulin growth factor levels. The second is a widespread loss of mechanical loading on bone. Lastly, the type of neural injury may have an effect, with SCI causing greater bone loss due presumably to a loss of spinal cord derived bone trophic factors.

17.6.2 Effects of Cerebral Palsy on Bone

Cerebral palsy (CP) is a developmental neurological disorder characterized by spastic or flaccid paralysis in some muscles and sensory and motor abnormalities [64, 120]. The definition of CP has recently been revised [112]. CP is now defined as "a group of permanent disorders of the development of movement and posture, causing activity limitation, attributed to a non-progressive disturbance that occurred in the developing fetal or infant brain. The motor disorders of cerebral palsy are often accompanied by disturbances of sensation, perception, cognition, communication, and behavior, by epilepsy, and by secondary musculoskeletal problems." The impairment of posture and movement control caused by the primary neural insult in CP includes altered muscle activation and function and spastic paralysis [88, 115, 117]. The changes lead to muscle atrophy and a decreased range of motion [89]. While the neurological lesion is nonprogressive, the musculoskeletal sequelae often increase over time and with growth [88, 107].

The myriad muscle changes in CP lead to secondary bone malformations because of the abnormal forces on the bones. Bone malformations include equinus foot, foot valgus or varus, knee valgus or varus, rotational malformation of the tibia or femur, and hip subluxation [25, 56, 95, 107]. The bone malformations include tibial shortening as a result of long-term gastrocnemius spasticity and shortening. The incongruent distribution of load on joints also leads to changes in articular cartilage, such as cartilage pitting, eburnations, and erosions [95]. Several radiological studies show tibial chondromalacia, recurvatum deformities, patella fragmentation, articular cartilage degeneration [25, 95, 107], and severe chondromalacia of most of the joints of the foot [107]. Children with CP also have low bone mineral content (BMC) and underdeveloped bone structure in the lower extremities [102, 103]. Central nervous system changes in the sensorimotor cortices contribute to these musculoskeletal malformations in a rat model of CP [34]; alterations in the central neural signaling systems on bone have yet to be explored in CP.

17.6.3 Current Treatments for Bone Loss After SCI and in Cerebral Palsy

The treatment of spasticity is often a primary therapeutic goal for children with CP or SCI. Many clinical interventions are currently employed to treat spasticity or the effects of spasticity associated with CP. However, the outcome of most interventions is highly variable and inconsistent [128]. Tendon lengthening and serial casting [81] are used to correct for the reduced range of motion around a given joint. Restricted movements from casting can also lead to bone and joint degradation [34].

Pharmacological interventions, such as injections of botulinum toxin [81], intrathecal injections, or oral antispasmodic medications, are in use to improve function by weakening or reducing the reflex activity of spastic muscles [97]. Botox is generally considered safe to reduce muscle spasticity and tone. Recent murine studies suggest that Botox causes substantial deterioration of muscle mass, bone mass, and bone structure [118, 142]. The use of this neuromuscular inhibitor led to profound atrophy of the quadriceps and gastrocnemius muscles, and a reduction of trabecular and cortical bone volume in the ipsilateral femur and tibia. Botox injections had a moderate effect in the contralateral noninjected limb, but loss of muscle and muscle atrophy were maximal at day 28 after treatment, with only partial recover by day 84 [118]. As yet studies have determined the effect of Botox treatment on bone in humans. The use of Botox A in children with CP is worrisome as the children already have low bone mineral content and structural changes of bone.

Cycling is being used to improve muscle strength in children with CP or SCI [76, 77], but no study to date has investigated the effects of cycling on bone in children with CP.

Vibration therapy using high-frequency, low-magnitude vibration and electrical stimulation of muscles to induce mechanical bone loading are fairly new therapies to treat bone to inpatients with SCI or CP [35, 39, 141].

17.7 Traumatic Brain Injury and Heterotopic Bone Formation/Fracture Repair

Patients who have sustained traumatic brain injury (TBI) exhibit increased osteogenesis associated with higher rates of heterotopic ossification [48, 49, 99, 127] and accelerated fracture healing [54, 106, 114, 133]. Inasmuch as blood is the link between traumatized brain tissue and peripheral sites of increased bone formation, a centrally mediated mechanism involving the release of osteogenic humoral factors may be involved, but the key factor(s) have not been identified [140]. There is also evidence that CSF collected from patients following TBI has increased osteogenic potential [52]. This supports the notion of a centrally mediated mechanism.

17.7.1 Incidence of Heterotopic Ossification After TBI

The incidence of heterotopic ossification following TBI has been reported to range between 5% and 40% of patients. This variability is likely due to differences in methods of patient selection, diagnosis, and management [48, 50, 51, 99, 127]. The most common site of heterotopic ossification (HO) is the hip joint, though many other joints are affected as well. The HO ranges from mild to severe, with ankylosis of the joint in the most severe cases.

The bone that is formed at heterotopic sites following TBI is histologically similar to mature bone and involves the recruitment, proliferation, and differentiation of osteoprogenitor cells into osteoblasts [82]. In a large study demonstrating an increased rate of fracture healing after TBI, the nature of the callus formed was found to be histologically different from normal callus

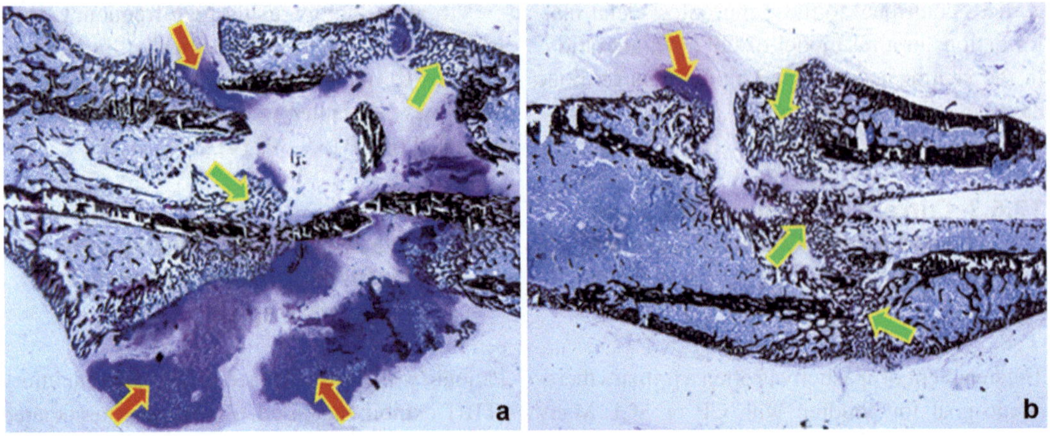

Fig. 17.2 Histology of fracture callus formation in adult (male) rat femurs at 1 week postfracture. Sections of undecalcified, methylmethacrylate-embedded control fracture (**a**) and TBI fracture (**b**) at 1 week postinduction. Sections were stained with von Kossa for visualization of mineralized bone and counterstained with toluidine blue to visualize cells and unmineralized tissues. There are distinct histological differences in the TBI (**b**) versus control fracture callus (**a**). After 1 week postfracture, a normal callus (**a**) contains a mix of soft tissue, cartilage (*red arrows*), and newly formed trabecular bone (*green arrows*). The callus in the TBI/fracture site (**b**) is primarily composed of new trabecular bone (*green arrows*) with little if any appearance of cartilage (*red arrows*). Bridging of the fracture site by the newly formed trabecular bone occurs substantially sooner in the TBI/fracture versus fracture only model (compare **b** with **a**). These results demonstrate that much of the bone formed at the fracture site following TBI is formed directly from mesenchymal cells rather than utilizing a cartilaginous precursor as in the process of endochondral bone formation characteristically observed in the normal fracture callus

formation [133]. On the basis of these observations, enhanced osteogenesis at the fracture callus may be representative of HO [133]. In a rodent model for TBI and fracture repair, young adult male rats were subjected to a standard closed femoral and a closed head trauma. This procedure led to a diffuse axonal injury resembling that in patients with TBI. The fracture callus was assessed histologically and by microCT analyses at several time points following the induction of TBI/fracture. Unpublished observations from our laboratories (Fig. 17.2) have confirmed that osteogenesis is enhanced at the fracture site. There were distinct histological differences in the TBI versus control fracture callus. After 1 week postinduction, a normal callus contains a mix of soft tissue, cartilage, and newly formed trabecular bone. The callus in the TBI/fracture site is primarily composed of new trabecular bone with little if any appearance of cartilage. Bridging of the fracture site by the newly formed trabecular bone occurs substantially sooner in the TBI/fracture. Our results suggest that much of the bone formed at the fracture site following TBI is formed directly from mesenchymal cells rather than through a cartilaginous intermediary as in endochondral bone formation.

17.7.2 Heterotopic Ossification After TBI May Be Induced by Centrally Released Humoral Factors

Most in vitro studies support the hypothesis that centrally released osteogenic factors mediate HO and the increase in fracture healing that follows TBI [16, 18, 41, 52, 85]. In these studies, the serum or CSF came from patients or rats with cultures of osteoblast cell lines or primary osteoblasts (mostly rat or human). Some were bone marrow stromal or mesenchymal cells, while others were committed to the osteoblast lineage, human fetal osteoblasts, or rat calvarial osteoblasts. In most studies, the serum or CSF following TBI promoted the growth of osteogenic cells particularly, if they were less mature, e.g., mesenchymal stem cells. The outcome of these experiments depended on the precise nature of the cell type and on the source of the serum/CSF. One study with neonatal rat calvarial cells actually showed that serum following TBI had no growth-promoting properties [119]. A link between serum-mediated effects on enhanced fracture healing was demonstrated in an in vivo rat model of traumatic brain injury in association with a standard closed fracture [18]. In that study, the healing fractures in the brain-injured group exhibited increased stiffness. Culture experiments demonstrated a significant increase in the proliferative response of mesenchymal stem cells, but not of fibroblasts or committed osteoblasts. In another study, serum from patients with severe TBI accelerated the proliferation of mesenchymal and osteoprogenitor cells, and supported the expression of osteoblast differentiation markers in primary cultures of skeletal muscle [22]. These studies lend support to the increase in osteogenic potential and fracture healing secondary to TBI and suggest that mitogenic factors in the serum can expand the pool of mesenchymal cells with osteogenic potential.

17.7.3 Other Novel Potential Central Mechanisms for Heterotopic Ossification After TBI

Aside from a central, humoral mechanism that mediates osteogenesis following TBI, other novel central mechanisms may mediate this effect. One mechanism involves the endocannabinoid system and the CB1 receptor (cf. the section on skeletal endocannabinoids). A centrally mediated mechanism involving the cannabinoid receptor CB1 appears to be present in sympathetic nerve terminals in the bone microenvironment [138]. In this study, the authors report that stimulation of bone formation following TBI is absent in CB1, but not CB2 null mice. They also demonstrated that TBI-stimulated osteogenesis is preceded by an increase in endocannabinoid, 2-arachidonoylglycerol (2-AG), and a concomitant decrease in the norepinephrine (NE) levels in the bone microenvironment. A previous study has shown that NE release from sympathetic terminals in bone produces a tonic inhibition of bone formation through activation of β2-adrenergic receptors [136]. Based on this finding, Tam and colleagues postulated that sympathetic control of bone formation is exerted by 2-AG regulation of prejunctional CB1 receptors that act to suppress the release of NE from sympathetic terminals. This in turn is thought to alleviate the sympathetic inhibition of bone formation, but there is no current evidence to support this mechanism of action.

Another study [8] was undertaken to assess the role of the peripheral nervous system in regulating bone metabolism. In this study, sensory denervation by capsaicin injection resulted in a decrease in cartilage and bone matrix formation, in a significantly larger callus, and in impaired mechanical strength of the callus. Although the precise mechanism of action is unclear, sensory denervation seems to negatively affect fracture healing and bone formation and resorption. Inasmuch as the capsaicin-induced denervation destroyed the CGRP and substance P-positive neurons, more studies are needed to determine how these neuropeptides regulate bone metabolism.

17.7.4 Current Treatments for Heterotopic Ossification After TBI

In the absence of conclusive identification of the key etiological factor(s) that mediate increased bone formation following TBI, current treatments for HO are aimed at inhibition of osteogenesis, at pain management, and at increasing joint mobility [31]. Treatments include the use of diphosphonates, an FDA approved treatment for HO to inhibit formation of the mineral phase of hydroxyapatite crystals in bone [11]. Nonsteroidal anti-inflammatory drugs (NSAIDS) have been used to minimize HO and patient discomfort especially in the presence of inflammation [12, 13, 84, 98]. Radiation may inhibit HO by disrupting mesenchymal cell differentiation [21, 126]. Physical therapy serves as an adjunct in HO prevention by maintaining joint mobility. Additional studies are clearly needed to identify the key factors that mediate increased osteogenesis following TBI to be able to develop therapeutic agents that selectively block the effects of these factors on bone formation. Ultimately, it may become possible to develop therapeutics that selectively stimulate fracture repair.

17.8 Conclusion/Perspectives

The links described above between bone and the peripheral and central nervous systems affect the interpretation of how bone metabolism modulates neurological disorders. This applies to the complex regional pain syndrome (also called reflex sympathetic dystrophy syndrome) with sympathetic hyperactivity and osteopenia; traumatic brain injury outcomes that are characterized by increased osteogenic activity and BMD; stroke, spinal cord injury, and peripheral neuropathies that are often associated with osteopenia, bone fragility, poor fracture healing; and robust neurogenesis during fracture healing [113].

Questions that need addressing include what signals feed information from osteoblasts to the brain or adipocytes [135]. Research is also needed to define the relative importance of central (neuronal) versus peripheral mechanisms whereby the endocannabinoid system regulates bone metabolism. Beta antagonists are attractive candidates for the treatment of osteoporosis and of the complex regional pain syndrome, but the signaling pathway from the hypothalamus still needs to be identified. Botox A has become a treatment to reduce muscle spasticity in children with CP. However, appropriate clinical trials are needed to determine long-term effects, as these patients already exhibit degradative bone changes. Also, additional studies are needed to identify the key factors that mediate increased osteogenesis following TBI. This knowledge may enable development of appropriate therapeutic agents.

References

1. Adam C, et al. Effects of capsaicin-induced sensory denervation on osteoclastic resorption in adult rats. Exp Physiol. 2000;85(1):62–6.
2. Adami S, et al. Bisphosphonate therapy of reflex sympathetic dystrophy syndrome. Ann Rheum Dis. 1997;56(3):201–4.
3. Adamus MA, Dabrowski ZJ. Effect of the neuropeptide substance P on the rat bone marrow-derived osteogenic cells in vitro. J Cell Biochem. 2001;81(3):499–506.
4. Albrecht PJ, et al. Pathologic alterations of cutaneous innervation and vasculature in affected limbs from patients with complex regional pain syndrome. Pain. 2006;120(3):244–66.
5. Allison SJ, Baldock PA, Herzog H. The control of bone remodeling by neuropeptide Y receptors. Peptides. 2007;28(2):320–5.
6. Amann R, Egger T, Schuligoi R. The tachykinin NK(1) receptor antagonist SR140333 prevents the increase of nerve growth factor in rat paw skin induced by substance P or neurogenic inflammation. Neuroscience. 2000;100(3):611–5.
7. Amann R, Lanz I, Schuligoi R. Effects of morphine on oedema and tissue concentration of nerve growth factor in experimental inflammation of the rat paw. Pharmacology. 2002;66(3):169–72.
8. Apel PJ, et al. Effect of selective sensory denervation on fracture-healing: an experimental study of rats. J Bone Joint Surg Am. 2009;91(12):2886–95.
9. Bab I, et al. Endocannabinoids and the regulation of bone metabolism. J Neuroendocrinol. 2008;20 Suppl 1:69–74.
10. Bab I, Zimmer A. Cannabinoid receptors and the regulation of bone mass. Br J Pharmacol. 2008;153(2):182–8.
11. Banovac K. The effect of etidronate on late development of heterotopic ossification after spinal cord injury. J Spinal Cord Med. 2000;23(1):40–4.
12. Banovac K, et al. Prevention of heterotopic ossification after spinal cord injury with indomethacin. Spinal Cord. 2001;39(7):370–4.
13. Banovac K, et al. Prevention of heterotopic ossification after spinal cord injury with COX-2 selective inhibitor (rofecoxib). Spinal Cord. 2004;42(12):707–10.
14. Bauman WA, Spungen AM. Metabolic changes in persons after spinal cord injury. Phys Med Rehabil Clin N Am. 2000;11(1):109–40.
15. Bergmann I, et al. Nerve growth factor evokes hyperalgesia in mice lacking the low-affinity neurotrophin receptor p75. Neurosci Lett. 1998;255(2):87–90.
16. Bidner SM, et al. Evidence for a humoral mechanism for enhanced osteogenesis after head injury. J Bone Joint Surg Am. 1990;72(8):1144–9.
17. Bjurholm A, et al. Substance P- and CGRP-immunoreactive nerves in bone. Peptides. 1988;9(1):165–71.
18. Boes M, et al. Osteogenic effects of traumatic brain injury on experimental fracture-healing. J Bone Joint Surg Am. 2006;88(4):738–43.
19. Brighton CT, Tadduni GT, Pollack SR. Treatment of sciatic denervation disuse osteoporosis in the rat tibia with capacitively coupled electrical stimulation. Dose response and duty cycle. J Bone Joint Surg Am. 1985;67(7):1022–8.
20. Buckley NE, et al. Immunomodulation by cannabinoids is absent in mice deficient for the cannabinoid CB(2) receptor. Eur J Pharmacol. 2000;396(2–3):141–9.

21. Burd TA, Lowry KJ, Anglen JO. Indomethacin compared with localized irradiation for the prevention of heterotopic ossification following surgical treatment of acetabular fractures. J Bone Joint Surg Am. 2001;83-A(12):1783–8.
22. Cadosch D, et al. Serum after traumatic brain injury increases proliferation and supports expression of osteoblast markers in muscle cells. J Bone Joint Surg Am. 2010;92(3):645–53.
23. Calvo W. The innervation of the bone marrow in laboratory animals. Am J Anat. 1968;123(2):315–28.
24. Cardozo CP, et al. Nandrolone slows hindlimb bone loss in a rat model of bone loss due to denervation. Ann N Y Acad Sci. 2010;1192:303–6.
25. Carter DR, Tse B. The pathogenesis of osteoarthritis in cerebral palsy. Dev Med Child Neurol. 2009;51 Suppl 4:79–83.
26. Chacur M, et al. A new model of sciatic inflammatory neuritis (SIN): induction of unilateral and bilateral mechanical allodynia following acute unilateral perisciatic immune activation in rats. Pain. 2001;94(3):231–44.
27. Cheng MZ, et al. Enhancement by sex hormones of the osteoregulatory effects of mechanical loading and prostaglandins in explants of rat ulnae. J Bone Miner Res. 1997;12(9):1424–30.
28. Chenu C. Role of innervation in the control of bone remodeling. J Musculoskelet Neuronal Interact. 2004;4(2):132–4.
29. Chenu C. Glutamatergic innervation in bone. Microsc Res Tech. 2002;58(2):70–6.
30. Cherruau M, et al. Chemical sympathectomy-induced changes in TH-, VIP-, and CGRP-immunoreactive fibers in the rat mandible periosteum: influence on bone resorption. J Cell Physiol. 2003;194(3):341–8.
31. Cipriano CA, Pill SG, Keenan MA. Heterotopic ossification following traumatic brain injury and spinal cord injury. J Am Acad Orthop Surg. 2009;17(11):689–97.
32. Coleman DL, Hummel KP. Effects of parabiosis of normal with genetically diabetic mice. Am J Physiol. 1969;217(5):1298–304.
33. Collet C, et al. The serotonin 5-HT2B receptor controls bone mass via osteoblast recruitment and proliferation. FASEB J. 2008;22(2):418–27.
34. Coq JO, et al. Impact of neonatal asphyxia and hind limb immobilization on musculoskeletal tissues and S1 map organization: implications for cerebral palsy. Exp Neurol. 2008;210(1):95–108.
35. Davis R, et al. The effects of whole body vibration on bone mineral density for a person with a spinal cord injury: a case study. Adapt Phys Activ Q. 2010;27(1):60–72.
36. DeLeo JA, Colburn RW, Rickman AJ. Cytokine and growth factor immunohistochemical spinal profiles in two animal models of mononeuropathy. Brain Res. 1997;759(1):50–7.
37. Denes A, et al. Central autonomic control of the bone marrow: multisynaptic tract tracing by recombinant pseudorabies virus. Neuroscience. 2005;134(3):947–63.
38. Ducy P, et al. Leptin inhibits bone formation through a hypothalamic relay: a central control of bone mass. Cell. 2000;100(2):197–207.
39. Dudley-Javoroski S, Shields RK. Dose estimation and surveillance of mechanical loading interventions for bone loss after spinal cord injury. Phys Ther. 2008;88(3):387–96.
40. Duncan CP, Shim SS, Edouard J. Samson address: the autonomic nerve supply of bone. An experimental study of the intraosseous adrenergic nervi vasorum in the rabbit. J Bone Joint Surg Br. 1977;59(3):323 30.
41. Eid K, et al. Systemic effects of severe trauma on the function and apoptosis of human skeletal cells. J Bone Joint Surg Br. 2006;88(10):1394–400.
42. Elefteriou F. Regulation of bone remodeling by the central and peripheral nervous system. Arch Biochem Biophys. 2008;473(2):231–6.
43. Elliott MB, et al. Performance of a repetitive task by aged rats leads to median neuropathy and spinal cord inflammation with associated sensorimotor declines. Neuroscience. 2010;170(3):929–41.
44. Elliott MB, et al. High force reaching task induces widespread inflammation, increased spinal cord neurochemicals and neuropathic pain. Neuroscience. 2009;158(2):922–31.
45. Elliott MB, et al. Peripheral neuritis and increased spinal cord neurochemicals are induced in a model of repetitive motion injury with low force and repetition exposure. Brain Res. 2008;1218:103–13.
46. Elliott RA, et al. The cost effectiveness of a telephone-based pharmacy advisory service to improve adherence to newly prescribed medicines. Pharm World Sci. 2008;30(1):17–23.
47. Erselcan T, et al. Carpal tunnel syndrome leads to significant bone loss in metacarpal bones. J Bone Miner Metab. 2001;19(5):317–20.
48. Flin C, et al. Heterotopic ossification and brain injury. Ann Readapt Med Phys. 2002;45(9):517–20.
49. Garland DE. Clinical observations on fractures and heterotopic ossification in the spinal cord and traumatic brain injured populations. Clin Orthop Relat Res. 1988;233:86–101.
50. Garland DE, Blum CE, Waters RL. Periarticular heterotopic ossification in head-injured adults. Incidence and location. J Bone Joint Surg Am. 1980;62(7):1143–6.
51. Garland DE, Rothi B, Waters RL. Femoral fractures in head-injuries adults. Clin Orthop Relat Res. 1982;166:219–25.
52. Gautschi OP, et al. Osteoinductive effect of cerebrospinal fluid from brain-injured patients. J Neurotrauma. 2007;24(1):154–62.
53. Gazda LS, et al. Sciatic inflammatory neuritis (SIN): behavioral allodynia is paralleled by peri-sciatic proinflammatory cytokine and superoxide production. J Peripher Nerv Syst. 2001;6(3):111–29.
54. Giannoudis PV, et al. Accelerated bone healing and excessive callus formation in patients with femoral fracture and head injury. Injury. 2006;37 Suppl 3:S18–24.
55. Gkonos PJ, et al. Biosynthesis of calcitonin gene-related peptide and calcitonin by a human medullary

thyroid carcinoma cell line. J Biol Chem. 1986; 261(31):14386–91.
56. Gormley Jr ME. Treatment of neuromuscular and musculoskeletal problems in cerebral palsy. Pediatr Rehabil. 2001;4(1):5–16.
57. Goto T, et al. Light- and electron-microscopic study of the distribution of axons containing substance P and the localization of neurokinin-1 receptor in bone. Cell Tissue Res. 1998;293(1):87–93.
58. Gronblad M, et al. Innervation of human bone periosteum by peptidergic nerves. Anat Rec. 1984;209(3):297–9.
59. Gros M. Note sur les nerfs des os. C R Acad Sci (Paris). 1846;23:1106–8.
60. Gu Y, et al. The NMDA type glutamate receptors expressed by primary rat osteoblasts have the same electrophysiological characteristics as neuronal receptors. Calcif Tissue Int. 2002;70(3):194–203.
61. Hara-IrieF,AmizukaN,OzawaH.Immunohistochemical and ultrastructural localization of CGRP-positive nerve fibers at the epiphyseal trabecules facing the growth plate of rat femurs. Bone. 1996;18(1):29–39.
62. Hill EL, Elde R. Distribution of CGRP-, VIP-, DβH-, SP-, and NPY-immunoreactive nerves in the periosteum of the rat. Cell Tissue Res. 1991;264(3):469–80.
63. Hill EL, Elde R. Calcitonin gene-related peptide-immunoreactive nerve fibers in mandibular periosteum of rat: evidence for primary afferent origin. Neurosci Lett. 1988;85(2):172–8.
64. Hill A, Volpe JJ. Perinatal asphyxia: clinical aspects. Clin Perinatol. 1989;16(2):435–57.
65. Hohmann EL, et al. Innervation of periosteum and bone by sympathetic vasoactive intestinal peptide-containing nerve fibers. Science. 1986;232(4752):868–71.
66. Holzer P, Lembeck F. Effect of neuropeptides on the efficiency of the peristaltic reflex. Naunyn Schmiedebergs Arch Pharmacol. 1979;307(3):257–64.
67. Hunt JL, et al. Repeated injury to the lumbar nerve roots produces enhanced mechanical allodynia and persistent spinal neuroinflammation. Spine. 2001; 26(19):2073–9.
68. Idris AI, et al. Regulation of bone mass, bone loss and osteoclast activity by cannabinoid receptors. Nat Med. 2005;11(7):774–9.
69. Idris AI, et al. Cannabinoid receptor type 1 protects against age-related osteoporosis by regulating osteoblast and adipocyte differentiation in marrow stromal cells. Cell Metab. 2009;10(2):139–47.
70. Imai S, et al. An ultrastructural study of calcitonin gene-related peptide-immunoreactive nerve fibers innervating the rat posterior longitudinal ligament. A morphologic basis for their possible efferent actions. Spine (Phila Pa 1976). 1997;22(17):1941–7.
71. Imai S, Matsusue Y. Neuronal regulation of bone metabolism and anabolism: calcitonin gene-related peptide-, substance P -, and tyrosine hydroxylase-containing nerves and the bone. Microsc Res Tech. 2002;58(2):61–9.
72. Imai S, et al. Calcitonin gene-related peptide, substance P, and tyrosine hydroxylase-immunoreactive innervation of rat bone marrows: an immunohistochemical and ultrastructural investigation on possible efferent and afferent mechanisms. J Orthop Res. 1997;15(1):133–40.
73. Irie K, et al. Calcitonin gene-related peptide (CGRP)-containing nerve fibers in bone tissue and their involvement in bone remodeling. Microsc Res Tech. 2002;58(2):85–90.
74. Jiang SD, Jiang LS, Dai LY. Spinal cord injury causes more damage to bone mass, bone structure, biomechanical properties and bone metabolism than sciatic neurectomy in young rats. Osteoporos Int. 2006;17(10):1552–61.
75. Jimenez-Andrade JM, et al. A phenotypically restricted set of primary afferent nerve fibers innervate the bone versus skin: therapeutic opportunity for treating skeletal pain. Bone. 2010;46(2):306–13.
76. Johnston TE, Lauer RT, Lee SC. The effects of a shank guide on cycling biomechanics of an adolescent with cerebral palsy: a single-case study. Arch Phys Med Rehabil. 2008;89(10):2025–30.
77. Johnston TE, et al. Exercise testing using upper extremity ergometry in pediatric spinal cord injury. Pediatr Phys Ther. 2008;20(2):146–51.
78. Jones KB, et al. Bone and brain: a review of neural, hormonal, and musculoskeletal connections. Iowa Orthop J. 2004;24:123–32.
79. Kawase T, et al. Diverse actions of calcitonin gene-related peptide on intracellular free Ca^{2+} concentrations in UMR 106 osteoblastic cells. Bone. 1995;16(4 Suppl):379S–84.
80. Kawase T, et al. Calcitonin gene-related peptide rapidly inhibits calcium uptake in osteoblastic cell lines via activation of adenosine triphosphate-sensitive potassium channels. Endocrinology. 1996;137(3):984–90.
81. Kay RM, et al. Botulinum toxin as an adjunct to serial casting treatment in children with cerebral palsy. J Bone Joint Surg Am. 2004;86-A(11):2377–84.
82. Keenan M, Haider T. The formation of heterotopic ossification after traumatic brain injury: a biopsy study with ultrastructural analysis. J Head Trauma Rehabil. 1996;11:8–22.
83. Kingery WS, et al. A substance P receptor (NK1) antagonist enhances the widespread osteoporotic effects of sciatic nerve section. Bone. 2003;33(6):927–36.
84. Kjaersgaard-Andersen P, Schmidt SA. Total hip arthroplasty. The role of anti-inflammatory medications in the prevention of heterotopic ossification. Clin Orthop Relat Res. 1991;263:78–86.
85. Klein BY, et al. Serum-mediated osteogenic effects of head injury on cultured rat marrow stromal cells. Calcif Tissue Int. 1999;65(3):217–22.
86. Kozin F, et al. The reflex sympathetic dystrophy syndrome. II. Roentgenographic and scintigraphic evidence of bilaterality and of periarticular accentuation. Am J Med. 1976;60(3):332–8.
87. Kozin F, et al. The reflex sympathetic dystrophy syndrome. I. Clinical and histologic studies: evidence for bilaterality, response to corticosteroids and articular involvement. Am J Med. 1976;60(3):321–31.
88. Lauer RT, et al. Age and electromyographic frequency alterations during walking in children with cerebral palsy. Gait Posture. 2010;31(1):136–9.

89. Lauer RT, et al. Lower extremity muscle activity during cycling in adolescents with and without cerebral palsy. Clin Biomech (Bristol, Avon). 2008;23(4):442–9.
90. Lembeck F, Holzer P. Substance P as neurogenic mediator of antidromic vasodilation and neurogenic plasma extravasation. Naunyn Schmiedebergs Arch Pharmacol. 1979;310(2):175–83.
91. Lerner UH. Deletions of genes encoding calcitonin/alpha-CGRP, amylin and calcitonin receptor have given new and unexpected insights into the function of calcitonin receptors and calcitonin receptor-like receptors in bone. J Musculoskelet Neuronal Interact. 2006;6(1):87–95.
92. Lerner UH. Neuropeptidergic regulation of bone resorption and bone formation. J Musculoskelet Neuronal Interact. 2002;2(5):440–7.
93. Levin AB, Sperling KB. Complications associated with infusion pumps implanted for spasticity. Stereotact Funct Neurosurg. 1995;65(1–4):147–51.
94. Lofvenmark I, Werhagen L, Norrbrink C. Spasticity and bone density after a spinal cord injury. J Rehabil Med. 2009;41(13):1080–4.
95. Lundy DW, et al. Pathologic morphology of the dislocated proximal femur in children with cerebral palsy. J Pediatr Orthop. 1998;18(4):528–34.
96. Mach DB, et al. Origins of skeletal pain: sensory and sympathetic innervation of the mouse femur. Neuroscience. 2002;113(1):155–66.
97. Maimoun L, et al. Bone loss in spinal cord-injured patients: from physiopathology to therapy. Spinal Cord. 2006;44(4):203–10.
98. McMahon JS, Waddell JP, Morton J. Effect of short-course indomethacin on heterotopic bone formation after uncemented total hip arthroplasty. J Arthroplasty. 1991;6(3):259–64.
99. Mendelson L, et al. Periarticular new bone formation in patients suffering from severe head injuries. Scand J Rehabil Med. 1975;7(4):141–5.
100. Merskey H, Bogduk N. Classification of chronic pain: descriptions of chronic pain syndromes and definitions of pain terms. 2nd ed. Seattle: IASP Press; 1994.
101. Milligan ED, et al. Spinal glia and proinflammatory cytokines mediate mirror-image neuropathic pain in rats. J Neurosci. 2003;23(3):1026–40.
102. Modlesky CM, Subramanian P, Miller F. Underdeveloped trabecular bone microarchitecture is detected in children with cerebral palsy using high-resolution magnetic resonance imaging. Osteoporos Int. 2008;19(2):169–76.
103. Modlesky CM, et al. Evaluation of the femoral midshaft in children with cerebral palsy using magnetic resonance imaging. Osteoporos Int. 2009;20(4): 609–15.
104. Morimoto R, Uehara S, Yatsushiro S, Juge N, Hua Z, Senoh S, Echigo N, Hayashi M, Mizofuchi T, Ninomiya T, Udagawa N, Omote H, Yamamoto A, Edwards R, Moriyama Y. Secretion of L-glutamate from osteoclasts through transcytosis. EMBO J. 2009;25(18):4175–86.
105. Moriyama Y, Omote H. Vesicular glutamate transporter acts as a metabolic regulator. Biol Pharm Bull. 2008;31(10):1844–6.
106. Morley J, et al. Does traumatic brain injury result in accelerated fracture healing? Injury. 2005;36(3): 363–8.
107. Morrell DS, Pearson JM, Sauser DD. Progressive bone and joint abnormalities of the spine and lower extremities in cerebral palsy. Radiographics. 2002;22(2):257–68.
108. Oaklander AL, et al. Evidence of focal small-fiber axonal degeneration in complex regional pain syndrome-I (reflex sympathetic dystrophy). Pain. 2006;120(3):235–43.
109. Oaklander AL, Fields HL. Is reflex sympathetic dystrophy/complex regional pain syndrome type I a small-fiber neuropathy? Ann Neurol. 2009;65(6): 629–38.
110. Ofek O, et al. Peripheral cannabinoid receptor, CB2, regulates bone mass. Proc Natl Acad Sci USA. 2006;103(3):696–701.
111. Offley SC, et al. Capsaicin-sensitive sensory neurons contribute to the maintenance of trabecular bone integrity. J Bone Miner Res. 2005;20(2):257–67.
112. World Health Organization. International classification of functioning, disability and health/World Health Organization. 2001 www.who.int/classifications/icf/en/.
113. Patel MS, Elefteriou F. The new field of neuroskeletal biology. Calcif Tissue Int. 2007;80(5):337–47.
114. Perkins R, Skirving AP. Callus formation and the rate of healing of femoral fractures in patients with head injuries. J Bone Joint Surg Br. 1987;69(4):521–4.
115. Pierce SR, et al. Roles of reflex activity and co-contraction during assessments of spasticity of the knee flexor and knee extensor muscles in children with cerebral palsy and different functional levels. Phys Ther. 2008;88(10):1124–34.
116. Pierce SR, et al. Examination of spasticity of the knee flexors and knee extensors using isokinetic dynamometry with electromyography and clinical scales in children with spinal cord injury. J Spinal Cord Med. 2008;31(2):208–14.
117. Pierce SR, et al. Comparison of percutaneous and surface functional electrical stimulation during gait in a child with hemiplegic cerebral palsy. Am J Phys Med Rehabil. 2004;83(10):798–805.
118. Poliachik SL, et al. Transient muscle paralysis disrupts bone homeostasis by rapid degradation of bone morphology. Bone. 2010;46(1):18–23.
119. Renfree KJ, et al. Evaluation of serum osteoblast mitogenic activity in spinal cord and head injury patients with acute heterotopic ossification. Spine (Phila Pa 1976). 1994;19(7):740–6.
120. Rosenbaum P, et al. A report: the definition and classification of cerebral palsy April 2006. Dev Med Child Neurol Suppl. 2007;109:8–14.
121. Rossi F, et al. The endovanilloid/endocannabinoid system in human osteoclasts: possible involvement in bone formation and resorption. Bone. 2009;44(3): 476–84.

122. Sabsovich I, et al. Effect of anti-NGF antibodies in a rat tibia fracture model of complex regional pain syndrome type I. Pain. 2008;138(1):47–60.
123. Sakai A, et al. Bone marrow capacity for bone cells and trabecular bone turnover in immobilized tibia after sciatic neurectomy in mice. Bone. 1996;18(5):479–86.
124. Sample SJ, et al. Functional adaptation to loading of a single bone is neuronally regulated and involves multiple bones. J Bone Miner Res. 2008;23(9):1372–81.
125. Sato S, et al. Central control of bone remodeling by neuromedin U. Nat Med. 2007;13(10):1234–40.
126. Sautter-Bihl ML, et al. Fractionated and single-dose radiotherapy for heterotopic bone formation in patients with spinal cord injury. A phase-I/II study. Strahlenther Onkol. 2001;177(4):200–5.
127. Sazbon L, et al. Widespread periarticular new-bone formation in long-term comatose patients. J Bone Joint Surg Br. 1981;63-B(1):120–5.
128. Scianni A, et al. Muscle strengthening is not effective in children and adolescents with cerebral palsy: a systematic review. Aust J Physiother. 2009;55(2):81–7.
129. Serre CM, et al. Evidence for a dense and intimate innervation of the bone tissue, including glutamate-containing fibers. Bone. 1999;25(6):623–9.
130. Sherman MS. The nerves of bones. J Bone Joint Surg Am. 1963;45:522–8.
131. Shih C, Bernard GW. Neurogenic substance P stimulates osteogenesis in vitro. Peptides. 1997;18(2):323–6.
132. Skerry TM. The role of glutamate in the regulation of bone mass and architecture. J Musculoskelet Neuronal Interact. 2008;8(2):166–73.
133. Spencer RF. The effect of head injury on fracture healing. A quantitative assessment. J Bone Joint Surg Br. 1987;69(4):525–8.
134. Szczesniak AM, et al. Mechanical loading modulates glutamate receptor subunit expression in bone. Bone. 2005;37(1):63–73.
135. Takeda S. Osteoporosis: a neuroskeletal disease? Int J Biochem Cell Biol. 2009;41(3):455–9.
136. Takeda S, et al. Leptin regulates bone formation via the sympathetic nervous system. Cell. 2002;111(3):305–17.
137. Tam J, et al. Involvement of neuronal cannabinoid receptor CB1 in regulation of bone mass and bone remodeling. Mol Pharmacol. 2006;70(3):786–92.
138. Tam J, et al. The cannabinoid CB1 receptor regulates bone formation by modulating adrenergic signaling. FASEB J. 2008;22(1):285–94.
139. Thurston TJ. Distribution of nerves in long bones as shown by silver impregnation. J Anat. 1982;134(Pt 4):719–28.
140. Toffoli AM, et al. From brain to bone: evidence for the release of osteogenic humoral factors after traumatic brain injury. Brain Inj. 2008;22(7–8):511–8.
141. Ward K, et al. Low magnitude mechanical loading is osteogenic in children with disabling conditions. J Bone Miner Res. 2004. doi:10.1359/JBMR.040129.
142. Warner SE, et al. Botox induced muscle paralysis rapidly degrades bone. Bone. 2006;38(2):257–64.
143. Wei T, et al. Pentoxifylline attenuates nociceptive sensitization and cytokine expression in a tibia fracture rat model of complex regional pain syndrome. Eur J Pain. 2009;13(3):253–62.
144. Willert RP, et al. Exploring the neurophysiological basis of chest wall allodynia induced by experimental oesophageal acidification – evidence of central sensitization. Neurogastroenterol Motil. 2007;19(4):270–8.
145. Woolf CJ, Salter MW. Neuronal plasticity: increasing the gain in pain. Science. 2000;288(5472):1765–9.
146. Wu G, et al. Early onset of spontaneous activity in uninjured C-fiber nociceptors after injury to neighboring nerve fibers. J Neurosci. 2001;21(8):RC140.
147. Zaidi M, et al. Effects of peptides from the calcitonin genes on bone and bone cells. Q J Exp Physiol. 1988;73(4):471–85.
148. Zhao J, et al. Effects of nandrolone on denervation atrophy depend upon time after nerve transection. Muscle Nerve. 2008;37(1):42–9.

Index

F. Bronner et al. (eds.), *Bone-Metabolic Functions and Modulators*, Topics in Bone Biology,
DOI 10.1007/978-1-4471-2745-1, © Springer-Verlag London 2012

MIX
Papier aus verantwortungsvollen Quellen
Paper from responsible sources
FSC® C105338

If you have any concerns about our products,
you can contact us on
ProductSafety@springernature.com

In case Publisher is established outside the EU,
the EU authorized representative is:
Springer Nature Customer Service Center GmbH
Europaplatz 3, 69115 Heidelberg, Germany

Printed by Libri Plureos GmbH
in Hamburg, Germany